# Integrative Addiction and Recovery

Integrative Medicine Library

Published and Forthcoming Volumes

SERIES EDITOR

Andrew Weil, MD

# Integrative Addiction and Recovery

EDITED BY

## Shahla J. Modir, MD

Chief Addiction Psychiatrist
Avalon Malibu Residential Treatment Center
Soba Malibu Treatment Center
Club Soba Intensive Outpatient Program
Los Angeles, CA

## George E. Muñoz, MD

Chief Medical Officer
The Oasis Institute
Integrative Medicine and Disease Prevention Clinic
Miami, FL
Chief, Integrative Rheumatology & Founding Board Member
AARA-American Arthritis & Rheumatology Associates
Miami & Boca Raton, FL

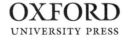

OXFORD
UNIVERSITY PRESS

# OXFORD
UNIVERSITY PRESS

Oxford University Press is a department of the University of Oxford. It furthers
the University's objective of excellence in research, scholarship, and education
by publishing worldwide. Oxford is a registered trade mark of Oxford University
Press in the UK and certain other countries.

Published in the United States of America by Oxford University Press
198 Madison Avenue, New York, NY 10016, United States of America.

CIP data is on file at the Library of Congress
ISBN 978-0-19-027533-4

1 3 5 7 9 8 6 4 2

Printed by Webcom, Inc., Canada

# CONTENTS

# CONTRIBUTORS

**Jeffrey Becker, MD, ABIHM**
Functional Psychiatrist
Los Angeles, CA

**Lisa Benson, PhD**
Clinical Psychologist I
Harbor-UCLA Medical Center
Torrance, CA

**Florian Birkmayer, MD**
Co-Founder AromaGnosis
Taos, New Mexico

**Karen E. Cardon, MD**
Director, Co-occurring
  Disorders Clinic
New Mexico Veterans Affairs Health
  Care System
Albuquerque, New Mexico

**Avghi Constantinides, D.Hom,
HMC, MA**
Founder, Homeopathy for Life—
  Homeopathic Practice
Director, Los Angeles School of
  Homeopathy
Los Angeles, CA

**Itai Danovitch, MD, MBA**
Chairman, Department of Psychiatry
  and Behavioral Neurosciences
Cedars Sinai Medical Center
Los Angeles, CA

**Timothy Fong, MD**
Professor of Psychiatry
Co-Director, UCLA Gambling Studies
  Program
Department of Psychiatry and
  Biobehavioral Sciences at UCLA
Los Angeles, CA

**Isabella Leoni Garcia, MS, LDN, CNS**
Licensed Nutritionist/Dietitian
Miami, FL

**Cynthia M. A. Geppert, MD, PhD**
Professor, Department of Psychiatry
Director of Ethics Education
University of New Mexico School of
  Medicine
Chief Consultation Psychiatry
  and Ethics
New Mexico Veterans Affairs Health
  Care System
Albuquerque, New Mexico

**Rick Ginsberg, PhD**
Clinical Psychologist
President, Beacon View
   Consulting LLC
Denver, CO

**Charles S. Grob, MD**
Professor, Departments of Psychiatry
   & Biobehavioral Sciences and
   Pediatrics
Director, Division of Child and
   Adolescent Psychiatry
UCLA School of Medicine
Los Angeles, CA

**Bettina Herbert, MD**
Instructor of Rehabilitation Medicine
   and Emergency Medicine
Jefferson-Myrna Brind Center of
   Integrative Medicine
Thomas Jefferson University Hospital
Philadelphia, PA

**Rachel Higier, PhD**
Clinical Psychologist I
Harbor-UCLA Medical Center
Torrance, CA

**Robert Krochmal, MD**
Founder M.D. Integrative
   Wellness Clinic
Woodland Hills, CA

**Bruce Y. Lee**
Departments of Medicine and
   Biomedical Informatics
University of Pittsburgh
Pittsburgh, Pennslyvania

**Walter Ling, MD**
Professor, Emeritus and Founding
   Director
Integrated Substance Abuse Programs
Department of Family Medicine
Center for Behavioral & Addiction
   Medicine
UCLA David Geffen School of
   Medicine
Los Angeles, CA

**David Martarano, MD**
Director Adult Psychiatry, Wyoming
   Behavioral Institute
Clinical Instructor, University of
   Washington, School of Medicine
Consult Liaison Psychiatrist, Wyoming
   Medical Center
Medical Director, Vistas Substance
   Abuse Center at WBI
Director, Wyoming Psychiatry
Casper, Wyoming

**Lynn McFarr, PhD**
Director, Cognitive Behavioral
   Therapy Clinic
Professor, Department of Psychiatry
   and Biobehavioral Sciences
UCLA David Geffen School of
   Medicine
Harbor UCLA Medical Center
Torrance, CA

**Edison de Mello, MD, PhD**
Founder, Board Certified Integrative
   Physician, Chief Medical Officer
Akasha Center for Integrative
   Medicine
Santa Monica, CA

**Andrew Mitton, MD**
Psychiatrist
Kaiser Permanente
Los Angeles, CA

**Shahla J. Modir, MD**
Chief Addiction Psychiatrist
Avalon Malibu Residential
    Treatment Center
Soba Malibu Treatment Center
Club Soba Intensive Outpatient
    Program
Integrative Psychiatrist at Centre
    for Life
Culver City, CA

**Larissa J. Mooney, MD**
Associate Clinical Professor
Director, UCLA Addiction
    Medicine Clinic
UCLA School of Medicine
Los Angeles, CA

**Joel Morris, MD**
Integrative Psychiatrist
Culver City, CA

**George E. Muñoz, MD**
Chief Medical Officer
The Oasis Institute
Integrative Medicine and Disease
    Prevention Clinic
Miami, FL
Chief, Integrative Rheumatology
    & Founding Board Member
AARA-American Arthritis &
    Rheumatology Associates
Miami & Boca Raton, FL

**Andrew B. Newberg, MD**
Department of Radiology and
    Psychiatry
University of Pennslyvania
    Health System
Thomas Jefferson University Hospital
Philadelphia, PA

**Lynette M. Pujol, PhD**
Assistant Professor of Psychiatry and
    Anesthesiology
Thomas Jefferson University
Philadelphia, PA

**Gayla Rees, MD**
Psychiatrist
Los Angeles, CA

**Meredith Sagan, MD**
Integrative Psychiatrist
Santa Monica, CA

**E. Hitchcock Scott, PhD**
Licensed Professional Clinical
    Counselor
Licensed Advanced Alcohol and Drug
    Counselor (LAADC)
Board Certified Registered Art
    Therapist (ATR-BC)
Registered Expressive Arts
    Therapist (REAT)
Board Member for The Global Art
    Project for Peace and Brass Tracks
    Recovery
Private Practice Psychotherapy and
    Consulting
Malibu, CA

**Benjamin Shapiro, MD**
Geriatric Psychiatry
UCLA School of Medicine
Los Angeles, CA

**Cathy Skipper**
Co-Founder AromaGnosis
Taos, New Mexico

**David E. Smith MD**
Chief, Addiction Medicine,
Muir Wood Adolescent & Family
  Services,
Petaluma, California
Medical Director,
Center Point, San Rafael, California
Chief, Addiction Medicine, Alta Mira
  Recovery,
Sausalito, California
Consulting Physician,
North Bay Recovery Center
San Francisco, California

**Julie Snyder, PsyD**
Clinical Director, CBT California
Volunteer Faculty
UCLA David Geffen School of
  Medicine
Los Angeles, CA

**Dean Taraborelli**
The Sanctuary at Sedona
Sedona, AZ

**Matthew Torrington, MD**
Board Certified Family Medicine and
  Addiction Medicine
Associate Clinical Professor, UCLA
  School of Nursing

Founder and Primary Provider,
  Common Ground Free Clinic
Venice, CA
Founding Chief of Addiction
  Medicine, Avalon Malibu
Malibu, CA
Addiction Medicine Private Practice
Culver City, CA

**John Tsuang, MD**
Director of Dual Diagnosis Treatment
  Program
Clinical Professor of Psychiatry
Harbor-UCLA Medical Center
Department of Psychiatry
Torrance, CA

**Alberto Villoldo, PhD**
Founder, The Four Winds Society
Book Author
Medical Antropologist, Healer,
  Shaman, Visionary
Miami, FL

**Jeff Wilkens, MD**
Lincy/Heyward-Moynihan Endowed
  Chair in Addiction Medicine
Department of Psychiatry and
  Behavioral Neurosciences
Cedars-Sinai Medical Center
Los Angeles, CA

# SECTION I

# Overarching View of Addiction

# 1

## Addiction: Definition, Epidemiology, and Neurobiology

### MATTHEW TORRINGTON

First the man takes a drink,
Then the drink takes a drink,
Then the drink takes the man.

*—old Japanese proverb*

Addiction is not a problem of personal weakness, a state of mind, or a personality trait. Addiction is a disorder of the innate learning and reward pathways in our brains. All addictions—from chemicals such as alcohol, prescription pills, drugs, tobacco, to behaviors such as gambling, food, work, shopping, sex, or gaming—are characterized ultimately by the loss of control. Addiction is often accompanied by obsession and compulsion along with this loss of control; often the addicted person engages in the behavior no longer to obtain pleasure but to relieve the discomfort created by withdrawal from the drug. Dysfunction in limbic and neocortical areas of the brain lead to a maladaptive cycle of dis-ease. This chronic disease of reward, motivation and memory, is rooted in complex biologic changes. Numerous survival systems are intertwined with genetics, early brain development, and learning pathways; these instincts are as basic as our aversion to pain and our desire to survive.

The severity and progression of addiction is highly variable across individuals. Some patients have mild forms with little propensity for misuse and loss of control while others cannot stop, even with the most intense and comprehensive treatment. Everyone suffering from addiction is on this continuum of susceptibility. Genetic vulnerability, exposure to addictive agents, psychosocial coping mechanisms, environment, and stressors combine to determine who develops an addictive disorder and how rapidly it evolves.

These disorders of maladaptive control are on the rise throughout our world. There is no doubt that we are all affected by addiction, and its epidemic proportion has infiltrated every income, educational, and social strata.

## Definition of Addiction

Addiction and substance-use disorders have been described as a pro-inflammatory, bio-psycho-social-environmental-spiritual disease state, characterized by compulsive engagement in rewarding stimuli despite adverse consequences. Addictions can be thought of as impulse control disorders that have biological, psychological, social, environmental, spiritual, and nutritional elements. Medication is often necessary to assist with detoxification or maintenance of sobriety. Using drugs or engaging in compulsive behaviors to deal with emotional or social issues are as inadequate strategies that only work in the short term. It is crucial to develop new psychological tools to facilitate adequate coping with both historically unprocessed emotional negativity as well as the normal ongoing emotional stress associated with contemporary life. Socially, if the environment is dysfunctional and unhealthy, users must disassociate themselves from those "people, places and things" associated with addictive behavior. Spiritually, the minimum faith requirement necessary to improve is faith in oneself: "You can't hit the bull's eye looking at the floor" or finish a marathon chanting "I can't, I can't, I can't." Whatever the individual's preferred spiritual outlet, some form of spirituality is definitively better than none. Nutritionally, taking command of and executively controlling what foods are going in the body is a crucial element of sustained success. Each case is distinct; each person requires a comprehensive individualized multimodal disease management approach. Evaluating and addressing the biological, psychological, social, spiritual, and nutritional gives individuals the best chance at complete and sustained recovery.

While the most qualified professionals in the addiction/recovery field ascribe to the bio-psycho-social-environmental-spiritual-nutritional disease model, there remains an abundance of unimodal or bimodal treatment. Many of those seeking treatment have access to only a fraction of the support they need to be successful: medication only, therapy only, group support only, spiritual only, nutritional only, and social only strategies remain popular. Without integrated, consistent, focused, multipronged therapy over time, many will unnecessarily succumb to their inability to control their impulse to use drugs.

Addiction is a disease characterized by relapse. Like other chronic diseases, addiction often involves cycles of relapse and remission. Although multiple discrete treatment attempts may be necessary to achieve lasting remission from substance-use disorders, treatment success, usually about 30%, is achieved with rates similar to other chronic disease states such as diabetes, hypertension, and hyperlipidemia. Unlike other disease states, mind-altering drugs can produce out-of-control behavior, unacceptable emotional responses, and continued exposure despite severe negative consequences. Progress can fluctuate with periods of intermittent remission, but addiction is generally progressive. Without treatment, it can result in death.

However, relapse in addictive disorders often results from premature failure to sustain treatment that was effective, such as when a necessary abstinence medication is impulsively discontinued or a patient leaves their outpatient program. Relapse in addictive diseases is not an inevitable intrinsic feature of the disease and may be "preventable" by sustained treatment.

Addiction is distinguished from drug use by a "lack of freedom of choice" as the individual loses control over the frequency, quantity, and other parameters of use. The pathologic pursuit of substance use coupled with the obsessive preoccupation, despite potential and accumulating adverse consequences, is characteristic of addiction. Use despite harm is the characteristic behavior of the user, whereas the addict is driven to use—the addict cannot "not"[1] use in the presence of drugs. These manifestations can occur compulsively or impulsively, as a reflection of impaired control. For instance, a person can exercise compulsively or binge watch videos beyond normal tolerance. But unless these actions are pathologic, the behavior might not be considered addictive.

With an addiction, reasoning is often impaired. Those with substance-use disorders often experience problems in perception, learning, impulse control, compulsivity, and judgment. They can be reticent to change their destructive and dysfunctional behaviors despite concerns of their friends and family, and usually, they lack the ability to see the magnitude of the cumulative problems and compounding ramifications of their behavior. The profound drive or craving to use substances or engage in what they view as rewarding behaviors underscores the compulsive or avolitional aspect of this disease.[2] The "powerlessness" over addiction and "unmanageability" of life while addicted is a central tenet of 12-step recovery programs.

The current diagnostic criteria, the *DSM-5* are divided into substance induced disorders and substance use disorders. Recent nomenclature has shifted away from "dependence" to "use disorder" for various substances and have developed modifying terms to describe the severity of illness, aka, "mild, moderate and severe." These criteria are broken into categories associated with impaired control (4 criteria), social impairment (3 criteria), risky use (2 criteria) and pharmacological criteria (2 criteria: tolerance and withdrawal).[3] The criteria are listed below:

# DSM-5 General Criteria for Substance Use Disorder

A minimum of 2–3 criteria are required for a mild substance use disorder diagnosis, while 4–5 is moderate, and 6–7 is severe (APA, 2013).

1. Taking the drug/alcohol in larger amounts and for longer than intended
2. Wanting to cut down or quit but not being able to do it
3. Spending a lot of time obtaining the drug/alcohol
4. Craving or a strong desire to use the drug/alcohol
5. Repeatedly unable to carry out major obligations at work, school, or home due to drug/alcohol use
6. Continued use despite persistent or recurring social or interpersonal problems caused or made worse by drug/alcohol use
7. Stopping or reducing important social, occupational, or recreational activities due to drug/alcohol use
8. Recurrent use of drugs/alcohol in physically hazardous situations
9. Consistent use of drugs despite acknowledgment of persistent or recurrent physical or psychological difficulties from using drugs/alcohol
10. *Tolerance as defined by either a need for markedly increased amounts to achieve intoxication or desired effect or markedly diminished effect with continued use of the same amount
11. *Withdrawal manifesting as either characteristic syndrome or the substance is used to avoid withdrawal.

## Drug Classes and Behavioral Addictions

There are four major classes of drugs. The first class includes stimulants that produce behavioral and central nervous system activation. These include drugs like amphetamines, cocaine, nicotine, and caffeine. The next class is the opioids which include natural, synthetic, and semi-synthetic drugs binding to the opioid receptor that produce pain analgesia and euphoria. The sedative/hypnotic class of drugs reduce anxiety and lower physiologic arousal or induce sleep such as benzodiazipines, alcohol, and barbiturates. Finally, the psychedelic/hallucinogenic class of drugs alter perception of time and space and may induce visual hallucinations and include drugs such as LSD (lysergic acid diethylamide), psilocybin, and cannabis. Behavioral addictions such as food addiction, best defined thru binge eating disorder, gambling disorder, and Internet/Gaming disorders all have the same underlying neurobiology as substance use disorders including activation of the ventral tegemental and nucleus accumbens reward areas of the brain. Love and sex addiction have not been included as behavioral addictions due to a paucity of evidence to support a consistent diagnostic profile at this time.

## Epidemiology of Addiction

According to the 2014 National Survey on Drug Use and Health, an estimated 27 million Americans aged 12 or older were current (past month) illicit drug users. Slightly more than 2.3 million adolescents aged 12–17 were current users, representing 9.4% of adolescents. Approximately 21.5 million people aged 12 or older in 2014 had SUDs (substance-use disorders) in the past year, including 17 million people with an alcohol use disorder and 7.1 million people with an illicit drug-use disorder.[4]

Addressing the impact of substance use alone is estimated to cost Americans more than $600 billion a year.[14] Direct and indirect costs from illicit drug use are evidenced in three principal areas—crime, health, and productivity.[5]

Tobacco use and its resulting addiction to nicotine is one of the costliest addictions in terms of general health. One study concluded that 8.7% of annual health-care spending (or $170 billion) in the United States will be linked to cigarette smoking.[6] An estimated 67 million people over age 12 were tobacco product users in 2014, including 55 million cigarette smokers. These numbers correspond to 25% and 21% of the population. Among the 32 million daily smokers, 40% smoke more than 16 cigarettes per day.[7] Statistics from a National Health Interview Survey reveal that, in 2015, the percentage of adults 18 and older who were current cigarette smokers was lower than 2014 (15% to almost 17%), and this number has been in a steady decline since 1997, when it was at 25% of all adults.[8]

Alcohol use and abuse is widespread throughout the United States. According to the National Institute of Alcohol Abuse and Alcoholism in a 2014 SAMHSA (Substance Abuse and Mental Health Services Administration) study, 88% of people aged 18 or older reported that they drank at some point in their lifetime with 71% saying they drank alcohol in the past year and 57% in the past month. One in four (24.7%) of people aged 18 or older reported that they engaged in binge drinking in the past month, and 6.7% reported that they engaged in heavy drinking in the past month.[9] The same study counted 16.3 million adults over age 18 with an alcohol-use disorder. Only 1.5 million adults received treatment at a specialized facility in 2014.[10]

In a study that evaluated the connection between excessive alcohol consumption and years of potential life lost (ypll) in the United States, alcohol contributed to 2.5 million ypll between 2006 and 2010. From this and other data, it was concluded that excessive drinking accounted for 1 in 10 deaths among working-age adults.[11] The US Department of Transportation National Highway Traffic Safety Administration (NHTSA) concluded that alcohol-impaired driving caused 31% of total car crash fatalities in 2014 (9,967 deaths). The percentage of alcohol-impaired deaths ranked higher than deaths due to speeding (28%), distracted driving (10%), and drowsy driving (2.6%).[12]

According to the Centers for Disease Control and Prevention (CDC) in the study of Alcohol-Related Disease Impact (ARDI), between 2006 and 2010 there were 38,253 deaths due to chronic abuse of alcohol and 49,544 deaths due to acute abuse, totaling 87,798 alcohol related deaths.[13] Drugs caused more than 47,000 deaths in 2013, according the CDC, accounting for more than alcohol- and firearm-related deaths. Males are more likely to die (18%) than females (11%) and white people (16.5%) more than black people (10%).[14]

Cannabis use disorder affected approximately 4.2 million people aged 12 and over in 2014, representing 1.6% of the population. An estimated 1.9 million people aged 12 and over had a opiate use disorder, and about 913,000 of this age group had a cocaine-use disorder.[15]

Addiction to sugar and food is also a major health concern; the link between obesity, diabetes, and heart disease is evident. An analysis of the data from the National Health and Nutrition Examination Survey 2005–2008 by the Center for Health Statistics found that about one-half of the population over the age of 2 consumes at least one sugary drink per day.[16] The National Center for Health Statistics analyzed the data collected from the Health and Nutrition Examination Survey, which examined the consumption of fast food in the United States. According to the data, 34.3% of all children between the ages of 2 and 19 consumed fast food on any given day in 2011–2012.[17]

Increasing evidence suggests that binge eating may lead to compulsive eating patterns due to the addictive potential of hyperpalatable foods. Studies on the prevalence of food addiction, however, are rare. Binge eating disorder closely resembles food addiction and there are mounting studies on the epidemiology of this disorder. Interestingly, an arguably high prevalence of food addiction can be found in underweight and normal-weight individuals. Future studies may investigate which factors are associated with addictive eating in non-obese individuals.[18]

Stimulant use is on the rise with the number of children taking medication for ADHD increasing by 28% between 2007 and 2011, as per the third National Survey of Children's Health. In 2011, 11% of children had been diagnosed with ADHD, with the percentage being much higher for high school boys (1 in 5) and lower for high school girls (1 in 11). In an analysis of the College Life Study by the Center for Substance Abuse Research (CESAR) to better understand the diversion of medically prescribed stimulants, researchers found that of the 44% of students that were prescribed amphetamine-dextroamphetaime, 70% diverted it at least once.[19]

Nonmedical stimulant use among adults aged 26 and older reached one million, according to the results from the 2014 National Survey on Drug Use and Health (NSDUH). Of that population, 438,000 (0.2%) were concurrent methamphetamine users. The most widely used stimulant, cocaine, affects individuals between the ages of 18 and 25 more than people aged 12 to 17 and 26 and older.[20]

Nonmedical sedative use is prevalent in at 330,000 people (0.1% of those over age 12), according to the 2014 National Survey on Drug Use and Health. This percentage was a bit higher (0.2%) for age groups 12–17 and 18–25, and lower for individuals aged 26 and older (0.1%).[21] According to the data from the National Comorbidity Survey, almost 1 in 10 adults have misused sedatives in their lifetime. Sedative consumption is associated with psychopathology, suicide risk, and specifically associated with parental abuse of prescription medications.[22] In an analysis of the National Health and Nutrition Examination Survey 2005–2010 by the Center for Disease Control and Prevention (CDC), researchers have found that about 4% of US adults aged 20 or older over used prescription sleep aids, and abuse in the past 30 days increased with age.[23]

Opioid use was higher among older adults (8.1% for adults aged 40–59 years). The CDC provided a data brief on research conducted by the National Health and Nutritional Examination Survey, confirming that 6.9% of adults aged 20 and over reported using opioid analgesic in the previous 30 days.[24]

National overdose deaths from benzodiazepines has been steadily increase also from 2001 to 2014, according to data by the National Center for Health Statistics at the CDC.[25]

## The Neurobiology of Addiction

According to the American Society of Addiction Medicine (ASAM):

> The neurobiology of addiction encompasses more than the neurochemistry of the reward. Addiction affects neurotransmission and interactions within reward structures of the brain, including the nucleus accumbens, anterior cingulate cortex, basal forebrain, and amygdala, such that motivational hierarchies are altered and addictive behaviors, alcohol, and other drug use, supplant self-care related behaviors. Addiction also affects neurotransmission and interactions between cortical and hippocampal circuits and brain reward structures, such that the memory of previous exposures to rewards (such as food, sex, alcohol, and other drugs) leads to a biological and behavioral response to external cues, in turn triggering craving and/or engagement in addictive behaviors.[26]

There's no doubt that addiction is prevalent and deadly. It is often referred to as "cunning" and "baffling," making it extremely difficult to understand why individuals suffer and even die from the "self administration" of substances seemingly against their own will. Why are we so susceptible to these disorders? The answer is complex but at its most basic level it can be thought of as an impulse control disorder that causes neuroadaptive and behavioral changes that can alter decision making capacity, adversely affect mood and impulse control and cause abstinence to be challenging.

The most anterior division of the brain, also called the pre-frontal cortex, is the part of the brain where humans develop executive and inhibitory control. This is part of the brain allows individuals to make decisions and assign priority to tasks. It also helps us to "apply the brakes" and say "no" to a desire that may not lead to a good outcome such as using drugs. It enables individuals to make these decisions weighing in a number of factors when it is working properly, and it's the part of the brain that is most affected when individuals start using drugs and alcohol. The pre-frontal cortex decision making capability is "hijacked" with repeated substance use which causes neuroadaptive changes to that region which in turn lead to disinhibition and impaired function, perpetuating faulty decision making and worsening impulse control.

The middle of the brain, the limbic brain, is a constellation of brain structures that includes (but is not limited to) the entorhinal complex, hippocampus, amygdala, nucleus accumbens, hypothalamus, and mammillary bodies. The nucleus accumbuns (NA) is referred to as the brain's "pleasure center." It is the major site of all reward stimulation in animals and humans. Addictive drugs highly stimulate the nucleus accumbens, far more directly than normal life rewards. Another major site in the mid-brain is associated with processing reward and known as the ventral tegemental area (VTA). The VTA is the most primitive part of the brain and located just below the nucleus accumbens. The brain cells in the VTA project to both the nucleus accumbens and the pre-frontal cortex and influence both pleasure and self-control. If the nucleus accumbens is tonically overstimulated as it is with regular drug use, it will modulate the stimulation it is receiving by releasing cAMP response element binding protein (CREB). In chronic drug use, CREB initiates a cascade of chemical interactions to release dynorphin. Dynorphin then inhibits stimulation of the nucleus accumbens. Thus in a person addicted to drugs who is over-stimulating the nucleus accumbens (NA), the NA will keep turning down the signal leading to less pleasure from the drug over time, which is the effect of tolerance requiring more of the drug to obtain the same reward. As drug use becomes chronic, this reward system dysfunction can lead to decreased pleasure from regular life rewards "anhedonia" that can create a vicious cycle of needing to use drugs to experience any reward and the use of drugs to avoid feeling bad instead of using them to get "high."

The limbic brain is able to affect and control both the neocortex (i.e., the way you think) and the midbrain (i.e., the way you feel.) The limbic brain responds to and is activated by dopamine, the currency of reward. Pleasurable activities make us feel good, and that is mediated by dopamine in the NA. Dopamine helps the limbic brain determine what is salient, what we need to do again, and what we can forgo. The more dopamine that is released, the more reinforcing the activity is to the limbic brain to a certain extent after which, it can cause anxiety, dysphoria, and psychosis. To further simplify the dopamine reward "economy" of the brain, imagine that the limbic brain gets $0.01 for a breath, $0.25 for food, $0.50 for sleep and about $2.00 for sex. This dopamine economy of "dollars and cents" works perfectly until we get exposed to some substance or activity that releases and abnormally large amount of dopamine. Think of alcohol as paying $5 per drink, cocaine as paying $300, concentrated opiates as paying $800, and methamphetamine paying $1,000 in dopamine. These and other inappropriately large dopamine releasers condition the limbic brain such that nothing else in life "matters" as much as the high- dopamine-releasing event.

The limbic brain has the ability to manipulate the way we think and feel. The intense physical withdrawal from substances of abuse—fever, chills, sweats, nausea, vomiting, diarrhea, muscle pain, joint pain, bone pain, restlessness, agitation, insomnia, irritability, depression—can be thought of as the limbic brain activating the brain stem and cerebellum to make the individual *feel* horrendous until the behavior in question is repeated. At the same time the limbic brain is able to affect the way that we *think*, convincing us that "it doesn't matter . . . I can stop later . . . no one can tell . . . I am still doing ok . . . " and on and on and overriding the messages from the pre-frontal cortex that are trying to use reason to stop this behavior. Additionally, using drugs will cause damage to the pre-frontal cortex over time, making inhibitory control more difficult and driving the train of addiction.

With chronic drug exposure, there is damage to the NA and diminished reward when trying to get high from drugs. However, this is not true for recalling the memory of using drugs—so-called "euphoric recall." Euphoric recall is extremely important in the cycle of drug addiction. External cues can trigger a craving through recall of previous drug-related euphoric experiences. While dopamine reward is reduced with the use of drugs chronically, there is sensitization that occurs with chronic dopamine stimulation. This makes the dopamine receptors "hypersensitive" to the cues of drug-related behavior and memories and causes craving. The brain will release elevated amounts of dopamine during a craving episode, allowing for a "high" beyond that which is achievable by using the drug itself. This was demonstrated by Nora Volkow, MD, at the National Institute for Drug Abuse (NIDA) in a recent study and is critical in understanding that the cycle of relapse has its roots in biology as well as psychology. It's also important for treatment, which will be discussed in later chapters with respect to naltrexone and its effect on decreasing euphoric recall for certain drugs and alcohol.

The solution lies in part by consistently using the pre-frontal cortex to guide behavior. Since the pre-frontal cortex can be manipulated by the limbic brain, it is essential that individuals develop a paradigm of "fact checking" their thoughts to make sure that they are not engaging in behaviors that are likely to lead to relapse. This can be accomplished with comprehensive individualized multimodal treatment over time, ongoing testing for drugs of abuse and contingency management strategies.

## Addiction Predispostion

Genetic sensitivity and vulnerability clearly plays a significant role in who will and who will not succumb to substance-use disorders. Similar to inheriting a predilection toward medical conditions such as high cholesterol or hypertension, addictions are moderately to highly heritable depending on the drug of abuse. According to several studies, addiction is attributed 50–60% to genetic predisposition. Family, adoption, and twin studies have shown that an individual's risk is proportional to the degree of genetic relationship to an addicted relative and there is a range of heritabilitiy of addictive disorders from 0.39 for hallucinogens to 0.72 for cocaine. One study looked at identical and non-identical twins and found when one identical twin was addicted to alcohol, the other twin had a high probability of being addicted, and this did not hold true for the non-identical twins.[27]

Adolescent exposure to substances contributes to the development of addiction. The frontal lobes are important in inhibiting impulsivity and in assisting individuals to appropriately delay gratification.[28] Frontal lobe morphology, connectivity, and functioning are still in the process of maturation during adolescence and young adulthood, while normal adolescent behaviors involving risk taking and novelty seeking are at a peak. This lack of myelination in pre-frontal cortex neurons, coupled with the teenage drive toward increased experimentation with drugs, is believed to be the reason that rates of substance abuse are the highest in those aged 18 to 25 years. In this regard, addiction can be regarded as a developmental illness.

Clearly the environment, exposure to drug related behavior and substances of abuse, as well as exposure to stress and a history of trauma all play significant roles in the development of substance use disorders. In contrast to the nature versus nurture argument, in this case, it is clearly nature *and* nurture, in addition to other modifying factors.

## Emotional Aspect of Addiction

The emotional aspects of addiction are complex. Many people use drugs and alcohol, or pathologically pursue rewards because they are seeking euphoria or a positive change in their mood or emotional state. Others self-medicate and act out to gain relief from dysphoric or negative emotional states.

According to the ASAM, emotional changes that occur in substance use disorder can include:

- increased anxiety, dysphoria and emotional pain
- increased sensitivity to stressors associated with the recruitment of brain stress systems, such that "things seem more stressful" as a result
- difficulty in identifying feelings, distinguishing between feelings and the bodily sensations of emotional arousal, and describing feelings to other people (sometimes referred to as alexithymia)[29]

It's interesting to note that withdrawal from virtually all pharmacological classes of addictive drugs leads to an anxious, agitated, dysphoric, and labile emotional experience. Tolerance develops to the "high" but not to the "low" of intoxication and withdrawal. While people who suffer from addiction repeatedly try and re-create a high, they mostly re-create deeper lows. This often changes their "desire" to get high into a "need" in order to avoid the mounting dysphoria that repeated substance use can create thru dynorphin related neuroadaptive mechanisms that alter the brain's reward system. There's not a simple solution to this complex condition. Remission and relapse are part of the disease. The 12 step program Alcoholics Anonymous, AA has saved the lives of millions and is a strong thread of community support for the recovery community. Inpatient and outpatient rehabilitation programs have spread around the United States, catering to both poor and wealthy patients creating a billion dollar industry. Most rehabilitation programs include individual and group therapy, 12-step programs, and a restructuring of social circles and habits. Addiction success rates are cited at about 30%. Due to the anonymity of the recovery programs, realistic statistics of long-term sobriety and success can only be estimated. In most cases, medication management can improve treatment outcomes.

Comprehensive, individualized multimodal treatment over time is most likely to help the greatest number of people not succumb to addictive illness. Consider the disease management strategies utilized for the treatment of diabetes. A normal diabetic getting treatment in contemporary medicine gets coordinated treatment plan that includes but may not be limited to: regular primary care, regular lab testing, regular ophthalmology follow-up, regular podiatry follow up, regular nutritional counseling, regular medication compliance assessments in addition to specialist intervention when necessary. The contemporary care of diabetes isn't seen as having an "end"; rather, it is seen as something that hopefully can be managed better over time. There isn't really a point where we discharge the diabetic and say "you are cured . . . bye." Contrast this with much of mainstream addiction treatment; many of these ill patients with a "life threatening brain disease," are given 30, 60, or 90 days of residential treatment or sometimes 6 to 12 weeks of outpatient treatment and then discharged. Some programs go as far as to advertise the selling "addiction cure." There is no known cure for addiction. Fortunately, helping patients develop and implement treatment plans that address the biological, psychological, social, spiritual, and nutritional aspects of their illness over time enhances outcomes and saves lives. Applying the disease management model to addiction remains the simplest and most cost-effective method of saving lives, reducing morbidity, and saving society's resources from being squandered by continuing to simply clean up the cycle of addiction.

## REFERENCES

1. http://www.addictionsandrecovery.org/is-addiction-a-disease.htm
2. http://www.addictionsandrecovery.org/is-addiction-a-disease.htm
3. *DSM-V APA, DSM* 5th ed., Arlington VA, APA, 2013.
4. http://www.samhsa.gov/data/.
5. National Drug Intelligence Center. National Threat Assessment: the Economic Impact of Illicit Drug Use on American Society. May 2011. Department of Justice, Washington, DC.
6. Xu X, Bishop EE, Kennedy SM, Simpson SA, Pechacek TF. Annual health-care spending attributable to cigarette smoking: An update. *American Journal of Preventive Medicine.* 2015;48(3):326–333.
7. http://www.samhsa.gov/data/.
8. "National Health Interview Survey 1997–2015 Sample Adult Core Component." *CDC.* CDC, n.d. Web. 25 May 2016.
9. Found at https://www.niaaa.nih.gov/alcohol-health/overview-alcohol-consumption/alcohol-facts-and-statistics, Substance Abuse and Mental Health Services Administration (SAMHSA). 2014 National Survey on Drug Use and Health (NSDUH). Table 2.41B—Alcohol use in lifetime, past year, and past month among persons aged 18 or older, by demographic characteristics: Percentages, 2013 and 2014. Available at: http://www.samhsa.gov/data/sites/default/files/NSDUH-DetTabs2014/NSDUH-DetTabs2014.htm#tab2-41b
10. found at https://www.niaaa.nih.gov/alcohol-health/overview-alcohol-consumption/alcohol-facts-and-statistics, Substance Abuse and Mental Health Services Administration (SAMHSA). 2014 National Survey on Drug Use and Health (NSDUH). Table 5.8B—Substance dependence or abuse in the past year among persons aged 18 or older, by demographic characteristics: Percentages, 2013 and 2014. Available at http://www.samhsa.gov/data/sites/default/files/NSDUH-DetTabs2014/NSDUH-DetTabs2014.htm#tab5-8b
11. Stahre M, Roeber J, Kanny D, et al. Contribution of excessive alcohol consumption to deaths and years of potential life lost in the United States. *Preventing Chronic Disease.* 2014;11:e109.
12. National Center for Statistics and Analysis. (2015, November). *2014 Crash Data Key Findings* (Traffic Safety Facts Crash Stats. Report No. DOT HS 812 219). Washington, DC: National Highway Traffic Safety Administration. Available at: http://www-nrd.nhtsa.dot.gov/Pubs/812219.pdf

13. http://www.ncbi.nlm.nih.gov/pmc/articles/PMC3207274/
14. CDC death information 2013—"National Vital Statistics System." *Centers for Disease Control and Prevention.* Centers for Disease Control and Prevention, n.d. Web site. http://www.cdc.gov/nchs/products/nvsr.htm
15. http://www.samhsa.gov/data/. Accessed February 15, 2016.
16. Ogden CL, Kit BK, Carroll MD, Park S. Consumption of sugar drinks in the United States, 2005–2008. In: NCHS data brief, no 71. Hyattsville, MD: National Center for Health Statistics; 2011.
17. Vikraman S, Fryar CD, Ogden CL. Caloric intake from fast food among children and adolescents in the United States, 2011–2012. In: NCHS data brief, no 213. Hyattsville, MD: National Center for Health Statistics. 2015.
18. Centers for Disease Control and Prevention (CDC). Alcohol and public health: Alcohol-related disease impact (ARDI). Available at: http://nccd.cdc. gov/DPH_ARDI/Default/Report.aspx?T=AAM&P=f6d7eda7-036e-4553-9968-9b17ffad620e&R=d7a9b303-48e9-4440-bf47-070a4827e1fd&M=AD96A9C1-285A-44D2-B76D-BA2AE037FC56&F=&D
19. Garnier L, Arria, A. Diversion of Medically Prescribed Stimulants and Analgesics by College Students. *Diversion of Medically Prescribed Stimulants and Analgesics by College Students* (n.d.): Web site.
20. Center for Behavioral Health Statistics and Quality. *Behavioral health trends in the United States: Results from the 2014 National Survey on Drug Use and Health* (HHS Publication No. SMA 15-4927, NSDUH Series H-50). 2015. Retrieved from http:// www.samhsa.gov/ data/
21. Center for Behavioral Health Statistics and Quality. *Behavioral health trends in the United States: Results from the 2014 National Survey on Drug Use and Health* (HHS Publication No. SMA 15-4927, NSDUH Series H-50). 2015. Retrieved from http:// www.samhsa.gov/ data/
22. Goodwin, RD, Hasin, DS. Sedative use and misuse in the United States. *Addiction.* 2002;97:555–562. doi: 10.1046/j.1360-0443.2002.00098.x
23. Chong Y, Fryar CD, Gu Q. Prescription sleep aid use among adults: United States, 2005–2010. In: NCHS data brief, no 127. Hyattsville, MD: National Center for Health Statistics; 2013.
24. Frenk SM, Porter KS, Paulozzi LJ. Prescription opioid analgesic use among adults: United States, 1999–2012. In: NCHS data brief, no 189. Hyattsville, MD: National Center for Health Statistics; 2015.
25. "Overdose Death Rates." National Institute on Drug Abuse (NIDA). Centers for Disease Control and Prevention. Web site. Accessed June 1, 2016.
26. http://www.asam.org/quality-practice/definition-of-addiction
27. Prescott, CA, Kendler KS. Genetic and environmental contributions to alcohol abuse and dependence in a population-based sample of male twins. *Am J Psychiatry.* 1999;156(1):34–40.
28. http://www.asam.org/quality-practice/definition-of-addiction
29. http://www.addictionsandrecovery.org/is-addiction-a-disease.htm

# 2

## Overview of the Addiction Recovery Industry

### MATTHEW TORRINGTON

We are living in an age where addiction is an expanding epidemic spreading at an alarming rate. A survey done by SAMHSA looked at people aged 12 years and older in need of treatment for drug and alcohol abuse and found that 23.5 million are in need of assistance. This is equivalent to about 10% of the US population and extraordinary in its own right. It is tragic that only 11% of these people are receiving treatment, which accounts for only 1% of the US population.

That said, the addiction recovery business is booming; SAMHSA and others report that it is a $35 billion industry. SAMHSA, in 2015, reported the number of residential programs, specifically broken down into Residential Detoxification (RD), Long-term Residential (RL), and Short-term Residential, at 2,792 facilities. The same study listed 6,822 facilities as intensive outpatient treatment (IOP) centers. The National Directory of Drug and Alcohol Abuse Treatment Facilities in 2015 cited 4,127 treatment programs accepted clients who were referred from the court/judicial system.[1] In 2015 the American Board of Addiction Medicine (ABAM) surveyed physicians in the United States and found there are 3,630 physicians board certified in addiction medicine.[2]

According to the National Institute on Drug Abuse, more than 23% of admissions to public rehab programs are due to alcohol abuse or substance-use disorders, while another 18% go for addiction to both alcohol and other substances.[3] The number of substance abuse treatment admissions for both narcotic pain reliever and benzodiazepine abuse increased 570% from 2000 to 2010, with 33,701 admissions. During the same period, admissions for all other substances decreased by nearly 10%.[4] Another study on facilities that report to state administrative data systems counted 1.8 million admissions, with most of those (41%) for alcohol abuse. Heroin and other opiates accounted for 20% and marijuana for 17%.[5]

The anonymous aspects of addiction, recovery, treatment, and the shame surrounding addiction makes it difficult to know how many people are actually struggling to recover from substance-use disorders. There is no accurate data that reflect how many people are recovering through 12-step programs or individual private counseling. Whichever set of numbers you choose to use or believe, the bottom line is that far too many people, especially the young, are using, abusing, or are addicted to alcohol, nicotine, and other drugs or combinations of substances; clearly only a fraction of those suffering are getting the help they need.

From the National Center on Addiction and Substance Abuse:

- 40 million Americans aged 12 and older—or more than 1 in 7 people—abuse or are addicted to nicotine, alcohol, or other drugs.[6]

From the World Health Organization:

- 76.3 million people worldwide have alcohol-use disorders, and at least 15.3 million have drug-use disorders.
- Use of injected drugs has been reported in 136 countries, of which 93 report HIV infection among this population.[7]

From the Center for Disease Control and SAMSHA:

- Prescription drug abuse, while most prevalent in the United States, is also a worldwide problem.
- More people died in the United States in 2015 from prescriptions drug overdose than motor vehical accidents, according to the 2015 National Drug Threat Assessment Summary, published by the DEA in 2015.
- The 2014 National Survey on Drug use and Health performed by SAMSHA found that 15 million people abuse prescription drugs in the United States alone, more than the combined number who reported abusing cocaine, hallucinogens, inhalants, and heroin.
- Prescription drug abuse causes the largest percentage of deaths from drug overdoses.
- According to Center for Disease Control's 2017 report, more than 64,000 Americans died from drug overdoses in 2016, including illicit drugs and prescription opioids. This is nearly a doubling of deaths in 1 decade.
- Among the more than 64,000 drug overdose deaths estimated in 2016, the CDC found the sharpest increase occurred among deaths related to fentanyl and fentanyl analogs (synthetic opioids) with over 20,000 overdose deaths in 2016.
- Nearly half of all teen drug users believe that prescription drugs are much safer than illegal street drugs, with 60–70% saying that their home medicine cabinets are their source of drugs.[8]

## Addiction in Animals

Addiction is not limited to humans. There is evidence of substance use and pleasure-seeking behavior in animals. Wallabies have been known to snack on opium poppies and dance around in circles. Dolphins have been recorded chewing on pufferfish and then looking very tranquil and dazed. Consider "catnip" and beef-liver dog treats, affectionately known as "doggie crack." Humans and other mammals are programmed to seek pleasure. It's as if it is our animal nature to seek out pleasure with experiences and substances that bring us an altered experience.

We have learned a great deal about the biology and pathophysiology of addiction and substance abuse from animal models. According to the National Center for Biotechnology Information (NCBI) and the National Institute of Health (NIH), animal studies often focus on the ability of drugs to directly alter an animal's behavior. Animal studies have demonstrated that the rewarding effect is not dependent on preexisting conditions and that exposure to a drug can be sufficient to motivate drug-taking behavior. Studies that allow the animals to self-administer drugs known to be abused by humans support the concept that drugs act as universal reinforcers. Animal models illustrate that some typical behaviors associated with drug abuse in humans involve biologic processes common to all mammals.[9]

## Historical Background of Addiction

There's no doubt that the use of intoxicants pre-dates the written word. References describing crops of hemp go back 10,000 years. Addiction is referenced in ancient Greek and Roman literature.

In the United States, from 1850 to 1915, marijuana was widely used throughout the nation as a medicinal drug and could be purchased easily in pharmacies and general stores.[10] The 18th Amendment, passed in 1920, banned the manufacture, sale, and transportation of alcohol and was an attempt to curb alcohol consumption that resulted in or from increased poverty, housing problems, and "immorality." The strategy didn't work; alcohol use was far from curtailed, and an era of rampant violent crime was facilitated by the "black market" for "booze". Prohibition was repealed in 1933 with the 21st Amendment.

## History of Treatment Evolution

The New York State Inebriate Asylum, which opened in 1864, was the first hospital dedicated to the treatment of alcoholism as a mental health condition. Seventy years later, in 1935, the Alcoholics Anonymous model was born, when Dr. Bob and Bill W. founded the first 12-step program. Using a spirituality-and-abstinence-based approach to rehabilitation, it set the stage for a huge industry of addiction treatment centers, sober housing, and all types of 12-step and other inpatient and outpatient programs for addicts and their families.

## History of US Drug Policy

One of the first sets of anti-drug laws was directed at Chinese immigrants in the 1870s and their use of opium. The anti-cocaine laws that cropped up in the 1900s targeted black men in the South who were the predominant users of that time. Marijuana use by Mexican migrants in the Midwest and Southwest became a focus in 1910–1920. In the 1960s, drugs became a symbol of social rebellion and political dissent, which led to President Nixon declaring a "war on drugs" in 1971. In 1973, New York State enacted the draconian Rockefeller laws, making the penalty for selling 2 ounces of heroin, morphine, opium, cocaine, or marijuana—or possessing 4 ounces or more of the same drugs—a minimum of 15 years to life in prison. These laws became the strictest in the country.

The introduction of "crack" cocaine in the 1980s led President Reagan to expand the drug war and criminalize all aspects of drug use, sale, and abuse. The number of people who entered US jails for non-violent drug law offenses increased from 50,000 in 1980 to over 400,000 in 1997.[11]

Focused on saving lives by decreasing driving under the influence, Mothers Against Drunk Drivers (MADD) rose to public attention in 1980s. They claim their efforts have saved 330,000 lives and halved the number of deaths due to drunk driving since then with the introduction of the "designated-driver," alcohol checkpoints, and a general awareness to the issue. Despite MADD, federal, state, and local efforts, arrests for driving under the influence of alcohol or narcotics still number over 1.1 million a year.[12]

Today, most Americans favor sensible reforms that expand health-based approaches to alcohol- and drug-related offenses, yet 700,000 people are still arrested annually for marijuana offenses, and almost 500,000 are still behind bars.[13] Historically we have not done a good job of integrating the delivery of substance-use identification and treatment with the rest of medical care, but this trend began to change with enactment of the Paul Wellstone and Pete Domenici Mental Health Parity and Addiction Equity Act of 2008 (MHPAEA) and the Affordable Care Act in 2010.[14,15] MHPAEA requires that the financial requirements and treatment limitations imposed by health plans and insurers for substance-use disorders be no more restrictive than the financial requirements and treatment limitations they impose for medical and surgical conditions. The Affordable Care Act required the majority of United States health plans and insurers to offer prevention, screening, brief interventions, and other forms of treatment for substance-use disorders.[16] As of 2016, it appears that the federal government is facing the issue head on with the publication of the first ever "Surgeon General's report: Facing Addiction in America." This 428-page resource provides a comprehensive overview and strategic blueprint for addressing the crisis.

## Cost to Society

The impact of tobacco, alcohol, and other drugs on crime, lost work productivity, and health care is estimated to cost the United States more than $700 billion annually. Tobacco leads at $295 billion, followed by alcohol at $224 billion and illicit drugs at $193 billion.[17] Injection drug use provides an efficient mechanism for transmitting blood-borne viruses, such as HIV and hepatitis C and B and is thought to be the vector of infection for more than one-fifth of American adults and adolescents currently living with HIV infections.[18]

The cost to society continues with prescription opioid abuse, which cost nearly $56 billion in 2009, with health-care costs at $25 billion.[19] And a recent study in the *American Journal of Preventive Medicine* showed that from 2012 to 2014 excessive drinking cost the United States $249 billion, based on the change in alcohol-attributable deaths and price or inflation rate in cost of medical care, with the government paying for $101 billion (40.4%) of these costs.[20]

## Drug-Related Deaths

According to the CDC's National Center for Health Statistics, from 2001 to 2014, deaths due to all types of drugs have risen in the past 14 years.[21]

- prescription drugs—up from 9,000 to 25,000
- prescription opioid pain relievers—up from 5,500 to 18,000
- benzodiazepines—up from 1,570 to 8,000
- cocaine—up from 3,750 to 5,000, with a spike to 7,500 in 2006
- heroin—up from 1,750 to 10,000

## Drug Emergencies

Many addictions lead to medical emergencies from a wide range of drugs that are commonly abused. The largest percentage of medical emergencies come from pharmaceutically produced benzodiazepines and opiates. Others come from a mixture of prescription and illicit drugs, such as heroin, cocaine, or methamphetamine.

Still others include alcohol in addition to prescription or illicit drugs. The largest percentage of emergency room visits involved the use of prescription drugs with no other substances. These statistics come from the Drug Abuse Warning Network (DAWN), a division of the SAMHSA,[22] from a study done from 2004 to 2009, published in 2013:

- Emergency room visits for nonmedical use of pharmaceuticals alone: 117% increase
- Emergency room visits for pharmaceuticals with illicit drugs: 97% increase
- Emergency room visits for pharmaceuticals with alcohol: 63% increase
- Emergency room visits for pharmaceuticals used with illicit drugs and alcohol: 76% increase

## Health Insurance's Part

As mentioned, drug, alcohol, and other addiction rehabilitation treatment in the United States is big business—$35 billion by 2012. There are now 14,000+ treatment facilities, and this number is growing. A total of 2.5 million persons received treatment, but many more need it, and facilities are filled to capacity. However, insurance coverage for rehabilitation is limited but improved with the ACA.

High-end niches have emerged for the self-funded cash payors, and new niches are emerging in areas such as: sex addiction, problem gambling, Internet addiction, and nicotine addiction. Facilities are also diversifying by specializing in treating people with anxiety disorders, eating disorders, trauma, and posttraumatic stress in Iraq and Afghanistan veterans.[23]

The Affordable Care Act has and will continue to increase the number of people who are eligible for health-care coverage through Medicaid and federal and state exchanges, and it includes parity for mental health and substance abuse services. More people have access to health care, and as screening for substance abuse and mental illness becomes more commonplace in primary care, more individuals in need of substance abuse care will get it. A program developed and propagated by the SAMHSA, SBIRT (screening, brief intervention, and referral to treatment) has helped to train primary care and other medical service providers to "Ask, Advise and Assist" patients to identify and treat substance-use disorders. Reimbursement codes have been developed and implemented to further encourage and compensate health-care providers to address this often-neglected issue. Regardless of these efforts, the ability to afford care, which was cited as the most significant barrier to receiving care for substance abuse disorder in 33% of those surveyed who needed services, remains a serious problem.[24]

# Physicians' Part

Historically physicians, knowingly and unknowingly, have played a massive role in this issue. They have been taught and trained to treat pain, the so-called fifth vital sign. In some states, such as California, laws mandate the treatment of pain. When a doctor was convicted of "battery" for the under-treatment of pain in 2002, it was like a "shot heard around the world." Numerous factors have compelled physicians to dole out medications, often powerful narcotics, in order to comply with the standard of care, to gain patient satisfaction, and to ensure their employment. The time required and the out-of-pocket costs of writing a prescription pale in comparison to those providing solid emotional support and helping patients develop and implement comprehensive multimodal treatment plans.

Most practicing physicians had little to no training on substance-use disorders and have not been trained to take an active role in preventing abuse. Over-reliance on prescription opioids, lack of training regarding recognizing early signs of prescription drug misuse, and limited coverage for non medical treatments (i.e., acupuncture, massage, physical therapy, mind body activities) all compounded the problem. In addition to the issues around getting doctors to address the fact that they are sometimes part of the problem, getting patients into treatment programs that are often unaffordable and inconvenient can be major challenges for frontline physicians.

As of this writing there is a major shift happening in our medical culture that focuses on changing the paradigm of pain management to include more multimodal treatment interventions and to more clearly delineate and disseminate guidelines about appropriate prescribing of opiate medications. The FDA now requires risk evaluation and mitigation strategies (REMS) for all newly approved drugs that are controlled substances. There is also mandatory training of medical students and medical residents about addiction and pain management as well as some states requiring all physicians to have access to prescription drug monitoring programs that allow health-care providers to see all the controlled substances that patients have been prescribed by other providers. In addition to these measures is the birth of the newest ACGME-recognized medical specialty: addiction medicine. At this time there are more than 20 brick-and-mortar fellowship programs in addiction medicine, and more are being added every year. The quality and quantity of targeted medical education, basic science, and clinical research focused on this emerging area of interest continues to increase.

In addition to medical specialists focused on the treatment of addiction, it is helpful to consider other treatment resources available in the environment. The American Society of Addiction Medicine publishes and updates the ASAM Criteria, formerly known as the patient placement criteria, which is the most widely used and comprehensive set of guidelines for placement, continued stay and transfer/discharge of patients with addiction and co-occurring conditions.[25] These criteria help to account for biological, psychological, social, and nutritional elements affecting those seeking treatment and help treatment professionals determine the most appropriate level of care. The criteria consider at six different domains (acute intoxication and withdrawal potential; biomedical conditions and complications; emotional, behavioral, or cognitive conditions and complications; readiness to change; relapse, continued use, or continued problem potential; recovery and living environment) (Figure 2.1) in order to best assess what intervention is most likely to help the patient.[26]

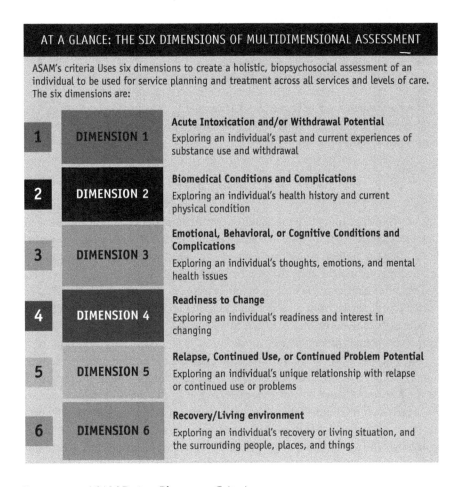

## AT A GLANCE: THE SIX DIMENSIONS OF MULTIDIMENSIONAL ASSESSMENT

ASAM's criteria Uses six dimensions to create a holistic, biopsychosocial assessment of an individual to be used for service planning and treatment across all services and levels of care. The six dimensions are:

**1   DIMENSION 1**
**Acute Intoxication and/or Withdrawal Potential**
Exploring an individual's past and current experiences of substance use and withdrawal

**2   DIMENSION 2**
**Biomedical Conditions and Complications**
Exploring an individual's health history and current physical condition

**3   DIMENSION 3**
**Emotional, Behavioral, or Cognitive Conditions and Complications**
Exploring an individual's thoughts, emotions, and mental health issues

**4   DIMENSION 4**
**Readiness to Change**
Exploring an individual's readiness and interest in changing

**5   DIMENSION 5**
**Relapse, Continued Use, or Continued Problem Potential**
Exploring an individual's unique relationship with relapse or continued use or problems

**6   DIMENSION 6**
**Recovery/Living environment**
Exploring an individual's recovery or living situation, and the surrounding people, places, and things

**FIGURE 2.1** ASAM Patient Placement Criteria.
http://www.asam.org/quality-practice/guidelines-and-consensus-documents/the-asam-criteria/about

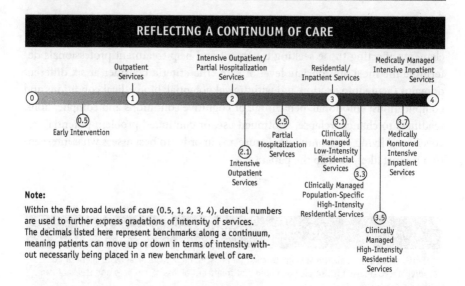

FIGURE 2.2  Continuum of Care in SUD Treatment.
http://www.asam.org/quality-practice/guidelines-and-consensus-documents/the-asam-criteria/about

# Conclusion

It is our challenge in society to change our attitudes about addiction and, on a societal level, to prevent the overwhelming epidemic of addiction we have created. With 1 in 7 (40 million Americans aged 12 and older) who abuse (or are addicted to) nicotine, alcohol, or other drugs, a new battle on addiction must be waged. The cycle of addiction must be broken before it leads to death. In 2014, the CDC reported 47,055 deaths from prescription analgesics and heroin, which was up from 38,000 in 2010. Add to this 29,000 alcohol-induced deaths and another 36,000 from liver-related ailments and cirrhosis.[27]

The solution won't be found by putting doctors or addicts in prison. More money needs to be directed at mental health and addiction recovery programs. As the National Center on Substance Abuse and Addiction reported in 2009, of the nearly half a trillion dollars per year we spend on substance-related costs, nearly 97 cents per dollar is spent "shoveling up the mess" as burden to public programs while less than 3 cents per dollar is spent on prevention, treatment, and research combined. We cannot afford to watch and wait for addiction to go away—it is here, and we are all responsible for addressing it. As they say in AA, the first step is admitting, in this case, that the system has become unmanageable.

## REFERENCES

1. Substance Abuse and Mental Health Services Administration, Center for Behavioral Health Statistics and Quality. *Behavioral Health Services Information Series: National Directory of Drug and Alcohol Abuse Treatment Facilities 2015*, HHS Publication No. (SMA) 16-4940.

2. Find a Doctor—American Board of Addiction Medicine. American Board of Addiction Medicine RSS. N.p., n.d. Web. June 15, 2016.

3. http://luxury.rehabs.com/alcohol-rehab/statistics/#Rehab.

4. Substance Abuse and Mental Health Services Administration, Center for Behavioral Health Statistics and Quality. (December 13, 2012). *The TEDS Report: Admissions Reporting Benzodiazepine and Narcotic Pain Reliever Abuse at Treatment Entry.* Rockville, MD: Center for Behavioral Health Statistics and Quality.

5. https://www.drugabuse.gov/publications/drugfacts/treatment-statistics.

6. http://www.centeronaddiction.org/addiction?gclid=CjwKEAjwgdSBRDA7fT68f6s8
zMSJADZwHmvBZKadLcJxoktp5hGnxWGvyoVsaatInRoTE3RRGObWx0Cn4vw.

7. http://www.ncbi.nlm.nih.gov/pmc/articles/PMC2890392/.

8. http://www.drugfreeworld.org/drugfacts/prescription/abuse-international-statistics.html.

9. http://www.ncbi.nlm.nih.gov/pmc/articles/PMC2890392/.

10. http://www.advancedholistichealth.org/history.html.

11. http://www.drugpolicy.org/new-solutions-drug-policy/brief-history-drug-war.

12. http://www.madd.org/drunk-driving/about/drunk-driving-statistics.html.

13. http://www.drugpolicy.org/drug-war-statistics.

14. Patient Protection and Affordable Care Act, 42 U.S.C. § 18001, H.R. 3590, Public Law No. 111-148, 124 Stat. 119 Stat. (2010).

15. Paul Wellstone and Pete Domenici Mental Health Parity and Addiction Equity Act of 2008, H.R. 6983 (2008).

16. Patient Protection and Affordable Care Act, 42 U.S.C. § 18001, H.R. 3590, Public Law No. 111-148, 124 Stat. 119 Stat. (2010).

17. https://www.drugabuse.gov/related-topics/trends-statistics.

18. Centers for Disease Control and Prevention. Monitoring selected national HIV prevention and care objectives by using HIV surveillance data—United States and 6 US-dependent areas—2010. HIV Surveillance Supplemental Report 2012;17 (No. 3, part A). http://www.cdc.gov/hiv/topics/ surveillance/resources/reports/. Published June 2012. Accessed [date].

19. Birnbaum HG, White, AG, Schiller M, Waldman T, Cleveland JM, Roland CL. Societal costs of prescription opioid abuse, dependence, and misuse in the United States. *Pain Medicine.* 2011;12(4):657–667. Web. 16 Feb. 2016.

20. Sacks JJ, Gonzales KR, Bouchery EE, et al. 2010 national and state costs of excessive alcohol consumption. *American Journal of Preventive Medicine.* 2015;49(5):e73–e79. PMID: 26477807.

21. https://www.drugabuse.gov/related-topics/trends-statistics/overdose-death-rates.
22. http://luxury.rehabs.com/drug-rehab/statistics/#treatment-program.
23. http://luxury.rehabs.com/alcohol-rehab/statistics/#Rehab.
24. http://store.samhsa.gov/shin/content/PEP13-RTC-BHWORK/PEP13-RTC-BHWORK.pdf.
25. http://www.asam.org/quality-practice/guidelines-and-consensus-documents/the-asam-criteria
26. http://www.asam.org/quality-practice/guidelines-and-consensus-documents/the-asam-criteria/about
27. http://www.drugwarfacts.org/cms/Causes_of_Death#sthash.SVgRSoRj.dpbs.

# SECTION II

# The Substances

# 3

## Food Addiction

EDISON DE MELLO

## Introduction

The alarming growth of the obesity epidemic in the United States and globally has created both controversy and burgeoning interest in the field of
food addiction.

The latest Center for Disease Control (CDC) data on obesity released in 2011
was extremely disturbing. It shows, for example, that 35% of American adults age
20 and over are obese (BMI > 30). When people categorized as overweight (BMI
of 25 to 29) are combined with those considered obese, the percentage skyrockets
to a startling 69%. These percentages have been equally and inexorably increasing
for both children and adolescents as well.[1]

How has the situation deteriorated so rapidly? The answer may lie in having
under-estimated the root of the problem. An impressive body of recent research strongly suggests that addiction-like processes, which impair satiety and
cause food-intake dysregulation, may actually underline obesity. Support for the
food addiction hypothesis comes from alterations in the neurochemistry of dopamine and endogenous opioids, the neuroanatomy of the limbic system, and
self-medication behaviors. Foods identified as having potential addictive properties include sweets, carbohydrates, fats, sweet/fat combinations, and possibly
processed and/or high salt foods. Eating topography is understood as a necessary
factor in neural pathway changes that promote addiction-like properties in response to some foods. Thus, chronic food cravings, compulsive overeating, and
binge eating may represent a phenotype of obesity.[2]

Unlike using drugs, eating is essential for survival and part of common daily
routine. Thus, diagnosing food addiction can present obstacles and challenges
in separating addictive behavior from normal biological imperatives. Social and
cultural influences on eating habits and person-to-person variability in feeling

satiated after eating make establishing baselines and discerning food-addiction from extraneous factors more challenging. Fortunately, however, a questionnaire developed by Yale University in 2009 to assess food addiction based on the *DSM-4* criteria for substance dependence has proven to be an effective tool in the initial diagnosis of food addiction. Known as the Yale Food Addiction Scale (YFAS), this 25-item, self-report scale measures food addiction symptoms such as tolerance, withdrawal, and loss of control. It uses the criteria for substance dependence established by the *DSM-4*. In addition, the scale contains 2 items that clinically assesses significant impairment or distress from eating. Food addiction, as per the YFAS, is diagnosed when 3 symptoms are present and are accompanied by clinically significant impairment or distress. While there is no uniformly accepted way to diagnose food addiction as of yet, the YFAS helps to identify individuals with signs and symptoms of dependency to some foods. As suspected, foods most notably identified to cause food addiction are those high in fat and high in sugar.[3] (See Table 3.1.)

Behavioral dependence criteria, in diagnostic terms, show that addiction is now referred to as "substance use disorder." The *DSM-4* defines SUD as having 2 or more of 11 symptoms occurring within 1 year, which include substances taken in larger amounts or for a longer duration than intended, building up tolerance, and having withdrawals. Based on these criteria, binge eaters, many chronic overeaters, and emotional eaters would meet the criteria for food addiction.

## Genetics

Research on physical craving and food addiction has come a long way since 1993, when G. Terence Wilson, a national authority on eating disorders and psychology professor at Rutgers University, concluded that the widely held belief that foods cause physical cravings was without convincing empirical support.[4] In 1994, however, Ernest Noble et al at UCLA contradicted Wilson and reported that some obese adults who were binging on dense carbohydrates and who were neither alcoholic nor drug addicted had the same D2 dopamine gene markers specific to alcoholism and other drug addictions. Subsequent research has supported Noble's findings, confirming that addiction to food in humans does indeed exist, and it is likely composed of a cluster of chemical dependencies that starts with physical craving.[5] Rather than eating from hunger, consumption of food and drug use is initially driven by rewarding properties that involve activation of mesolimbic dopamine (DA) pathways. As Nora Volkow and Roy Wise from NIDA demonstrated in their groundbreaking study in 2005, food and drug abuse both activate DA pathways, albeit differently. Using positron emission tomography, they demonstrated the role of DA in the nucleus accumbens in drug addiction and obesity and proposed a common thread for both. While food activates brain reward circuitry

**Table 3.1 Yale Food Addiction Scale**

| In the Past 12 Months: | Never | Once a Month | 2–4 Times a Month | 2–3 Times a Week | 4 or More Times or Daily |
|---|---|---|---|---|---|
| 1. I find that when I start eating certain foods, I end up eating much more than planned | 0 | 1 | 2 | 3 | 4 |
| 2. I find myself continuing to consume certain foods even though I am no longer hungry | 0 | 1 | 2 | 3 | 4 |
| 3. I eat to the point where I feel physically ill | 0 | 1 | 2 | 3 | 4 |
| 4. Not eating certain types of food or cutting down on certain types of food is something I worry about | 0 | 1 | 2 | 3 | 4 |
| 5. I spend a lot of time feeling sluggish or fatigued from overeating | 0 | 1 | 2 | 3 | 4 |
| 6. I find myself constantly eating certain foods throughout the day | 0 | 1 | 2 | 3 | 4 |
| 7. I find that when certain foods are not available, I will go out of my way to obtain them. For example, I will drive to the store to purchase certain foods even though I have other options available to me at home. | 0 | 1 | 2 | 3 | 4 |
| 8. There have been times when I consumed certain foods so often or in such large quantities that I started to eat food instead of working, spending time with my family or friends, or engaging in other important activities or recreational activities I enjoy. | 0 | 1 | 2 | 3 | 4 |
| 9. There have been times when I consumed certain foods so often or in such large quantities that I spent time dealing with negative feelings from overeating instead of working, spending time with my family or friends, or engaging in other important activities or recreational activities I enjoy. | 0 | 1 | 2 | 3 | 4 |
| 10. There have been times when I avoided professional or social situations where certain foods were available, because I was afraid I would overeat. | 0 | 1 | 2 | 3 | 4 |
| 11. There have been times when I avoided professional or social situations because I was not able to consume certain foods there. | 0 | 1 | 2 | 3 | 4 |

(continued)

**Table 3.1 Continued**

| In the Past 12 Months: | Never | Once a Month | 2–4 Times a Month | 2–3 Times a Week | 4 or More Times or Daily |
|---|---|---|---|---|---|
| 12. I have had withdrawal symptoms such as agitation, anxiety, or other physical symptoms when I cut down or stopped eating certain foods. (Please do NOT include withdrawal symptoms caused by cutting down on caffeinated beverages such as soda pop, coffee, tea, energy drinks, etc.) | 0 | 1 | 2 | 3 | 4 |
| 13. I have consumed certain foods to prevent feelings of anxiety, agitation, or other physical symptoms that were developing. (Please do NOT include consumption of caffeinated beverages such as soda pop, coffee, tea, energy drinks, etc.) | 0 | 1 | 2 | 3 | 4 |
| 14. I have found that I have elevated desire for or urges to consume certain foods when I cut down or stop eating them. | 0 | 1 | 2 | 3 | 4 |
| 15. My behavior with respect to food and eating causes significant distress. | 0 | 1 | 2 | 3 | 4 |
| 16. I experience significant problems in my ability to function effectively (daily routine, job/school, social activities, family activities, health difficulties) because of food and eating. | 0 | 1 | 2 | 3 | 4 |

| In the Past 12 Months: | NO | YES |
|---|---|---|
| 17. My food consumption has caused significant psychological problems such as depression, anxiety, self-loathing, or guilt. | 0 | 1 |
| 18. My food consumption has caused significant physical problems or made a physical problem worse. | 0 | 1 |
| 19. I kept consuming the same types of food or the same amount of food even though I was having emotional and/or physical problems. | 0 | 1 |
| 20. Over time, I have found that I need to eat more and more to get the feeling I want, such as reduced negative emotions or increased pleasure. | 0 | 1 |

| 21. I have found that eating the same amount of food does not reduce my negative emotions or increase pleasurable feelings the way it used to. | 0 | 1 |
|---|---|---|
| 22. I want to cut down or stop eating certain kinds of food. | 0 | 1 |
| 23. I have tried to cut down or stop eating certain kinds of food. | 0 | 1 |
| 24. I have been successful at cutting down or not eating these kinds of food. | 0 | 1 |

25. How many times in the past year did you try to cut down or stop eating certain foods altogether?

| 1 time | 2 times | 3 times | 4 times | 5 or more times |
|---|---|---|---|---|

26. Please circle ALL of the following foods you have problems with:

| *Ice cream* | *Chocolate* | *Apples* | *Doughnuts* | *Broccoli* | *Cookies* | *Cake* | *Candy* |
|---|---|---|---|---|---|---|---|
| White Bread | Rolls | Lettuce | Pasta | Strawberries | Rice | Crackers | Chips |
| Pretzels | French Fries | Carrots | Steak | Bananas | Bacon | Hamburgers | Cheese burgers |
| Pizza | Soda Pop | None of the above | | | | | |

27. Please list any other foods that you have problems with that were not previously listed:

through palatability, increases in glucose, and insulin concentrations, drugs activate this same circuitry via their pharmacological effects directly on DA cells or indirectly through neurotransmitters that modulate DA cells, such as: opiates, nicotine, gamma aminobutyric acid (GABA) or cannabinoids.[6]

The study of genetic inheritance of specific biochemical traits in SUD, initially based on the theory of alcoholism, has also come a long way since 1993. Until then, it was assumed that less than 10% of the US population was alcoholic. However, empirical studies have since shown that in single families with 1 diagnosed alcoholic, at least half of the blood relatives are frequently found to be alcoholics or otherwise addicted.[7] Similar statistical evidence has continuously supported the existence of genetic factors with regard to compulsive overeating and food addiction. Two studies in particular exemplify the advances that have been made in this regard. A survey of Overeaters Anonymous members conducted in the early 1990s found similar percentages of people who identified as compulsive overeaters or food addicts who had at least one blood relative also addicted to food or alcohol. In a paper published in the *International Journal of Eating Disorders* in 1994, Dr. Ernest Noble and colleagues tested a sample of non-alcoholic individuals who were obese and who craved and binged on simple carbohydrates. They concluded that these individuals had the same genetic aberration that had previously been established as a genetic marker for alcoholism and other drug addictions. This finding was heralded at that time as the obesity gene. However, at the First Annual Food Addiction Conference, Noble clarified that the genetic marker identified was not for the external presence of obesity but rather from an underlying internal chemical dependency on food.

In 2013, however, Dr. Belinda Lennerz and colleagues at the University of Boston wanted to know if sugar-laden junk food activates the same region of the brain affected by heroin and cocaine. They conducted a study that involved creating 2 milkshakes—one with a high, and one with a low glycemic index. The milkshakes were otherwise identical, with similar calories and taste. The drinks were then given to 12 otherwise healthy, overweight men on different days and in random order. Four hours after the high glycemic index shake, participants were hungrier than those who had consumed the low glycemic index shake. They then used functional MRI imaging on all participants. The images revealed intense activation of the nucleus accumbens, specifically in the dopaminergic, mesolimbic system that mediates pleasure eating, reward, and craving. Similar activation patterns have been found in people after consumption of addictive substances, such as heroin and cocaine. Dr. Lennerz concluded that her findings provided further qualified support for the possibility of food addiction and stated that more research is needed to examine the concept of food addiction.[8] The fact that food affects addiction centers in the brain, independent of calories or pleasure, provides the basis to rethink the current approach to food addiction and dietary recommendations.

## Binge Eating and the Nucleus Accumbens

Binge eating has also recently been viewed as a food disorder associated with food addiction. This has sparked more research geared toward finding both the cause and triggers of binge eating. Substantial evidence supports the fact that binge eating is linked to the nucleus accumbens, which is believed to be a key component of the brain's reward pathway.[9] The nucleus accumbens plays a role in reinforcing eating habits, which can lead to binge eating. In 2004, Gene-Jack Wang and Nora Volkow reported that DA release in the nucleus accumbens was associated with the reinforcing effects of food.[10] The findings provide further evidence that the nucleus accumbens has a direct effect on food intake and reward.

In 2006, Dana Smith and Trevor Robbins reported that food scaled consumption increased significantly when low doses of dopamine receptor antagonists were injected into the nucleus accumbens. The study, based on the Yale Food Addiction Scale (YFAS), was designed to identify those exhibiting signs of addiction toward certain types of foods, such as high fat and high sugar. That is, food consumption triggers dopamine receptors in the nucleus accumbens, which prompting an individual to keep eating even when satiated.[11] The nucleus accumbens, therefore, doesn't just effect drug users and alcoholics but food addicts as well.

In addition, through microdialysis studies in the brains of addicted animals, we now know that both food reward and addiction to cocaine increase extracellular dopamine (DA) in the nucleus accumbens. When rats self-administered injections of amphetamine or cocaine, extracellular dopamine increased five-fold in the nucleus accumbens, demonstrating that amphetamine and cocaine increase dopamine in a behavior reinforcement system that is normally activated by eating.[12]

Research continues to postulate that overeating is perpetuated by processed food, especially those with a high glycemic index. High glycemic index foods, such as refined starches and concentrated sugar, cause a rapid rise and fall in blood sugar after consumption. This triggers hunger and, similarly to drug dependence, an occasional sense of desperation when food is not available.[13]

Sadly, it has been speculated that the food industry has utilized the effects of the high glycemic index, taking advantage of the fact that refined starches, sugars, and fat have reinforcing effects on the brain. Michael Moss, a Pulitzer Prize winning reporter for the New York Times who has researched big food companies for many years, reported that the big food industry companies produce foods that are essentially engineered for taste, not nutrition, in his 2014 book entitled, *Salt Sugar Fat: How the Food Giants Hooked Us.* Moss postulated that the common goal of these food companies is to create as much dependency as possible in people who cannot stop eating foods such as potato chips, cookies, and caffeinated sodas. This, he states, likely explains the alarming growth in the number and variety of convenience foods in the last 3 decades. The convenience of fast foods is increasingly relied upon as the number of American households with 2 working parents increases. Fast food is now the norm. Today, the thirty big food manufacturers produce over 60,000 different products and employ over 1.4 million people; a dramatic shift from an industry that began around a century ago with the production of packaged cereals. Moss's research further revealed that the other goal of these big companies is to increase their profits or "stomach share," an inside term used to describe the profits obtained from a total estimated revenue of over 1 trillion dollars annually.[14]

## The Microbiome Connection

Integrative medicine has put forth a plethora of hypotheses for the root causes of unhealthy eating, food addiction, and obesity. Noteworthy among them are: lack of willpower, environmental mismatch, psycho-emotional trauma, the existence of genetic variables, and nutrient shortage. However, a growing amount of research has proposed, and many addiction specialists seem to agree, that bacterial imbalance (microbial dysbiosis) may be a driving factor in food addiction.[15] Moreover, it does not appear to be mutually exclusive of other hypotheses, meaning the benefits of this field of research can be applied in addition to, not in place of, other approaches to food addiction.[16,17]

Through an impressive body of research, we now know that the vast number of intestinal bacteria—the microbiome—plays a complex and essential function in everyday life, with microbial genes outnumbering human genes by a ratio of one hundred to one.[16,18,19] Since the microbiome performs essential functions for the host, such as strengthening immunity, digestion, and metabolism, some leading experts have proposed that the microbiome be conferred a higher status and be referred to as a "microbial organ." To perform these functions, as well as survive, microbes in the gastrointestinal tract are under selective pressure to manipulate host-eating behavior. The microbiota ensure we fed them essential nutrients needed for survival, sometimes at the expense of the host. They do so by generating cravings and inducing dysphoria until an individual eats. This is why those with food addiction may eventually succumb, despite their attempts to use willpower to deny what their microbiome is demanding. Microbes can exert powerful influences on reward and satiety pathways, mood-altering toxins, taste receptors, and control of the vagus nerve—the neural axis connection between the gut and the brain.[18] Evidence shows that microbes can have dramatic effects on behavior through this microbiome-gut-brain axis. Food addicts, therefore, are at an extreme disadvantage with such imperious internal forces working against them.

In addition, recent research also bolsters the notion that the microbiome may be a major factor in obesity. In 2004, Backhed and colleagues displayed that mice that were genetically predisposed to obesity remained lean when they were raised without microbiota and were germ-free. These germ-free mice quickly transformed into obese mice after being fed a fecal pellet from a conventionally raised obese mouse. In short, populating the lean mice's microbiomes with microbiota from obese mice had an undeniable, obesity-inducing effect on them. Inoculation of germ-free mice with microbiota from an obese human produced similar results. Mice lacking the receptor being studied became obese and developed altered gut microbiota, hyperphagia, insulin resistance, and pro-inflammatory gene expression.[19]

What does this mean for humans? It is now accepted that the gut microbes of obese individuals are less diverse when compared to non-obese individuals. This validates the hypothesis that lower diversity may affect eating behavior and satiety. Since eating behavior and satiety are seminal to obesity and food addiction, the microbiome's diversity is clearly a factor deserving and requiring greater attention. The good news is that prebiotics, probiotics, antibiotics, fecal transplants, and dietary changes easily manipulate microbiota. In fact, restoring the microbiome is a viable approach to the overwhelming number of problems that often follow unhealthy eating, food addiction, and obesity.

The idea that particular foods strengthen the microbiome and increase the proliferation of good bacteria in our microbiota is not new. Nobel Prize–winning microbiologist Elie Metchnikoff introduced this theory more than a century ago, hypothesizing that lactic acid bacteria were important to gut health and longevity. Regarded by many as the father of probiotics, Metchnikoff observed a connection between fermented milk and life-span among Bulgarian peasant. In 1907, he hypothesized that replacing the number of bad bacteria in the gut with lactic acid bacteria, like the kind found in yogurt and kefir, could normalize bowel health and prolong life.[20]

The discovery of penicillin, however, pushed Metchnikoff's ideas aside for decades as research focused on a paradigm of killing off harmful bacteria with antibiotics. The importance of beneficial bacteria has only recently reemerged, as an increasing body of research compellingly shows that beneficial microorganisms play a critical role in the functioning of our bodies and brains.[21] It is now well-documented and increasingly-accepted that the mix of bacteria that populate the gut not only play a significant role in susceptibility and immunity, but may also drastically influence emotional health.[22]

How does this burgeoning field of consuming beneficial microbes relate to the mechanisms of food addiction? Admittedly, the growing amount of evidence that commensal gut microbiota affect the central nervous system (CNS) is still mostly indirect, with only a few studies being conducted in humans. For example, a major CNS-inhibitory neurotransmitter, gamma aminobutyric acid (GABA), is significantly involved in regulating physiological and psychological conditions believed to be strong triggers in food addiction, such as anxiety and depression. Since it has now been shown that alterations in central GABA receptor expression can lead to anxiety and depression, a link between the pathogenesis of food addiction and anxiety and depression can therefore be established.

Research is now focused on further clarifying this link between microbiotic factors, neurotransmitters, and behavioral drivers of food addiction. In 2012 Cryan et al designed an experiment to observe behavior changes secondary to gut bacteria in laboratory mice. They fed a strain of Lactobacillus rhamnosus to one group of mice every day for a month. They found that this group was significantly less anxious compared to the group that was fed a regular broth. It appears that treatment with *L. rhamnosus* induced alterations in GABA in the brains of the Lactobacillus-consuming mice. There were increases of GABA in the cortical regions (cingulate and prelimbic) and concomitant reductions in expression in the hippocampus, amygdala, and *locus ceruleus* compared to the control group. In addition, while *L. rhamnosus* also reduced GABA expression in the prefrontal cortex, it increased it in the hippocampus. Therefore, *L. rhamnosus* was shown to play a significant role in the mechanism of stressed eating. *L. rhamnous* reduced stress-induced corticosterone and anxiety- and depression-related behavior, suggesting a strong tie between microbiotics and subject moods and behaviors.[17,20,25]

Furthermore, neurochemical and behavioral effects were not found in vagotomized mice, regardless of microbiota. This identifies the vagus as a major modulatory, constitutive communication pathway between the bacteria in the gut and the brain. Because of the increasingly clear role of bacteria in bidirectional gut-brain axis communication, we may infer that certain microbiota would be impactful therapeutic adjuncts when treating stress-related disorders such as anxiety and depression.

Such findings have encouraged further research into the essential function of the very active, collective communication pathway between the gastrointestinal tract and the brain.[3,25] Some of the information provided by this gut-brain axis must travel via the vagus nerve, which extends from the GI tract to the brain. According to Cryan, the interconnection of these 2 regions should not be a surprise. "Think of phrases in our everyday language," Cryan says. We have "gut instincts" and "gut feelings," he notes—or if we're brave, then we're "gutsy." We refer to butterflies in our tummy if we're feeling a bit anxious. So we portray a raft of human emotions directly in our gut. Cryan expounded on this potential in a recent NPR article, where he stated that the mood-alerting and behavioral effects of the microbiota were so profound that "the mice behaved almost as if they were on Valium or Prozac." The possibilities available through understanding our own gastrointestinal system and its interrelations with other systems in our body, such as the central nervous system, holds great potential for both science and integrative medicine.

The logical and exciting extension of these findings is to explore how these effects may be seen in humans. To date, there have been a handful of small studies. For example, researchers at Leiden University in The Netherlands recently preformed a double-blind study on 40 healthy volunteers.[1] In this study, 20 volunteers (half) took a probiotic containing a mix of eight strains of bacteria for one month. The other 20 volunteers took a placebo, which looked identical. All 40 participants filled out questionnaires at the beginning and end of the study to assess their vulnerability to sad moods. They rated how strongly they agreed with statements such as, "When I'm in a sad mood, I think how my life could be different." and "When I'm down, I more often feel overwhelmed by things."[23] Steenbergen and her colleagues found that the ratings of the participants taking the probiotics were significantly different at the end of the study than they were at the beginning. They reported less aggressive and less ruminative thoughts. They were also less reactive to negative thoughts and feelings.

Drawing scientific evidence from such subjective measures can be problematic given the many variables involved. This is especially true when the results of a particular experiment, such as that of Steenberger's group, attempts to measure subtle, subjective awareness, then expects participants to accurately communicate such changes. However, as the interest in the microbiome's potential benefits on physical and mental health continues to grow, it seems clear that the effects of the "good bacteria" will continue to bring into the spotlight the very concept that Elie Metchnikoff proposed over one hundred years ago. Perhaps this is an idea whose time has come.[25,27]

Certainly, from the perspective of the suffering food addict or overeater, this could be game changing. Instead of having to rely on mustering enough lasting willpower to continually deny themselves forbidden cravings and food items, an integrative and comprehensive treatment approach to their condition can be designed. It would include teaching the afflicted person how to incorporate dietary changes and take notional supplements into a regiment that will reduce their gut's overpowering microbial messages and cravings. As good microbes begin to replace and balance the bad microbes in their gut, the moods and behaviors contributing to the addiction could be alleviated.[21,25,27] As their gut sends fewer addiction-triggering impulses to the brain, it could also become easier to have a healthier, appropriate relationship with food.[9,11,20,24] Instead of the old stereotype of the long-suffering dieters, grimly forcing themselves to struggle against their own urges, there is hope that an integrative approach addressing the powerful connection between satiety and the microbiome can make the journey to their health-goals less difficult and more promising.[20] The importance of this new approach holds the possibility for a potentially viable solution—one that is more sustainable and offers a higher chance of long-term success and less suffering.

---

1. It was funded in part by a probiotics manufacturer, though not designed or executed by the manufacturer.

# Withdrawal

Similar to drug addiction, food addicts can experience withdrawal symptoms after detoxing. Withdrawal is defined as the development of physiological or cognitive symptoms in response to periods of abstinence or reduced consumption of a substance.[3] Although there is debate as to whether food can actually create withdrawal symptoms, recent studies do support the fact that food withdrawal can indeed occur. In 2004, Karen Von Deneen, in a piece called "Food Addiction, Obesity, and Neuroimaging," reported that withdrawal resulting from the addictive food is likely caused by alterations in the opioid system.[17] It was postulated that withdrawal symptoms are experienced by 2 distinct alterations in the reward system. The first consists of DA decreases from the nucleus accumbens and the second is based on the release of acetylcholine (ACh) from Nucleus Accumbens (NA).[20] Von Deneen also found that sugar was capable of triggering the production of DA, ACh, and opioids similar to most narcotic substances and that withdrawal was followed by anxiety and depression.[17] This evidence helps to validate the fact that food addiction does fall into a similar category as drug addiction and alcoholism and perhaps should be treated as such.[18,21,25]

Further evidence that food addiction can result in withdrawal symptoms is shown in lab rats. At a symposium on food addiction in 2005, Corwin and Grigson described how withdrawal from a high-fat diet leads to neurochemical responses comparable to those induced by withdrawal from drugs. They reported that psychological states can play a major role in food withdrawal and that depression, which often accompanies drug withdrawal, can modify endogenous signals involved in food intake regulation.[18]

# Treatment Approaches

## RESTORING THE MICROBIOTA

A significant and impressive body of research points to the fact that prebiotics, probiotics, antibiotics, fecal transplant, and diet changes can alter the microbiota and lead to changes in eating behavior.[20] In order to successfully treat food addiction, a treatment plan must be integrative, person-oriented (as opposed to disease-based) and must induce a personalized dietary program geared toward restoring the microbiome.

We now know that microbial diversity can affect food choices and satiety and that certain features of microbial ecology, such as population size, are believed to influence a microbe's capacity to manipulate the host. Microbial communities with low diversity might be more prone to overgrowth by one or more species, giving those organisms increased ability to manufacture behavior-altering neurochemicals and hormones. In contrast, highly diverse gut microbiotas tend to be more resistant to invasion by pathogenic species than less diverse microbiotas. Supporting the hypothesis that a more diverse microbiota causes fewer cravings, gastric bypass surgery has a twofold effect: increasing alpha diversity in the gut microbiota as well as reducing preference for high-fat and high-carbohydrate foods. Food preferences of germ-free mice inoculated with low- versus high-diversity microbial communities have provided a test of this prediction. In humans, probiotics that increase microbiota diversity are also believed to reduce cravings.[21]

It has been shown that neurochemical and behavioral effects mediated via the vagus nerve is the result of a very effective communication pathway between the bacteria in the gut and the brain. Given this essential bidirectional role of bacteria in gut-brain axis communication, restoring the microbiota can have a powerful and impactful therapeutic effect when treating stress-related disorders, such as anxiety and depression, that often accompanies food addiction.[20,21]

## AMINO ACIDS: BIOCHEMICAL RESTORATION VIA NUTRITION AND IV THERAPY

When combined with other treatment modalities, amino acids, the molecular basis for neurotransmitters and neuropeptides, are believed by many to be the key to appetite control, minimizing overeating and hence reduce the urge to binge.[26] For example, appetite disturbances may develop when abnormally low neurotransmitter and neuropeptide levels of serotonin, GABA, dopamine, L-lysine, L-arginine, and norepinephrine occur. Supplementing the diet of a person afflicted with food addiction with the proper regimen of neurotransmitter precursors and amino acids, such as 5-hydroxytryptophan (5-HTP) and tryptophan, can be successful in decreasing binging and sugar cravings, improving mood, diminishing anxiety, and optimizing appetite control.[27]

Serotonin, whose roles in appetite reduction, satiety and mood have led to an impressive body of research, is synthesized from tryptophan through 5-HTP via the enzyme tryptophan hydroxylase.[28] 5-HTP has been shown to be so reliable in increasing serotonin levels that it has been used as a test to evaluate the potency of drugs that affect serotonin levels and thus can cause serotonin syndrome. The test pairs an experimental drug with 5-HTP to induce "serotonin syndrome," or serotonin toxicity to see the dose of 5-HTP required to induce the syndrome.[29]

5-HTP supplements are made from extracts of the seeds of the African tree *Griffonia simplicifolia* and has been shown to be very effective in controlling appetite, especially cravings for carbohydrates. Furthermore, it has been well documented that the serotonergic system plays a role in macronutrient selection particular in obese persons with a craving for carbohydrates[30] and that enhancing its transmission reduces these cravings and increases satiety.[31] For example, in

2012, Rondanell et al demonstrated in a 2-month double-blind, placebo controlled study trial that the 5-HTP group experienced a significantly greater increase in satiety over an 8-week period than the placebo group. They found that 5-HTP supplementation led individuals to feel more satiated after eating and therefore ate less. When compared to the control group during a diet and non-diet period, those taking 5-HTP had a loss of 2% of body weight during the non-diet period and 3% when they dieted. Those taking placebo did not lose any weight loss. The study concluded that 5-HTP was safe and effective to help control appetite in overweight women.[32,33]

In 1989, Cecil et al studied 19 obese women with body mass index between 30 and 40 to whom they gave either placebo or 8 mg/kg daily of 5-HTP for 5 weeks without any concurrent dietary recommendations. 5-HTP treatment was associated with a decrease in appetite and food intake, resulting in weight loss without significantly affecting mood state.[34] This study noted that food intake was reduced from an average of 2,903 kcal to 1,819 kcal (62% of baseline) while placebo only reduced calories to 80%, and the 0.5 kg weight loss in placebo was outperformed by a near 1.5 kg loss with 5-HTP. Weight loss has also been noted with 750 mg 5-HTP over 2 weeks in overweight diabetics and over 12 weeks in obese persons given 900 mg 5-HTP daily.[35,36] A decrease in both carbohydrate and dietary fat has also been seen with 750 mg 5-HTP daily for 2 weeks in non-dieting diabetics, but appeared to be reduced to a similar degree as calories overall.

Ceci et al differentiated between "an increase in satiety" defined as a sensation of fullness and a "decrease in appetite" as less desire to eat. They noted that 5-HTP causes an increase in satiety without a concomitant decrease in appetite. Although there are few studies conducted in men, there appears to be a consensus that 5-HTP benefits both genders.[38]

Further pharmacological, biochemical, and behavioral evidence have demonstrated that, in addition to its role as a regulator of appetite and nutrient preference, serotonin also plays an important role in mood in both animals and humans. Serotonin-releasing brain neurons were described in 1995 by authors Richard and Judith Wuthman in their book *Brain Serotonin, Carbohydrate-Craving, Obesity and Depression* as unique because the amount of neurotransmitter they release is normally controlled by food intake. They wrote that carbohydrate consumption has the ability to increase insulin secretion, coined the "plasma tryptophan ratio," and is therefore often the trigger. They concluded that the ability of neurons to couple neuronal signaling properties to food consumption is a link in the feedback mechanism that normally keeps carbohydrate and protein intakes more or less constant, and that since serotonin release is also involved in sleep onset, pain sensitivity, blood pressure regulation, and mood stability, patients learn to overeat carbohydrate-rich foods such as potato chips and pastries to make themselves feel better. This tendency to use certain foods as mood-enhancing drugs is a frequent cause of weight gain often seen in patients who become fat when exposed to stress, in women with premenstrual syndrome, and in patients with season affective disorder.[37]

Although several publications recommend a 150 mg daily dose of 5-HTP, appetite reduction has been shown to occur with dosages of 600 to 900 mg.[42,43] Because 5-HTP can be toxic at high doses, however, caution is advised. It is recommended to start with a dose of 50 mg twice a day and titrate upwards.[36] In addition, 5-HTP can also be found in many multivitamin and herbal preparations. Caution is advised when prescribing it because the patient may be already unknowingly taking it.[41]

For the most part, the side effects of 5-HTP are mild, such as nausea, heartburn, gas, and rumbling sensations. However, serotonin syndrome has been reported at doses as low as 200 mg a day with symptoms ranging from mild shivering and diarrhea to severe, such as muscle rigidity, fever and seizures. If not immediately treated, serotonin syndrome can lead to multiple organ failure and death.[41] As such, SSRIs, tricyclic, monoamine oxidase inhibitors (MAOIs) should be avoided or at best used with caution with patients taking 5-HTP. Some antidepressant medications can also interact with 5-HTP.

Likewise, the pain medication used for fibromyalgia, Robitussin, meperidine, and the triptans used to treat migraines can also cause serotonin syndrome if taken with high doses of 5-HTP. Caution is therefore strongly recommended and patients must be asked if they are taking any supplements that might contain 5-HTP.[41]

Once the potential side effects of medication and nutraceuticals combination have been ruled out, addiction treatment experts and nutritionists agree that the single most important (but often most ignored) factor in treating addiction is treating the nutritional deficiencies that often accompany it.[29]

Recovering addicts tend toward highly palatable foods that can provide a temporary reprieve from negative feelings. These foods, known as hyperpalables, are almost invariably processed foods with added sugar, salt, vegetable oil fats, refined carbohydrates, and caffeine. They are known to destabilize blood sugar, spur inflammation, deplete essential neurotransmitters that play a large role in stabilizing moods, and induce cravings by directly modulating the brain reward center.[38]

It was shown in a recent study at the University of Michigan that our understanding of people's inability to resist hyperpalable foods is of fundamental importance when treating food addiction. In the study, Shulte et al used the Yale Food Addiction Scale to assess food habits. Individuals were asked to score foods between 1 and 7 based on resistibility, with 1 being the easiest to resist and 7 being the most difficult. Not surprisingly, the study's ten most addictive foods were pizza, potato chips, chocolate chip cookies, ice cream, French fries, cheeseburgers, soda, cake, and cheese. If possible, these foods should be avoided if not completely eliminated.[39]

In contrast, from a nutritional perspective, an individual in early recovery can improve mood and fight off depression, anxiety, and stress by incorporating foods that contain an ample amount of omega-3 essential fatty acids, complete proteins, and antioxidant and anti-inflammatory vitamins and minerals.[45]

This combination type of treatment aims to repair the biochemical imbalances that cause cravings, depression, anxiety, and the unstable moods that contribute to addiction behavior. Biochemical imbalances of neurotransmitters, nutrient deficiencies, amino acid imbalances, hypoglycemia, inflammatory and oxidative stress, and adrenal fatigue are believed to be improved by nutrient therapy that usually includes IV Meyer's cocktail and its many individualized forms.[45]

## HERBS AND NUTRACEUTICALS

In the last few decades, increasing interest in nutraceuticals, also known as dietary supplements, to treat food addiction has lead to increased research on their effectiveness as part of integrative treatment approach.[45] A *PubMed* review for this chapter revealed a significant amount of data supporting the effectiveness of a selected number of dietary supplements. Although the evidence varies depending on the supplement, health-care practitioners, in collaboration with patients, should integrate dietary supplement strategies that maximize benefits into a comprehensive treatment plan.[40] Inositol, for example has been shown to have modest effects in patients with panic disorder or obsessive-compulsive disorder.[47]

Studies have also shown that chromium picolinate improves insulin function and may be beneficial as an adjunct in the treatment of depression, carbohydrate cravings, and weight gain. It may also take the edge off cravings. Magnesium fights insulin resistance and depression, while glucomannan, a sugar made from the root of the konjac plant *(Amorphophallus konjac)* can reduce the spikes in sugar and insulin that are know to drive cravings and hunger.[30,41]

An impressive body of research has validated the important role that vitamins play in the treatment of food addiction. Both low vitamin D and B levels have been implicated in mood and appetite control. Vitamin B6, for example, is a factor in serotonin synthesis, while inositol, a close relative to the B family that is produced in plants and animals, enhances insulin sensitivity. Using supplements of inositol and folate are effective adjuncts in the treatment of depression.[48] Testing for the methyl-tetrahydrofolate reductase (MTHFR) genetic mutation can help determine what form of folate and B vitamins are appropriate. Niacin, also known as vitamin B3, is a precursor to nicotinamide adenine dinucleotide (NAD), a coenzyme derivative of vitamin B3 that is found in all living cells and essential in ATP production in the mitochondria. NAD stimulates the production of dopamine, serotonin, and noradrenaline, and NAD deficiency is now recognized as a key feature of depression, anxiety, addiction, memory disturbance, focus, and concentration. IV therapy with NAD has become a valuable resource for helping patients with addiction to detox. It is thought to reduce cravings and withdrawal symptoms in patients using lower amounts or no replacement therapies. Studies have indicated that NAD has been used successfully to treat addictions in that it improves mental clarity, increases cognitive function, focusand concentration, and improves mood.[45]

A systematic reviews of research for this chapter revealed that there is strong evidence for the use of herbal supplements to reduce the stress, anxiety, and insulin spikes that are associated with overeating. For example, *Gymnema sylvester* (*Gurmar*), a tropical plant of the milkweed family with an ancient Sanskrit name meaning "destroyer of sugar," has been clinically shown to reduce blood glucose and glycoside hemoglobin in type 1 and type 2 diabetics. First used in Ayurvedic medicine to treat a variety of conditions, including diabetes, constipation and weight loss facilitation, the gymnemic acids, found in *Gurmar* have been shown to decrease the absorption of glucose from the small bowel, among many other benefits.[42]

In addition, research has demonstrated that this powerful herb blocks the sensation of sweetness on the tongue, which may minimize the demand for insulin and in turn decreases sugar cravings. *Gurmar* also leads to increases in insulin by decreasing the absorption of glucose by the intestines and by restoring damaged pancreatic beta cells. The effectiveness of this herb is so profound that practitioners using it to treat insulin-dependent diabetics are advised to be very cautious as it can lead to hypoglycemia.[43]

In 1990 Baskaran studied the effectiveness of *Gurmar* in controlling hyperglycemia in 22 patients with type 2, non-insulin dependent diabetes. They found that using 400 mg of a water-soluble *Gurmar* supplement for 18 to 20 months lead to a significant reduction in blood glucose, hemoglobin AIC, and glycosylated plasma proteins. Five of the 22 diabetic patients were able to discontinue their conventional drug and maintain their blood glucose homeostasis with *Gurmar* alone. Their data showed raised insulin levels in the serum of type 2 diabetic patients taking *Gurmar* supplementation and suggested that the beta cells may be either newly regenerated or repaired in these patients.[44]

As with most herbs and nutraceuticals, the appropriate dose of *Gurmar* depends on several factors such as the patient's overall health, age, and use of other herbs and supplements that may cause undesirable interactions. In general, however, the recommended dose of *Gurmar* is between 400 to 600 mg daily, with the starting dose being no higher than 400 mg to ascertain that no side effects, such as hypoglycemia, occurs.[49,50]

Bitter melon may be effective by enhancing the uptake of glucose, promote the release of insulin, and increase insulin sensitivity. In addition, it also increases glycogen synthesis inside cells and tissues. Similar to *Gurmar*, bitter melon increases the number of beta cells in the pancreas.[45]

Fenugreek seed, another herb often used in Ayurvedic medicine, is fiber-rich and has properties shown to support insulin insensitivity and slow the absorption of glucose following a meal, therefore reducing fasting blood sugar levels.[46]

Stress reducing herbs such as golden rose (*rhodiola rosea*), kava (*Piper methysticum*), valerian root (*Valeriana officinalis*), lemon balm (*Melissa officinalis*), and passionflower (*Passiflora incarnata*) have also shown impressive results.[30] Passionflower, for example, which is used to treat anxiety and insomnia, is believed to work by increasing GABA levels in the brain. Studies have shown that passionflower is as effective as benzoadezipine oxazepam (Serax) for treating symptoms for generalized anxiety disorder.[47] Although passionflower did not work as quickly as oxazepam (day 7 compared to day 4), it produced less impairment on job performance when compared with oxazepam.

In another study, patients given passionflower before surgery had less anxiety than those given a placebo and recovered from anesthesia just as quickly.[54] Similarly, kava seems to have greater benefits than harm in those with mild to moderate anxiety, while St. John's-wort monotherapy has someevidence for use as an effective anxiolytic treatment.[48]

## PSYCHOTHERAPY

People suffering from food addiction are believed to be motivated to overeat by a desire to escape from self-awareness. Binge eaters often exhibit high standards and expectations, especially an acute sensitivity to the demands of others. An often rash and aversive pattern of high self-awareness, unflattering views of self generally occur when they believe they have failed the expectations of others.[49,50] Emotional distress, including anxiety and depression, follows and can be accompanied by a desire to escape from their unpleasant reality. Overeating is used as an attempt to avoid their internalized conflict and suffering.[51]

There is an impressive body of research attesting the effectiveness of psychotherapy in the treatment of food addiction. CBT has demonstrated substantial improvements in the short- and long-term improvement of core symptomatology and associated psychosocial conflict that characterizes eating disorders and food addiction, including binge-eating disorder (BED).[53,54] This chapter will focus on the therapeutic approaches that have been used with promising results.

## Cognitive Behavioral Therapy

There has been significant progress in the development and evaluation of evidence-based psychological treatments for eating disorders over the past 30 years. Of those CBT is the treatment of choice for eating disorders and BED.[52,53] CBT, also used in the treatment of drug and alcohol addictions, is based on social-behavioral learning theory that addictive behaviors are learned.[57] The first stage of CBT treatment plan is a detailed evaluation of thoughts, feelings, and beliefs that contribute to overeating or binging. The goals of CBT treatments for addictions is to teach patients to modify thoughts and feelings, develop skills for recognizing and coping with cravings, triggers, and pressures, and plan ahead for situations that increase risk for use.[54] Relapse prevention is an important component of CBT as well.[55]

For the treatment of overeating, binge eating and obesity, the 3 most important components generally include dietary change, increased physical activity, and behavior therapy techniques, such as goal-setting, self-monitoring, stimulus control, and behavioral contracting.[55,56] In addition to weight loss itself, these lifestyle changes are believed to increase the likelihood that weight loss will be maintained. Similar to CBT for drug addictions, patients are taught to identify thoughts and feelings that contribute to overeating and effective skills for preventing and dealing with relapse. Studies on cognitive behavioral interventions and weight loss have demonstrated efficacy and long lasting results.[57,58,59,60]

For example, in a study completed in 1995, Agras et al examined the effectiveness of group interpersonal therapy (IPT) with BED patients who did not stop binge eating after 12 weeks of group cognitive-behavioral therapy (CBT). Participants were randomly allocated to either the CBT group or to an assessment-only control group. After 12 weeks of treatment with CBT, 55% of participants met criteria for improvement and began 12 weeks of weight loss therapy, whereas the non-responders began 12 weeks of group IPT. Over the 24-week period, participants who received treatment reduced binge eating and weight significantly more than the weight-loss control group. However, IPT led to no further improvement for those who did not improve with CBT.[61]

## Overeaters Anonymous (OA)

Overeaters Anonymous (OA) is a 12-step program that, like AA, views compulsive overeating as an addictive disease. However, despite popularity of OA, there is little published research examining its effectiveness.[62] Similar to AA and other 12-step programs, OA also emphasizes the mental and spiritual aspects of compulsive overeating and focuses on community building, recognizing the limits of willpower and thus surrendering to a higher power, learning self-acceptance, and identifying interpersonal issues that leads to loss of control of eating by taking a "moral inventory." While total abstinence from alcohol is the uncompromising goal in AA, this is not a possible approach in OA. Therefore, the definition of control over addiction to food is hence more flexible. One of the main goals in OA is to encourage program participants to abstain from foods believed to trigger overeating and to refrain from bingeing or overeating.[63]

Research designed to evaluate the effectiveness of OA showed that the majority of OA members are middle-aged, college-educated, and white females. In a nationwide study in 1992, Spitzer et al found that 44.5% of the OA participants were identified as compulsive overeaters, 40.7% as bulimic, and 14.8% as anorexic.[53] In 1988, Malenbaum et al found that the outcome of OA intervention in the treatment of 40 bulimics evaluated on measures of length and consistency was very significant. For an average of 3 years after the study, participants had remained abstinent from binge or overeating and continued to attend meetings, call their sponsors, and sponsor others. The study demonstrated that participant's awareness in those attending OA meetings was essential when addressing their food addiction behaviors, which was of paramount importance before they could confront more core psychological issues that lead to the addiction in the first place.[75]

## Contingency Management

Based on the Operant Conditioning principles to induce behavioral changes, Contingency Management (CM) programs provide tangible reinforcements for target behaviors, such as abstinence from drugs or binge eating. The key components of CM are to identify a target behavior and objectively measure it, such as weight loss as a direct result of eating less. The ultimate objective is to provide reinforcement each time the target behavior is detected. The use of vouchers exchangeable for goods and services has been highly efficacious in promoting addictions treatment retention and extending duration of abstinence from a range of substances in CM.[64,65]

Given its proven efficacy when used to treat addictive disorders, CM is believed to be an effective treatment for reducing overeating, binge eating, and promoting weight loss. Advocates of CM believe that reinforcement can be given when participants achieve weight loss and for activities associated with weight loss, such as decreasing calorie intake, exercising, keeping a food diary, and preparing healthy meals.[66,67]

## Other Integrative-Based Approaches

### NEUROFEEDBACK

Used for over 3 decades, mostly in the treatment of PTSD, neurofeedback trains individuals to gain control over electro-physiological processes in the human brain and has been increasingly used in the treatment of SUD.[68,69] A speciality of biofeedback, neurofeedback uses information from an electroencephalogram (EEG) to show the individual current patterns in his or her cortex. It enables individuals to learn how to change physiological activity to improve health and performance.[70,71] Users claim that neurofeedback helps them cope with many symptoms, most importantly anger, anxiety, insomnia, and depression, all believed to be triggers to addiction and relapse.[72]

## EXERCISE

Daily exercise is known to help balance mood, which is an essential component to most recovering food addicts. Exercise, whether aerobic or otherwise, has well-known health benefits, including improvements in the function of the cardiovascular, pulmonary, and endocrine systems. Exercise increases neurotransmitter levels, improves oxygen and nutrient delivery, and increases neurogenesis in the hippocampus. It has a positive effect on learning and memory, executive control processes, working memory, multitasking, and planning. Exercise has been shown to be an effective treatment for depression as well.

## ACUPUNCTURE

Acupuncture, a form of complementary and alternative medicine in the West, is a key component of Traditional Chinese Medicine (TCM). It has been shown to be helpful in treating addictions like alcohol and opiate use.

## MEDITATION/MINDFULNESS PRACTICES

Mindfulness meditation has been shown to help regulate mood by lowering cortisol, increase interleukin, and enhance neurotransmitter receptors.[73] Vipassana, one of the most widely used forms of meditation, teaches the mind not to react to the emotions and thoughts that result in harmful behavior. Meditation experts believe that it is possible to become permanently free of all negative behavior, including addiction, through a commitment to a daily meditation practice. The Transcendental Meditation Organization (tm.org) reports that controlled studies have demonstrated that TM, when compared to other forms of meditation and relaxation, can significantly reverse the physiological and psychological factors that lead to abuse, including alcohol, cigarettes, and illicit drugs in the general population. The TM association's studies have demonstrated that abstinence was maintained over time.[74]

In addition, an increasing number of studies have indicated that mindfulness-based relapse prevention techniques do reduce cravings and prevent relapse as well as, if not better than, traditional treatment. The journal *Substance Use & Misuse* published an entire special issue in April 2014, focused on mindfulness-based interventions for SUDs. Katie Witkiewitz, an associate professor of psychology at the University of New Mexico, published 2 studies in 2015 that found that mindfulness-based relapse prevention was more effective than a traditional relapse prevention program in decreasing substance use and heavy drinking up to 1 year later.[83] There have been several randomized clinical trials, as well as smaller controlled studies, that have found meditation to be as effective or more effective than existing treatments for addiction.

## YOGA

Yoga, which means "union" in Sanskrit, combines 3 aspects: physical postures, breathwork, and meditation. The philosophy of yoga is to integrate mind, body, and spirit. In doing so, yoga can promote a state of inner peace that can prevent relapse in recovering addicts. Many studies indicate that yoga can relieve anxiety, stress, and depression,[75] all of which are indicated as factors in food addiction.

One of the goals of yoga is to teach bodily awareness so that pent-up emotions can be released. Because disassociation from the body through the use of drugs, alcohol, food, or other substances is common in addicts, practicing the physical poses of yoga, also called *asanas*, can increase awareness of their outdated behavioral patterns and thus lead to a clearer and more grounded decision to change.[92]

Breathwork and meditation, which are major components of yoga, are believed by addiction experts to be a key aspect of healing and recovery from addiction. Both promote a deeper sense of self-awareness and help individuals struggling with addiction become less influenced by the world around them and embrace their inner strength without the dependence for external validation through substances, including food. The lungs, the link between the circulatory and nervous systems, are believed by practitioners of yoga and meditation to be fundamentally important in detoxification, energy, and as a built-in relaxation response.[45] Slow, deep-breathing increases activity of the parasympathetic system activity—the "break" of the nervous system, while concurrently decreases the activity of the sympathetic system—the "gas" or fight-or-flight survival response of the nervous system. In essence, the functions of the parasympathetic system and sympathetic system are similar to the concepts of the yin and yang balance that yoga and breathwork seek to achieve. Each system is essential for survival, and a deep sense of well-being is achieved when the 2 are perfectly balanced.[76]

## ANIMAL CONTACT/PET THERAPY

The ultimate goal of pet therapy is to help addicts develop self-nurturing skills and the ability to be responsible for the welfare of others. Petting, hugging, and loving an animal can fulfill the basic human need to touch. Current evidence shows that pet therapy can increase the levels of serotonin and dopamine and thus lower stress, reduce anxiety and depression, lower blood pressure and heart rate, increase self-esteem, and reduce the severity of painful physical symptoms of illness. In addition, dog owners have been shown to be more motivated to exercise with their dogs and thus benefit from exercise-induced endorphins.[94]

Equine therapy, another type of pet therapy, is believed to benefit recovering addicts through the interaction and bonding with horses, which builds confidence, increases trust, patience, and self-esteem. Horses are believed to be naturally responsive to humans and to possess similar interactive communication styles to humans, such as nuzzling.[77]

## HYPNOSIS

The word hypnosis is derived from the Greek word *hypnos*, which means sleep. Hypnotherapists use techniques that enhance deep relaxation and lead individuals to an altered state of consciousness, known as a hypnotic trance. The goal of hypnosis is to help individuals find an internal calm, natural state of focused attention so that the mind is receptive to ideas and suggestions compatible with the person's goals. Hypnosis teaches people how to master their own states of awareness of bodily functions and psychological responses.[78]

## GARDENING/HORTICULTURE THERAPY

Horticulture therapy (HT), commonly known as gardening therapy, is now utilized in many treatment settings including prisons, psychiatric hospitals, mental health programs, and addiction rehab. Similar to animal therapy, gardening therapy offers a caregiving role to the recovering addict.

Research has shown that gardening can have a positive effect on a range of problems by reducing aggression, lowering cortisol levels, improving self-esteem, helping people feel less anxious, reducing the severity of depression, and improving concentration in people who are depressed.[79]

## VIRTUAL REALITY THERAPY

Virtual reality therapy (VRT), sometimes referred to as immersive multimedia, is a form of exposure therapy that uses virtual reality technology to simulate real-life experiences. Often used to train pilots, it has also been used to treat patients with anxiety disorders and phobias, specifically as a treatment for PTSD. Now, newer applications are allowing it to be used for treating addiction and other behavioral problems, due in part to its ability to generate virtual sensory experience for all 5 senses.

Researchers are building realistic virtual worlds at the University of Houston that re-create triggers as a way to help participating addicts beat cravings for nicotine, alcohol, marijuana, and heroin.[80] The treatment can be likened to exposure therapy, which deliberately triggers the addicts into their addiction behavior while being guided by a therapist.[81] Proponents of VRT have used some supporting evidence to show that VRT is more effective than simply encouraging addicts to avoid the people, places, or things that can trigger a desire to use.[82]

## ART-BASED THERAPY

Considered an activity-based therapy such as animal therapy and gardening, art therapy employs art through music therapy or certain construction projects to encourage addicts to externalize their emotions. Studies have shown that art therapy can build self-esteem and self-confidence, helping reduce relapse rates for several psychiatric disorders, including food addiction. Likewise, music therapy has been shown to lower depression, stress, anxiety, and anger in patients attending rehab for substance abuse.[83]

## PHARMACOLOGICAL INTERVENTION

While not equivalent to CBT, antidepressant drug therapy has proven to curtail binge-purge frequency and lower scores on depression inventories. Drugs studied thus far for the treatment of food addiction have focused on individuals with BED. Randomized, placebo-controlled studies are being conducted primarily with antidepressants, anti-obesity agents, and antiepileptic drugs. Anti-addiction agents and stimulants are the 2 other classes of drugs being studied.

Medications that are effective in reducing substance use are also effective for reducing food intake. Topiramate is thought to inhibit dopamine release in the mesocorticolimbic system, thus dampening the rewarding effects of alcohol and modulating glutamate over-excitation.[84] Topiramate similarly appears to be effective in producing weight loss in obese individuals.[85]

Rimonabant, a drug that blocks the cannabinoid receptors, was tested as a treatment for both substance use disorders and obesity.[86] Preliminary findings suggested it was effective as a treatment for nicotine and alcohol dependence, as well as reducing food intake and improving lipid and blood sugar levels in obese patients.[87] However, rimonabant was associated with a high incidence of serious psychiatric side effects, leading the US Food and Drug Administration to deny its approval.[88]

As of February 2015, the FDA approved the psychostimulant Vyvanse (*Lisdexamfetamine*) for the treatment of BED. In recent years, the popularity of Vyvanse to treat Attention Deficit Disorder (ADD) has skyrocketed. Because it has been shown to reduce appetite and improve impulse control and cognitive function, Vyvanse is now also popular for weight loss and sports performance. The "pro-drug" benefit of Vyvanse is believed to result in smoother absorption and a longer-lasting effect (up to 12 hours in some people).[89] In addition to decreasing appetite and cravings, and thus promoting weight loss, Vyvanse has also been shown to be effective in controlling impulses by boosting cognition and hence an increase in the understanding of one's tendencies to overeat.[89] In 1 of the double-blind, placebo-controlled government sponsored clinical trials to demonstrate efficacy before approval, 724 participants between the ages of 18 and 55 were randomly assigned a fixed-dose of Vyvanse or a placebo (at a 1:1 ratio). Those that received the fixed doses of Vyvanse were given 30 mg, 50 mg, or 70 mg per day. The trial was designed to determine the safety, efficacy, and tolerability of Vyvanse among individuals meeting criteria for BED (as defined by the *DSM-4*). The patients were then screened at various intervals throughout 12 weeks of treatment to determine whether the drug had reduced the number of binge-eating days and episodes. Both males and females were involved in the study and BMIs (body mass indexes) ranged between 25 and 45. Results demonstrated that the patients receiving the 50 mg and 70 mg of daily Vyvanse experienced a statistically significant reduction in the number of binge-eating days in comparison to a placebo. Approximately 50% of those taking 70 mg of Vyvanse stopped binge eating for the 4-week study compared to 21% of those taking the placebo. Most of the people taking the drug also ended up losing weight.[90]

Like other amphetamines, Vyvanse use has also been associated with abuse and other side effects.[91] While most research reveals that amphetamines tend to be relatively safe over the long-term, at this time it is unknown if taking Vyvanse for an extended period could cause psychological dependence. There is a risk, however, that Vyvanse users may not be able to resist further use due to the initial feelings of euphoria, increased pleasure, and improved performance. Rebound binge eating, although not common, has also been reported to occur if patients are not slowly weaned off the drug.[98]

Due to increased activity in the central nervous system, other side effects such as high anxiety, heart palpitations, jitters, and insomnia are reported. Similar to other amphetamines, more serious adverse effects, including myocardial infarction, stroke, mania, and psychosis, can potentially occur. Cautions should therefore be used in any patients with a previous history of heart disease and psychiatric conditions. If a patient has a heart conditions and/or defects, Vyvanse could exacerbate the condition.

## REFERENCES

1. Yanovski SZ, Yanoviski JA. Obesity prevalence in the United States—up, down, or sideways? *The New England Journal of Medicine.* 2011;364:987–989.
2. Corsica JA, Pelchat ML. Food addiction: true or false? *Current Opinion in Gastroenterology.* 2010;26:16:5–169.
3. Gearhardt AN, Corbin WR, Brownell KD. Food addiction: an examination of the Diagnostic Criteria for Dependence. *Addict Med.* 2009;3(1):1–7.
4. Fariburn CG, Wilson T. *Binge Eating: Nature, Assessment, and Treatment.* New York: Guilford Press; 1996.
5. Noble EP, et al. D2 dopamine receptor gene and obesity. *International Journal of Eating Disorders.* 1994;15(3):205–217.
6. Volkow ND, Wise RA. How can drug addiction help us understand obesity? *Nature Neuroscience.* 2005;8(5):555–560.
7. Werdell P. Science of Food Addiction. ACORN Food Dependency Recovery Services Web site. http://foodaddiction.com/resources/science-of-food-addiction/. Accessed June 5, 2015.
8. Renter E. Processed Foods Similarly Addictive As Illicit Drugs, Another Study Finds. Natural Society Transform your health naturally Web site. http://naturalsociety.com/processed-foods-addictive-drugs-study-finds/. September 26, 2013. Accessed June 5, 2015.
9. Roitman MF, Wheeler RA, Carelli RM. Nucleus accumbens neurons are innately tuned for rewarding and aversive taste stimuli, encode their predictors, and are linked to motor output. *Neuron.* 2005;45:587–597.
10. Wang GJ, Volkaw ND, Thanos PK, Fowler JS. Similarity between obesity and drug addiction as assessed by neurofunctional imaging: a concept review. *Eating Disorders, Overeating, and Pathological Attachments to Food.* 2004;23(3):39–53.
11. Smith DG, Robbins TW. The neurobiological underpinnings of obesity and binge eating: a rationale for adopting the food addiction model. *Society of Biological Psychiatry.* 2013;804–810.

12. Willuhn I, Wanat MJ, Clark JJ, Phillips PE. Dopamine signaling in the nucleus accumbens of animals self-administering drugs of abuse. *Behavioral Neurosciences of Drug Addiction.* 2009;3:29–71.

13. Lennerz BS, et al. Effects of dietary glycemic index on brain regions related to reward and craving in men. *American Journal of Clinical Nutrition.* 2013;98(3):641–647.

14. Moss M. *Salt Sugar Fat: How the Food Giants Hooked Us.* New York: Random House; 2013.

15. Goyette P, et al. Human methylenetetrahydrofolate reductase: isolation of cDNA, mapping and mutation identification. *Nature Genetics.* 1994;7(2):195–200.

16. Von Deneen KM, Liu Y. Food addiction, obesity and neuroimaging. *Addictions— From Pathophysiology to Treatment.* 2012;59:290.

17. Corwin RL, Grigson PS. Symposium overview. Food addiction: fact or fiction? *The Journal of Nutrition.* 2009;139:617–619.

18. Alcock J, Maley CC, Aktipis A. Is eating behavior manipulated by the gastrointestinal microbiota? Evolutionary pressures and potential mechanisms. *BioEssays.* 2014;36(10):940–949.

19. Backhead F, et al. The gut micobiota as an environmental factor that regulates fat storage. *The National Academy of Sciences.* 2004;101(44):15718–15723.

20. Anukam KC, Reid G. Probitoics: 100 years (1907–2007) after Elie Metchnikoff's observation. *Communicating Current Research and Educational Topics and Trends in Applied Microbiology.* 2007:466–474.

21. Doucleff M. How Modern Life Depletes Our Gut Microbes. Goats and Soda—Stories of Life in a Changing World. Web site. http://www.npr.org/sections/goatsandsoda/2015/04/21/400393756/how-modern-life-depletes-our-gut-microbes. Accessed July 20, 2015.

22. Bravo JA, et al. Ingestion of Lactobacillus strain regulates emotional behavior and central GABA receptor expression via the vagus nerve. *Proceedings of The National Academy of Sciences of The United States of America-Physical Sciences.* 2011;108(38):16050–16055.

23. Steenbergen L, et al. A randomized controlled trial to test the effect of multispecies probiotics on cognitive reactivity to sad mood. *Brain, Behavior, and Immunity.* 2015;48:258–264.

24. Heyes D, Carlander A. The Ibogaine Experience: A Miracle Cure or a Bad Trip? the fix addiction and recovery, straight up. Web site. http://www.thefix.com/content/buying-into-ibogaine-treatment. Accessed June 5, 2015.

25. Wiss D. Self-efficacy and nutrition: promoting behavior change in substance abuse recovery. *Behavioral Health Nutrition.* 2013:11–12.

26. Lakhan SE, Vieira KF. Nutritional and herbal supplements for anxiety and anxiety-related disorders: systematic review. *Nutrition Journal.* 2010;9:42.

27. Greenblatt J. Mine the complexities of treating food addiction. Addiction Professional-Driving Clinical Excellence. Web site. http://www.addictionpro.com/article/mine-complexities-treating-food-addiction. Accessed July 14, 2015.

28. Turner EH, Loftis JM, Blackwell AD. Serotonin a la carte: supplementation with the serotonin precursor 5-hydroxytryptopham. *Pharmacology & Therapeutics.* 2006;109(3):325–338.

29. O'Neill MF, Moore NA. Animal models of depression: are there any? *Hum Psychopharmacology.* 2003;18(4):239–254.

30. Wurtman RJ, Hefti F, Melamed E. Precursor control of neurotransmitter synthesis. *Pharmacological Reviews.* 1981;32(4):315–331.

31. Routh VH, Stern JS, Horwitz BA. Serotonergic activity is depressed in the ventro-medial hypothalamic nucleus of 12-day-old ovese Zucker rats. *American Journal of Physiology.* 1994;267(3–2):R712–R719.

32. Rondanelli M, et al. Relationship between the absorption of 5-hydroxytryptophan from an integrated diet, by means of *Griffonia simplicifolia* extract, and the effect on satiety in overweight females after oral spray administration. *Eat Weight Disord.* 2012;17(1):e22–e28.

33. Rondanelli M, et al. Satiety and amino-acid profile in overweight women after a new treatment using a natural plant extract sublingual spray formulation. *International Journal of Obesity* (London). 2009;33(10):1174–1182.

34. Ceci F, et al. The effects of oral 5-hydroxytryptophan administration on feeding behavior in obese adult female subjects. *Journal of Neural Transmission.* 1989;76(2):109–117.

35. Cangiano C, et al. Effects of oral 5-hydroxytryptophan on energy intake and macro-nutrient selection in non-insulin dependent diabetic patients. *International Journal of Obesity Relations Metabolism Disorders.* 1998;22(7):648–654.

36. Cangiano C, et al. Eating behavior and adherence to dietary prescriptions in obese adult subjects treated with 5-hydroxytryptophan. *American Journal of Clinical Nutrition.* 1992;56(5):863–867.

37. Wurtman RJ, Wurtman JJ. Brain Serotonin, Carbohydrate-Craving, Obesity and Depression. North American Association for the Study of Obesity (NAASO). 6 September 2012. doi: 10.1002/j.1550-8528.1995.tb00215.x.

38. Swanson J. 13 Valuable Alternative Treatments for Addiction. The Fix-addiction and recovery, straight up Web site. http://www.thefix.com/content/therapies-outside-box?page=all. Accessed June 5, 2015.

39. Schulte E, Avena N, Gearhardt A. Which foods may be addictive? The roles of processing, fat content, and glycemic load. *PLos One.* 2015. doi: 10.1371/journal.pone.0117959

40. Saeed SA, Bloch RM, Antonacci DJ. Herbal and dietary supplements for treatment of anxiety disorders. *American Family Physician.* 2007;76(4):549–556.

41. Hyman M. Food Addiction: Could It Explain Why 70 Percent of America is Fat? D. Mark Hyman Web site. http://drhyman.com/blog/2011/02/04/food-addiction-could-it-explain-why-70-percent-of-america-is-fat/. Accessed July 14, 2015.

42. Kumar SN, Mani UV, Mani I. An open label study on the supplementa-tion of *Gymea sylvestre* in type 2 diabetics. *Journal of Dietary Supplements.* 2010;7(3): 273–282.

43. Pothuraju R, et al. A systematic review of *Gymnema sylvestre* in obesity and diabetes management. *Journal of the Science of Food and Agriculture.* 2014;94(5):834–840.

44. Baskaran K, et al. Antidiabetic effect of a leaf extract from *Gymnema sylvestre* in non-insulin-dependent diabetes mellitus patients. *Journal of Ethnopharmacology.* 1990;30(3):295–305.

45. Grover JK, Yadav SP. Pharmacological actions and potential uses of *Momordica charantia*: a review. *Journal of Ethnopharmacology.* 2004;93(1):123–132.

46. Gupta A, et al. Effect of *Trigonella foenum-graecum* (fenugreek) seeds on glycemic control and insulin resistance in type 2 diabetes mellitus: a double blind placebo controlled study. *Journal of Association of Physicians of India.* 2001;49:1057–1061.

47. Akhondzadeh S, et al. Passionflower in the treatment of generalized anxiety: a pilot double-blind randomized controlled trial with oxazepam. *Journal of Clinical Pharmacy and Therapeutics.* 2001;26(5):363–367.

48. Oliveira AI, et al. Neuroprotective activity of *Hypericum perforatum* and its major components. *Frontiers in Plant Science.* 2016;7:1004.

49. Fabricatore AN. Behavior therapy and cognitive-behavioral therapy of obesity: is there a difference? *Journal of the American Dietetic Association.* 2007;107:92–99.

50. Brownell KD, Heckerman CL, Westlake RJ. The behavioral control of obesity: a descriptive analysis of a large-scale program. *Journal of Clinical Psychology.* 1979;35:864–869.

51. Heatherton TF, Baumesiter RF. Binge eating as escape from self-awareness. *Psychological Bulletin.* 1991;110(1):86–108.

52. Carroll KM. A cognitive-behavioral approach: treating cocaine addiction. Vol 1. Rockville, MD: National Institute on Drug Abuse; 1998.

53. Kadden R, et al. Cognitive-behavioral coping skills therapy manual. Rockville, MD: National Institutes of Health; 1994.

54. Monti, et al. Treating alcohol dependence: a coping skills training guide. 2nd ed. New York: Guilford; 2002.

55. Fabricatore AN. Behavior therapy and cognitive-behavioral therapy of obesity: is there a difference? *Journal of the American Dietetic Association.* 2007;107:92–99.

56. Brownell KD, et al. The behavioral control of obesity: a descriptive analysis of a large-scale program. *Journal of Clinical Psychology.* 1979;35:864–869.

57. Ashley JM, et al. Weight control in the physician's office. *Archives of Internal Medicine.* 2001;161:1599–1604.

58. Brownell KD, et al. Weight reduction at the work site: a promise partially fulfilled. *American Journal of Psychiatry.* 1985;142:47–52.

59. Gardner CD, et al. Comparison of the Atkins, Zone, Ornish, and LEARN diets for change in weight and related risk factors among overweight premeno-pausal women: the A TO Z Weight Loss Study: a randomized trial. *JAMA.* 2007;297:969–977.

60. Marchesini G, et al. Effects of cognitive-behavioural therapy on health-related quality of life in obese subjects with and without binge eating disorder. *International Journal of Obesity Relations Metabolism Disorders.* 2002;26:1261–1267.

61. Agras WS, et al. Does interpersonal therapy help patients with binge eating disorder who fail to respond to cognitive-behavioral therapy? *Journal of Consulting and Clinical Psychology.* 1995;63(3):356–360.

62. Weiner S. The addiction of overeating: self-help groups as treatment models. *Journal of Clinical Psychology.* 1998;54:163–167.

63. Barry D, Clarke M, Petry NM. Obesity and its relationship to addictions: is overeating a form of addictive behavior? *American Journal on Addictions.* 2009;18(6):439–451.

64. Higgins ST, et al. Contigent reinforcement increases cocaine abstinence during outpatient treatment and 1 year of follow-up. *Journal of Consulting and Clinical Psychology.* 2000;68:64–72.

65. Lussier JP, et al. A meta-analysis of voucher-based reinforcement therapy for substance use disorders. *Addiction.* 2006;101:192–203.

66. Epstein LH, Masek BJ, Marshall WR. A nutritionally based school program for control of eating in obese children. *Behavior Therapy.* 1978;9:766–778.

67. Jason LA, Brackshaw E. Access to TV contingent on physical activity: effects on reducing TV-viewing and doby-weight. *Journal of Behavior Therapy and Experimental Psychiatry.* 1990;30:145–151.

68. Evans JR, Abarbanel A. *Introduction to Quantitative EEG and Neurofeedback.* San Diego, CA: Acadamic Press; 1999.

69. Thompson M, Thompson L. *The neurofeedback book: An introduction to basic concepts in applied psychophysiology.* Wheat Ridge, CO: Association for Applied Psychophysiology: 2003.

70. Gilbert C, Moss D. Biofeedback and biological monitoring. In: Moss D, McGrady A, Davies T, Wickramasekera I, eds. Handbook of Mind-Body Medicine for Primary Care. Thousand Oaks, CA: SAGE, 2003:109–122.

71. Schwartz M, Andrasik F. *Biofeedback: A Practitioner's Guide.* 3rd ed. New York: Guilford; 2003.

72. Scott WC, Kaiser D, Othmer S, et al. Effects of an EEG biofeedback protocol on a mixed substance abusing population. *American Journal of Drug and Alcohol Abuse.* 2005;31(3):455–469.

73. Alexander R. Mindfulness Meditation & Addiction—Causes for addiction and how mindfulness meditation can help with them. *Psychology Today* Web site. https://www.psychologytoday.com/blog/the-wise-open-mind/201004/mindfulness-meditation-addiction. Accessed August 7, 2015.

74. Thompson N. Vipassana Meditation Helps Addicts Stay Clean. The Fix-addiction and recovery, straight up Web site. http://www.thefix.com/content/vipassana-meditation-addiction9914. Accessed June 5, 2015.

75. Yoga for anxiety and depression. Harvard Health Publications-Harvard Medical School Web site. http://www.health.harvard.edu/mind-and-mood/yoga-for-anxiety-and-depression. April 1, 2009. Accessed August 7, 2015.

76. Williams M. Take a Deep Breath: The Physiology of Slow Deep Breathing. Mindfulness, MD Web site. http://www.mindfulnessmd.com/2015/06/27/neuroscience-of-mindfulness-take-a-deep-breath/. Accessed September 20, 2015.

77. Wesley MC, Minatrea NB, Watson JC. Animal-assisted therapy in the treatment of substance depedence. *Anthrozoös: A Multidisciplinary Journal of the Interactions of People and Animals.* 2009;22(2):137–148.
78. Hypnotherapy. University of Maryland Medical Center Web site. http://umm.edu/health/medical/altmed/treatment/hypnotherapy#ixzz3hLhPYKIL. Accessed August 7, 2015.
79. Wahrborg P, Annerstedt M. Nature-assisted therarpy: systematic review of controlled and observational studies. *Scandinavian Journal of Public Health.* 2011;39:371–388.
80. Pearson J. Virtual Reality Is Being Used to Treat Heroin Addiction. *Motherboard* Web site. http://motherboard.vice.com/read/virtual-reality-is-being-used-to-treat-heroin-addiction. Accessed June 5, 2015.
81. Horvath TA. Exposure Therapy: A New Look at Conquering Cravings. The Fix-Addiction and Recovery, Straight Up Web site. http://www.thefix.com/content/exposure-therapy-cravings-triggers-CBT8915. Accessed June 5, 2015.
82. Gorini A, et al. A second life for eHealth: prospects for the use of 3-D virtual worlds in clinical pyschology. *Journal of Medical Internet Research.* 2008;10(3).
83. Mills KL, et al. Integrated exposure-based therapy for co-occurring Posttraumatic Stress Disorder and substance dependence: a randomized controlled Trial. *JAMA.* 2012;308(7):690–699.
84. Chiu YH, Lee TH, Shen WW. Use of low-dose topiramate in substance use disorder and bodywedight control. *Psychiatry and Clinical Neurosciences.* 2007;61:630–633.
85. Bray GA, et al. A 6-month randomized, placebo-controlled, dose ranging trial of topiramate for weight loss in obesity. *Obesity Research.* 2003;11:722–733.
86. Muccioli GG. Blocking the cannabinoid receptors: drug candidates and therapeutic promises. *Chemistry & Biodiversity.* 2007;4:1805–1827.
87. Janero DR, Makriyais A. Targeted modulators of the endogenous cannabinoid system: future medications to treat addiction disorders and obesity. *Current Psychiatry Reports.* 2007;9:365–373.
88. Stapleton JA. Trial comes too late as psychiatric side effects end hope for rimonabant. *Addiction.* 2009;104:277–278.
89. Goodman, DW. Lisdexamfetamine dimesylate (Vyvanse), a prodrug stimulant for Attention-Deficit/Hyperactivity Disorder. *P T.* 2010;35(5):273–276, 282–287.
90. FDA expands uses of Vyvanse to treat binge-eating disorder. FDA News Release. http://www.fda.gov/newsevents/newsroom/pressannouncements/ucm432543.htm. Accessed January 30, 2015.
91. Heal DJ, et al. Amphetamine, past and present—a pharmacological and clinical perspective. *Journal of Pyschopharmacology.* 2013;27(6):479–496.

# 4

# Integrative Approach to Alcohol Use Disorder

## JEFF WILKENS AND SHAHLA J. MODIR

## Introduction

This chapter reviews the medical and neurobehavioral effects of alcohol and alcohol-use disorders (AUDs) within the context of traditional medical treatment and integrative medicine. The chapter focuses on how alcohol impacts the brain and body, the influence of genetics on an individual's sensitivity (or insensitivity) to alcohol, how alcohol's effects vary according to the duration of alcohol use over time, and whether an individual's drinking patterns include heavy episodic drinking. In addition, the chapter defines the diagnostic criteria for alcohol-use disorders, as well as the physical, mental, and behavioral disorders that commonly co-occur with alcohol-use disorders. Also, the chapter describes how evidence-based use of select medications and psychosocial treatments can be combined with exercise, healthy diet, meditation, yoga, mindfulness, acupuncture, and neurofeedback to provide care to individuals who struggle with heavy episodic drinking (HED) and/or alcohol-use disorders.

Ethanol is a relatively small, two-carbon and two-hydroxyl (oxygen + hydrogen) molecule that has amused and tormented the human species for at least 9,000 years.[1] Seventy-one percent of people in the United States reported drinking during 2014, while in the same year 16.3 million adults (18 and over), and close to 700,000 adolescents (12 to 17 years of age), had signs of an AUD[2]—all consistent with alcohol-use disorders. These disorders rank third in the United States in preventable causes of morbidity and mortality.[3] Of note, the majority of the adolescents were females, representing 3% of all US females in this age group; the males with an AUD represented 2.5% of US males 12 to 17 years of age.[2] The cost of alcohol-related problems to US society is approximately $240 billion per year.[4]

# Epidemiology

## PREVALENCE

There are a number of different surveys used to assess the prevalence of alcoholism in the United States and globally. The goal of these varied surveys is to show a difference between social normative drinking patterns and problematic drinking along a continuum. These surveys often include binge drinking, HED, and heavy drinking to elucidate a spectrum of drinking related to consequences medically, socially, and legally. The *DSM-4* (APA, 1994) previously used the criteria of alcohol abuse and alcohol dependence but has subsequently revised the diagnostic system in the *DSM-5* to include alcohol use disorders with varying levels of severity scaled to criteria in 2013.

SAMHSA defines HED as having 5 or more standard drinks on onesingle occasion in the past year. According to the World Health Organization's global status report on alcohol and health from 2014, the Americas have the highest rate of HED (22.0%) while South east Asia has the lowest (12.4%).[5] Worldwide, HED is more common in young people between the ages of 15 and 19 (12%) than the total population over the age of 15 (7.5%).[6] The rates of HED for adolescents are highest in Europe, the Americas, and the Western Pacific region. The highest rate of HED among older individuals is found in Southeast Asian countries.

Wealthier countries have higher rates of alcohol consumption and HED than poor countries. However, approximately 40% of all alcohol consumption in poor and middle-income countries is unrecorded, most likely because unrecorded alcohol is often cheaper.[7]

In the United States, HED is defined as the consumption of 5 drinks or more for males or 4 or more drinks for females in the past year. In data published from a national health survey interview conducted from 2008–2010, The Center for Disease Control reported that 64.9% of adults drink and 5.4% are classified as heavy drinkers. One in 4 adults have had more than 5 drinks in 1 day at least once during the past year.[8]

Drinking rates are influenced by sex, age, race, educational status, economics, and marital status. According to the CDC and multiple surveys, the prevalence of AUD is consistently higher in men than women. This difference is two-fold in some reports. In the CDC report, 70.8% of male adults drink compared to 59.5% of female adults. Whereas 26.5% of women abstain from alcohol, men have an abstention rate of 14.7%. Men are twice as likely as women to have consumed at least 5 drinks in 1 day at least once in the past year.[9]

In the United States, alcohol consumption is most prevalent (73.1%) in the 25 to 44 age group and starts to decline in the 45 to 64 age group.[10] HED is strongly associated with age. The prevalence of HED ranges from 35.1% in the 18 to 24 age group to 2.3% in adults over the age of 75.[11] A similar finding was published in the 2009 National Survey on Drug Use and Health (NSDUH; SAMHSA, 2010) where the prevalence of current alcohol use increased with age up to 21 to 25 years, and the highest rates of binge drinking and heavy drinking occurred during that same time period.[12]

Whites (67.8%) are more likely to be current consumers of alcohol than any other race. The lifetime abstinence rate is highest among Asians (42.5%). HED is also highest in whites (26.0%), followed by blacks (14.0%) and Asians (11.2%).[13]

The prevalence of current drinking increases with educational status. 46.8% of adults with less than a high school diploma consume alcohol compared to 77.3% of adults with graduate degrees.[14] Similarly, income level affects alcohol consumption, as 48.5% of adults below the poverty line are current drinkers compared to 76.5% of adults who drink and make 4 times the poverty level.[15] Adults below the poverty line are twice as likely to abstain from alcohol as adults with incomes 4 times the poverty line. Furthermore, adults with high incomes were more likely to have more than 5 drinks per day at least once in the past year than adults in lower income groups.[16]

National epidemiologic data on the most recent classification of AUD in the *DSM-5* (involving 36,309 subjects over the age of 18) showed that the 1 year prevalence of AUD was 13.9%, and lifetime prevalence was 29.1%. Prevalence of AUD was highest for white and Native American men who were either never married or previously married. The 1 year and lifetime prevalence of AUD was greatest for individuals in the lowest income bracket (1.8% and 1.5%). Less than 20% of respondents with lifetime AUD were treated.[17]

## COMORBIDITIES

Alcohol use disorder (or alcohol abuse) is associated with many psychiatric illnesses, as well as occupational, financial, and relationship problems. The combination of heavy alcohol consumption and comorbid conditions is associated with higher rates of morbidity and mortality, despite seeking treatment. There is a very strong association between individuals whose death was related to excessive alcohol consumption and previously failed interventional attempts by their physicians, family members, and friends.[18] There is also a strong association between losing one's job due to problems with alcohol consumption and a heightened risk of mortality (HR = 1.36, 95% CI: 1.11, 1.65).[19] Social risks surrounding alcohol consumption are either more strongly or equally linked to mortality risk compared to the physiological effects of alcohol abuse.

There is a strong association with alcohol abuse and psychiatric illnesses, especially bipolar disorder, borderline personality disorder, antisocial disorder, and major depression. In the adult population over age 65 who engage in hazardous or harmful drinking, symptoms of depression and anxiety are much more prevalent in females.[20] Among adolescent girls and boys aged 12 to 17, AUD and it's spectrum are significantly associated with separation anxiety, generalized anxiety, depression, oppositional defiant disorder, and conduct disorder.[21] There is also a strong association between AUD and both panic disorder and obsessive-compulsive disorder in adolescent females.[22] A history of traumatic events or posttraumatic stress disorder is associated with alcohol abuse, especially in immigrant populations relocating to a new country.[23] War veterans who are diagnosed with both AUD and major depression have higher rates of other comorbidities, such as bipolar disorder, drug abuse, liver disease, and higher rates of homelessness.[24]

Alcohol abuse is often associated with other substance abuse. Alcohol abuse is associated with tobacco use 32.4% of the time and is associated with tobacco, cannabis, cocaine, or other illicit drug use 25.3% of the time.[25] The later association has a stronger correlation with major depression, generalized anxiety, borderline personality disorder, antisocial disorder, and histrionic personality disorder than alcohol abuse by itself.[26]

AUD and bipolar disorder have a high rate of comorbidity. In fact, bipolar disorder is the *DSM* Axis 1 disorder most significantly associated with alcohol abuse.[27] Specifically, alcohol use disorderaffects one-third of individuals diagnosed with bipolar disorder.[28] Bipolar disorder and AUD'sare known to have similar etiological traits, including similarities on the genetic, neurochemical, and neuroanatomic level.[29]

There is also a high rate of physical comorbidities with AUD, including liver disease, pancreatic disease, airway diseases, neurological diseases, gastrointestinal diseases, kidney disease, cellulitis, iron deficiency anemia, and femur fractures.[30]

## GENETICS

Current research strongly suggests that genetics plays just as much a role as environmental factors in the etiology of alcohol abuse. Both family and twin studies indicate genetics is a key risk factor for AUD, and specific genes and genetic polymorphisms have been linked to alcohol abuse. A thorough meta-analysis of twin and adoption studies concluded that alcohol use disorders are at least 50% heritable.[31] Two single nucleotide polymorphisms of the gene for GRM8, a glutamate receptor, are significantly linked to alcohol dependent symptoms, particularly in European American young adults.[32] A similar genetic association was not found in black Americans.

The association between many gene candidates and alcohol use disorders is currently unclear and more research is needed. For example, a large, comprehensive meta-analysis of six candidate genes involved in neuroplasticity (BDNF,

DRD1, DRD3, DRD4, GRIN2B, and MAOA) did not show a significant association for AUD.[33]

AUD and its most common associated comorbidities may be linked to the same genetic variations. For example, a large, robust population-based twin study involving 12,000 pairs of twins showed that shared genetic factors accounted for 64% of the overlap of attention deficit hyperactivity disorder and alcohol dependence.[34] Furthermore, single nucleotide polymorphisms have been significantly linked to alcohol abuse and comorbid drug problems.[35]

# Diagnosis: AUD

According to the *DSM-5*, in order for an individual to be diagnosed with AUD, he or she must display 2 of the following 11 symptoms within a 1-year period: (1) consuming more alcohol than originally planned; (2) worrying about stopping or consistently failing to control one's use; (3) spending an exorbitant amount of time using alcohol or doing whatever it takes to obtain alcohol; (4) using alcohol instead of fulfilling major role obligations at home, work, and school; (5) craving alcohol; (6) continuing the use of alcohol despite health problems caused or worsened by it (including psychological problems or worsening physical health); (7) continuing the use of alcohol despite it creating relationship problems; (8) repeated use of alcohol in a dangerous situation; (9) giving up or reducing activities in a person's life because of alcohol; (10) building up tolerance to alcohol; (11) experiencing withdrawal symptoms after stopping use. Moderators are included in the current diagnostic system to reflect mild, moderate, and severe based on the number of criteria present.[36]

## DIAGNOSTIC SCREENING TOOLS

There are several screening tools for AUD. These include the CAGE questionnaire, MAST, and AUDIT. The CAGE questionnaire consists of four questions, making it a very quick and convenient screening tool. Two positive responses indicate that alcoholism may be present. The four questions are: (1) Have you ever felt you needed to Cut down on your drinking? (2) Have people Annoyed you by criticizing your drinking? (3) Have you ever felt Guilty about drinking? (4) Have you ever felt you needed a drink first thing in the morning (Eye-Opener)?

The Michigan Alcoholism Screening Test (MAST) is one of the oldest alcohol screening test and constructed to effectively screen the general population. The MAST contains 25 questions and is rated on a point system. One disadvantage to the MAST screening tool is that it can be timely and inconvenient for busy primary care physicians.

The Alcohol Use Disorders Identification Test (AUDIT) is a 10-question, point-based screening tool for alcohol dependence. AUDIT was developed by the World Health Organization and can effectively screen for hazardous or dependent drinking patterns. A score of 8 or higher on the AUDIT indicates that alcohol dependence may be present.

### PHYSICAL FINDINGS: LABS/PHYSICAL EXAM

There are several biomarkers that serve as indicators for AUD. These lab markers can be especially helpful since there is a tendency for individuals to underreport alcohol use. Alcohol-use biomarkers are classified as indirect and direct. Indirect biomarkers indicate the damage alcohol is having on organ systems. They include elevated levels of: Aspartate aminotransferase (AST), Alanine aminotransferase (ALT), Gamma glutamyltransferase (GGT), Mean corpuscular volume (MCV), and Carbohydrate-deficient transferrin (CDT). As a screening tool for alcohol dependence, CDT tends to have the highest specificity and sensitivity. For diagnosing purposes, the combination of GGT and CDT has the highest sensitivity, specificity, and the strongest correlation to the actual amount of alcohol consumed. Direct biomarkers are from the metabolism of alcohol itself. Direct biomarkers for alcohol-use disorders include elevations in alcohol and ethyl glucuronide (EtG).[37] A blood alcohol level of 300 mg/dL or higher indicates alcohol abuse. A blood alcohol level of 150 mg/dL or higher without symptoms of intoxication indicate alcohol abuse. A blood alcohol level of 100 mg/dL at a routine examination can indicate alcoholism as well.

Alcohol has a short half-life, which limits its ability as a reliable biomarker for AUD EtG is a direct metabolite of alcohol and is a reliable biomarker for alcohol-abuse, because it can be detected in the urine for up to 5 days following heavy drinking. On physical exam, there are several indications of alcohol-use disorders. An elevated blood pressure or heart rate, an enlarged or tender liver, or a tremor may be indicators of alcoholism. Certain skin changes may be noticeable. Erythema on the palms of the hands and spider veins or broken capillaries may be visible on the face or abdomen. A patient's balance may be affected by alcohol as well as his/her cognitive function, both of which can be assessed during a neurological exam. If a patient is acutely intoxicated, either the smell of alcohol or mouthwash may be detected in the mouth.

Signs of alcohol-induced portal hypertension may be discovered during a physical exam. These include ascites, or an enlarged, fluid-filled abdomen, confusion due to a malfunctioning liver and possibly bloody stools or blood in one's vomit.

# Neurobiology

The neurobiology of AUD has recently been described as a 2-stage process: an initial positive reinforcement stage (behavior is driven by the seeking of a reward), and a subsequent negative reinforcement stage (behavior is driven by seeking a reduction of a negative emotional state, and as a response to alcohol cravings—both of which are linked to stress regulatory systems within the brain).[38] Thus, the drinking of alcohol can produce pleasure and gratification or relief.[38] The positive reinforcement that occurs from alcohol use is mediated by alcohol-stimulated mu-opioid receptors that produce increases in dopamine-based reward mechanisms in the ventral striatum of the brain.[41,42] Consistent heavy use of alcohol then leads to changes in the brain that establish the second stage, or negative reinforcement condition.[38,39,40] The negative reinforcement process is mediated by progressive decreases in the alcohol-induced reward process (e.g., decreased dopamine), coupled with alterations in stress and emotional regulatory systems, including in the extended amygdala that produce the negative emotional state, and contribute to the development of alcohol cravings.[38,39,40]

Included in the sections that follow are discussions of the pharmacotherapy treatment of AUDs, as well as descriptions of integrative medicine interventions and their impact on AUD and addiction—including yoga, exercise, meditation and mindfulness, and acupuncture. We hypothesize that positive treatment effects secondary to medication treatments may share a neurobiological basis with integrative interventions that appear to be effective. For example, as discussed in the sections below, meditation, and particularly practice of mindfulness, may stimulate the healing of alcohol-induced pathological alterations in the brain's stress regulatory systems.

# Medical Complications from Alcohol

It is estimated that 3.8% of all deaths worldwide are attributable to problematic alcohol use[43] The Center for Disease Control (CDC) has reported that 88,000 people (approximately 62,000 men and 26,000 women) die from alcohol-related causes annually, making it the third leading preventable cause of death in the United States. AUD is a chronic, relapsing disorder that includes compulsive alcohol use, including continuing to drink despite known harmful consequences. There is also the development of withdrawal syndrome upon stopping drinking. Regarding the impact of alcohol on liver function, of the 71,713 liver disease deaths among individuals aged 12 and older in the US in 2013, 46.4% involved alcohol. Among males, 48.9% of the 46,240 liver disease deaths involved alcohol. Among females, 42.7% of the 25,433 liver disease deaths involved alcohol (CDC, 2013).

Further, one in three liver transplants in the United States in 2009 were attributable to alcohol-related liver disease.[44] Also, alcohol is linked to increases in the risk of cancers of the mouth, esophagus, pharynx, larynx, liver, and breast (National Cancer Institute, 2012). Finally, with respect to trauma, alcohol-impaired driving fatalities accounted for 10,076 deaths (30.8% of overall driving fatalities).[45]

Whereas the extraordinary number of medical consequences of alcohol cannot be sufficiently covered in this chapter, Box 4.1 provides the reader with a perspective on the scope of alcohol-induced medical complications.

# Treatment of AUD

## MEDICATIONS FOR THE TREATMENT OF ALCOHOL WITHDRAWAL

The alcohol withdrawal syndrome was not established until 1953, when Victor and Adams reported their findings related to the effects of "alcohol on the nervous system" through careful observations of close to 300 patients admitted to a metropolitan hospital.

Medication regimens for the treatment of alcohol withdrawal follow one of three methodologies, a fixed schedule, withdrawal symptom triggered dosing, or the establishment of a loading dose until the patient manifest a state of light sleep/sedation (Table 4.1).

## MEDICATIONS FOR THE TREATMENT OF AUD

Disulfiram (Antabuse™) was the first Food and Drug Administration (FDA)—approved medication to stop or decrease alcohol use; it was approved in 1949. Over 50 years later, naltrexone (ReVia™) became the second in 1994, acamprosate (Campral™) was approved in 2004, and a depot formulation of naltrexone (Vivitrol™) was approved in 2006;[46] the mechanisms of action of these 3 classes of medications are described below. In addition to the FDA-approved medications, other medications that are not FDA approved have been shown to reduce various measures of alcohol use in persons with AUD—these medications include anticonvulsants, including topiramate (Topamax™) and gabapentin (neurontin™), baclofen, a GABA-B receptor agonist, select serotonin reuptake blockers (SSRIs), especially fluoxetine, citalopram, and sertraline—with sertraline and the 5-HT3 receptor antagonist ondansetron potentially offering pharmacotherapy for select subtypes of persons with alcohol use disorders (Table 4.2).

Disulfiram shifts the metabolism of alcohol to achieve a build-up of toxic metabolic products, creating a disturbing biological sensitization to the user of alcohol,

## Box 4.1  MEDICAL CONSEQUENCES OF ALCOHOL

- *Heart*: heart muscle failure (Cardiomyopathy), so-called holiday heart (atrial fibrillatiion), high blood pressure (hypertension), heart rate irregularities (dysrhythmia), masks heart related chest pain (angina) symptoms, coronary artery spasm, heart attack (myocardial ischemia), coronary artery disease, sudden death
- *Liver*: fatty liver (Steatosis), alcoholic hepatitis, cirrhosis, liver failure secondary to blood vessel blockage, venous enlargement (varices), and additional hepatic infections
- *Kidneys*: combined kidney and liver failure, muscle breakdown and acute failure of kidneys, blood volume depletion, biochemical failures throughout the body secondary to kidney failure
- *Stomach and Bowels*: infections of the stomach, esophagus, and pancreas (pancreatitis), diarrhea, folic acid and lactase deficiency, enlargement of the parotid gland, specific cancers, bleeding of the stomach and bowels
- *Brain and nervous system*: nerve dysfunction (Peripheral neuropathy), seizures, delirium, Korsakoff's dementia, Wernicke's syndrome, cerebellar dysfunction, Marchiafava-Bignami syndrome, central pontine myelinolysis, myopathy, amblyopia, stroke, withdrawal delirium, hallucinations, toxic leukoencephalopathy, subdural hematoma, intracranial hemorrhage
- *Infections*: hepatitis C, pneumonia, tuberculosis (including meningitis), HIV, sexually transmitted diseases, spontaneous bacterial peritonitis, brain abscess, meningitis
- *Sleep*: apnea, periodic limb movements of sleep, insomnia, disrupted sleep, daytime fatigue
- *Trauma*: motor vehicle crash, fatal and nonfatal injury, physical and sexual abuse
- *Prenatal and perinatal*: fetal alcohol effects and syndrome
- *Hematologic*: macrocytic anemia, pancytopenia because of marrow toxicity and/or splenic sequestration, leukopenia, thrombocytopenia, coagulopathy because of liver disease, iron deficiency, folate deficiency, spur cell anemia, burr cell anemia
- *Musculoskeletal*: striatal muscle destruction (Rhabdomyolysis), gout, fracture, osteopenia, osteonecrosis
- *Nutritional*: vitamin and mineral deficiencies (B1, B6, riboflavin, niacin, vitamin D, magnesium, calcium, folate, phosphate, zinc)

(Adapted from Saitz, R. Medical and Surgical Complications of Addiction, The ASAM Principles of Addiction Medicine (Fifth Edition, R. K. Ries, Editor, 2014).)

### Table 4.1 Medication Regimens

| Type of Dosing Regime | Patient Group | Dosing Regime |
|---|---|---|
| Fixed schedule | Appropriate for clients at risk of complicated withdrawal who are not in a hospital or other supervised environment (eg, community-based withdrawal) | Specified doses at fixed intervals, tapered over a set number of days |
| Symptom-triggered dosing | Appropriate for alcohol withdrawal clients in a medically supervised setting | Doses administered according to Individually experienced symptoms of alcohol withdrawal |
| Loading dose | Appropriate for alcohol withdrawal clients in a medically supervised setting | Large doses until alcohol withdrawal subsides or light sedation is reached |

characterized by flushing of the upper areas of the body, palpitations, increased heart rate, nausea, vomiting, and other experiences. However, the effective use of disulfiram has been shown to generally require a second person, often spouse or family member, to administer the medication on a daily basis.[47]

Naltrexone, a mu-opioid receptor blocker, was first reported to produce fewer drinking days and less craving for alcohol than placebo.[48] Shortly thereafter,

### Table 4.2 Medication-Assisted Treatment of Alcohol Use Disorders

| Mu Opioid Antagonists | Glutamate Antagonists | GABA Agonists | Aversive Agent | Serotonin |
|---|---|---|---|---|
| Naltrexone[‡] (Revia®, Vivitrol®, Naltrel®) | Acamprosate[‡] (Campral®) | Baclofen (Lioresal®) | Disulfiram[†] (Antabuse®) | Serotonin Reputake Inhibitors (SSRI's) (fluoxetine, sertraline, others) |
| | Topiramate* (Topamax®) | Gabapentin* (Neurontin®) | | 5-HT3 receptor antagonist Ondansetron (Zofran®) |

‡ FDA Approved
* Impacts multiple systems

naltrexone's efficacy was demonstrated to be enhanced by the addition of cognitive-behavioral therapy (CBT), or supportive therapy.[49] Further study demonstrated naltrexone's ability to decrease relapses to heavy drinking,[50] and subsequently reducing heavy drinking among patients who continued to drink.[51] Naltrexone is known to produce dizziness and nausea in patients[46] and is contraindicated in patients with acute hepatitis or liver failure since it has the capacity to cause damage to the cells of the liver if given in doses equal to, or exceeding 300 mg/day.[52] Yet this contrasts with the traditional 50 mg/day of naltrexone.

Acamprosate, an amino acid derivative, that produces a favorable neurotransmission ratio between gamma-aminobutyric acid (GABA) and that of glutamate, a excitatory amino acid glutamate with harmful effects. Acamprosate has been predominately evaluated in European clinical studies that have demonstrated consistent positive effects.[53,54,55] But a recent meta-analysis of pharmacotherapy of AUDs performed a subgroup analysis for return to any drinking for acamprosate. The analysis of a pooled effect of studies rated as low risk of bias found no significant difference between acamprosate and placebo.[56] In addition, a 4-month, multicenter study, placebo-controlled study of close to 1,400 abstinent alcohol dependent subjects (per *DSM-4*) conducted at 11 sites in the United States, compared naltrexone, acamprosate, and their combination in subjects who were also randomized to receive either medical management or a combined behavioral intervention.[57] The patients receiving naltrexone with medical management had the best drinking outcomes, while acamprosate showed no efficacy when compared to placebo.[57]

Anticonvulsants, including topiramate,[58,59] have been found to produce positive outcomes in study subjects with alcohol use disorders, presumably through their GABA agonist and glutamate antagonism.[58,59] Thus, these medications again impact the neurotransmission balance between GABA and glutamate. Baclofen, though not an anticonvulsant, is a GABA-B agonist that has FDA approval as a antispasmodic.[60] Another anticonvulsant, gabapentin, has been evaluated in a 16-week study of 150 alcohol-dependent subjects who were randomly assigned to receive naltrexone 50 mg/day, or naltrexone plus gabapentin (up to 1,200 mg/day). The combination of both medications was shown to lengthen the interval to heavy drinking, had fewer heavy drinking days when compared to naltrexone, and fewer drinks when drinking when compared to placebo.[61] A recent study, also of 150 male and female study participants provided placebo and doses of either 900 mg per day of gabapentin or 1,800 mg/day plus manual-guided counseling.[62] In this study, gabapentin significantly increased the rates of abstinence (17% in the 1,800 mg group versus 4% in the placebo group) while persons achieving no heavy drinking was 45% (1,800 mg gabapentin) versus 23% (placebo).[62]

A multitude of serotonin reuptake inhibitors (SRIs) have been evaluated to determine their utility for AUD. The serotonergic system plays a significant role in alcohol intake and dependence, and low serotonin has been associated with increased alcohol consumption and an increased risk of alcohol dependence. In the short term, alcohol consumption increases extracellular concentrations of serotonin (5-HT), but chronic alcohol consumption causes an overall decrease in 5-HT neurotransmission.[63]

5-HTT, a transmembrane monoamine neurotransporter that controls the concentration of 5-HT at central and peripheral sites, plays a significant role in how alcohol affects the serotonergic system. The 5-HTT gene is located on chromosome 17 and has a polymorphic region (5-HTTLPR) that alters 5-HTT transcription and has been linked to alcohol dependence.[64] The 5 HTTLPR polymorphisms are designated L (for long) and S (for short). The 5-HTTLPR polymorphism has been linked to alcohol cravings, alcohol neurotoxicity, withdrawal symptoms, antisocial behavior and impulsivity.[65] Specifically, alcoholics are 15% to 18% more likely to have an S allele, and S-allele carriers are 18% more likely to developAUD.[65] S-allele carriers are more likely to be alcohol-dependent individuals who have an earlier onset of alcohol use, a more severe dependence on alcohol, and a higher occurrence of comorbid psychiatric conditions.[65] Specifically, these findings are more common in Type 2 or Type B alcoholics, or those individuals characterized as having an early onset of alcohol use, weak environmental influences, more severe dependence, and a higher frequency of antisocial and impulsive traits.[66] (Type A or Type 1 alcoholics are individuals characterized as having a later onset of alcohol use, a lower rate of comorbidities, and less severe substance dependence.)

Some research indicates that the efficacy of SRIs for treating alcoholism depends on whether the individuals being treated are Type 2 (Type B) or Type 1 (Type A) alcoholics. One study analyzed the effects of an SRI, fluoxetine, in Type B alcoholics verses Type A alcoholics. Results showed that Fluoxetine resulted in poorer drinking-related outcomes than placebo in the Type B alcoholics, or more severe alcoholics. Type B alcoholics on fluoxetine were more likely to relapse on alcohol than those on placebo. The same effect was not observed in the Type A alcoholics. Therefore, it was recommended that fluoxetine not be used to achieve abstinence or reduce drinking in high-risk alcoholics (Type B) and should be used with caution for any on label use for this same reason.[67]

A 12-week, double-blind, randomized, placebo-controlled trial analyzed the SRI, sertraline, for alcohol dependence in both late onset (age >25) and early onset (age <25) alcoholics. Results showed that in the late onset group, treatment with sertraline resulted in less heavy drinking, whereas in the early onset group, treatment with a **placebo** resulted in less heavy drinking.[68] This study implies that SRIs may be an effective treatment for alcohol-dependent individuals who started drinking later in life, but not for those individuals with an earlier onset. And in fact, sertraline can increase relapse rates in the early onset alcoholic again showing the need for caution for using it with this type of alcoholic even for on label indications. A review of several double-blind, placebo-controlled trials on the usefulness of SRIs in AUD's was conducted by Pettinati et al. Results showed that SRIs provided only a minimum advantage in reducing the number of drinks per day, and this advantage was witnessed only when the drugs were prescribed at much higher doses than recommended. The authors also note that more recent research suggests that SRIs may be most useful in subpopulations of alcohol-dependent individuals, such as those individuals who have clear symptoms of comorbid depression and anxiety, or clear signs of serotonin dysfunction.[69]

## DIET

Alcohol-use disorder puts a person at risk for a variety of nutrient, mineral, and vitamin deficiencies. The best diet for alcoholics is one that is balanced, gets the majority of calories from whole foods, and does not include alcohol. Nutrient and vitamin levels should be measured, monitored, and supplemented if low. Alcoholics often eat poorly and often substitute drinking for eating for as much as 50% of their daily caloric intake. Alcohol interferes with digestion, storage, utilization, and excretion of foods.[70] For example, alcohol interferes with the ability of the pancreas to secrete digestive enzymes and break down food, and it damages the lining of the stomach, which affects nutrient absorption. Alcohol can impair insulin secretion and cause hyperglycemia, but it can also result in hypoglycemia when a fasting individual consumes alcohol. Alcohol can also impair absorption of proteins due to impaired processing of amino acids by the intestines and liver and impaired secretion of proteins by the liver. Vitamin deficiencies are common in alcoholics, especially the fat-soluble vitamins, because alcohol inhibits fat absorption. Hence, deficiencies in fat-soluble vitamins A, E, D, and K are often noted. Deficiencies in vitamin B are also common. Mineral deficiencies occur as well, especially for calcium, magnesium, iron, and zinc. Thiamine deficiencies can occur in chronic alcoholics and can lead to severe neurological problems and memory loss (Wernicke-Korsoff syndrome). There is not a "cure-all" diet for alcoholics, and not every alcoholic will have the same nutrient/vitamin deficiencies or comorbidities. Still, a nutritious diet is necessary for recovery, and medical professionals should work with their alcoholic patients to ensure all dietary needs are being met. For a more complete discussion of the optimal use of food as functional medicine in the treatment of addiction, we invite the reader to explore the "Nutrition and Nutraceuticals" chapters of this book.

## YOGA

In most scientific literature, yoga is the generalized term for a variety of postures, stretches, breathing techniques, and meditation. As of yet, there is no robust body of evidence suggesting that yoga is an effective complementary treatment for alcohol addiction, but smaller studies have concluded that yoga can be effective. The breathing techniques, self-awareness, spiritual philosophy, and self-discipline cultivated through yoga can target the psychological, stressful, and behavioral factors, including cravings, linked to alcohol addiction. While there are many different kinds of yoga, the most effective approach to addiction is most likely integrated yoga, which involves meditation, exercise, and spiritual teachings. Integrated yoga has been shown to reduce cortisol, the stress hormone, by 31%.[71] Since stress is a huge risk factor for alcohol abuse and relapse, incorporating integrated yoga as part of a holistic treatment plan may be helpful.

One study analyzing a 12-session yoga intervention for veteran and civilian women with posttraumatic stress disorder (PTSD) showed that yoga was effective at reducing the symptoms of PTSD and reducing the risk for alcohol and drug abuse.[72] A small pilot study analyzing the effects of a 10-week yoga intervention as part of a treatment plan for AUD showed that yoga was highly accepted by the alcohol-dependent participants and that alcohol consumption decreased more in the group using yoga as part of their treatment plan than the control group.[73] Qualitative data from the same study showed that yoga helped participants postpone drinking and slept better; and most participants attributed these to the stress reduction and mood enhancing effects of yoga.[73]

The Mindfulness-Based Relapse Prevention (MBRP) program is an 8-week, group-based alternative treatment that teaches mindful movement in addition to prevention strategies and meditation. Mindful movement is similar to yoga in that it includes light stretching and gentle movement. This type of movement may be more conducive for individuals with AUD since many of them also have physical disabilities and limitations. One study involving 168 adults and MBRP showed that compared to the treatment-as-usual group, the MBRP group had statistically significant lower rates of substance abuse at the 2-month follow-up and attributed this improvement to a decreased association between depressive symptoms and cravings.[74] At this point, the beneficial effect yoga has on alcohol-addiction needs further exploration.

## EXERCISE

Physical exercise is known to be a beneficial adjunct therapy for individuals diagnosed with mental disorders, especially depression, and generalized anxiety disorder. While to date there is a paucity of interventional trials, physical exercise may also be beneficial for substance-abuse disorders, although much more research is needed to decipher the type of exercise that is most beneficial and the demographics of individuals who respond best. A large systematic review of how physical activity relates to individuals diagnosed with AUD showed that increased rates of smoking, obesity, anxiety, depression, and low self-efficacy may limit his/

her ability to be physically active.[75] Comorbidities and physical diseases caused by excess alcohol use can certainly limit one's ability to exercise as well. Still, the evidence for the theoretical and practical benefits of exercise, including psychological, behavioral, and neurobiological benefits; reduced cravings; and overall health effects support its use for alcohol-abuse disorders.[76]

In one randomized, placebo-controlled study analyzing the effects of aerobic exercise intervention on alcohol-dependent participants, the alcohol-dependent participants assigned to the exercise group reported less drinking and fewer heavy drinking days than the treatment-as-usual group.[77] A large population-based study involving 9,415 participants between the ages of 30–60 and analyzing the effects of exercise on substance use showed that at the 10-year follow-up mark, a greater reduction in binge drinking in the exercise group than the control group. However, there were no changes in the average alcohol consumption per week.[78]

## MEDITATION

Meditation is the deliberate act of spending time in quiet thought or relaxation. Meditation is an exercise in mindfulness that is designed to increase self-awareness, self-control, and an improved capability for managing negative emotions. Cravings and negative emotions are strong predictors of relapse and alcohol-abuse, and meditation may be an effective tool for addressing them.

MBRP is a new type of cognitive behavioral therapy designed to target cravings and negative emotions. MBRP uses mindfulness meditation exercises along with cognitive behavioral prevention and coping skills. Specifically, MBRP teaches addicted individuals how to become more aware of their external triggers, their internal thought process, and how to better tolerate physical and emotional experiences. In essence, MBRP teaches individuals struggling with alcohol and substance use to experience negative feelings and thoughts without giving in to the conditioned response: a craving. Some studies suggest that the mindful meditation component of MBRP leads to increased attention and ability to control one's actions, mostly by teaching addicted individuals to notice uncomfortable cravings and negative emotions and not automatically react to them.[79] MBRP teaches an approach rather than an avoidance type of coping by cultivating a sense of curiosity and encouraging individuals to notice and investigate their thoughts and feelings without habitually responding to them.

One systematic review of the effectiveness of MBRP showed that individuals who used MBRP reported reduced substance use, reduction in cravings, and reduced reactivity to environmental cues.[79] The MBRP group also reported a significantly higher level of awareness and self-acceptance, as well as significant decreases in cravings over a 4-month follow up period.[79] A large randomized clinical trial showed that compared to treatment as usual, MBRP led to lower risk of relapse to substance use and heavy drinking, and amongst participants who continued to use substances, significantly fewer days of substance use and drinking at the 6-month follow-up. At the 12-month follow-up, the MBRP group reported statistically significant fewer days of substance use and significantly decreased heavy drinking compared to the treatment-as-usual group.[80]

Consistent with these findings, research suggests that meditation may actually change certain brain structures, thereby attenuating the symptoms of alcohol addiction. For example, compared to non-meditators, meditators have greater cortical thickness in the right anterior insula, which may correlate to greater awareness of bodily sensations and emotions.[81] Another study showed that 8 weeks of meditation resulted in increased gray matter in the hippocampus, the cerebellum and cortical regions responsible for emotional regulation, body awareness, and awareness of one's self.[82]

## ACUPUNCTURE

Acupuncture is an alternative therapy rooted in traditional Chinese medicine that has been in existence for over 5,000 years. Acupuncture involves the insertion of needles into the body at specific points, to stimulate nerves, relieve pain, treat a disease, and reduce inflammation. Some doctors and therapists are using acupuncture as an adjunct therapy for AUD.

Acupuncture has been used to help alleviate cravings in patients with alcohol dependence. A recent randomized, placebo-controlled study showed a significant reduction in alcohol cravings in the group receiving acupuncture therapy.[83] The group was given acupuncture twice a week for 4 weeks. The type of acupuncture delivered is called Zhubin acupuncture, which is unique for its map of body points used for delivery.

Specifically, auricular (or ear) acupuncture has been tried as an adjunct therapy for alcohol withdrawal and shown to be effective.[84] One randomized, placebo-controlled study showed that alcohol-dependent participants assigned to an orthodox acupuncture treatment group, treated for a total of 10 treatments over a 2-week period, had better outcome results and fewer withdrawal symptoms.[85]

## NEUROFEEDBACK

Neurofeedback is a type of biofeedback tool that utilizes conventional displays of brain activity to teach individuals how to manipulate their breathing and behavior to self-regulate brain function. This type of biofeedback often involves electroencephalography (EEG) or functional magnetic resonance imaging

(MRI). Using either of these two technologies, brain activity is measured and recorded and then a signal (often a sound or a video reminder) is used to condition an individual to self-regulate his or her own brain function in a positive, desirable way. Neurofeedback has been used for a variety of physical and psychiatric illnesses but also as a coping mechanism for stress, anxiety, and depression. It has also been used effectively as an adjunct therapy for treating alcohol addiction.

Alcohol-related environmental triggers are known to activate the ventral striatum are of the brain. Activation of the ventral striatum, or the reward-related area of the brain, is theorized to create cravings. One study using neurofeedback with functional magnetic resonance imaging and non-addicted, heavy social drinkers showed that the treatment was significantly effective for reducing ventral striatum activity due to alcohol triggers.[86]

Several studies have shown that EEG neurofeedback has a positive effect on decreasing drug use, treatment compliance, and alcohol-dependent user's responses to environmental triggers. Alcohol-dependent individuals have also shown decreased cravings after EEG neurofeedback sessions, which could be a key interventional therapy in the future, since cravings play a significant role in why many alcoholics relapse.[87,88]

## REFERENCES

1. McGovern PE. *Wine: The Search for the Origins of Viniculture.* Princeton, NJ: Princeton University Press; 2002.
2. National Institute on Alcohol Abuse and Alcoholism. Alcohol Facts and Statistics. http://pubs.niaaa.nih.gov/publications/AlcoholFacts&Stats/Alcohol Facts& Stats.pdf
3. US Preventive Services Task Force. http://www.uspreventiveservicestaskforce. org
4. Rehm J, Mathers C, Popova S, et al. Global burden of disease and injury and economic cost attributable to alcohol use and alcohol-use disorders. *Lancet.* 2009b;373(9682):2223–2233.
5-10. World Health Association. *Global Status Report on Alcohol and Health.* 2014: 1–57.
10-17. Center For Disease Control. *Health Behaviors of Adults: United States, 2008–2010. Data from the National Health Interview Survey.* Feb 2014. Hyattsville, Maryland. DHHS Publication No. 2014-1588.
18-19. Rogers R, Boardman J, Pendergast P, Lawrence E. Drinking problems and mortality risk in the United States. *Drug and Alcohol Dependence.* 2015;151:38–46.
20. Wilson S, Knowles S, Huang Q, Fink A. The prevalence of harmful and hazardous alcohol consumption in older U.S. adults: data from the 2005–2008

National Health and Nutrition Examination Survey (NHANES). *Journal of General Internal Medicine.* 2014;29(2):312–319.

21-22. Harford T, Hy Y, Chem C, Grant B. Psychiatric symptom clusters as risk factors for alcohol use disorders in adolescence: a national study. *Alcoholism, Clinical and Experimental Research.* 2015;39(7):1174–1185.

23. Szaflarski M, Cubbins L, Ying J. Epidemiology of alcohol abuse among US immigrant populations. *Journal of Immigrant and Migrant Health.* 2011;13(4):647–658.

24. Yoon G, Petrakis I, Rosenheck R. Correlates of major depressive disorder with and without comorbid alcohol use disorder nationally in the veterans health administration. *American Journal on Addictions.* 2015;24(5):419–426.

25-26. Moss H, Goldstein R, Chen C, Yi H. Patterns of use of other drugs among those with alcohol dependence: associations with drinking behavior and psychopathology. *Addictive Behaviors.* 2015;50:192–198.

27-29. Vicent B, Crespo-Facorro B, Gonzalez-Pinto A, Vieta E. Bipolar disorder co-morbid with alcohol use disorder: focus on neurocognitive correlates. *Frontiers in Physiology.* 2015;6:108.

30. Schoepf D, Heun R. Alcohol dependence and physical comorbidity: increased prevalence but reduced relevance of individual comorbidities for hospital-based mortality. *European Psychiatry.* 2015;30(4):459–468.

31. Verhulst B, Neale M, Kendler K. The heritability of alcohol use-27 disorders: a meta-analysis of twin and adoption studies. *Psychological Medicine.* 2015;45(5):1061–1072.

32. Long E, Fazil A, Wang J, et al. Further analyses of genetic association between GRM8 and alcohol dependence symptoms among young adults. *Journal of Studies on Alcohol and Drugs.* 2015;76(3):414–418.

33. Forero D, Loepz S, Doo Shin H, Park B, Kim D. Meta-analysis of six genes (BDNF, DRD1, DRD2, DRD4, GRIN 2b and MAOA) involved in neuroplasticity and the risk for alcohol dependence. *Drug and Alcohol Dependence.* 2015;149(1):259–263.

34. Capusan A, Bendtsen P, Marteinsdottir I, Kuja-Halkola R, Larsson H. Genetic and environmental contributions to the association between attention deficit hyperactivity disorder and alcohol dependence in adulthood: a large population-based twin study. *American Journal of Medical Genetics Part B-Neuropsychiatric Genetics.* 2015;168(6):414–422.

35. Palmer R, Brick L, Nugent N, Bidwell C, McGeary J, Knopik V, Keller M. Examining the role of common genetic variants on alcohol, tobacco, cannabis and illicit drug dependence: genetics of vulnerability to drug dependence. *Addiction.* 2015;110(3):530–537.

36. *Diagnostic and statistical manual of mental disorders* (5th ed.). Washington, DC: American Psychiatric Association. 2013.

37. Jatlow PI, Agro A, Wu R, et al. Ethylglucuronide and ethyl sulfate assays in clinical trials, interpretation and limitations: results of a dose ranging alcohol challenge study and two clinical trials. *Alcoholism-Clinical and Experimental Research.* 2014;38:2056–2065.

38. Koob GF. Theoretical frameworks and mechanistic aspects of alcohol addiction: alcohol addiction as a reward deficit disorder. *Current Topics in Behavior Neuroscience.* 2013;13:3–30.
39. Wise RA, Koob GF. The development and maintenance of drug addiction. *Neuropsychopharmacology.* 2014;39:254–262.
40. Koob GF, Volkow ND. Neurocircuitry of Addiction. *Neuropsychopharmacology Reviews.* 2010;35:217–238.
41. Gilpin NW, Koob GF. Neurobiology of alcohol dependence. *Alc Res & Health.* 2008;31:185–195.
42. Volpicelli JR, Alterman AI, Hayashida M, O'Brien CP. Naltrexone in the treatment of alcohol dependence. *Archives of General Psychiatry.* 1992;49:876–880.
43. Rehm Colin Mathers, Svetlana Popova, Montarat Thavorncharoensap, Yot Teerawattananon, Jayadeep Patra. Global burden of disease and injury and economic cost attributable to alcohol use and alcohol-use disorders. *Lancet.* 2009;373:2223–2233.
44. Singal A. *World Journal of Gastroenterology.* 2013 Sep 28;19(36):5953–5963.
45. National Highway Traffic Safety Administration. Traffic Safety Facts Research Note. 2014; NHTSA's National Center for Statistics and Analysis. Publication 812101;1–6.
46. Myrick H, Kranzler HR, Ciraulo DA, Saxon AJ, Jaffe JH. *The ASAM Principles of Addiction Medicine.* 4th ed. 2014.
47. Johnson BA. Medication treatment of different types of alcoholism. *American Journal of Psychiatry.* 2010;167:630–639.
48. Volpicelli JR, Alterman AI, Hayashida M, et al. Naltrexone in the treatment of alcohol dependence. *Archives of General Psychiatry.* 1992;49:876–880.
49. O'Malley SS, Jaffe AJ, Chang G, et al. Naltrexone and coping skills therapy for alcohol dependence. A controlled study. *Archives of General Psychiatry.* 1992;49:881–887.
50. Kranzler HR, Armeli S, Tennen H, et al. Targeted naltrexone for early problem drinkers. *Journal of Clinical Psychopharmacology.* 2003;23:294–304.
51. Heinala P, Alho H, Kiianmaa K, et al. Targeted use of naltrexone without prior detoxification in the treatment of alcohol dependence: a factorial double-blind, placebo-controlled trial. *Journal of Clinical Psychopharmacology.* 2001;21:287–292.
52. Center for Substance Abuse Treatment. Treatment Improvement Protocol (TIP) Series, No. 49. Substance Abuse and Mental Health Services Administration (US). 2009. http://www.ncbi.nlm.nih.gov/books/NBK64041/pdf/Bookshelf_NBK64041.pdf
53. Kranzler HR, Van Kirk J. Efficacy of naltrexone and acamprosate for alcoholism treatment: a meta-analysis. *Alcoholism-Clinical and Experimental Research.* 2001;25:1335–1341.
54. Bouza C, Angeles M, Muñoz A, et al. Efficacy and safety of naltrexone and acamprosate in the treatment of alcohol dependence: a systematic review. *Addiction.* 2004;99:811–828.
55. Mann K, Lehert P, Morgan MY. The efficacy of acamprosate in the maintenance of abstinence in alcohol-dependent individuals: results of a meta-analysis. *Alcoholism-Clinical and Experimental Research.* 2004;28:51–63.

56. Jonas DE, Amick HR, Feltner C, et al. Pharmacotherapy for adults with alcohol use disorders in outpatient settings: a systematic review and meta-analysis. *JAMA.* 2014;311(18):1889–1900.

57. Anton RF, O'Malley SS, Ciraulo DA, et al. Combined pharmacotherapies and behavioral interventions for alcohol dependence: the COMBINE study: a randomized controlled trial. *JAMA.* 2006;295:2003–2017.

58. Johnson BA, Ait-Daoud N, Bowden CL, et al. Oral topiramate for treatment of alcohol dependence: a randomised controlled trial. *Lancet.* 2003;361:1677–1685.

59. Johnson BA, Rosenthal N, Capece JA, et al. Topiramate for treating alcohol dependence: a randomized controlled trial. *JAMA.* 2007;298:1641–1651.

60. Addolorato G, Leggio L, Ferrulli A, et al. Effectiveness and safety of baclofen for maintenance of alcohol abstinence in alcohol-dependent patients with liver cirrhosis: randomised, double-blind controlled study. *Lancet.* 2007;370:1915–1922.

61. Anton RF, Myrick H, Wright TM, et al. Gabapentin combined with naltrexone for the treatment of alcohol dependence. *American Journal of Psychiatry.* 2011;168(7):709–7171.

62. Mason, BJ, Quello, S, Goodell, V, Shadan, F, Kyle, M, Begovic, A. Gabapentin treatment for alcohol dependence: A randomized clinical trial. *JAMA Internal Medicine.* 2014;174:70–77.

63-65. Youssef S, Verity J, Weedman J. Role of the serotonergic system in alcohol dependence: from animal models to clinics. *Progress in Molecular Biology and Translational Science.* 2011;98:401–443.

66. Youssef S, Verity J, Weedman J. Role of the serotonergic system in alcohol dependence: from animal models to clinics. *Progress in Molecular Biology and Translational Science.* 2011;98:401–443.

67. Kranzler H, Burleson J, Brown J, Thomas F. Fluoxetine treatment seems to reduce the beneficial effects of cognitive-behavioral therapy in Type B alcoholics. *Alcoholism: Clinical and Experimental Research.* 1996;20(9):1534–1541.

68. Kranzler H, Armeli S, Tennen H, et al. A double-blind, randomized trial of sertraline for alcohol-dependence: moderation by age of onset and 5-HTTLPR genotype. *Journal of Clinical Psychopharmacology.* 2011;31(1):22–30.

69. Pettinati H, Oslin D, Decker K. Role of serotonin and serotonin-selective pharmacotherapy in alcohol dependence. *CNS Spectrums.* 2000;5(2):33–46.

70. US Dept. of Health and Human Services. Alcohol alert. *National Institute on Alcohol Abuse and Alcoholism.*Oct 1993:No. 22;PH 346.

71. Khanna S, Greeson, J. A narrative review of yoga and mindfulness as complementary therapies for addiction. *Complementary Therapies in Medicine.* 2013;21(3):244–252.

72. Reddy, S., Dick, A., Gerber, M., Mitchell, K. The effect of a yoga intervention on alcohol and drug abuse risk in veteran and civilian women with posttraumatic stress disorder. *Journal of Alternative and Complementary Medicine.* 2014;20(10):750–756.

73. Halligren M, Romberg K, Bakshi A, Andreasson S. Yoga as an adjunct treatment for alcohol dependence: a pilot study. *Complementary Therapies in Medicine.* 2014;22(3):441–445.

74. Khanna S, Greeson J. A narrative review of yoga and mindfulness as complementary therapies for addiction. *Complementary Therapies in Medicine.* 2013;21(3):244–252.5454.

75. Vancampfort D, De Hert M, Stubbs B. A systematic review of physical activity correlates in alcohol use disorders. *Archives of Psychiatric Nursing.* 2015;29(4):196–201.

76. Linke S, Ussher M. Exercise-based treatments for substance use disorders: evidence, theory and practicality. *The American Journal of Drug and Alcohol Abuse.* 2015;41(1):7–15.

77. Brown R, Abrantes A, Minami H, et al. A preliminary, randomized trial of aerobic exercise for alcohol dependence. *Journal of Substance Abuse Treatment.* 2014;47(1):1–9.

78. Baumann S, Toft S, Aadahl M., Jorgensen T, Pisinger C. The long-term effect of a population-based lifestyle intervention on smoking and alcohol consumption. The Inter99 Study-a randomized controlled trial. *Addiction.* 2015;110(11):1853–1860.

79. Witkiewitz K, Lustyk K, Bowen S. Re-training the addicted brain: a review of hypothesized neurobiological mechanisms of mindfulness-based relapse. *Psychological Addictive Behavior.* 2013;27(2):351–365.

80. Bowen S, Witkiewitz K, Clifasefi S, et al. Relative efficacy of mindfulness-based relapse prevention, standard relapse prevention, and treatment as usual for substance use disorders: a randomized clinical trial. *JAMA Psychiatry.* 2014;71(5):547–556.

81. Lazar S, Kerr C, Wasserman R. Meditation experience is associated with increased cortical thickness. *Neuroreport.* 2005;16(17):1893–1897.

82. Holzel BK, Carmody J, Vangel M, Congleton C, Lazar S. Mindfulness practice leads to increases in regional brain gray matter density. *Psychiatry Research: Neuroimaging.* 2011;191:36–42.

83. Lee JS, Kim SG, Jung TG, Jung WY, Kim SY. Effect of Zhubin acupuncture in reducing alcohol cravings in patients with alcohol dependence: a randomized placebo-controlled trial. *Chinese Journal of Integrative Medicine.* 2015;21(4):307–311.

84. Kunz S, Schulz M, Lewitzky M, Driessen M, Rau H. Ear acupuncture for alcohol withdrawal in comparison with aromatherapy: a randomized-controlled trial. *Alcoholism, Clinical and Experimental Research.* 2007;31(3):436–442.

85. Karst M, Passie T, Friedrich S, Wiese B, Schneider U. Acupuncture in the treatment of alcohol withdrawal symptoms: a randomized, placebo-controlled inpatient study. *Addiction Biology.* 2002;7(4):415–419.

86. Kirsch M, Gruber I, Ruf M, Kiefer F, Kirsch P. Real-time functional magnetic resonance imaging neurofeedback can reduce striatal cue-reactivity to alcohol stimuli. *Addiction Biology.* 2015;21(4):982–992.

87. Luigies J, Breteler R, Vanneste S, Ridder D. Neuromodulation as an intervention for addiction: overview and future prospects. *Tijdsch Psychiatry.* 2013;55(11):841–852.

88. Karch S, Keeser D, Hummer S, et al. Modulation of craving related brain responses using real-time fMRI in patients with alcohol use disorder. *PloS One.* 2015;10(7):1–18.

# 5

## Integrative Approach to Sedative-Hypnotic Use Disorder

### GAYLA REES, BENJAMIN SHAPIRO, DAVID E. SMITH, AND MATTHEW TORRINGTON

### Introduction

Sedatives, hypnotics, and anxiolytics comprise a chemically diverse group of agents with related brain activity that are used to manage anxiety, panic, insomnia, spasticity, seizures, restless legs syndrome, alcohol withdrawal, and anesthesia. Much like alcohol, these substances are CNS depressants with risks for substance use and substance-induced disorders, including lethal intoxication and withdrawal that like all substances of abuse are potentially habit forming due to their activity in brain reward pathways. Unlike most street drugs, which are manufactured and distributed illegally, sedatives, hypnotics, and anxiolytics are largely products of the pharmaceutical industry obtained either by prescription or through diversion in drug black markets. They are among the most highly used pharmaceuticals worldwide; diazepam alone was the most widely prescribed drug in the United States from 1969 to 1982, and the prevalence of it and its benzodiazepine siblings remains high, only tempered by the development of serotonin reuptake inhibitors and the z-drug hypnotics.[1,2]

Clinically appropriate use of sedatives, hypnotics, and anxiolytics should reflect a judicious balance between their medical uses and their considerable risk potential. Sedatives, hypnotics, and anxiolytics create substantial morbidity and mortality due to inappropriate prescribing, frequent over-prescribing, and widespread diversion use. They are central players in the drug overdose epidemic with benzodiazepines (BZD) being involved in approximately 31% of all fatal overdoses.[3] Though not all individuals who use these medications as prescribed develop sedative-hypnotic or anxiolytic-use disorders, a substantial number do, with an estimated two-thirds of prescriptions in various populations being inappropriate in indication or in length of use.[4]

This chapter reviews the medical and neurocognitive effects of sedatives, hypnotics, and anxiolytics and also defines the diagnostic criteria for sedative, hypnotic, and anxiolytic-use disorders and their associated risks and public health impact. We highlight the challenges of diagnosing these disorders in patients with certain premorbid conditions and the importance of careful risk assessment and ongoing surveillance of use. The chapter concludes with evidence-based pharmaceutical and psychosocial treatments for sedative-hypnotic and anxiolytic-related disorders and reviews the potential benefit of exercise, healthy diet, meditation, yoga, mindfulness, and acupuncture.

## Sedative-, Hypnotic-, and Anxiolytic-Related Disorders

Patterns of sedative, hypnotic, and anxiolytic abuse vary depending on the properties of the agent and culture of its abuse. Short-acting barbiturates may be injected for a "rush" or may be ingested to produce a state of disinhibition and mild euphoria similar to that achieved with alcohol. BZDs are often taken in combination with other primary intoxicants to intensify the desired effects, to alleviate withdrawal symptoms (e.g., heroin), or to reduce unpleasant side effects (e.g., cocaine or methamphetamine).

The *DSM-5* divides sedative-, hypnotic-, or anxiolytic-related disorders into two groups: (1) sedative-, hypnotic-, or anxiolytic-use disorders, and (2) sedative-, hypnotic-, or anxiolytic-induced disorders, including intoxication, withdrawal, sexual dysfunctions, sleep disorders and other substance- or medication-induced mental disorders.

### SEDATIVE-, HYPNOTIC-, OR ANXIOLYTIC-USE DISORDERS

Sedative, hypnotic, or anxiolytic use qualifies as a use disorder when the individual continues using despite clinical and functional impairment from cognitive, behavioral, and physiologic symptoms. As in the case of other substances of abuse, the *DSM-5* diagnostic criteria fit within overall groupings of (1) impaired control, (2) social impairment, (3) risky use, and (4) pharmacological symptoms.[5]

A. *Sedative, hypnotic, or anxiolytic intoxication.* Signs of sedative-hypnotic or anxiolytic intoxication are similar to those of alcohol intoxication and include sedation, behavioral disinhibition, and occasionally, paradoxical excitation. Signs of toxicity include slurred speech, incoordination, ataxia, sustained nystagmus, impaired cognition, and when severe,

**Table 5.1  Commonly Used Sedative-Hypnotic and Anxiolytic Medications, Therapeutic Use and Half Life**

| Generic Name | Trade Name/s | Therapeutic Use | Therapeutic Dose Range (mg/d) | Half Life (Hrs) [Active Metabolite] |
|---|---|---|---|---|
| **Benzodiazepines** | | | | |
| Alprazolam | Xanax | Anxiolytic | 0.75–6 | 6–12 |
| Chlordiazepoxide | Librium | Anxiolytic | 15–100 | 5–30 [36–200] |
| Clonazepam | Klonopin | Anticonvulsant/ Anxiolytic | 0.5–4 | 18–50 |
| Clorazepate | Tranxene | Anxiolytic | 15–60 | [36–200] |
| Diazepam | Valium | Anticonvulsant/ Antianxiety | 5–40 | 20–100 [36–200] |
| Estazolam | ProSom | Hypnotic | 1–2 | 10–24 |
| Flunitrazepam | Rohypnol | Hypnotic | 1–2 | 18–26 [36–200] |
| Flurazepam | Dalmane | Hypnotic | 15–30 | [40–250] |
| Halazepam | Paxipam | Anxiolytic | 60–160 | [30–100] |
| Lorazepam | Ativan | Anxiolytic | 1–16 | 10–20 |
| Midazolam | Versed | Anesthetic | – | 1.5–2.5 |
| Oxazepam | Serax | Anxiolytic | 10–120 | 4–15 |
| Prazepam | Centrax | Anxiolytic | 20–60 | [36–200] |
| Quazepam | Doral | Hypnotic | 15 | 25–100 |
| Temazepam | Restoril | Hypnotic | 7.5–30 | 8–22 |
| Triazolam | Halcion | Hypnotic | 0.125–0.5 | 2 |
| **Non-benzodiazepine Hypnotics** | | | | |
| Eszopiclone | Lunesta | Hypnotic | 1–3 | 6 (9 in elderly) |
| Zaleplon | Sonata | Hypnotic | 5–20 | 2 |
| Zolpidem | Ambien | Hypnotic | 5–10 | 2 |
| **Barbiturates** | | | | |
| Amobarbital | Amytal | Sedative | 50–150 | 10–40 |
| Butabarbital | Butisol | Sedative | 45–120 | 35–50 |
| Butalbital | Fiorinal, Sedapap | Sedative/ analgesic | 100–300 | 35–88 |
| Pentobarbital | Nembutal | Hypnotic | 50–100 | 35–88 |
| Secobarbital | Seconal | Hypnotic | 50–100 | 22–29 |
| Phenobarbital | Luminal | Sedative/ anticonvulsant | 30–320+ | 80–120 |

progressive respiratory depression, coma, and death. Toxicity may result from a large single dose, or from accumulation of a smaller dose or doses in those with impaired metabolism.

B. *Sedative, hypnotic, or anxiolytic withdrawal.* Sedative, hypnotic, or anxiolytic withdrawal results from a precipitous decrease in or discontinuation of regular use of sedatives, hypnotics, or anxiolytics, producing a constellation of symptoms, typically opposite to their primary action. Two or more of these symptoms are diagnostic and include autonomic hyperactivity (e.g., increases in heart rate, respiratory rate, blood pressure, or body temperature, sweating), hand tremor, insomnia, nausea, vomiting, transient visual, tactile, or auditory hallucinations or illusions, anxiety, psychomotor agitation, and/or generalized tonic-clonic seizures. The syndrome causes clinically significant distress or impairment in social, occupational, or other important areas of functioning and cannot be attributed to another medical or mental disorder. Relief of withdrawal symptoms with administration of any sedative-hypnotic agent would support a diagnosis of sedative, hypnotic, or anxiolytic withdrawal.

Physiological dependence on sedatives, hypnotics, or anxiolytics occurs not only after long-term use of amounts greater than normally prescribed or recommended but also after use of therapeutic doses. The abstinence syndrome is qualitatively similar for all sedative hypnotics or anxiolytics, although the time course of symptoms depends on the particular drug. Withdrawal from short-acting medication (e.g., pentobarbital, secobarbital, alprazolam) typically begins 12 to 24 hours after the last dose and peaks in intensity between 24 and 72 hours, while withdrawal syndrome from long-acting drugs (e.g., phenobarbital, diazepam, and chlordiazepoxide) typically peaks on the fifth to eighth day.

The literature describes 4 different kinds of withdrawal syndromes:

a. *High-dose withdrawal syndromes*—triggered by discontinuation or dose reduction of not only high dosages of barbiturates,[6] but also of benzodiazepines.[7,8]

   i. *Minor withdrawal*—characterized by anxiety, insomnia and/or nightmares.[9]

   ii. *Major withdrawal*—manifested by generalized tonic-clonic seizures, delirium, hyperpyrexia, and possibly death.

b. *Low-dose withdrawal syndrome*—follows discontinuation of long-term, low-dose treatment, and may include muscle twitches, abnormal perception of movement, depersonalization or derealization, anxiety, headache, insomnia, diaphoresis, difficulty concentrating, tremor, fear, fatigue, dysphoria, and lowered threshold to perception of sensory stimuli.[10] Low-dose withdrawal syndromes can occur when substituting short acting BZDs with long-acting benzodiazepines,[11] and rebound sleep disturbances have been reported after only 7 to 10 days of treatment with BZDs.[12] When low-dose BZDs are gradually tapered, the low-dose withdrawal syndrome becomes most pronounced and most difficult to tolerate as the individual drops to 10–20% of their prior peak dose. Distinguishing reemergence of the target symptoms for which the medication was prescribed (e.g., insomnia, panic attacks, generalized anxiety) from symptom rebound (transient worsening of symptoms typically lasting 1 to 2 weeks) and from low-dose withdrawal syndrome can be challenging. Those symptoms that are particularly suggestive of low-dose withdrawal are those that are new, including increased sensitivity to sound, light, and touch as well as paresthesias.

   c. *Protracted withdrawal syndrome*—lasting months and ranging from mild symptoms, such anxiety or insomnia, to those that are severe and disabling. Symptoms may be non specific and difficult to differentiate from symptom reemergence or comorbidities. A diagnosis is supported by waxing and waning symptom intensity that gradual improves with continued abstinence.

C. *Other sedative-, hypnotic-, or anxiolytic-induced disorders.* An episode of psychosis, mania, hypomania, depression, anxiety, insomnia, hypersomnia, neurocognitive dysfunction (dementia, amnestic disorders), obsessions, compulsions, sexual dysfunction, or delirium can result alone or in combination from exposure to or withdrawal from a sedative, hypnotic, or anxiolytic. These psychiatric states are deemed sedative, hypnotic, or anxiolytic-induced when there is a supportive pattern to the symptom onset and time course as well as a lack of other clear etiologic factors.

# Neurobiology and Epidemiology

## BENZODIAZEPINES

Benzodiazepines ("Benzos") share the chemical structure of a fused benzene and diazepine rings with most having a phenyl ring substituted on the latter.[13] BZDs increase the frequency of the channel's opening and thus the chloride ion flux, thereby enhancing neuronal inhibition by GABA and producing sedation, muscle relaxation, as well as hypnotic, anxiolytic, and anticonvulsant actions.[14] The GABA-A receptor has 5 different subunits, with 12 different isoforms, each with small differences in amino acid composition. While GABA binds to 2 sites on all GABA receptors, benzodiazepines bind to only 1 subunit of the receptor. This subunit has several different isoforms that are concentrated in different brain areas resulting in at least two phenotypically distinct benzodiazepine receptors that respond differentially to different benzodiazepines. The sedative effects of this class are closely associated to the α1 isoform, which is distributed in the cortex, thalamus, and cerebellum, while the α2 isoform mediates the anxiolytic and myorelaxant effects due to its segregation to the limbic system, motor neurons, and dorsal horn of the spinal cord.[15] These different isoforms and receptor properties are non-trivial in sedative, hypnotic, and anxiolytic disorders as abstinence and long-term treatment with different agonists can modulate differential expression of different GABA receptor subunit isoforms. This differential receptor subunit expression is thought to underlie prolonged withdrawal phenomenon, tolerance to specific agonists, and the temporal evolution of GABA withdrawal syndrome in the absence of particular agonists.[16] Though tolerance to clinical effects such as sedation and motor impairment has been established[17,18] tolerance to the benzodiazepine anxiolytic has not been clearly shown.[19]

The habit-forming activity of BZDs is mediated by both the acute effect on GABA A as wells as their interactions with other brain networks, though the precise mechanism remains unknown. Reward can be attenuated by depletion of dopamine from the nucleus accumbens[20] and administration of AMPa/Kainate receptor antagonists.[21] Unlike other drugs of abuse, such as morphine and cocaine that increase dopamine signaling in the nucleus accumben,[22] the administration of BZDs reduces dopamine concentrations.[23,24] Benzodiazepines have an intermediate abuse potential compared to other addictive substances as they more directly target anxiety and/or dysphoric states and counteract side effects and withdrawal symptoms from other agents rather than produce the intense euphoria common to most substances with high abuse potential.[25] Benzodiazepines with a rapid onset and short duration pose the highest risk for abuse, especially among subjects with a history of a substance-use disorder[26,27,28] and anxiety.[29]

Benzodiazepines have supplanted the older tranquilizers such as barbiturates for treatment of anxiety and insomnia due to their wider therapeutic index and an early misconception that these medications could not cause dependence. However, barbiturates remain an important alternative in managing alcohol and benzodiazepine withdrawal syndrome, with particular benefit for severe withdrawal in the intensive care unit as well as when benzodiazepine-resistant withdrawal occurs.[30]

*Epidemiology:* The epidemiology of BZDs use reflects the high prevalence of the disorders that BZDs are use to treat, particularly those of anxiety and sleep disorders. Prevalence estimates range from 0.7% to 4.3% throughout Europe, the United States, and Australia.[31] Use in psychiatric patients is considerably higher, ranging 17–36.9%.[32] Use disorders and BZD-induced disorders have risen to the point of being epidemic,[33] as even therapeutic doses of BZDs can cause physiological dependence and an abstinence syndrome.[34,35,36] Furthermore, there is increasing concern over their toxicity in even in normal use. This is particularly true of older adults who have increased risk for falls following any administration,[37] impaired cognition from chronic use, and probable increase in dementia risk.[38,39,40]

In 2011, 20.4% of drug-related emergency department visits involved BZDs, sedatives, and/or hypnotics.[41] In fact, from 2004–2011 there was an estimated 149% increase in non-medical use of BZDs and a 64.2% increase in the number of non-suicidal deaths related to BZDs in 2004–2007.[42] Particularly alarming is their estimated 29.3% involvement in suicide attempts in 2011, also reflecting an increasing trend.[43] According to the 2014 National Survey on Drug Use and Health,[44] 1.9 million people aged 12 or older are nonmedical users of tranquilizers in 2014, of which nearly a third met *DSM-4* criteria for substance abuse and/or dependence. Rates of nonmedical use and abuse were nearly 3 times higher in patients who had a major depressive episode in the past year.

*Polydrug Use/Abuse:* Benzodiazepines are rarely used alone for recreational purposes. More commonly, they are used in combination with an opiate, alcohol, or a combination of drugs. The SAMHSA Treatment Episodes Data Set[45] indicates that admissions for BZD use disorders are increasing, particularly among patients 55 and older, despite the historical pattern that they are not typically primary or secondary drugs of abuse triggering treatment. From 2004 to 2011 patient seeking detoxificationfrom BZDs more than tripled, exceeding 56,000. More then 20% of the patients in drug treatment centers use BZDs, with a high degree of concurrent use by opiate users,[46,47] both due to their synergistic effect on reinforcement[48] and for non-medical management of opiate withdrawal symptoms. Roughly 10–20% of individuals in treatment for alcohol use disorders abuse BZDs.[49] Lastly, 40–60% of chronic pain patients have been estimated to use BZDs,[50] though no clear effect on pain has been demonstrated.

Importantly, while BZDs are remarkably safe when taken in overdose alone, when combined with alcohol, other sedative hypnotics drugs, methadone, or even buprenorphine, BZDs can be lethal. Clinical and public awareness of the risks associated with opiate prescription is well supported by hundreds of published studies and is rising, however, the awareness of the risk associated BZD remains limited. Despite BZDs' frequent contribution to multidrug overdose and potentially life-threatening withdrawal, current literature on benzodiazepine-related disorders is scarce, and toxicology screens are often insufficient; yet, prescriptions are rising, especially among the elderly.[51]

## Z-DRUGS

The non-benzodiazepine hypnotics (zolpidem, zaleplon, eszopiclone, and zopiclone [or "Z-drugs"]) were introduced in the late 1980s and early 1990s as safer alternatives for the treatment of insomnia; they are slowly replacing the BZDs as the most commonly prescribed hypnotics. These medications are chemically unrelated to the BZDs but bind the same modulatory site on the GABA A receptor, thus sharing the same pharmacodynamic profile. The pharmacodynamic and pharmacokinetic of the Z-drugs approach that of an ideal anti-insomnia medication due to their rapid onset of ~30 minute, short half-life of 1 to 7 hours, and limited residual effect. In addition, unlike the benzodiazepines, they fundamentally do not disturb sleep architecture. However, the "z" class of drugs are not without risk. The longer half life z drugs are associated with risk of psychomotor impairment, falls, and hip fractures especially when they are abused at higher-than-recommended doses and when mixed with other psychoactive substances including alcohol. Additionally z drugs are associated with complex sleep behaviors like sleepwalking, sleep-driving, and hallucinations. Specifically, zopiclone and zolpidem have an increased risk of motor vehicle collisions, beyond double that of unexposed drivers.

Similar to the BZDs, Z-drugs are considered relatively safe in overdose. Sudden cessation of therapeutic use can produce rebound insomnia, more intense dreams, and even seizures, although seizure risk is considerably lower than with benzodiazepines. The abuse potential of non-benzodiazepine hypnotics is also postulated to be lower than that of BZDs.

Long-term effectiveness and safety data of non-benzodiazepine hypnotics remains limited and at times, conflicting. The 2014 National Survey on Drug Use and Health[52] estimated 330,000 people aged 12 or older were nonmedical users of sedatives in 2014. Diversion and abuse are common in other countries as well.[53] Tolerance as well as withdrawal syndromes are similar to that of other sedative-hypnotics[54,55,56,57,58,59] including some potential for withdrawal seizures[60,61]. Case reports of transient psychosis with visual hallucinations have been described from therapeutic doses of Zolpidem, even from an the initial dose[62,63,64,65]. Zolpidem alone accounted for more than 30,000 ED visits involving illicit prescription drug and was identified in more than 14,000 suicidal overdose attempts in 2011.[66] Despite its reported safety, Zolpidem toxicity often leads to ICU admission, especially when co-ingested with over the counter cold and flu medications, preparations, other psychotropic medication, or ethanol.[67] Finally, lethal toxicity of Z-drugs may not differ from that of BZDs, as indicated by death by poisoning data from NZ,[68] forensic cases, and motor vehicle accidents statistics.[69]

## BARBITURATES

Barbiturate use and abuse has declined markedly since the introduction of BZDs. Today, Barbiturates are primarily used for anesthesia, to manage seizures, and to treat migraines and cluster headaches. They may also be used, where legal, for physician assistant suicide, euthanasia, and capital punishment. Barbiturates are derived from barbituric acid and produce CNS depression, from mild sedation to anesthesia, via GABA-induced inhibition and other mechanisms. Ultra-short acting barbiturates, such as Thiopental and Methohexital, are primarily used as anesthetics and administered intravenously, while short to intermediate onset agents (amobarbital, butabarbital, sodium pentobarbital, and secobarbital) are used as anxiolytics, and long-acting agents (phenobarbital and mephobarbital) are used as anxiolytics or as anticonvulsants. Most barbiturate abusers abuse other illicit drugs, yet they still account for an appreciable role in ED visits, accounting for more than 18,000 visits in 2011.[70]

## TREATMENT OF SEDATIVE-HYPNOTICS AND ANXIOLYTIC-USE DISORDERS

### Prevention

Strategies to prevent sedative, hypnotic, or anxiolytic misuse and its consequences include (a) reducing reliance on sedatives, hypnotics, and anxiolytics by optimization of alternative treatments, (b) patient risk assessment, (c) limiting dose and early refills, and (d) use of a treatment agreement. A large retrospective cohort study reported an increased (3.4 hazard ratio) risk of mortality in patients taking anxiolytic and hypnotic drugs.[71] Once a diagnosis of sedative-hypnotic dependence is manifested it is unlikely that a patient will be able to return to controlled, therapeutic use of sedative-hypnotics. All sedative-hypnotics, including alcohol, are cross-tolerant, and physical dependence and tolerance are quickly reestablished if a patient resumes use of sedative-hypnotics. If after sedative-hypnotic withdrawal the patient has another primarily psychiatric disorder such as generalized anxiety disorder, panic attacks, or insomnia, alternate treatment strategies should be employed.

Treatment of a sedative-, hypnotic-, or anxiolytic-use disorder that has developed as a result of treatment of an underlying psychiatric disorder is usually protracted and prone to complications. Establishing the substance-use disorder diagnosis and, to the extent possible, the comorbid psychiatric diagnoses as well as establishing a therapeutic relationship with the patient are important initial goals. A discerning clinician may defer instituting drug withdrawal until a strong therapeutic alliance develops. Insurance utilization reviewers may present further difficulties by failing to authorize inpatient treatment of "low-dose" BZD dependence or by attributing symptoms arising during withdrawal in the inpatient setting to mismanagement of symptom reemergence.

## DETOXIFICATION PROTOCOLS FOR SEDATIVE, HYPNOTIC, OR ANXIOLYTIC MEDICATIONS

Detoxification is indicated in the following cases: (1) Patients on therapeutic dosages of medications for a long period of times for whom a trial off medications is desired; (2) Patients on supra-therapeutic dosages of BZDs; and (3) Mixed substance use cases.

### Detoxification of Therapeutic Doses and Low-Dose Withdrawal

Patients taking BZDs as prescribed for long periods of time, either to treat a diagnosed anxiety disorder or as careless continuation of treatment of a long-resolved acute problem often present a management dilemma. Justifying the continued benefit from long-term BZD use can be challenging and often requires discontinuation of the drug. Unfortunately, symptom reemergence, rebound symptoms, and discontinuation syndrome are often hard to differentiate and frequently lead to re-initiation of the treatment. In general, emergence of symptoms similar to those that the patient was having before sedative hypnotic treatment was started suggests symptom reemergence, while new symptoms such as paresthesias or sensitivity to light or sound typically indicate a withdrawal syndrome.

Detoxification of therapeutic doses of BZDs can usually be accomplished using the BZDs that the patient was already taking, although this may prove more difficult for short-acting BZDs. A gradual taper of therapeutic doses of BZDs by no more than 25% per week is typically better tolerated than an abrupt taper. Withdrawal from short-acting benzodiazepines typically occurs earlier, in the first 2 to 3 days and is often more severe and than withdraw from long-acting benzodiazepines. Tapering the last 25% of short acting benzodiazepines, such as the last 1 mg of alprazolam,[72] is characteristically challenging and may require a prolonged gradual taper, switching to a long-acting agent, or addition of adjunctive medications, such as Gabalpentin or Pregabalin for better symptom control.

### High-Dose Benzodiazepine Detoxification/Withdrawal

Patients on supra-therapeutic doses of benzodiazepines are at great risk of having severe withdrawal symptoms including seizures, psychoses, and delirium. Though a slow outpatient dose reduction of 5% per week may be successful in motivated patients with a strong therapeutic alliance and close follow-up,[73] inpatient detoxification is often safest and most successful in this population, especially in patients with a prior history of severe withdrawal symptoms.

Three detoxification algorithms are commonly used for patients taking supra-therapeutic doses of BZDs: (1) substitution followed by gradual taper off a long-acting BZD (see above), (2) substitution followed by gradual taper off a long-acting barbiturate (see Table 2),[74,75] and (3) gradual reduction of the agent of dependence. The preferred withdrawal strategy depends on the particular BZD, the involvement of other drugs of dependence, and the clinical setting in which the detoxification program takes place.

## EMERGING ALTERNATIVE PHARMACOTHERAPY FOR TREATMENT OF BENZODIAZEPINE DEPENDENCE

1. *Flumazenil*: Several small studies have explored the use of the benzodiazepine antagonist, flumazenil for managing symptoms that emerged after benzodiazepine discontinuation. In an early, open-label pilot study, Lader and Morton[76] used a single flumazenil injection administered by slow intravenous infusion of dosages between 0.2 and 2.0 mg) in 11 patients to assess the effect on persistent symptoms following withdrawal. Because of concern about precipitating benzodiazepine withdrawal, all patients had been off benzodiazepines from between 1 month to 5 years before flumazenil treatment. Current package inserts for flumazenil caution that insufficient data exist to support the use of flumazenil for treatment of benzodiazepine dependence.

2. *Pregabalin*: A growing body of evidence supports the use of pregabalin for the treatment of BZD withdrawal and use disorders. Pregabalin binds to the α2 delta subunit isoform or the presynaptic voltage-gated calcium channel, causing a decrease in release of neuroexcitatory neurotransmitterns, including glutamate, substance P, calcitonin gene-related peptide, and monoaminergic neurotransmitters.[77] Pregabalin has no clinically significant effects at GABA receptors, although tolerance, dose escalation, and withdrawal can occur. Oulis, et al[78] transitioned 15 patients with a mean of 13 years of BZD dependence fully from BZD to pregabalin over 5.5 weeks with 50% improvement in measures of depression and anxiety and nearly 10% improvement in MMSE and various other cognitive measures. These findings were replicated in later studies with additional findings of improved subjective sleep quality with some investigators finding benefits to super-therapuetic dosages up to 900mg per day, 300mg over the FDA limit.[79] However, current literature has also revealed the potential for misuse and abuse of Pregabalin (and Gabapentin) due to more recently identified action in reward pathways as well as a GABAergic withdraw syndrome, although not typically as intense as those associated with BDZ and barbiturates.[80,81]

## PSYCHOTHERAPY AND PSYCHOSOCIAL INTERVENTIONS

Psychotherapy is one of the few modalities that has clear interventional studies of tapering or discontinuing BZD use, although the majority of these studies focus on management of rebound symptoms of underlying conditions where BZD and hypnotics were being used or have direct indication. In these studies BZD use is typically conceptualized around the underlying disorder rather than as a particular use disorder. Efficacy is typically highest for psychotherapeutic alternatives to BZD for anxiety disorders, which can be particularly effective for helping taper use. Rebound symptoms are extremely common to individuals with anxiety disorders attempting to taper BZD and frequently cause aborted attempts to discontinue. In the late 1980s several studies characterized these difficulties, noting for example 60% of patients with panic disorder experienced symptoms equal or worse than prior to BZD treatment, and 64% failed the discontinuation attempt with global symptom recurrence being the rule rather than the exception.[82] In the example of panic disorder, CBT uses the emergence of discontinuation symptoms as a central focus to restructure patients' response to these symptoms in a manner that dismantles the cycle of anxiogenic responses that characterizes panic disorder and subsequent dependence on BZD. Using techniques such as interoceptive exposure, arousal management, and cognitive restructuring over ten sessions of CBT discontinuation success at 3 months improved from 25% without adjunctive CBT to 77% with adjunctive CBT for a slow taper of 6 months or greater management with BZD with follow-up studies showing equal or greater efficacy.[83]

Several other psychosocial interventions have been studied as a means to decrease chronic BDZ use, including motivational interviewing, relaxation therapy, e-counseling, and PCP advice-based interventions, among others. The Cochrane Collaboration assessed 25 such psychosocial interventions involving 1666 subjects. Similar to the findings of Otto, Hong, and Safren[84] in panic disorder, the greatest efficacy was found for CBT augmentation of a conservative BDZ taper up to 3 months post-treatment.[85] Unfortunately, these benefits did not persist from 6 to 24 months. Furthermore, studies or psychosocial interventions to reduce BZD use 50% or greater, including those employing CBT, failed to provide adequate evidence of benefit. However, a separate metanalysis by Gould, et al[86] concluded that supervised withdrawal with psychotherapy at post-intervention made the odds of not using benzodiazepines 5.06 times greater than for control interventions among older adults trying to taper BDZ use.

## COMPLEMENTARY ALTERNATIVE MEDICINE

The study of complementary alternative medicine (CAM) interventions to manage BZD use disorders similarly suffers from the conceptual overlaps discussed above for psychotherapy and psychosocial interventions. Again, the focus of study is typically the underlying syndrome that benzodiazepines were prescribed to treat rather than identifying BZD use disorder as a focus. Further complicating this dichotomy is that BZD disorders straddle a wide spectrum from iatrogenic BZD use disorders evolving from management of an underlying disorder where there is limited dose escalation to excessive use of BDZ in an individual conspicuously seeking out their reinforcing effects and more likely to be engaged in abusing other substances. This broad spectrum reflects different patient populations and psychologies of use and would be anticipated to diverge in response to both traditional and alternative therapies for substance-use disorders. Given these factors, there is a conspicuous absence of literature on CAM approaches to sedative-hypnotic and anxiolytic-use disorders.

Research has demonstrated that hypnotics-dependent insomnia, versus insomnia alone, can have significant benefits from elements of traditional Chinese medicine (TCM), which in this study included acupuncture, Tuina massage, Chinese medicine psychotherapy, and Chinese herbal medicine, limiting REM sleep rebound, increasing delta sleep, decreasing sympathetic outflow.[87] Furthermore, a variety of herbal medicines have varying evidence and rational for benefitting alcohol use disorders. Since alcohol use disorder shares pathophysiology with BDZ use disorder and they demonstrate cross-tolerance, all of these alternative agents warrant further study with reasonable speculation that some may ultimately benefit management of BDZ use disorder. Traditional herbal medicines that may have efficacy in alcohol use disorder include: *Radix Puerariae* or *Pueraria lobata* (Kudzu), *Withania somnifera* (Ashwagandha), *Thumbergia laurifolia Linn* (Rang Jert, Acanthaceae), *Salvia miltiorrhiza* (Danshen, Red Sage root), *Banisteriopsis caapi* (ayahuasca, yage, caapi), and *Lophophora williamsii* (peyote).[88,89] For further information on the integrative management of primary anxiety and insomnia, The *Integrative Psychiatry* publication from the Weil medical library provides detailed information on complementary approaches to the treatment of these conditions.

## YOGA

No literature exists that directly explores the potential benefits that yoga can provide in the treatment of sedative-hypnotic and anxiolytic-use disorders. However, there are studies of yoga indicating that yoga asana sessions increase GABA levels in participants' brains.[90]

## MINDFULNESS-BASED RELAPSE PREVENTION

While the literature for mindfulnessbased relapse prevention (MBRP) directly managing sedative-hypnotic and anxiolytic-use disorders is woefully inadequate, the practice of MBRP holds promise and is particularly apt for their treatment given that iatrogenic use disorders arise due to limited psychological resources and/or resilience to manage underlying symptoms, such as insomnia and various forms of anxiety. The Western allopathic tradition typically conceptualizes addiction and cravings as aberrant secondary pathological entities that arise and need to be diminished through some sort of imposed treatment regimen. In contrast, mindfulness meditation has roots in Buddhism and relegates addiction and cravings as manifestations of excessive attachment and thus as a root of suffering, where attachment is more fluid than addiction and the individual is more self-determined. More colloquially, it is the lack of acceptance of transient pain and discomfort that ultimately leads one to pathological manifestations of desire and the experience of suffering; once one accepts ones experience, those elements that seem noxious become more tolerable. Thus, MBRP is ideally suited to address elements of sedative-hypnotic and anxiolytic use disorders, both in helping to tolerate the symptom rebound of withdrawal and abstinence as well as the symptoms of underlying disorders when there is an iatrogenic use disorder. As argued earlier, the overlap between alcohol dependence and BDZ dependence and the substantial literature for MBRP in alcohol addiction creates an argument that MBRP may benefit treatment of BDZ-use disorders. A study by Kitkiewitz, et al,[91] found that MBRP participants had significantly reduced self-reported cravings for any substance both before and after treatment; the "latent factor" that mediated subjects' lower levels of cravings related to increased measures of acceptance, awareness, and non-judgment. This finding and the overall approach of MBRP could have considerable relevance to the treatment of sedative-hypnotic and anxiolytic use disorders, as it uniquely supports self-efficacy and broadens the interpretation and experience of cravings as something beyond just cognitive, affective, and biological, integrating ideas about intention and equanimity.

## REFERENCES

1. Kurko T, Saastamoinen L, Tähkäpää S, Tuulio-Henriksson A, Taiminen T, Tiihonen J., et al. Long-term use of benzodiazepines: Definitions, prevalence and usage patterns—a systematic review of register-based studies. *Eur Psychiatry.* 2015;30(8):1037–1047

2. Lader M. Benzodiazepines revisited—will we ever learn? *Addiction.* 2011;106(2): 2086–2109.

3. Bachhuber M, Hennessy S, Cunningham C, Starrels J. Increasing benzodiazepine prescriptions and overdose mortality in the United States, 1996-2013. *Am J Public Health.* 2016;106(4):686–688.

4. Lader M. Benzodiazepines revisited—will we ever learn? *Addiction.* 2011;106(2): 2086–2109.

5. American Psychiatric Association. Diagnostic and statistical manual of mental disorders. 5th ed. Arlington, VA: American Psychiatric Publishing; 2013.

6. Isbell H, Altschul S, Kornetsky CH, Eisenman AJ, Flanary HG, Fraser HF. Chronic barbiturate intoxication: An experimental study. *Arch. Neurol. & Psychiat.* 1950;64:1–28.

7. Hollister LE, Motezenbecker FP, Degan RO. Withdrawal reactions from chlordiazepoxide ("Librium"). *Psychopharmacologia.* 1961;2:63–68

8. Hollister LE, Bennett JL, Kimbell I, Jr, Savage C, Overall JE. Diazepam. In newly admitted schizophrenics. *Dis Nerv Syst.* 1963;24:746–750

9. Smith DE, Wesson DR. Benzodiazepine dependency syndromes. *J Psychoactive Drugs.* 1983;15(1-2):85–95.

10. Wesson DR, Smith DE, Ling W, Sabnani S. Substance abuse: Sedative, hypnotic, or anxiolytic use disorders, psychiatry. 3rd ed. (2008): 1186–1200[[

11. Conell LJ, Berlin RM. *JAMA.* 1983;250(20):2838–2840.

12. Vgontzas AN, Kales A, Bixler EO. Benzodiazepine side effects: role of pharmacokinetics and pharmacodynamics. *Pharmacology.* 1995;51(4):205–223.

13. Griffin, C. E., Kaye, A. M., Bueno, F. R., & Kaye, A. D. (2013). Benzodiazepine Pharmacology and Central Nervous System–Mediated Effects. The Ochsner Journal, 13 (2), 214–223.

14. Ibid.

15. Ibid.

16. Calixto E. GABA withdrawal syndrome: GABAA receptor, synapse, neurobiological implications and analogies with other abstinences. *Neuroscience.* 2016;28(313):57–72.

17. File SE, Pellow S. The effects of triazolobenzodiazepines in two animal tests of anxiety and in the holeboard. *British Journal of Pharmacology.* 1985;86(3):729–735.

18. Miller LG, Greenblatt DJ, Barnhill JG, Shader RI. Chronic benzodiazepine administration. I. Tolerance is associated with benzodiazepine receptor downregulation and decreased gamma-aminobutyric acidA receptor function. *J Pharmacol Exp Ther.* 1988;246(1):170–176.

19. Rickels K. Benzodiazepines in emotional disorders. *J Psychoactive Drugs.* 1983;15(1–2):49–54

20. Spyraki C, Fibiger HC. A role for the mesolimbic dopamine system in the reinforcing properties of diazepam. *Psychopharmacology react-text* 55. 1988;94(1):133–137.

21. Gray AM, Rawls SM, Shippenberg TS, McGinty JF. The kappa-opioid agonist, U-69593, decreases acute amphetamine-evoked behaviors and calcium-dependent dialysate levels of dopamine and glutamate in the ventral striatum. *J Neurochem.* 1999;73(3):1066–1074.

22. Pontieri FE, Tanda G, Di Chiara G. Intravenous cocaine, morphine, and amphetamine preferentially increase extracellular dopamine in the "shell" as

compared with the "core" of the rat nucleus accumbens. *Proc Natl Acad Sci U S A.* 1995;92(26):12304–12308.

23. Di Chiara G, Imperato A. Drugs abused by humans preferentially increase synaptic dopamine concentrations in the mesolimbic system of freely moving rats. *Proc Natl Acad Sci U S A.* 1988;85(14):5274–5278.

24. Finlay JM, Damsma G, Fibiger HC. Benzodiazepine-induced decreases in extracellular concentrations of dopamine in the nucleus accumbens after acute and repeated administration. *Psychopharmacology.* 1992;106(2):202–208.

25. Griffiths RR, Weerts EM. Benzodiazepine self-administration in humans and laboratory animals—implications for problems of long-term use and abuse. *Psychopharmacology* 1997;134(1):1–37.

26. Ciraulo DA, Sarid-Segal O, Knapp C, et al: Liability to alprazolam abuse in daughters of alcoholics. *Am J Psychiatry.* 1996;153(7):956–958.

27. Mumford GK, Rush CR, Griffiths RR. Abecarnil and alprazolam in humans: behavioral, subjective and reinforcing effects. *J Pharmacol Exp Ther.* 1995;272(2):570–580.

28. Roache JD, Griffiths RR. Diazepam and triazolam self-administration in sedative abusers: concordance of subject ratings, performance and drug self-administration. *Psychopharmacology.* 1989;;99(3):309–315.

29. Roache JD, Stanley MA, Creson DR, Shah NN, Meisch RA. lprazolam-reinforced medication use in outpatients with anxiety. *Drug Alcohol Depend.* 1997;45(3):143–155.

30. Martin K, Katz A. The Role of Barbiturates for Alcohol Withdrawal Syndrome. *Psychosomatics.* 2016;57(4):341–347.

31. Lader M. Benzodiazepines revisited—will we ever learn? *Addiction.* 2011;106(2):2086–2109.

32. Wesson DR, Smith DE, Ling W, and Sabnani S, 64. Substance Abuse: Sedative, Hypnotic, or Anxiolytic Use Disorders, Psychiatry, Third Edition (2008), pp.1186–1200.

33. Yu HY. The prescription drug abuse epidemic. *Clin Lab Med.* 2012;32(3):361–377.

34. Lader M. Dependence and withdrawal: comparison of the benzodiazepines and selective serotonin re-uptake inhibitors. *Addiction.* 2012;107(5):909–910.

35. Busto U, Sellers EM, Naranjo CA, Cappell H, Sanchez-Craig M, Sykora K. Withdrawal reaction after long-term therapeutic use of benzodiazepines. *N Engl J Med.* 1986;315(14):854–859.

36. Nielsen M, Hansen EH, Gøtzsche PC. What is the difference between dependence and withdrawal reactions? A comparison of benzodiazepines and selective serotonin re-uptake inhibitors. *Addiction.* 2012;107(5):900–908.

37. Cumming RG, Le Couteur DG. Benzodiazepines and risk of hip fractures in older people: a review of the evidence. *CNS Drugs.* 2003;17(11):825–837.

38. Barker MJ, Greenwood KM, Jackson M, Crowe SF. Cognitive effects of long-term benzodiazepine use: a meta-analysis. *CNS Drugs.* 2004;18(1):37–48.

39. Islam MM, Iqbal U, Walther B, et al. Benzodiazepine use and risk of dementia in the elderly population: A systematic review and meta-analysis. *Neuroepidemiology.* 2016;47(3–4):181–191.

40. Takada M, Fujimoto MI, Hosomi K. Association between benzodiazepine use and dementia: Data mining of different medical databases. *Int J Med Sci.* 2016;13(11):825–834.

41. Substance Abuse and Mental Health Services Administration. Drug Abuse Warning Network, 2007: Area Profiles of Drug-Related Mortality. Rockville, MD: Sub-stance Abuse and Mental Health Services Administration; 2009. http://dawninfo.samhsa. gov/pubs/mepubs. Accessed June 10, 2010.

42. Ibid.

43. Ibid.

44. Center for Behavioral Health Statistics and Quality. *Behavioral Health Trends in the United States: Results from the 2014 National Survey on Drug Use and Health.* 2016. Retrieved from http://www.samhsa.gov/data/.

45. http://wwwdasis.samhsa.gov/webt/information.htm

46. Iguchi MY, Handelsman L, Bickel WK, Griffiths RR. Benzodiazepine and sedative use/abuse by methadone maintenance clients. *Drug Alcohol Depend.* 1993;32(3):257–266.

47. Stitzer ML, Griffiths RR, McLellan AT, Grabowski J, Hawthorne JW. Diazepam use among methadone maintenance patients: patterns and dosages. *Drug Alcohol Depend.* 1981;8(3):189–199.

48. Darke S, Ross J, Teesson M, Lynskey M. Health service utilization and benzodiazepine use among heroin users: findings from the Australian Treatment Outcome Study (ATOS). *Addiction.* 2003;98(8):1129–1135.

49. Ross HE. Benzodiazepine use and anxiolytic abuse and dependence in treated alcoholics. *Addiction.* 1993;88(2):209–218.

50. Kouyanou K, Pither CE, Wessely S. Medication misuse, abuse and depen- dence in chronic pain patients. *J. Psychosom. Res.* 1997;43:497–504.

51. Olfson M, King M, Schoenbaum M. Benzodiazepine use in the United States. *JAMA Psychiatry.* 2015;72(2):136–142.

52. Center for Behavioral Health Statistics and Quality. *Behavioral health trends in the United States: Results from the 2014 National Survey on Drug Use and Health.* 2015. Retrieved from http://www.samhsa.gov/ data/

53. Report of the International Narcotics Control Board for 2006 (March 2007). International Narcotics Control Board, United Nations, New York, NY.

54. Aragona M. Abuse, dependence, and epileptic seizures after zolpidem withdrawal: review and case report. *Clin Neuropharmacol.* 2000;23(5):281–283.

55. Rush CR, Frey JM, Griffiths RR. Zaleplon and triazolam in humans: acute behavioral effects and abuse potential. *Psychopharmacology.* 1999;145(1):39–51.

56. Ator NA, Weerts EM, Kaminski BJ, Kautz MA, Griffiths RR. Zaleplon and triazolam physical dependence assessed across increasing doses under a once-daily dosing regimen in baboons. *Drug Alcohol Depend.* 2000;61(1):69–84.

57. Griffiths RR, Johnson MW. Relative abuse liability of hypnotic drugs: a conceptual framework and algorithm for differentiating among compounds. *J Clin Psychiatry.* 2005;66(Suppl 9):31–41.

58. Jones IR, Sullivan G. Physical dependence on zopiclone: case reports. *BMJ*. 1998;316(7125):11.
59. Hajak G, Müller WE, Wittchen HU, Pittrow D, Kirch W. Abuse and dependence potential for the non-benzodiazepine hypnotics zolpidem and zopiclone: a review of case reports and epidemiological data. *Addiction*. 2003;98(10):1371–1378.
60. Aranko K, Henriksson M, Hublin C, Seppäläinen AM. Misuse of zopiclone and convulsions during withdrawal. *Pharmacopsychiatry*. 1991;24(4):138–140.
61. Flynn A, Cox D. Dependence on zopiclone. *Addiction*. 2006;101(6):898.
62. Ansseau M, Pitchot W, Hansenne M, Gonzalez Moreno A. Psychotic reactions to zolpidem. *Lancet*. 1992;339(8796):809.
63. Iruela LM, Ibañez-Rojo V, Baca E. More on zolpidem side-effects. *Lancet*. 1993;342(8885):1495–1496.
64. Markowitz JS, Brewerton TD. Zolpidem-induced psychosis. *Ann Clin Psychiatry*. 1996;8(2):89–91.
65. Pitner JK, Gardner M, Neville M, Mintzer J. Zolpidem-induced psychosis in an older woman. *J Am Geriatr Soc*. 1997;45(4):533–534.
66. Drug Abuse Warning Network: The DAWN Report. August 7, 2014. Emergency Department Visits Attributed to Overmedication That Involved the Insomnia Medication Zolpidem. https://www.samhsa.gov/data/sites/default/files/DAWN-SR150-Zolpidem-2014/DAWN-SR150-Zolpidem-2014.pdf. Accessed on March 10, 2017.
67. Zosel A, Osterberg EC, Mycyk MB. Zolpidem misuse with other medications or alcohol frequently results in intensive care unit admission. *Am J Ther*. 2011;18(4):305–308.
68. Reith DM, Fountain J, McDowell R, Tilyard M. Comparison of the fatal toxicity index of zopiclone with benzodiazepines. *J Toxicol Clin Toxicol*. 2003;41(7):975–980.
69. Gunja N. In the Zzz zone: the effects of Z-drugs on human performance and driving. *J Med Toxicol*. 2013;9(2):163–171.
70. Coupey SM. Barbiturates. *Pediatr Rev*. 1997;18(8):260–264.
71. Weich S, Pearce HL, Croft P, et al. Effect of anxiolytic and hypnotic drug prescriptions on mortality hazards: retrospective cohort study. *BMJ*. 2014;348:g1996.
72. Ciraulo DA, Antal EJ, Smith RB, et al. The relationship of alprazolam dose to steady-state plasma concentrations. *J Clin Psychopharmacol*. 1990;10(1):27–32.
73. Alexander B, Perry PJ. Detoxification from benzodiazepines: schedules and strategies. *J Subst Abuse Treat*. 1991;8(1–2):9–17.
74. Smith DE, Wesson DR, Lannon RA. New developments in barbiturate abuse. *Clin Toxicol*. 1970;3(1):57–65.
75. Smith DE, Wesson DR. Phenobarbital technique for treatment of barbiturate dependence. *Arch Gen Psychiatry*. 1971;24(1):56–60.
76. Lader MH, Morton SV. A pilot study of the effects of flumazenil on symptoms persisting after benzodiazepine withdrawal. *J Psychopharmacol*. 1992;6(3):357–363.
77. Sabioni P, Bertram J, Le Foll B. Off-label use of medications for treatment of benzodiazepine use disorder. *Curr Pharm Des*. 2015;21(23):3306–3310.

78. Oulis P, Konstantakopoulos G, Kouzoupis AV, et al. Pregabalin in the discontinuation of long-term benzodiazepines' use. *Hum Psychopharmacol.* 2008;23(4):337–340.
79. Ibid.
80. Sabioni P, Bertram J, Le Foll B. Off-label use of medications for treatment of benzodiazepine use disorder. *Curr Pharm Des.* 2015;21(23):3306–3310.
81. Schifano F. Misuse and abuse of pregabalin and gabapentin: cause for concern? *CNS Drugs.* 2014;28(6):491–496.
82. Otto M, Hong J, Safren S. Benzodiazepine dependence alternative treatment. *Current Pharmaceutical Design.* 2002;8(1):75–80.
83. Ibid.
84. Otto MW, Hong JJ, Safren SA. Benzodiazepine discontinuation difficulties in panic disorder: conceptual model and outcome for cognitive-behavior therapy. *Curr Pharm Des.* 2002;8(1):75–80.
85. Darker C, Sweeney B, Barry J, Farrell M, Donnelly-Swift E. Psychosocial interventions for benzodiazepine harmful use, abuse or dependence. *Cochrane Database of Systematic Reviews.* 2015;5, i–108.
86. Gould RL, Coulson MC, Patel N, Highton-Williamson E, Howard, RJ. Interventions for reducing benzodiazepine use in older people: meta-analysis of randomised controlled trials. *The British Journal of Psychiatry.* 2014;204(2):98–107.
87. Xuanzi Z, Fang W, Weidong W. Chinese medicine treatment of hypnotics-dependent insomnia. *Sleep Medicine.* 2015(16);S2–199.
88. Lu L, Liu Y, Zhu W, Shi J, Liu, Y, Ling, W, et al. Traditional Medicine in the Treatment of Drug Addiction. *The American Journal of Drug and Alcohol Abuse.* 2009;(35):1–11.
89. Keung WM, Vallee BL. Kudzu root: an ancient Chinese source of modern antidipsotropic agents. *Phytochemistry,* 1998;47(4):499–506.
90. Streeter C, Jensen J, Ruth M, et al. (2007). Yoga asana sessions increase brain GABA levels. *The Journal of Alternative and Complementary Medicine.* 2007;13(4):419–426.
91. Kitkiewitz K, Brown S, Douglas H, Hsu, SH. Mindfulness-based relapse prevention for substance craving. *Addictive Behaviors.* 2013;38:1563–1571.

# 6

## Integrative Approach to Cannabis-Use Disorder

### ITAI DANOVITCH AND SHAHLA J. MODIR

## Introduction

C annabis is a flowering plant, whose stem, leaves, and flowers have been cultivated by humans over millennia for varying purposes (Figure 6.1). The female plant produces resin-secreting flowers with elevated concentrations of cannabinoids, including tetrahydrocannabinol (THC), a lipophilic hydrocarbon that can produce intoxication when ingested. Cannabis cultivated for intoxication can be prepared in many different ways and goes by many different names. The most common preparations include collection of loose leaves and seeds (weed), pruning and harvesting the flowering buds (sensemilla), or extraction of the resin (hashish) where THC is most concentrated. Cannabis is also referred to, interchangeably, as marijuana.

In recent years the cultivation and hybridization of cannabis has generated many variants of the most common species—Cannabis indica, Cannabis sativa, and Cannabis ruderalis. Technological developments in the extraction, preparation, and formulation of cannabinoids derived from the cannabis plant have also generated a wide range of products consumed for medicinal and recreational purposes. The objective of this chapter is to review the diagnosis, epidemiology, assessment, and treatment of cannabis-use disorder, an addictive disorder that may develop in some users of cannabis and cannabis-related products.

### DIAGNOSIS

Reliable and valid diagnostic criteria have been established for the 3 most common cannabis diagnoses, see Table 6.1.

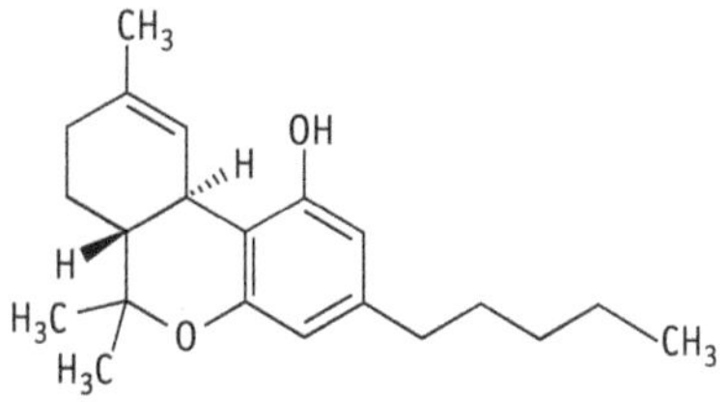

FIGURE 6.1   Parts of the Cannabis Plant.
https://www.leafly.com/news/cannabis-101/cannabis-anatomy-the-parts-of-the-plant,
accessed August 10, 2014.

## Cannabis Intoxication

Cannabis intoxication is a syndrome that develops within several minutes of smoking or 1 to 2 hours of ingesting cannabis products. The syndrome has both psychological and behavioral (euphoria, relaxation, increased appetite, impaired memory, and concentration) and physical (motor incoordination, tachycardia, orthostatic hypotension) manifestations. Intoxication is usually mild and self-limited, but occasionally markedly distressing effects can develop, such as intense anxiety, panic attacks, or psychosis.

## Cannabis Withdrawal

Cannabis withdrawal is a syndrome that develops upon abrupt reduction of heavy and prolonged cannabis use. The most common symptoms are dysphoric mood (anxiety, irritability, depression, restlessness), disturbed sleep, gastrointestinal symptoms, and decreased appetite. Most symptoms begin during the first week of abstinence and resolve within 4 weeks.[1] Up to half of patients in treatment for cannabis-use disorders report symptoms of a withdrawal syndrome. Although not medically serious, cannabis withdrawal should be addressed, because it may serve as negative reinforcement for relapse to cannabis use in individuals trying to abstain.

## Cannabis-Use Disorder

Cannabis-use disorder is a problematic pattern of cannabis use leading to significant distress and characterized by symptoms across several possible dimensions, including physical dependence, loss of control over use, harmful consequences, and compulsivity. See Table 6.1 for a summary of *DSM-5* diagnostic criteria. The

**Table 6.1 Cannabis-Use Disorder**

| Cannabis-Use Disorder | Cannabis Intoxication | Cannabis Withdrawal |
|---|---|---|
| A. A problematic pattern of cannabis use leading to clinically significant impairment or distress, as manifested by at least 2 of the following, occurring within a 12-month period: <br> 1. Use in larger amounts or over a longer period than was intended. <br> 2. Persistent desire or unsuccessful effort to cut back <br> 3. A great deal of time is spent in activities necessary to obtain, use, or recover effects. <br> 4. Cravings or persistent desire to use <br> 5. Failure to fulfill major role obligations at work, school, or home. <br> 6. Use despite recurrent social or interpersonal problems <br> 7. Important social, occupational, or recreational activities are given up or reduced <br> 8. Recurrent use in situations in which it is physically hazardous. <br> 9. Persistent use despite knowledge of physical or psychological problems caused or exacerbated by using <br> 10. Tolerance <br> 11. Withdrawal (refer to Criteria A and B of the criteria set for cannabis withdrawal). | A. Recent use of cannabis. <br> B. Clinically significant problematic behavioral or psychological changes (e.g., impaired motor coordination, euphoria, anxiety, sensation of slowed time, impaired judgment, social withdrawal) that developed during, or shortly after, cannabis use. <br> C. Two (or more) of the following signs or symptoms developing within 2 hours of cannabis use: <br> 1. Conjunctival injection. <br> 2. Increased appetite <br> 3. Dry mouth <br> 4. Tachycardia <br> D. The signs or symptoms are not attributable to another medical condition and are not better explained by another mental disorder, including intoxication with another substance. | A. Cessation of cannabis use that has been heavy and prolonged <br> B. Three (or more) of the following signs and symptoms develop within approximately 1 week after Criterion A: <br> 1. Irritability, anger, or aggression. <br> 2. Nervousness or anxiety <br> 3. Sleep difficulty (e.g., insomnia disturbing dreams). <br> 4. Decreased appetite or weight loss. <br> 5. Restlessness. <br> 6. Depressed mood. <br> 7. At least one of the following physical symptoms causing significant discomfort: abdominal pain, shakiness/tremors, sweating, fever, chills, or headache. <br> C. The signs or symptoms in Criterion B cause clinically significant distress or impairment in social, occupational, or other important areas of functioning. <br> D. The signs or symptoms are not attributable to another medical condition and are not better explained by another mental disorder, including intoxication or withdrawal from another substance. |

*Source:* American Psychiatric Association. (2013). Diagnostic and statistical manual of mental disorders (5th ed.). Washington, DC.

syndrome is specified to be mild if there are 2 to 3 symptoms, moderate if there are 4 to 5 symptoms, and severe if there are 6 or more symptoms. By in large, the severity of cannabis use disorder tends to be mild, with subtle but significant impairments in occupational functioning, school performance, or social relationships that may be detected by concerned family and friends before the user. Heavy cannabis users have also been characterized as having low levels of motivation, which is likely the result of repeated cycles of use (intoxication) followed by recovery from use (withdrawal). Because these consequences may be subtle, particularly in comparison to other substance-use disorders, there is a tendency to minimize the significance of cannabis-use disorders. Consistent with this, compared with other drugs, persons who present for treatment of cannabis-use disorder are much more likely to espouse a goal of reduced use rather than abstinence.

## EPIDEMIOLOGY

### Patterns of Use

Worldwide, cannabis is the most commonly used illicit substance, with 2.8% to 4.5% of persons aged 15–64 having used at least once in the past year.[2] In the United States, 42% of persons over the age of 12 have used cannabis at least once in their life, and 11.5% have used in the past year.

Among persons who have ever used cannabis, approximately 9% will develop a cannabis-use disorder at some point in their life, and 1.8% will meet diagnostic criteria for cannabis-use disorder within the previous year. These rates are lower than many other drugs of abuse, but they are nonetheless significant considering the high prevalence of cannabis use across the population. The risk of developing a cannabis-use disorder is highest among persons who first use cannabis before the age of 18, an observation that has stimulated research into the role of cannabinoids during brain development and maturation.

### Comorbidities

Not all users of cannabis develop cannabis-use disorder; thus, when evaluating comorbidities it is important to distinguish associations with cannabis use from associations with cannabis-use disorder. Cannabis use has been linked with several comorbidities, particularly among persons who began to use it at an early age. An association with the development of psychotic disorders, such as schizophrenia, has been repeatedly observed in large, well-controlled population studies. Cannabis increases the risk of developing a psychotic disorder by 1.5 to 2 times, though this risk appears to be concentrated among persons with genetic vulnerabilities.[3]

Persons with cannabis-use disorder are 6 times more likely to have a co-morbid mood or anxiety disorder.[4] Cannabis-use disorder is also associated with other substance-use disorders, and development of cannabis-use disorder before the age of 18 is strongly linked with risk of developing other substance-use disorders. However, the consequences of cannabis-use disorder tend to be subtler than other substance-use disorders (commonly reported problems include perceived memory problems, lower productivity at school or work, and inability to cut back despite efforts to do so), such that when persons with cannabis-use disorder seek treatment they infrequently endorse abstinence as a goal.

Heavy use of cannabis prior to the age of 18 is linked with subtle impairments in cognitive functions, including demonstrable impairments in executive function, processing speed, memory, perceptual reasoning, verbal comprehension, and cognitive efficiency. These impairments cannot be explained by residual intoxication because they persist beyond the period of cannabis intoxication or withdrawal. There is also evidence that use of cannabis during brain maturation is associated with dose-dependent reductions in IQ, though this particular finding has yet to be replicated.

Many of the compounds found in cannabis, including THC, readily cross the placenta and pass into breast milk. This observation, coupled with animal studies demonstrating that THC impairs early embryonic development, implantation, and fetal growth raises concern about the impact of cannabis during pregnancy or breastfeeding. In human studies, cannabis use has been associated with low birth weight, developmental delay, and behavioral problems; however, these problems may be attributable to other risk factors, such as tobacco use. Evidence regarding teratogenic effects is inconclusive to-date, nevertheless during the perinatal period caution is advised and abstinence recommended.[5]

## Genetics

Several studies have evaluated the heritability of cannabis-use disorders. Studies suggest that approximately 30% to 80% of the variance in risk for developing cannabis-use disorder is attributable to genetic factors. These genetic factors likely also confer risk to other substance-use disorders. The genes that are most closely associated are linked to regions on chromosomes 3 and 9, though candidate genes also exist on chromosomes 1, 4, 14, and 18.

## NEUROBIOLOGY

### Endocannabinoid System

Cannabinoid receptors, their ligands, and the related metabolic pathways are known collectively as the endocannabinoid system. Two cannabinoid receptors have been described. The CB1 receptor is predominantly located in the central nervous system, particularly cortical, subcortical areas, and the spinal cord. It is a presynaptic receptor that appears to attenuate the release of other neurotransmitters, such as GABA, glutamate, serotonin, and dopamine. CB1 receptors are mostly highly concentrated at brain areas involved in executive function, memory, mood regulation, motor function, food intake, and pain sensitivity. CB2 receptors are predominantly located in the periphery, particularly on cells involved in immune function.

The natural ligands for the cannabinoid receptors are 2 fatty-acid derived neurotransmitters, anandamide and 2-arachidonoylglycerol, which are synthesized on demand and released from the postsynaptic cell. After release these neurotransmitters travel to the presynaptic cell, where they bind to cannabinoid receptors and reduce neurotransmitter release. Thus, the system appears to serve in a feedback role, modulating the release of other neurotransmitters. Over the last several decades research into the cannabinoid receptors and their endogenous neurotransmitters has grown from an obscure scientific niche to a burgeoning area of discovery. The endocannabinoid system is involved in wide-ranging brain functions, but we remain only at the cusp of understanding its significance.

### THC

The primary psychoactive compound in cannabis is delta-9-THC (Figure 6.2). The effects of THC, however, may be augmented or mitigated by any of the 60 to 80 other cannabinoids found in the cannabis plant. These other cannabinoids may act independently or in concert with THC, such that the psychoactive effects of cannabis cannot be reduced to THC. Nevertheless, because current evidence suggests that THC is responsible for the reinforcing effects of cannabis, it is the focus of this section on the neurobiology of cannabis-use disorder.

THC is a highly lipophilic hydrocarbon that rapidly crosses the blood brain barrier and binds to cannabinoid receptors, where it produces an intoxication syndrome. THC is rapidly metabolized, primarily by the liver, into active and inactive metabolites that are excreted in the feces and urine. Because THC and several of its metabolites are stored and slowly released from lipid compartments, the half-life of THC is prolonged. THC metabolites can be detected after a single use for 1 week and after heavy use for over 1 month.[6]

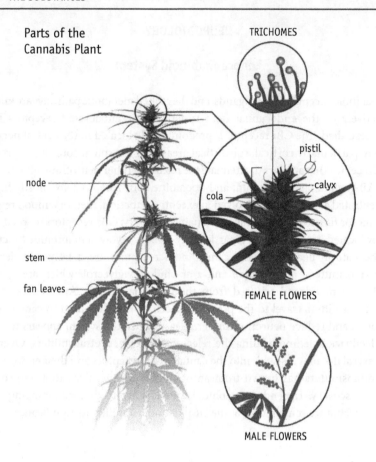

Parts of the Cannabis Plant

TRICHOMES

pistil

node

cola

calyx

stem

fan leaves

FEMALE FLOWERS

MALE FLOWERS

FIGURE 6.2 Tetrahydrocannabinol (THC).
https://commons.wikimedia.org/wiki/File:Tetrahydrocannabinol.svg, accessed
August 24, 2015 form public domain.

THC and its active metabolites exert effects by stimulating cannabinoid receptors at the locations described above. The reinforcing effects of THC are attributed to its effects in the mesolimbic region and nucleus accumbens, where it potentiates release of dopamine, one of the cardinal neurobiological features of addictive substances.

## TREATMENT OF CANNABIS-USE DISORDERS

### Therapy

Psychotherapy is a general term that encompasses many distinct "types" of therapy. Dozens of randomized trials have evaluated specific psychotherapies and demonstrated effectiveness in children and adults; however, the heterogeneity of these studies makes it difficult to compare their outcomes.[7] See Table 6.2 for a summary of the most commonly utilized therapies, almost all of which have been evaluated in clinical trials and for which manualized protocols are available.

Table 6.2  Summary of Clinical Trials Evaluating Medications for Cannabis-Use Disorders

| Class | Medication | Dose | Effect |
|---|---|---|---|
| **Anti-Depressants** | Bupropion | 150 mg, 300 mg | Worsened withdrawal |
| | Nefazodone | 450 mg | Improved anxiety |
| | Fluoxetine | 20–40 mg | Small reduction in cannabis use |
| | Escitaloporam | 10 mg | No clear benefit |
| | Mirtazapine | 30 mg | No clear benefit |
| | Fluoxetine | 20 mg | No clear benefit |
| | Venlafaxine | 375 mg | No clear benefit; possibly increased cannabis use |
| **Anxiolytic** | Buspirone | 30 to 60 mg | Small benefit in craving and irritability |
| **Mood Stabilizers** | Lithium | 50–900 mg | Reduced withdrawal symptoms |
| | Divalproex | 1500 mg | Increased withdrawal symptoms |
| | Gabapentin | 1200 mg | Reduced cannabis use and withdrawal symptoms |
| **Antipsychotic** | Quetiapine | 200 mg | No benefit and possibly worse outcomes |
| **Cannabis Agonist** | Oral THC | 10–90 mg | Reduced withdrawal symptoms |
| | Dronabinol | 10–120 mg | Reduced withdrawal symptoms |
| | Nabiximols | 86.4/80 | Reduced withdrawal symptoms |
| | Nabilone | 6–8 mg | Reduced withdrawal symptoms |

*(continued)*

**Table 6.2 Continued**

| Class | Medication | Dose | Effect |
|---|---|---|---|
| **Cannabis Antagonist** | SR141716 | 3–90 mg | Reduced pleasurable effects of intoxication |
| | Rimonabant | 90 mg | Reduced pleasurable effects of intoxication |
| **Opiate Antagonists** | Naltrexone | 12–200 mg | No benefit and possibly enhanced pleasurable effects of intoxication |
| **Dopamine** | Entacapone | 200 mg | Small reduction in craving |
| **Glutamate** | N-acetylcysteine | 1200 mg | Small reduction in cannabis use |
| **Norepinephrine** | Atomoxetine | 25–80 mg | Small reduction in use but poorly tolerated |

*Source*: Generated by authors.

The collective body of work suggests that there are generic and specific factors involved in facilitating change across different therapies. Generic factors include the development of a therapeutic alliance, support for self-efficacy, establishment of goals, and monitoring progress over time. Specific factors include the particular goals and approach facilitated by the therapy. For instance, motivational enhancement therapy focuses on helping individuals resolve ambivalence and make commitment to self-directed change; CBT teaches a model for understanding the relationship between thoughts, feelings, and behavior, and thus seeks to enhance the use of health coping mechanisms; contingency management uses external reinforcers to help motivate behavior change and prevent relapse; and family and systems therapies work with an individual's family or community to overcome obstacles, bolster supports, and facilitate interpersonal and intrapersonal change.

Varying lengths of sessions have been evaluated, with a trend toward longer courses of treatment showing greater efficacy. In addition, psychotherapies have been evaluated in combinations, typically involving an initial course of motivational enhancement therapy followed by cognitive behavioral therapy–based skills acquisition, and use of contingency management to encourage adherence to treatment. Such multifaceted approaches are promising, as are emerging technologies, such as computer- and phone-based systems, which may enable some individuals who would otherwise avoid treatment to benefit from it.

# Medications

There are no FDA-approved medications for the treatment of cannabis-use disorders. Medications that show promise are summarized in several recent systematic reviews,[8] to which readers are referred for greater details. See Table 6.3 for a summary of evidence from clinical trials, though few studies have been replicated and the sample size for most studies is small.

Cannabis intoxication is best treated supportively by offering verbal reassurance and containment in a safe and comforting setting until intoxication resolves. For severe symptoms, treatment with anxiolytic medication, or in the

**Table 6.3 Summary of Evidence Based Therapies for Cannabis-Use Disorders**

| Therapy | Overview | Administration (Rough Guidelines) |
|---|---|---|
| Motivational Enhancement Therapy (MET) | MET views readiness to change as a dynamic process involving multiple stages: pre-contemplation, contemplation, preparation, action, and maintenance, and proposes that the role of the therapist is to create the conditions that promote the patient's intrinsic motivation | Flexible; In studies MET sessions are typically 60–90 minutes long, with treatment occurring over 1 to 4 sessions |
| Cognitive Behavioral Therapy (CBT) | CBT views drug use as a learned behavior. CBT posits that by identifying the associative links and chain of events precipitating use, patients can identify opportunities to alter their behavioral repertoire and use alternative, healthy coping mechanisms | Administered alone as well as in combination with MET and CM. CBT is typically provided over 6–12 individual or group sessions |
| Contingency Management (CM) | CM posits that behaviors will increase or decrease as a function of immediate and directly associated consequences. By manipulating the quality and immediacy of external consequences, contingency management attempts to systematically increase the likelihood of desired behaviors, and minimize undesired behaviors | Typically used in combination with MET and CBT to enhance motivation and reinforce adaptive behaviors |

*(continued)*

**Table 6.3 Continued**

| Therapy | Overview | Administration (Rough Guidelines) |
| --- | --- | --- |
| Supportive Expressive Psychotherapy (SEP) | SEP seeks to establish a helpful, optimistic, encouraging, and empathic relationship between the patient and therapist. SEP posits that the development of a strong therapeutic alliance enables an expressive component, in which the therapist utilizes reflective listening and interpretation to explore the patient's subjective experience, point out patterns that manifest within the therapeutic relationship, and facilitate development of self-awareness, insight, and adaptive coping | Flexible; Typically 1–2x/wk 60 min sessions |
| Family Support Network (FSN) | FSN is an outpatient substance abuse treatment program targeting youth ages 10–18 years, and incorporating MET/CBT, as well as case management, home visits, and family education meetings | Individual MET/CBT sessions; 6 parent education sessions; 4 home visits; Didactic family session; Case Management; 3–6mo duration |
| Adolescent Community Reinforcement Approach (ACRA) | ACRA is a multisystem behavioral therapy that seeks to integrate cognitive behavioral skills training with collaborative community support, and contingency management | 10 individual sessions with patient; 4 sessions with caregivers including 2 family sessions; Case Management; 3–6mo duration |
| Multi-Dimensional Family Therapy (MDFT) | MDFT is a comprehensive systems therapy that targets the functioning of the individual within the context of his or her environment by integrating individual therapy, parent coaching, family systems therapy, and engagement of key community stakeholders such as school, medical supports, juvenile justice, and social services | 6 sessions with adolescent; 3 parent sessions; 6 whole family sessions; Case Management; 3–6mo |

*Source*: Generated by authors.

case of psychosis, a neuroleptic medication may be indicated under appropriate supervision.

Cannabis withdrawal is reliably alleviated with substitution therapy, either with cannabis derivatives or synthetic cannabis agents (e.g., dronabinol) that have been FDA approved for other indications. In practice, patients with distressing symptoms of withdrawal may benefit from time-limited treating with nonreinforcing anxiolytics to attenuate anxiety and non-reinforcing sedatives to reduce insomnia.

The search for a medication that can reliably treat cannabis-use disorder is ongoing. Several psychotropic medications have been studies in small trials, with disappointing results to date.[9] Gabapentin and buspirone have shown the greatest promise, though effect sizes have been small, and more studies are needed. Thus, the practicing clinician is left to use clinical judgment in deciding how to empirically treat distressing symptoms associated with cannabis cessation.

## Supplements

1) N-Acetyl Cysteine

N-Acetyl Cysteine (N-AC) is a derivative from the amino acid L-Cysteine. While N-AC has many uses in medicine, most notably to treat acetaminophen poisoning, it has been used as a supplement for treating cannabis-use disorder. Its proposed mechanism of action is modulation of the glutamate system in the nucleus accumbens. It is generally well tolerated with little to no side effects.

In addition to substance-use disorders, N-AC has been used for pathological gambling, obsessive-compulsive disorder, schizophrenia, unipolar depression, autism, and neurodegenerative diseases such as Alzheimer's and Parkinson's disease.[1] In addition to its ability to modulate glutamate, N-AC has many antioxidant properties. Oxidative stress has been linked to causing psychiatric disorders, which is another reason N-AC is an alternative treatment of interest.[2]

A double-blind, randomized controlled trial on the use of N-AC for treating cannabis-dependent adolescents showed that the group supplementing with N-AC had more than twice the odds of having cannabis-negative urine tests.[3] All study participants were treated for 8 weeks, with 1 group taking 1,200 mg of N-AC daily and 1 group taking a placebo.[4] The group taking N-AC also showed more favorable abstinence outcomes; however, the results were not statistically significant.

In a smaller study analyzing N-AC and cannabis use over a month's time, study participants supplementing with 1,200 mg of N-AC a day reported less daily "hits" of cannabis than the group not taking N-AC.[5] Cravings for cannabis, as measured by the Marijuana Craving Questionnaire (MCQ) decreased for 3 out of the 4 domains: emotionality (anticipation of using cannabis to improve negative mood), purposefulness (intention and planning to use cannabis for positive outcomes), and compulsivity (inability to control cannabis use).[6]

While more research is needed to determine the specific of using N-AC as an alternative treatment for substance-use disorders, research has shown that its use may be limited by its poor oral bioavailability, which ranges from 4–10%.[7] The current recommended dose of N-AC for substance-use disorders is 1200–2400 mgs a day, and it is usually administered as 2 to 4 pills over the course of the day. This medication plan may need to be revised, as it can be particularly burdensome for individuals with substance-abuse disorder, especially for individuals with comorbidities.

## 2) Bacopa Monnieri

*Bacopa monnieri* is a vigorously growing aquatic plant originally from the wetlands of southern India, Australia, and South America. While it has many uses in Ayurvedic medicine, its most notable use is for the improvement of memory and cognitive decline. Cannabis-use disorder is linked to memory difficulties and cognitive impairments, which is why it is reasoned that Bacopa may be helpful.[1]

One animal study showed that *Bacopa monnieri* extract improved memory function in rats previously given Okadaic Acid to impair memory.[2] In the same study, Bacopa was also shown to improve oxidative stress, neuro-inflammation, and neuronal loss. A double-blind, placebo-controlled randomized trial involving 76 individuals between the ages of 40 and 45 showed that supplementing with *Bacopa monnieri* increased retention of new information and decreases the rate of forgetting.[4]

A meta-analysis of 9 randomized controlled trials measuring the effects of standardized Bacopa extract on memory (for 12 weeks or longer) showed that Bacopa has significant potential to improve memory, especially the speed of attention.[5]

The precise mechanism of action for the ability of Bacopa to enhance cognition and improve memory is not clear. It seems to have multiple effects on the cellular level, including both anti-oxidant and anti-inflammatory effects. In Ayurvedic medicine, Bacopa is used to help clear the mind and as a tonic for the nervous system. It is a helpful tool for calming the anxiety and the weakening of the nervous system caused by regular cannabis use.

## 3) Tusli

Tulsi, or Holy Basil, is a medicinal plant from India. It has been used for a variety of ailments, including the common cold, diabetes, asthma, stomach ulcers, and the flu. Research has shown that Tulsi possesses anti-inflammatory, antipyretic, analgesic, antidiabetic, hepatoprotective, and anti-stress properties.[1] Because of its analgesic properties, it has been suggested that Tulsi may be an effective substitute to medical cannabis for treating cancer, AIDS, or other pain-related diseases. Long-term cannabis use can result in pulmonary, cardiovascular, and liver damage, as well as signs of cannabis withdrawal, namely anxiety, and irritability.[2] Long-term cannabis use can also result in impaired attention span, difficulty learning, and decreased motor ability. By substituting Tulsi for medical cannabis, it is possible to minimize those physical and mental consequences of long-term cannabis use. One of the active components of Tulsi, BCP (or beta-caryophyllene) has similar anti-inflammatory properties to cannabis, without the negative side effects.[3]

Research also suggests that holy basil may be beneficial for cannabis-use disorders due to its antioxidant properties. Several research studies involving animals have shown that Tulsi demonstrates more beneficial antistress activity than placebo.[4]

4) Gotu-Kola

Gotu-Kola, or *Centella asiatica*, may help attenuate the memory impairment, cognitive difficulties, and anxiety associated with cannabis withdrawal. Gotu-Kola is a tropical medicinal plant native to Southeast Asian countries such as India, Sri Lanka, China, Indonesia, and Malaysia. It has been studied for numerous medicinal effects, including anti-inflammatory, antiulcer, immunostimulant, cardioprotective, antidiabetic, antitumor, and antioxidant properties and as a treatment for venous insufficiency.[1] However, its researched neuroprotective effects may most relate to its usefulness in treating persons with cannabis-use disorder. The active chemical parts in Gotu-Kola are triterpenesaponosides.

Several animal studies have shown positive results for the neuroprotective and memory-boosting effects of Gotu-Kola supplementation. One study showed that giving rats 200 mg/kg/day of Gotu-Kola extract improved memory in a dose-dependent relationship.[2] The same study showed that significant oxidative stress was responsible for the neuro-degeneration observed in the rats' brains, and linked the strong antioxidant properties of Gotu-Kola to improving memory.[3]

Laboratory studies have shown that the hydroalcoholic component of Gotu-Kola can inhibit the enzyme acetylcholinesterase (which breaks down acetylcholine) and interfere with the cognitive decline associated with diseases such as Alzheimer's.[4] Another study showed that extracts of Gotu-Kola stimulate phosphorylation of cAMP, which has neuroprotective effects.[5]

A double-blind clinical study on children with mental deficiencies showed that supplementing with Gotu-Kola caused a statistically significant improvement in cognitive ability at both the third and sixth month follow-up marks.[6] Another double-blind, randomized, placebo-controlled study on 28 elderly volunteers showed that supplementing at the highest dose of Gotu-Kola, 759 mg daily, improved cognitive abilities.[7] A similar study on 60 volunteers showed that supplementing with 500 mg of Gotu-Kola twice daily for 6 months improved outcomes on the Mini Mental State Examination.[8]

Smaller clinical and animal studies suggest that the triterpenoids in Gotu-Kola may help reduce anxiety, a common withdrawal symptom; however, more research is needed to substantiate these conclusions.

5) L-Theanine

L-Theanine is derived from green tea leaves and is part of the *Theaceae* evergreen family native to East Asia. Green tea, itself, has been consumed for years for its subjective relaxation effect. L-Theanine as a supplement may help attenuate the anxiety symptoms and stress associated with cannabis withdrawal, although more research is needed to verify this theory. One animal study showed that L-Theanine, extracted from green tea, had a synergistic or additive effective with midazolam for reducing anxiety in rats.[1] The researchers also noted that this anxiolytic effect is not achieved by modulation of the GABA receptor, as was once thought, and due to a yet unknown mechanism of action.

A study involving human subjects showed that L-theanine may induce relaxation under resting conditions but not in an anticipatory state.[2] A smaller human study showed that L-theanine promotes alpha brain waves, which are associated with a state of relaxed wakefulness.[3] Another animal study on gene modifications and PTSD showed that administering L-theanine to rats with lab-generated PTSD significantly modifies certain genes.[4] PTSD is a common comorbid diagnosis with cannabis-use disorder (and all substance abuse disorders) so this study warrants future exploration.

## Diet

It is well known that cannabis use increases appetite and food consumption.[1] THC, the psychoactive component in cannabis, mimics the structure and function of endocannabinoids and is responsible for activating appetite through CB1 receptors.[2] Cannabis withdrawal is associated with changes in appetite. The majority of studies find that cannabis withdrawal leads to a reduced appetite and thus may result in reduced caloric intake, nutritional deficiencies, and weight loss. An individual trying to abstain from cannabis should ensure he or she is consuming a healthy, balanced diet.

Insomnia is an extremely common withdrawal symptom.[3] Therefore, research and experts recommend avoiding all caffeinated beverages.

Micronutrient supplements, especially amino acids, have also been shown to attenuate cannabis-use disorder, as well as substance-use disorder in general.[4] Research has shown that broad-spectrum micronutrient formulas help with many psychiatric symptoms, including stress-induced anxiety, depression, and mood irregularity.[5] Studies have shown that supplementing with an amino acid micronutrient can reduce cannabis use, as well as nicotine use.[6] Micronutrients may help attenuate associated psychiatric symptoms with substance use and withdrawal, such as mood irregularity, irritability, and anxiety. Micronutrients may also directly affect the brain reward circuitry by providing the appropriate cofactors and coenzymes needed for adequate neurotransmitter synthesis.[7]

## Yoga

Yoga is the ancient practice of combining body postures, stretches, and deep breathing exercises to promote health, relaxation, and stress reduction. Several research reports indicate its effectiveness as a complimentary treatment for substance-use disorder. One 90-day residential group study examined the effects of Kundalini yoga (a type of yoga that combines traditional yoga poses with meditation and mantras) on substance abuse. Participants showed improvements on both the behavior and symptom identification scale and the quality of recovery index.[1]

A meta-analysis of 8 randomized controlled trials showed that hatha yoga (HY), Iyengar yoga, nidra yoga, and the combination of cognitive behavioral therapy and vinyasa yoga resulted in more favorable results for addiction than the control interventions.[2]

Another study compared changes in the levels of y-aminobutyric (GABA) after 60 minutes of yoga to 60 minutes of reading. A 27% increase in GABA levels was seen in the group practicing yoga while no change occurred in the reading group.[3] Since anxiety is a common withdrawal symptom and low GABA is associated with anxiety, this mechanism of action of yoga for substance abuse is worth more exploration.

Yoga may also be an effective approach for individuals with cannabis-use disorder (and other substances) because it may help ease comorbid psychiatric symptoms and withdrawal symptoms. One study on psychiatric inpatients showed that those who participated in yoga class reported less tension, reduced anxiety, less depression, reduced anger, reduced fatigue, and less confusion.[4] Of course, a more recent trend is combining cannabis use with yoga class, which serves to highlight the complexities and gray areas that will arise as more states legalize cannabis use.

## Meditation and Mindfulness

Meditation is the practice of thoughtful contemplation with the intent to increase awareness without judgment. Some research supports the use of meditation for substance abuse; however, the evidence at this point is inconclusive. A large systematic review of 25 studies, including 8 randomized controlled trials, showed that meditation is safe and may be effective for addressing substance abuse. However, the authors also pointed out that methodological limitations existed in many of the studies, the data was not conclusive, and more research needs to be conducted to determine which type of substance abuse and/or individual responds to meditation and which do not.[1] Transcendental meditation is a technique for detaching oneself from anxiety and promoting happiness and self-awareness via meditation, mantra repetition, and basic yoga breathing. A retrospective study of 1,862 persons who practiced transcendental meditation for a duration of 20 months showed a decrease in cannabis use among the participants.[2] More research is warranted to determine if one kind of meditation, such as transcendental meditation, is more effective than another at addressing substance abuse.

Mindfulness is defined as a systematic development of attention to the present moment without judgment. Unlike traditional approaches to substance abuse, mindfulness exercises encourage an individual to stay in touch with the present moment, rather than remove oneself from uncomfortable situations or escape from unpleasant feelings. This approach allows for an individual to become more consciously aware of his or her habitat, triggers, and low-level cravings that can eventually become so disruptive and cause a relapse. A large meta-analysis involving 24 studies showed that mindfulness-based interventions (MBIs) can reduce consumption of cannabis, as well as alcohol, cocaine, amphetamines, nicotine, and opiates to a significantly greater extent than controls.[3] The same study noted that MBIs may be beneficial at reducing cravings.

One study involving neuro-imaging showed that even 1 mindfulness session can cause changes in brain structures and activation so as to reduce ruminations associated with cravings and relapse.[4,5] Another study showed that mindfulness-based therapies may be beneficial for disorders of behavioral dysregulation, for example, drug abuse and aggression or drug abuse and gambling. These types of disorders often involve more than 1 dysregulated behavior. The study compared mindfulness to treatment as usual for a 20-week period involving self-referred women. The mindfulness group showed significant decreases in verbal aggression, physical aggression, and both drug and alcohol usage.[6]

The preliminary research on mindfulness treatments for substance abuse suggests that it is effective; however, more research needs to be conducted to determine its practical application, including the minimal "dose" of mindfulness that is most effective and for how long one requires a mindfulness intervention to maintain positive results.

## Exercise

Physical exercise can be a great additional therapeutic approach to cannabis-use disorder. Since cannabis-use disorder is often accompanied with both physical and mental comorbidities, an effective exercise program will need to be tailored to each individual's ability and health status. The programs may need to be less strenuous than normal, focusing on light cardio and stretching exercises. Not only can a steady exercise program improve a substance abuser's overall health, but it can also be a great way to help manage the symptoms of withdrawal and maintain abstinence.

One cross-sectional and prospective study in young male substance abusers showed that sport and exercise was negatively associated with at-risk use of cigarettes and cannabis.[1] A thorough systematic review of 17 longitudinal studies suggests that sports participation during high school may help prevent cannabis and illicit drug use. Eighty percent of the studies showed a negative relationship between sport participation and illicit drug use, and 50% of the studies showed a negative relationship between sport participation and cannabis use.[2] A study analyzing the effects of an interventional group exercise program for individuals with substance-use disorder showed that participating in group exercise significantly improves their quality of life.[3]

While exercise has its benefits, it is important to remember that epidemiological studies have shown that individuals diagnosed with substance-use disorder and individuals who abuse substances are less likely to meet physical activity guidelines.[4] As a result, it is difficult to recommend a type and duration of exercise that is most beneficial for overcoming substance abuse. However, there is overwhelming evidence that supports the theoretical and practical reasons for including individuals with substance abuse disorders in exercise interventional programs. These reasons include: psychological benefits, behavioral improvements, neurobiological benefits, and overall positive health effects.

## Acupuncture

Acupuncture is a type of treatment where needles are inserted in the body at certain points. The points are designated along "energy channels" that theoretically connect the surface of the body to internal organs. The exact mechanism of how acupuncture benefits various ailments is unknown, including any beneficiary effects for substance abuse. Research suggests that auricular ear acupuncture may be effective for cannabis-use disorder, as well as alcohol, nicotine, cocaine, methadone, heroin, and caffeine addiction. Most practitioners of auricular acupuncture follow the National Acupuncture Detoxification Association (NADA) treatment protocol. This protocol uses 5 ear acupuncture points on each ear, specifically for addiction (Sympathetic point, Shenmen point, Kidney point, Liver point, and Lung point). While auricular acupuncture is widely used for treating addictions, it remains a controversial treatment that lacks a supportive body of research.[1]

One study that systematically analyzed the neurochemical and behavioral evidence for acupuncture's ability to suppress reinforcing effects of abused drugs shows that acupuncture modulates mesolimibic dopamine neurons.[2] The study further showed that acupuncture's modulation of dopamine release affects other neurotransmitters implicated in addiction pathways, such as serotonin and GABA.

A community-based study in Vancouver analyzed acupuncture's ability to reduce drug use in a marginalized, transient population. Results show that acupuncture helped lower rates of substance use and decreased the intensity of withdrawal symptoms, including: the shakes, stomach cramps, hallucinations, and insomnia.[3] Another study showed that acupuncture can significantly reduce the cravings and anxiety associated with substance-use withdrawal.[4] Other studies have shown that acupuncture is effective at reducing cravings and drug use in cocaine and heroin addicted populations, but much more research is needed to determine dose and overall efficacy.[5]

## Neurofeedback

Neurofeedback is a computer-aided training method in which areas of an individual's brain activity (brain waves) are made visible to the individual via monitors, graphs, and speakers. This type of feedback allows the individual to associate specific behaviors and thought patterns to brain activity and then self-regulate their behavior, physiological responses, and thoughts. This type of feedback is most useful for individuals addicted to substances in teaching him or her how to recognize the physiological response of cravings and withdrawal symptoms and to ultimately help him or her overcome them through self-regulation. This mode of treatment is growing in popularity because it is medication free and technological advances are allowing individuals to conveniently monitor their physiological state in convenient ways. The 3 most common systematic neurofeedback approaches to substance abuse are: the Peniston Protocol, the Scott-Kaiser Modification, and the Quantitative EEG Guided Training. (Both the Peniston Protocol and the Scott-Kaiser Modification approach teach individuals how to increase alpha and theta brainwave activity, both of which are associated with relaxed wakefulness.) One systematic review showed that alpha theta brainwave training in combination with beta brainwave training, along with residential treatment programs, is efficacious as a complimentary treatment for substance abuse.[1] Another review showed that EEG neurofeedback lowers feelings of depression associated with substance use and increases rates of abstinence.[2] Other studies show that neurofeedback, as a complimentary treatment to substance abuse, can improve somatic symptoms, reduce depression, decrease cravings, and improve overall mental health scores.[3] Another systematic review focusing on adolescents, neurofeedback, and substance abuse showed that neurofeedback is a significantly promising treatment modality for adolescents, especially those with comorbid attention and conduct problems.[4]

More research is needed to determine the most effective kind of neurofeedback, the duration of treatment that is needed for best results, and the substance abuse disorders and comorbid disorders that are most susceptible to treatment with positive outcomes.

## CANNABIS CHAPTER REFERENCES

### REFERENCES

1. Budney AJP. Review of the validity and significance of cannabis withdrawal syndrome. *American Journal of Psychiatry*. 2004 Nov;161(11):1967–77.
2. UNODC. Undoc.org., Drug report, 2011. http://www.unodc.org/documents/data-and-analysis/WDR2011/The_cannabis_market.pdf
3. Moore. Cannabis use and risk of psychotic or affective mental health outcomes: a systematic review. *Lancet*. 2007 Jul 28;370(9584):319–28.
4. Stinson R. Cannabis-use disorders in the USA: prevalence correlates and comorbidity. *Psychological Medicine*. 2006 Oct;36(10):1447–60.
5. ACOG Statement. 2015. Accessed August 24, 2015. http://www.acog.org/-/media/Committee-Opinions/Committee-on-Obstetric-Practice/co637.pdf?dmc=1&ts=20150824T1922212982
6. Huestis, M. A. (2007). Human Cannabinoid Pharmacokinetics. *Chemistry & Biodiversity*, 4(8), 1770–1804. http://doi.org/10.1002/cbdv.20079015
7. Cooper K. Psychological and psychosocial interventions for cannabis cessation in adults: a systematic review short report. *Health Technology Assessment*. 2015;19(56):1–130. doi:10.3310/hta19560.
8. Marshall K, Gowing L, Ali R, Le Foll B. Pharmacotherapies for cannabis dependence. *Cochrane Database of Systematic Reviews*. 2014;12:CD008940. doi: 10.1002/14651858.CD008940.pub2
9. Danovitch I, Gorelick DA. State of the art treatments for cannabis dependence. *Psychiatric Clinics of North America*. 2012;35(2):309–326.
10. Danovitch I, Gorelick DA. State of the art treatments for cannabis dependence. *Psychiatric Clinics of North America*. 2012;35(2):309–326.

## TREATMENT OF CANNABIS-USE DISORDER REFERENCES

### N-AC

1. McClure EA, Gipson CD, Malcolm RJ, Kalivas PW, Gray KM. Potential role ofN-Acetylcysteine in the management of substance use disorders. *CNS Drugs*. 2014;28(2):95–106. doi:10.1007/s40263-014-0142-x.

2. Ibid.
3. Gray KM, Carpenter MJ, Baker NL, et al. A double-blind randomized controlled trial of N-acetylcysteine in cannabis-dependent adolescents. *The American Journal of Psychiatry*. 2012;169(8):805–812. doi:10.1176/appi.ajp.2012.12010055.
4. Ibid.
5. Gray KM, Watson NL, Carpenter MJ, LaRowe SD. N-Acetylcysteine (NAC) in young marijuana users: An open-label pilot study. *The American Journal on Addictions/ American Academy of Psychiatrists in Alcoholism and Addictions*. 2010;19(2):187–189. doi:10.1111/j.1521-0391.2009.00027.x.
6. Ibid.
McClure EA, Gipson CD, Malcolm RJ, Kalivas PW, Gray KM. Potential role ofN-Acetylcysteine in the management of substance use disorders. *CNS Drugs*. 2014;28(2):95–106. doi:10.1007/s40263-014-0142-x.

## BACOPA

1. Hoch E, Bonnet U, Thomasius R, Preuss U. Risks associated with the non-medicinal use of cannabis. *DuetschesArzteblatt*. 2015;112(16):271–278.
* Hoch E, Bonnet U, Thomasius R, Ganzer F, Havemann-Reinecke U, Preuss UW. Risks associated with the non-medicinal use of cannabis. *Deutsches Ärzteblatt International*. 2015;112(16):271–278. doi:10.3238/arztebl.2015.0271.
2. Dwivedi S, Nagarajan R, Hanif K, Siddiqui HH, Nath C, Shukla R. (2013). Standardized Extract of *Bacopa monniera* Attenuates Okadaic Acid Induced Memory Dysfunction in Rats: Effect on Nrf2 Pathway. *Evidence-Based Complementary and Alternative Medicine : eCAM, 2013*, 294501. http://doi.org/10.1155/2013/294501
3. Ibid.
4. Roodenrys S, Booth D, Bulzomi S, Phipps A, Micallef C, Smoker J. Chronic effects of Bacopamonnieri on human memory. *Neuropsychopharmacology*. 2002;27:279–81.
5. Kongkeaw C, Dilokthornsakul P, Thanarangsarit P, Limpeanchob N, Scholfield N. Meta-analysis of randomized controlled trials on cognitive effects of Bacopamonnieri extract. *Journal of Ethnopharmacology*. 2014;151(1):528–35.

## TULSI

1. Manjeshwar B, Rosmy J, Karadika R, Venkatesh S, Bhat N, Palatty P. Special issue:recent advances in chemoprevention of cancer by dietary molecules. *Nutrition and Cancer*. 2013;65(1).
2. Volkow N, Baler R, Compton W, Weiss S. Adverse health effects of marijuana use. *New England Journal of Medicine*. 2014;2219–27.
* Volkow ND. Adverse health effects of marijuana use. *The New England Journal of Medicine*. 2014;370:2219–2227.

3. Hoffmann, David (2003). *Medical herbalism: the science and practice of herbal medicine.* Healing Arts Press, Rochester, Vermont.
4. Jvoti S, Satendra S, Sushma S, Anjana T, Shashi S. Antistressor activity of Ocimum sanctum (Tulsi) against experimentally induced oxidative stress in rabbits. *Methods Find ExpClinPharmacology.* 2007; 29(6):411–6.

## GOTU-KOLA

1. Orhan I. Centella asiatica urban: from traditional medicine to modern medicine with neuroprotective potential. *Evidence Based Complimentary and Alternative Medicine.* 2012. Article ID 946259, 8 pages. doi:10.1155/2012/946259
2. Veerendra Kumar MH, Gupta YK. Effect of different extracts of *Centella asiatica* on cognition and markers of oxidative stress in rats. *Journal of Ethnopharmacology.* 2002;79(2):253–60.
3. Ibid.
4. Orhan G, Orhan I, Şener B. Recent developments in natural and synthetic drug research for Alzheimer's Disease. *Letters in Drug Design and Discovery.* 2006;3(4):268–74.
5. Xu Y, Cao Z, Khan I, Luo Y. Gotu Kola (*Centella Asiatica*) extract enhances phosphorylation of cyclic AMP response element binding protein in neuroblastoma cells expressing amyloid beta peptide. *Journal of Alzheimer's Disease.* 2008;13(3):341–9.
6. Appa Rao MVR, Srinivasan K, Koteswara Rao T. The effect of *Centella asiatica* on the general mental ability of mentally retarded children. *Indian Journal of Psychiatry.* 1977;19(4):54–9.
7. Dev RDO, Mohamed S, Hambali Z, Samah BA. Comparison on cognitive effects of *Centella asiatica* in healthy middle age female and male volunteers. *European Journal of Scientific Research.* 2009;31(4):553–65.
8. Tiwari S, Singh S, Patwardhan K, Gehlot S, Gambhir IS. Effect of *Centella asiatica* on mild cognitive impairment (MCI) and other common age-related clinical problems. *Digest Journal of Nanomaterials and Biostructures.* 2008;(3):215–20.

## L-THEANINE

1. Heese T, Jenkinson J, Love C, et al. Anxiolytic effects of L-theanine-a component of green tea-when combined with midazolam, in the male Sprague-Dawley rat. *AANA Journal.* 2009;77(6):445–9.
2. Lu K, Gray MA, Oliver C, et al. The acute effects of L-theanine in comparison with alprazolam on anticipatory anxiety in humans. *Human Psychopharmacology.* 2004;19(7):457–65.
3. Eschenauer G, Sweet BV. Pharmacology and therapeutic uses of theanine. *American Journal of Health-System Pharmacy.* 2006;63(1):26, 28–30.

4. Ceremuga TE, Martinson S, Washington J, Revels R, Wojcicki J, Crawford D, . . . Bentley M. Effects of L-Theanine on Posttraumatic Stress Disorder Induced Changes in Rat Brain Gene Expression. *The Scientific World Journal.* 2014, 419032. http://doi.org/10.1155/2014/419032.

## DIET

1. Kogan N, Mechoulam, R. Cannabinoids in health and disease. *Dialogues in Clinical Neuroscience.* 2007;9(4).
2. Khamsi R. How safe is recreational Marijuana? *Scientific American.* 308(6).
3. Haney M, Ward A, Comer S, Foltin R, Fischman M. Abstinence symptoms following smoked marijuana in humans. *Psychopharmacology.* 1999;141(4).
4. Harrison RJ, Rucklidge J, Blampied N. Use of micronutrients attenuates cannabis and nicotine abuse as evidenced from a reversal design: a case study. *Journal of Psychoactive Drugs.* 2013;45(2).
5. Rucklidge J, Kaplan B. Broad-spectrum micronutrient formulas for the treatment of psychiatric symptoms: a systematic review. *Expert Review of Neurotherapeutics.* 2013;13(1).
6. Ibid.
7. Ibid.

## YOGA

1. Khalsa S, Gurucharan K, Hargopal K, Mukta K. Evaluation of a residential Kundalini yoga lifestyle pilot program for addiction in India. *Journal of Ethnicity in Substance Abuse.* 2008;7(1).
2. Posadzki P, Choi J, Lee M, Ernst E. Yoga for addictions: a systematic review of randomized clinical trials. *Focus on Alternative and Complementary Therapies.* 2014;19(1).
3. Streeter C, Jensen E, Perimutter R, Cabral H, Tian H, Domenic T, Renshaw P. Yoga Asana sessions increase brain GABA levels: A pilot study. *The Journal of Alternative and Complementary Medicine.* 2007;13(4).
4. Lavey R, Sherman T, Mueser K, Osborne D, Currier M, Wolfe R. The effects of yoga on mood in psychiatric inpatients. *Psychiatric Rehabilitation Journal.* 2005;28(4).

## MINDFULNESS AND MEDITATION

1. Zglerska A, Rabago D, Chawla N, Kushner K, Koehler R, Marlatt A. Special issue: mindfulness-related treatments and addiction recovery. *Substance Abuse.* 2009;30(4).

2. Telles S, Naveen KV. Yoga for rehabilitation: An overview. *Indian Journal of Medical Sciences*. 1997;51(4).

3. Chiesa A, Serretti A. Are mindfulness-based interventions effective for substance use disorders? A systematic review of the evidence. *Substance Use and Misuse*. 2014;49(5).

4. Holzel B, Carmody J, Vangel M, et al. Mindfulness practice leads to increases in regional brain gray matter density. *Psychiatry Research*. 2011;191(1):36–43.

5. Westbrook C, Creswell J, Golnaz T, Julson E, Kober H, Tindle, H. Mindful attention reduces neural and self-reported cue-induced craving in smokers. *Social, Cognitive and Affective Neuroscience*. 2011;8(1):73–84.

6. Wupperman P, Cohen M, Haller D, Flom P, Litt L, Rounsaville B. Mindfulness and modification therapy for behavioral dysregulation: a comparison trial focused on substance use and aggression. *Journal of Clinical Psychology*. 2015;71(10):964–78.

## EXERCISE

1. Henchoz Y, Dupuis M, Deline S, et al. Associations of physical activity and sport and exercise with at-risk substance use in young men: a longitudinal study. *Preventive Medicine*. 2014;64:27–31.

2. Kwan M, Bobko S, Faulker G, Donnelly P, Cairney J. Sports participation and alcohol and illicit drug use in adolescents and young adults: a systematic review of longitudinal studies. *Addiction Behavior*. 2014;39(3):497–506.

3. Muller AE, Clausen T. Group exercise to improve quality of life among substance use disorder patients. *Scand J Public Health*. 2015;43(2):146–52.

4. Linke SE, Ussher M. Exercise-based treatments for substance use disorders: evidence, theory, and practicality. *American Journal of Drug and Alcohol Abuse*. 2015;41(1):7–15.

## ACUPUNCTURE

1. Black S, Carey E, Webber A, Neish N, Gilbert R. Determining the efficacy of auricular acupuncture for reducing anxiety in patients withdrawing from psychoactive drugs. *Journal of Substance Abuse Treatment*. 2011;41(3):279–87.

2. Yang C, Lee B, Sohn S. A possible mechanism underlying the effectiveness of acupuncture in the treatment of drug addiction. *Evidence-based Complimentary and Alternative Medicine*. 2008;5(3):257–66.

3. Janssen P, Cemorest L, Whynot E. Acupuncture for substance abuse treatment downtown eastside of Vancouver. *Journal of Urban Health*. 2005;82(2):285–95.

4. Chang B, Sommers E. Acupuncture and relaxation response for craving and anxiety reduction among military veterans in recovery from substance use disorder. *American Journal of Addiction*. 2013;23(2):129–36.

5. Yoon S, Yang E, Lee, B, Jang E, Kim H, Steffensen S. Effects of acupuncture on stress-induced relapse to cocaine-seeking in rats. *Psychopharmacology*. 2012;222(2):303–11.

## NEUROFEEDBACK

1. Sokhadze T, Cannon R, Trudeau D. EEG biofeedback as a treatment for substance use disorders: review, ratings of efficacy, and recommendations for further research. *Applied Psychophysiology and Biofeedback*. 2008;33(1):1–28.
2. Shepard J. Neurofeedback for substance use disorders: a review of the applicability of treatment. VISTAS Online. Retrieved from http://www.counseling.org/docs/default-source/vistas/article_68a05a22f16116603abcacffoooobee5e7.pdf?sfvrsn=4
3. Dehghani-Arani F, Rostami R, Nadali H. Neurofeedback training for opiate addiction: improvement of mental health and craving. *Applied Psychophysiology and Biofeedback*. 2013;38(2):133–41.
4. Trudeau D. Applicability of brain wave biofeedback to substance use disorder in adolescents. *Child and Adolescent Psychiatric Clinics of North America*. 2005;14(1):125–36.

# 7

# Integrative Approach to Stimulant-Use Disorder

ANDREW MITTON AND LARISSA J. MOONEY

## Cocaine Use: Physical Effects and Public Health Impacts

Cocaine use remains a significant public health problem in the United States and throughout the world. In 2014, there were 1.5 million past-month users of cocaine in the United States, including 354,000 users of crack cocaine, and 0.9 million individuals age 12 or older met criteria for a cocaine-use disorder.[1] SAMHSA's 2014 National Survey of Drug Use and Health (NSDUH) estimated that 39.2 million Americans age 12 and over have used cocaine at least once in their lifetime, and 9.4 million have used crack, with over 40% of drug-related emergency department visits involving cocaine use.[2] Cocaine-use disorder accounts for 27% of all residential treatment admissions,[3] suggesting considerable potential for improving treatment methods for cocaine dependence. Cocaine stimulates the central nervous system and the cardiovascular system, increasing blood pressure, body temperature, and heart rate, occasionally inducing arrhythmia that can contribute to heart attack and stroke. Users experience euphoria, hyper-vigilance, increased energy, and appetite suppression. Cocaine may be snorted with rapid ability to cross the blood-brain barrier, or smoked when acquired in its crystalline form, also known as crack cocaine.[4]

Considerable effort and research has gone into investigating treatment modalities for cocaine users, effective medications to treat cocaine dependence have not been established. It is well known that individuals with cocaine-use disorder exhibit reduced dopaminergic function, which may contribute to dysphoria and relapse.[5] Increased activity of endogenous kappa agonist systems after chronic drug use may contribute to this dysfunction[6] and enhance stress-induced relapse.[7] Additionally elevated levels of dynorphin, the primary endogenous kappa receptor ligand involved in a feedback loop that suppresses dopaminergic activity, have been implicated in chronic cocaine users.[8]

## Methamphetamine Use: Physical Effects and Public Health Impacts

Methamphetamine and other amphetamine-type stimulants (ATS) are the world's second most widely used group of illicit substances (after cannabis), with prevalence varying by world region and by locales within nations. The highest prevalence rates are in North America, Western and Central Europe, and Southeast and East Asia. The United Nations estimates that up to 55 million people aged 15 to 64 had used ATS substances worldwide in the past year, with the highest rates of use in North America, Southeast and East Asia, and Western and Central Europe.[9] As many as 28 million people worldwide have used MDMA ("Ecstasy"), an ATS popular among younger users.[9] In the United States, recent estimates include 0.6 million current MA users, or 0.2% of the population.[2]

ATS remains a substantial contributor to global disease burden and accounts for the majority of drug treatment demand in many countries, including regions of Asia and the Middle East.[9] Variations in route of administration of MA produce differing consequences in terms of medical co-morbidities as well as potential for addiction. When administered via smoking or injection, MA enters the brain in seconds, whereas snorting and oral ingestion produce effects within several minutes to half an hour, respectively. The rapid uptake and effects of MA are attributable to its ability to cross the blood-brain barrier and enter cellular structures to inhibit dopamine storage and elicit release of dopamine, the primary mechanism of MA effects, in addition to stimulation of the cardiovascular system by increased norepinephrine.[10]

Methamphetamine stimulates the central nervous system and the cardiovascular system, increasing blood pressure, body temperature, and heart rate, and occasionally inducing arrhythmia that can contribute to heart attack and stroke. Users experience euphoria, hyper-vigilance, appetite suppression, and increased libido. Binge use is common to sustain the euphoria and other reinforcing effects that subside with rapidly developing tolerance. In the context of binge use, resultant elevated MA blood levels may lead to emergence of psychotic symptoms such as hallucinations, delusions, paranoia, mood disturbance, and repetitive activities. Acute psychosis may be associated with violence and other injurious behaviors that result in contact with law enforcement and medical emergency departments. It is well documented that extended use of MA can result in tremor, rapid tooth decay (known as "meth mouth"), insomnia, panic attacks, confusion, depression, irritability, and impairments in memory and other cognitive processes.[10]

# Pharmacotherapy for Cocaine-Use Disorder

Despite decades of research, there are currently no FDA approved medications for the treatment of SUD. In prior studies, the $GABA_B$ agonist baclofen attenuated cocaine-induced DA release in the nucleus accumbens,[11] and a double-blind, placebo-controlled study demonstrated reductions in cocaine use associated with baclofen treatment relative to placebo.[12] Findings were not replicated, however, in a subsequent study of severely dependent cocaine users.[13]

Other GABAergic medications that have been studied for the treatment of cocaine dependence include the anticonvulsants topiramate, gabapentin, tiagabine, and gamma-vinyl GABA.[14–16] Topiramate demonstrated preliminary efficacy in a 13-week randomized controlled clinical trial in which individuals who received topiramate for 8 weeks were more likely to be abstinent from cocaine than those who received placebo.[17] A more recent 12-week study yielded similar findings, including reduced cocaine use days observed in the topiramate group than the placebo group.[18]

Disulfiram, a medication approved for the treatment of alcohol dependence, has demonstrated preliminary efficacy in reducing cocaine use; effects on cocaine may be related to increased dopamine levels secondary to inhibition of dopamine beta hydroxylase and enhancement of adverse effects of cocaine. Disulfiram treatment has been associated with reduced cocaine use in several clinical trials,[19-22] and benefits have been found to be independent of its effects on alcohol use.[23] Nevertheless, results of a meta-analysis indicate insufficient evidence in support of the use of disulfiram as a treatment for cocaine addiction.[24]

Modafinil, a wakefulness-promoting medication approved for the control of daytime sleepiness in patients with certain sleep disorders, enhances glutamatergic activity and has been studied as a treatment for cocaine users with mixed results. Though an investigation of 400 mg/day modafinil vs. placebo demonstrated preliminary benefit in reducing cocaine use and prolonging abstinence,[25] findings were not replicated in a larger study comparing two doses and placebo.[26] Another study reported no difference in the primary outcome of weekly cocaine use over time between individuals receiving modafinil and placebo, but the 200 mg group demonstrated reduced cravings and maximum number of consecutive cocaine-free days relative to the 400 mg and placebo groups, and significant treatment effects were demonstrated in a post-hoc analysis of individuals without comorbid alcohol dependence.[27]

Preliminary evidence has supported efficacy of the mu opioid receptor antagonist naltrexone in reducing cocaine use.[28,29] Naltrexone given in combination with buprenorphine may also be associated with cocaine-use reduction;[30,31] the combination blocks mu agonist effects of buprenrophine, creating a functional kappa receptor antagonist that may counter elevated endogenous kappa activation associated with dysphoria and relapse risk after chronic drug use.[5] The combination of extended-release naltrexone and buprenorphine has been recently studied in a larger randomized trial of adults with cocaine dependence and a prior history of opioid use.[32]

A cocaine vaccine has been under investigation in clinical trials. The vaccine produces anti-cocaine antibodies that limit cocaine entry into the brain and have been shown to reduce brain cocaine levels following intravenous or intranasal cocaine administration.[33] Clinical trials for efficacy in humans have demonstrated safety and few side effects. Individuals who develop a sufficient antibody response demonstrate significant reductions in cocaine use, but progress has been hindered by development of non-uniform levels of antibody response among individuals receiving the vaccine and requirement for multiple dosing.[34,35]

## Pharmacotherapy for MA Use Disorder

Several medications have shown initial promise in reducing MA use, though findings have not been robust. GABAergic medications have been studied as potential agents including baclofen, which demonstrated potential benefit in reducing MA use relative to placebo in a post-hoc analysis in individuals who reported high medication adherence rates.[36] Gamma-vinvl GABA (GVG) has also been associated with stimulant use reduction in two open-label trials.[14,15]

Bupropion, an antidepressant with noradrenergic and dopaminergic effects, has shown some potential benefit in reducing MA use among less severe users.[37–39] The antidepressant mirtazapine has also demonstrated efficacy in reducing MA use relative to placebo.[40] Methylphenidate, a stimulant approved for the treatment of attention deficit hyperactivity disorder has been shown to reduce MA use relative to placebo in a European sample of amphetamine injectors who had attained abstinence in a residential program.[41] Results were not replicated in a recent study by Miles et al (2013),[42] but methylphenidate was associated with reductions in self-reported days of MA use relative to placebo in another trial.[43] Though no difference in MA use was demonstrated in a study comparing effects of dextroamphetamine 60 mg/day and placebo, diminished craving and withdrawal symptoms were observed in the dextroamphetamine group.[44]

Current evidence does not support the use of SSRI antidepressants for methamphetamine dependence, even though depression is common among individuals dependent on methamphetamine. A 12 week, randomized placebo-controlled trial testing the effectiveness of sertraline (SSRI) on methamphetamine cravings and use showed that individuals taking sertraline had **increased** methamphetamine cravings and use than individuals taking placebos.[45] A similar, randomized, placebo-controlled trial on sertraline and contingency management for methamphetamine abuse showed that methamphetamine-dependent individuals treated with sertraline had more adverse effects and craving than the group treated with placebos and did not experience a reduction in cravings or usage.[46] The authors of the study go as far to say sertraline is contraindicated for methamphetamine dependence because it can increase craving in these individuals.

Studies of modafinil as a treatment for MA dependence have yielded mixed results. Differences in MA use were not demonstrated in a prior study comparing modafinil 400 mg daily to placebo, but a trend toward reduction of use was observed among individuals in the modafinil group who reported a higher frequency MA use at baseline.[47] In a more recent study, beneficial effects of modafinil associated with MA abstinence were only observed in the subset of participants who demonstrated greater medication adherence as measured by urine assay.[48] Similar to the rationale for the use of modafinil in treating cocaine users, the stimulant properties of modafinil may counter dysphoria and fatigue associated with MA withdrawal and early abstinence,[49] and improvement in cognitive performance[50,51] and impulse control[51] associated with modafinil may confer additional benefit in stimulant using populations.[52]

The opioid receptor antagonist, naltrexone is approved for the treatment of both alcohol and opioid dependence and may function to modulate neural systems involved in craving and relapse. Reductions in subjective effects of MA and in relapse to MA use have been demonstrated in prior studies.[53,54] Results of a recent open-label study of extended-release naltrexone in combination with bupropion for the treatment of MA use disorder suggest potential utility of this combination warranting further study.[55]

## Cognitive Behavioral Therapy (CBT)

CBT is a behavioral treatment intervention with significant evidence base in the treatment of SUD. CBT can be utilized in individual or group sessions and focuses on learning and implementing relapse prevention skills that may be used in combination with pharmacotherapy and/or 12-step support. Specific lessons include identification of relapse triggers, strategies to reduce cravings, time management, and engagement in alternative healthy, non-drug related activities.[56] Coping skills are emphasized, including utilization of adaptive behaviors when faced with relapse triggers, and may be related to the effectiveness of CBT in reducing relapse to substance use.[57] CBT has been extensively studied in stimulant using populations, including the Matrix Model, a 16-week manualized CBT approach that was associated with reductions in MA use relative to standard treatment in a multisite trial of adults with MA dependence.[58] Computer-based CBT training has been developed and has demonstrated similar benefits in facilitating stimulant use reduction; this may enable more widespread dissemination of evidence-based behavioral treatments to areas or programs in need.[59]

## Contingency Management

Contingency management is a behavioral approach that incorporates tangible (often monetary) rewards for positive behaviors such as treatment attendance or abstinence. Incentive-based rewards have been shown to be highly effective in improving treatment adherence and reducing substance use. Utilization of voucher-based rewards for negative urine drug screens has been extensively studied in stimulant using populations, and the approach has demonstrated efficacy in improving abstinence rates in both cocaine and MA users.[56,60,61] CM may also be combined with CBT to augment treatment effectiveness.[62]

# Complementary and Alternative Medicine (CAM) Treatments

Given the lack of effective treatment options for stimulant use disorder currently in the traditional Western medical model, an evaluation of complementary and alternative approaches to treatment can further expand the options that care providers can offer as part of treatment planning for patients. Research on complementary and alternative medicine (CAM) treatments for SUD is mixed in regards to efficacy. Interpretation of study findings is limited by design and methodology, including small sample sizes in many studies. However many of these preliminary studies should be viewed as stepping stones for further inquiry, and use of various modalities in combination may warranted in some cases to provide a range of approaches to help individuals struggling with stimulant addiction.

## Yoga and Meditation

The term yoga comes from a Sanskrit word which means yoke or union. Yoga has its origins in in Ayurvedic practice developed in India, in which physical and mental exercises are designed to help stimulate and cultivate the spiritual aspects of the individual, culminating in self-transcendence, or enlightenment. There remain many different forms of yoga practice, each with different goals and philosophies. On the purely physical level, yoga postures are designed to tone, strengthen, and align the body. On the mental and spiritual level, yoga uses breathing techniques and meditation to quiet, clarify, and discipline the mind.

Yoga has been traditionally used to alleviate a diversity of problems including high blood pressure, high cholesterol, migraine headaches, asthma, lower back pain, constipation, diabetes, menopause, multiple sclerosis, varicose veins, carpal tunnel syndrome, and many chronic illnesses. Yoga has also been studied and championed for its ability to promote relaxation and reduce stress. Meditation and yoga practices have the ability to "strengthen self-soothing and executive practices."[63] The cultivation of these skills/capabilities have been postulated to correlate with greater resilience in the face of addiction, however there is currently limited research for these practices in acute treatment of the disorders as well as relapse prevention. With regard to SUD, a recent pilot study has shown some positive findings with regard to Yoga/meditation impacting quality of life markers for HIV+ patients who also use crack cocaine.[64]

Mindfulness meditation is a western form of meditation derived from the Buddhist practice of Vipassana. It is a practice designed to develop the skill of focused and nonjudgmental awareness of one's immediate experience and has been previously studied as an intervention to alleviate stress, depression, and chronic pain conditions. Given the established link between negative affect states and relapse risk,[65] mindfulness meditation has been used as a tool to reduce cravings, anxiety, and dysphoria that may be experienced by substance users. Mindfulness Based Relapse Prevention (MBRP) is a treatment intervention specifically adapted for substance using populations to provide skills to cope with cravings and psychological discomfort that may be associated with relapse, and preliminary evidence has accumulated in support of this approach to help reduce substance use and negative affect states.[66] The goal of MBRP is to monitor internal states and effectively process cues and triggers in order to facilitate healthy behavior choices. In a recent study of individuals with SUD who were randomized to receive MBRP or a health education control, MBRP was effective in reducing depression and anxiety relative to health education, and stimulant use reduction was demonstrated in the MBRP group among cocaine and methamphetamine users with co-occurring anxiety and major depressive disorder at baseline.[67] Another study enrolled 56 cocaine dependent patients who were randomized to receive either an integrative intervention with meditation with ear acupressure (IMEA) or outpatient treatment as usual (TAU). Participants in the IMEA group had higher rates of treatment retention and abstinence, in addition to greater reductions in cravings and anxiety relative to those maintained in TAU.[68]

## Exercise

Aerobic and resistance exercise have been studied as treatment interventions for substance use disorders including SUD.[69-71] Exercise has been shown to ameliorate depression and anxiety[72,73] via effects on dopamine transmission and the endogenous opioid system.[74] These negative affect states have been demonstrated in withdrawal and early abstinence from stimulant use[75] and have been associated with relapse risk.[65] Furthermore, exercise improves sleep and performance on cognitive tasks, and may be used as a healthy alternative non-drug behavior within a treatment plan focused on relapse prevention. Recent data has demonstrated improvement in physical health outcomes associated with exercise in a sample of methamphetamine users in a residential treatment setting randomized to receive an 8-week aerobic and resistance exercise program or health education control.[76] Improvements in depression and anxiety were demonstrated in the exercise group relative to health education,[77] and exercise was associated with recovery of striatal dopamine receptor deficits in MA users.[78] Furthermore, participation in the exercise intervention was associated with reduced rates of relapse to MA use post-residential treatment in individuals with less severe MA use at baseline,[79] suggesting potential utility of exercise as a treatment approach in stimulant users.

## Acupuncture

Acupuncture is a form of CAM and a key component of traditional Chinese medicine. It involves the insertion of thin needles at noted points in the body and can be associated with the application of heat, pressure, or electric stimulation to these same points. Acupuncture is based on the theory of manipulating and harnessing the *qi*, or what is understood as the essential life force or energy that exists both inside and outside the body. Acupuncture seeks to manipulate the status of the *qi* at certain surface points on the body. Acupuncture is commonly used for pain relief; however, there is an expanding interest in its application for the treatment of such targets as anxiety and depression to SUDs.

In one of the larger reviews of the cocaine-use disorder using treatment with acupuncture, sufficient evidence was not found to recommend the use of acupuncture for treatment. This detailed 7 studies that included a total of 1,433 participants.[80] In a subsequent large review that included existing trials in both the United States and Great Britain, results from 9 studies that enrolled 1,747 participants also did not demonstrate convincing evidence to support treatment of cocaine-use disorder with acupuncture. It was noted in this review that findings from most of the studies were limited by significant loss patients to follow up.[81]

There is some limited evidence that acupuncture can play a role in treating methamphetamine withdrawal syndrome. In a recent Chinese study it was found that electroacupuncture and auricular acupuncture can play a therapeutic role in the treatment of methamphetamine withdrawal by improving patients experience of anxiety and depression.[82] As of now there is not sufficient evidence to support the use of acupuncture to ameliorate cravings or prevent relapse in patients who use methamphetamine.

# N-acetylcysteine

L-cysteine is an essential amino acid, one of only 3 sulfur-containing amino acids. Cysteine plays a role in the sulfation cycle, acting as a sulfur donor in phase II detoxification and as a methyl donor in the conversion of homocysteine to methionine. Cysteine also helps synthesize glutathione, which is the body's most important intracellular antioxidant and a vital detoxifier.

N-acetyl-L-cysteine (NAC) is the acetylated form of L-cysteine. It is very efficiently absorbed and has been shown to have a low side-effect burden and is well tolerated by patients. NAC is an antioxidant and a free radical-scavenging agent that increases intracellular glutathione at the cellular level. NAC can act as a precursor for glutathione synthesis as well as a stimulator of the cytosolic enzymes involved in glutathione regeneration. NAC has been shown to protect against oxidative stress-induced neuronal death. Current uses of NAC include prevention of chronic obstructive pulmonary disease exacerbation, prevention of contrast-induced kidney damage during imaging procedures, attenuation of illness from the influenza virus when started before infection, treatment of pulmonary fibrosis, as well as for the treatment of picking disorders and trichotillomania.

The use of N-acetylcystine (NAC) has shown some preliminary evidence supporting its use in the treatment of MA cravings in MA users. NAC has been shown to be a well-tolerated intervention with a low side effect profile. In a recent Iranian study that followed 23 patients, positive results showed that NAC was associated with reduction in craving, self-reported use, and time spent using cocaine.[83] In another recent US study, one that followed 111 participants, limited efficacy of NAC was observed;[84] however, NAC did show some promise when administered at a higher than standard dose of 2,400 mg to patients who had already achieved abstinence. In this group of patients, NAC was associated lower overall cravings and longer time to relapse when compared to placebo.[85] Improvement in relapse rates was also demonstrated in an additional study, and beneficial effects of NAC were still present even after treatment was discontinued. This led the authors to posit that NAC may have a longer-term protective effect.[86]

# Transcranial Magnetic Stimulation

Transcranial magnetic stimulation (TMS) is a non-invasive, physical approach to treatment that involves the application of a fluctuating magnetic field through the skull into the brain. This application generates electrical currents which are then able to modulate neuronal firing. Multiple TMS pulses given consecutively are referred to as rTMS. Because TMS is applied directly to the brain, it may be better tolerated than systemic medications by some patients including the elderly, pregnant women, or those with severe medical conditions. The theoretical underpinnings of the treatment suggest that by focused application of current, neurons, and neuronal pathways can be manipulated to achieve therapeutic results in the patient without invasive and potentially harmful side effects.

While still early in research and trials, rTMS has shown some preliminary evidence for treatment of cocaine cravings. Application of high frequency rTMS to the Dorsal Lateral Prefrontal Cortex (DLPFC) showed a reduction in cravings in participants. In particular, results demonstrated that application to the left DLPFC had greater efficacy then when applied to the right DLPFC. In addition, participants "experienced a reduction of anxiety and an increase in happiness after the session" which may also play into the positive outcomes for the treatment modality.[87] It was noted that at least one week of daily treatment was needed to show positive finding for treatment with more than one week of treatment yielding better results.[88]

# Conclusions

Cocaine and ATS use are is associated with medical, psychiatric, and public health consequences; yet robust, effective treatment options for SUD are still lacking. Though new treatments are on the horizon, the prevalence of addiction to stimulants and the clear negative impacts on individuals and society demand that we expand the scope of treatment to include CAM approaches in addition to behavioral and pharmacological treatment interventions for the treatment of SUD. As initially noted, research on CAM treatments for SUD is mixed with regard to efficacy, but we must remember to temper these preliminary findings as being limited by design and methodology, including small sample sizes often reflective of nascent research. With this in mind, these studies should be viewed as stepping stones for further inquiry. And use of various modalities in combination (both mainstream and CAM) may be warranted in some cases to provide a range of approaches to help diverse individuals struggling with stimulant addiction.

## REFERENCES

1. Center for Behavioral Health Statistics and Quality. *2014 National Survey on Drug Use and Health: Detailed tables*. Rockville, MD: Substance Abuse and Mental Health Services Administration; 2015.
2. Substance Abuse and Mental Health Services Administration. *Results from the 2013 National Survey on Drug Use and Health: Summary of National findings*. NSDUH Series H-48, HHS Publication No. [SMA] 14-4863. Rockville, MD: Substance Abuse and Mental Health Services Administration; 2014.

3. Substance Abuse and Mental Health Services Administration, Center for Behavioral Health Statistics and Quality. *Treatment Episode Data Set (TEDS): 2003–2013. National Admissions to Substance Abuse Treatment Services.* BHSIS Series S-75, HHS Publication No. (SMA) 15-4934. Rockville, MD: Substance Abuse and Mental Health Services Administration; 2015.

4. National Institute on Drug Abuse. Drug facts: Cocaine. Retrieved February 28, 2016 from https://www.drugabuse.gov/publications/drugfacts/cocaine.

5. Little KY, Ramssen E, Welchko R, Volberg V, Roland, CJ, Cassin B. Decreased brain dopamine cell numbers in human cocaine users. *Psychiatry Research.* 2009;168(3):173–180.

6. Spanagel R, Herz A, Shippenberg, TS. Opposing tonically active endogenous opioid systems modulate the mesolimbic dopaminergic pathway. *Proceedings of the National Academy of Sciences USA.* 1992; 89(6):2046–2050.

7. Beardsley P, Pollard G, Howard J, Carroll F. Effectiveness of analogs of the kappa opioid receptor antagonist (3R)-7-Hydroxy-N-((1S)-1-{[(3R,4R)-4-(3-hydroxyphenyl)-3,4-dimethyl-1-piperidinyl]methyl}-2-methylpropyl)-1,2,3,4-tetrahydro-3-isoquinolinecarboxamide (JDTic) to reduce U50,488-induced diuresis and stress-induced cocaine reinstatement in rats. *Psychopharmacology.* 2010;210(2):189–198.

8. Frankel PS, Alburges ME, Bush L, Hanson GR, Kish SJ. Striatal and ventral pallidum dynorphin concentrations are markedly increased in human chronic cocaine users. *Neuropharmacology.* 2008;55(1):41–46.

9. United Nations Office on Drugs and Crime. *World drug report.* (United Nations publication, Sales No. E.15.XI.6). Vienna: United Nations Office on Drugs and Crime; 2015.

10. Rawson RA, Ling W, Mooney LJ. Clinical management: Methamphetamine. In: Galanter, M, Kleber HD, Brady K, eds., *The American Psychiatric Publishing Textbook of Substance Abuse Treatment.* 5th ed. Arlington, VA: American Psychiatric Publishing; 2015.

11. Fadda P, Scherma M, Fresu A, Collu M, Fratta W. Baclofen antagonizes nicotine-, cocaine-, and morphine-induced dopamine release in the nucleus accumbens of rats. *Synapse.* 2003;50(1):1–6.

12. Shoptaw S, Yang X, Rotheram-Fuller EJ, et al. Randomized placebo-controlled trial of baclofen for cocaine dependence: Preliminary effects for individuals with chronic patterns of cocaine use. *Journal of Clinical Psychiatry.* 2003;64(12):1440–1448.

13. Kahn R, Biswas K, Childress AR, et al. Multi-center trial of baclofen for abstinence initiation in severe cocaine-dependent individuals. *Drug and Alcohol Dependence.* 2009;103(1–2):59–64.

14. Brodie JD, Figueroa E, Dewey SL. Treating cocaine addiction: From preclinical to clinical trial experience with gamma-vinyl GABA. *Synapse.* 2003;50:261–265.

15. Brodie JD, Figueroa E, Laska EM, Dewey SL. Safety and efficacy of {gamma}-vinyl GABA (GVG) for the treatment of methamphetamine and/or cocaine addiction. *Synapse.* 2005;55(2):122–125.

16. González G, Desai R, Sofuoglu M, et al. Clinical efficacy of gabapentin versus tiagabine for reducing cocaine use among cocaine dependent methadone-treated patients. *Drug and Alcohol Dependence.* 2007;87(1):1–9.

17. Kampman, K. M., Pettinati, H., Lynch, K. G., Dackis, C., Sparkman, T., Weigley, C., O'Brien, C. P. A pilot trial of topiramate for the treatment of cocaine dependence. *Drug and Alcohol Dependence.* 2004;75(3):233–240.

18. Johnson BA, Ait-Daud N, Wang XQ, et al. Topiramate for the treatment of cocaine addiction: A randomized controlled clinical trial. *JAMA Psychiatry.* 2013;70(12):1338–1346.

19. Carroll KM, Nich C, Ball SA, McCance E., Rounsaville BJ. Treatment of cocaine and alcohol dependence with psychotherapy and disulfiram. *Addiction.* 1998;93(5):713–727.

20. Carroll KM, Nich C, Ball SA, McCance E, Frankforter TL, Rounsaville BJ. One-year follow-up of disulfiram and psychotherapy for cocaine-alcohol users: Sustained effects of treatment. *Addiction.* 2000;95(9):1335–1349.

21. Oliveto A, Poling J, Mancino MJ, et al. Randomized, double blind, placebo-controlled trial of disulfiram for the treatment of cocaine dependence in methadone-stabilized patients. *Drug and Alcohol Dependence.* 2011;113(2–3):184–191.

22. Petrakis IL, Carroll KM, Nich C, et al. Disulfiram treatment for cocaine dependence in methadone-maintained opioid addicts. *Addiction.* 2000;95(2):219–228.

23. Carroll KM, Fenton LR, Ball SA, et al. Efficacy of disulfiram and cognitive behavior therapy in cocaine-dependent outpatients: A randomized placebo-controlled trial. *Archives of General Psychiatry.* 2004;61(3):264–272.

24. Pani PP, Trogu E, Vacca R, Amato L, Vecchi S, Davoli M. Disulfiram for the treatment of cocaine dependence. *Cochrane Database of Systematic Reviews.* 2010;20(1): CD007024.

25. Dackis CA, Kampman KM, Lynch KG, Pettinati HM, O'Brien CP. A double-blind, placebo-controlled trial of modafinil for cocaine dependence. *Neuropsychopharmacology.* 2005;30(1):205–211.

26. Dackis CA, Kampman KM, Lynch KG, et al. A double-blind, placebo-controlled trial of modafinil for cocaine dependence. *Journal of Substance Abuse Treatment.* 2012;43(3):303–312.

27. Anderson AL, Reid MS, Li SH, et al. Modafinil for the treatment of cocaine dependence. *Drug and Alcohol Dependence.* 2009;104(1–2):133–139.

28. Oslin DW, Pettinati HM, Volpicelli JR, Wolf AL, Kampman KM, O'Brien, CP. The effects of naltrexone on alcohol and cocaine use in dually addicted patients. *Journal of Substance Abuse Treatment.* 1999;16(2):163–167.

29. Schmitz JM, Stotts AL, Rhoades HM, Grabowski J. Naltrexone and relapse prevention treatment for cocaine-dependent patients. *Addictive Behaviors.* 2001;26(2):167–180.

30. Gerra G, Fantoma A, Zaimovic A. Naltrexone and buprenorphine combination in the treatment of opioid dependence. *Journal of Psychopharmacology.* 2006;20(6):806–814.

31. Rothman RB, Gorelick DA, Heishman SJ, et al. An open-label study of a functional opioid kappa antagonist in the treatment of opioid dependence. *Journal of Substance Abuse Treatment.* 2000;18(3):277–281.
32. Ling W, Hillhouse M, Saxon A, et al. Buprenorphine + naloxone plus naltrexone for the treatment of cocaine dependence: The Cocaine Use Reduction with Buprenorphine (CURB) study. *Addiction.* 2016;111(8):1416–1427.
33. Fox BS. Development of a therapeutic vaccine for the treatment of cocaine addiction. *Drug and Alcohol Dependence.* 1997;48(3):153–158.
34. Kosten TR, Rosen M, Bond J, et al. Human therapeutic cocaine vaccine: safety and immunogenicity. *Vaccine.* 2002;20(7–8):1196–1204.
35. Shen XY, Orson FM, Kosten TR. Vaccines against drug abuse. *Clinical Pharmacology & Therapeutics.* 2011;91(1):60–70.
36. Heinzerling K, Shoptaw S, Peck J, et al. Randomized, placebo-controlled trial of baclofen and gabapentin for the treatment of methamphetamine dependence. *Drug and Alcohol Dependence.* 2006;85(3):177–184.
37. Elkashef A, Rawson R, Anderson A, et al. Bupropion for the treatment of methamphetamine dependence. *Neuropsychopharmacology.* 2008;33(5):1162–1170.
38. McCann DJ, Li SH. A novel, nonbinary evaluation of success and failure reveals bupropion efficacy versus methamphetamine dependence: reanalysis of a multisite trial. *CNS Neuroscience & Therapeutics.* 2012;18(5):414–418.
39. Shoptaw S, Heinzerling KG, Rotheram-Fuller E, et al. Randomized, placebo-controlled trial of bupropion for the treatment of methamphetamine dependence. *Drug and Alcohol Dependence.* 2008;96(3):222–232.
40. Colfax GN, Santos GM, Das, M., et al. Mirtazapine to reduce methamphetamine use: A randomized controlled trial. *Archives of General Psychiatry.* 2011;68(11):168–1175.
41. Tiihonen J, Kuoppasalmi K, Föhr J, et al. A comparison of aripiprazole, methylphenidate, and placebo for amphetamine dependence. *American Journal of Psychiatry.* 2007;164(1):160–162.
42. Miles SW, Sheridan J, Russell B. Extended-release methylphenidate for treatment of amphetamine/methamphetamine dependence: A randomized, double-blind, placebo-controlled trial. *Addiction.* 2013;108(7):1279–1286.
43. Ling W, Chang L, Hillhouse M. Sustained-release methylphenidate in a randomized trial of treatment of methamphetamine use disorder. *Addiction.* 2004;109(9):1489–1500.
44. Galloway GP, Buscemi R, Coyle JR. A randomized, placebo-controlled trial of sustained-release dextroamphetamine for treatment of methamphetamine addiction. *Clinical Pharmacology and Therapeutics.* 2011;89(2):276–282.
45. Zorick T, Sugar C, Hellemann G, Shoptaw S, London E. Poor response to sertraline in methamphetamine dependence is associated with sustained craving for methamphetamine. *Drug and Alcohol Dependence.* 2011;118(2–3):500–503.
46. Shoptaw S, Huber A, Peck J. Randomized placebo-controlled trial of sertraline and contingency management for the treatment of methamphetamine dependence. *Drug and Alcohol Dependence.* 2006;85(1):12–18.

47. Heinzerling K, Swanson AN, Kim S. Randomized, double-blind, placebo-controlled trial of modafinil for the treatment of methamphetamine dependence. *Drug and Alcohol Dependence.* 2010;109(1–3):20–29.
48. Anderson AL, Li SH, Biswas K. Modafinil for the treatment of methamphetamine dependence. *Drug and Alcohol Dependence.* 2012;120(1–3):135–141.
49. Peck JA, Reback CJ, Yang X, Rotheram-Fuller E, Shoptaw, S. Sustained reductions in drug use and depression symptoms from treatment for drug abuse in methamphetamine-dependent gay and bisexual men. *Journal of Urban Health: Bulletin of the New York Academy of Medicine.* 2005;82(Suppl 1): i100–i108.
50. Turner DC, Clark L, Dowson J, Robbins TW, Sahakian BJ. Modafinil improves cognition and response inhibition in adult attention-deficit/hyperactivity disorder. *Biological Psychiatry.* 2004b;55(10):1031–1040.
51. Turner DC, Clark L, Pomarol-Clotet E, McKenna P, Robbins TW, Sahakian BJ. Modafinil improves cognition and attentional set shifting in patients with chronic schizophrenia. *Neuropsychopharmacology.* 2004;29(7):1363–1373.
52. Dean AC, Sevak RJ, Monterosso JR, Hellemann G, Sugar CA, London ED. Acute modafinil effects on attention and inhibitory control in methamphetamine-dependent humans. *Journal of Studies on Alcohol and Drugs.* 2011;72(6):943–953.
53. Jayaram- Lindström N, Wennberg P, Beck O, Franck J. An open clinical trial of naltrexone for amphetamine dependence: compliance and tolerability. *Nordic Journal of Psychiatry.* 2005;59:167–171.
54. Jayaram-Lindström N, Hammarberg A, Beck O, Franck, J. Naltrexone for the treatment of amphetamine dependence: a randomized, placebo-controlled trial. *American Journal of Psychiatry.* 2008;165:1442–1448.
55. Mooney LJ, Hillhouse MP, Thomas, C. Utilizing a two-stage design to investigate the safety and potential efficacy of monthly naltrexone plus once-daily bupropion as a treatment for methamphetamine use disorder. *Journal of Addiction Medicine.* 2016;10(4):236–243.
56. Vocci FJ, Montoya ID. Psychological treatments for stimulant misuse, Comparing and contrasting those for amphetamine dependence and those for cocaine dependence. *Current Opinion in Psychiatry.* 2009;22(3):263–268.
57. Kiluk BD, Nich C, Babuscio T, Carroll KM. Quality versus quantity: Acquisition of coping skills following computerized cognitive-behavioral therapy for substance-use disorders. *Addiction.* 2010;105(12):2120–2127.
58. Rawson RA, Marinelli-Casey P, Anglin, MD. A multi-site comparison of psychosocial approaches for the treatment of methamphetamine dependence. *Addiction.* 2004;99(6):708–717.
59. Carroll KM, Kiluk BD, Nich C, Gordon MA. Computer-assisted delivery of cognitive-behavioral therapy: Efficacy and durability of CBT4CBT among cocaine-dependent individuals maintained on methadone. *American Journal of Psychiatry.* 2014;171(4):436–444.
60. Rawson RA, McCann MJ, Flammino F. A comparison of contingency management and cognitive-behavioral approaches for stimulant dependent individuals. *Addiction.* 2006;101(2):267–274.

61. Roll JM, Petry NM, Stitzer ML. Contingency management for the treatment of methamphetamine use disorders. *American Journal of Psychiatry.* 2006;163(11): 1993–1999.

62. Petitjean SA, Dursteler-MacFarland KM, Krokar MC. A randomized, controlled trial of combined cognitive-behavioral therapy plus prize-based contingency management for cocaine dependence. *Drug and Alcohol Dependence.* 2014;145:94–100.

63. Kissen M, Kissen-Kohn DA. Reducing addictions via the self-soothing effects of yoga. *Bulletin of the Menninger Clinic.* 2009;73(1):34–43.

64. Agarwal RP, Kumar A, Lewis JE. A pilot feasibility and acceptability study of yoga/ meditation on the quality of life and markers of stress in persons living with HIV who also use crack cocaine. *Journal of Alternative and Complementary Medicine.* 2005;21(3):152–158.

65. Marlatt GA. Taxonomy of high-risk situations for alcohol relapse: Evolution and development of a cognitive-behavioral model. *Addiction.* 1996;91(Suppl):37–S49.

66. Bowen S, Chawla N, Collins S, Witkiewitz K, Hsu S, Grow J. Mindfulness-based relapse prevention for substance use disorders: a pilot efficacy trial. *Substance Abuse.* 2009;30:205–305.

67. Glasner-Edwards S, Mooney LJ, Ang, A. Mindfulness based relapse prevention for stimulant dependent adults: a pilot randomized clinical trial. *Mindfulness (N Y).* 2017;8(1):126–135.

68. Chen KW, Berger CC, Gandhi D, Weintraub E, Lejuez CW. Adding integrative meditation with ear acupressure to outpatient treatment of cocaine addiction: a randomized controlled pilot study. *Journal of Alternative and Complementary Medicine.* 2013;19(3):204–210.

69. Brown RA, Abrantes AM, Read JP. A pilot study of aerobic exercise as an adjunctive treatment for drug dependence. *Mental Health and Physical Activity.* 2010;3(1):27–34.

70. Trivedi MH, Greer TL, Grannemann BD. Stimulant reduction intervention using dosed exercise (STRIDE)—CTN 0037: Study protocol for a randomized controlled trial. *Trials.* 2011;12:206.

71. Mooney LJ, Cooper C, London E. Exercise for methamphetamine dependence: Rationale, design, and methodology. *Journal of Contemporary Clinical Trials.* 2014;37(1):139–147.

72. Zschucke E, Gaudlitz K, Ströhle, A. Exercise and physical activity in mental disorders: clinical and experimental evidence. *Journal of Preventive Public Health.* 2013;46: S12–S21.

73. Martinsen EW. Physical activity in the prevention and treatment of anxiety and depression. *Nordic Journal of Psychiatry.* 2008;62(Suppl 47):25–29.

74. Meeusen R. Exercise and the brain: Insight in new therapeutic modalities. *Annals of Transplantation.* 2005;10:49–51.

75. Newton TF, Kalechstein AD, Duran S, Vansluis N, Ling W. Methamphetamine abstinence syndrome: Preliminary findings. *American Journal of Addiction.* 2004;13(3):248–255.

76. Dolezal BA, Chudzynski J, Storer TW. Eight weeks of exercise training improves fitness measures in methamphetamine-dependent individuals in residential treatment. *Journal of Addictive Medicine*. 2013;7:122–128.

77. Rawson RA, Chudzynski J, Gonzales R. The impact of exercise on depression and anxiety symptoms among abstinent methamphetamine-dependent individuals in a residential treatment setting. *Journal of Substance Abuse Treatment*. 2015;57:36–40.

78. Robertson CL, Ishibashi K, Chudzynski J. Effect of exercise training on striatal dopamine D2/D3 receptors in methamphetamine users during behavioral treatment. *Neuropsychopharmacology*. 2015;41(6):1629–1636.

79. Rawson RA, Chudzynski J, Mooney L. Impact of an exercise intervention on methamphetamine use outcomes post-residential treatment care. *Drug and Alcohol Dependence*. 2015;156:21–28.

80. Gates S, Smith LA, Foxcroft, DR. Auricular acupuncture for cocaine dependence. *Cochrane Database of Systematic Reviews*. 2006;1:CD005192.

81. Mills EJ, Wu P, Gagnier J, Ebbert JO. Efficacy of acupuncture for cocaine dependence: A systematic review & meta-analysis. *Harm Reduction Journal*. 2005;2(1):4.

82. Liang Y, Xu B, Zhang XC, et al. Comparative study on effects between electroacupuncture and auricular acupuncture for methamphetamine withdrawal syndrome. *Zhongguo Zhen Jiu = Chinese Acupuncture & Moxibustion*. 2014;34(3):219–224.

83. Salehi M. The efficacy of N-acetylcysteine in the treatment of methamphetamine dependence: a double-blind controlled, crossover study. *Archives of Iranian Medicine*. 2015;18(1):28.

84. LaRowe SD, Kalivas PW, Nicholas JS, Randall PK, Mardikian PN, Malcolm R. A double-blind placebo-controlled trial of N-acetylcysteine in the treatment of cocaine dependence. *American Journal on Addictions*. 2013;22(5):443–452.

85. LaRowe SD, Mardikian P, Malcolm R, et al. Safety and tolerability of N-acetylcysteine in cocaine-dependent individuals. *American Journal on Addictions*. 2006;15(1):105–110.

86. Reichel CM, Moussawi K, Do PH, Kalivas PW, See RE. Chronic N-acetylcysteine during abstinence or extinction after cocaine self-administration produces enduring reductions in drug seeking. *Journal of Pharmacology and Experimental Therapeutics*. 2011;337(2):487–493.

87. Protasio MI, da Silva JP, Arias-Carrión O, Nardi AE, Machado S, Cruz, MS. Repetitive transcranial magnetic stimulation to treat substance use disorders and compulsive behavior. *CNS & Neurological Disorders Drug Targets*. 2015;14(3):331–340.

88. Polti E, Fauci E, Santoro A, Smeraldi E. Daily sessions of transcranial magnetic stimulation to the left prefrontal cortex gradually reduce cocaine craving. *American Journal on Addictions*. 2008;17(4):345–346.

# 8

## Integrative Approach to Opiates, Opioids, and Opiate Use Disorder

### WALTER LING AND MATTHEW TORRINGTON

## Definition and History

Opiates are natural alkaloid compounds derived from the opium poppy *Papaver somniferum*. Opioids are chemicals or drugs that behave like opiates in the body. Opiates such as morphine and heroin are therefore opioids; however, not all opioids, like methadone, meperidine, and fentanyl, as well as the endogenous opioids endorphin and enkephalin, are opiates. In practice, the terms are used interchangeably, and people often use the term that sounds natural in the particular circumstance. All opioids, whether natural, synthetic, or semi-synthetic, bind to the opioid receptors and, depending on their intrinsic activity and strength of binding, produce results designating them as agonists, antagonists, or partial agonists. Opioid agonists produce effects roughly proportional to their doses; antagonists bind to the same receptors but produce no physiological effects and prevent, depending on the binding strength, other administered opioids from occupying the same receptors. Partial agonists, formerly known as mixed agonists/antagonists, such as buprenorphine and pentazocine, can act as agonists or antagonists depending on the level of background receptor opioid activities.[1,2] Partial agonists are largely employed therapeutically for their agonist properties. But their antagonistic properties can precipitate symptoms of opioid withdrawal in circumstances of high-background opioid activity: these symptoms could be triggered in individuals maintained, for example, on a high dose of an agonist such as methadone.[3]

The medicinal use of opiates to treat pain, coughs, and diarrhea dates back more than 5,000 years. Morphine remains one of the best painkillers available. Other principal effects of opioids are sedation, respiratory suppression (which could result in overdose deaths), and euphoria (which causes addiction). For several millennia, opiates were available as opium and in the form of other crude preparations made from the poppy. Morphine, named after the Greek god of dreams, Morpheus, was isolated from opium in 1805 and became widely popular. The invention of the hypodermic needle in 1853 allowed the drug to be injected directly into the circulatory system and heightened its use and abuse. The first opioid addiction epidemic in the United States occurred during the Civil War; so many soldiers had become addicted that morphine addiction was known as the "soldiers' disease."[4] The early attempts by medical professionals to cure morphine addiction largely failed and for the century that followed the civil war, opioid addiction had been largely regarded as a criminal matter and left in the hands of law enforcement.[5] The second opioid addiction epidemic can be dated to the Vietnam War when many soldiers returning from Vietnam were addicted to heroin.[6] This led to the introduction of the methadone maintenance, the current addiction treatment system, as well as the growth of the addiction treatment industry. The current prescription opioid addiction epidemic is thus, rightly, the third opioid addiction epidemic in the United States.[7]

## Some Specific Opioids

### MORPHINE

Morphine is the principal ingredient that accounts for the pharmacological effects of opium. Its mysterious power over pain extends beyond the reduction of pain perception and has a qualitative effect on the person's reaction to pain. Morphine reduces pain so that it is experienced in a less distressful way. This special characteristic makes morphine an excellent therapeutic agent in acute pain where the source of pain is obvious; caution is needed, however, where the cause is obscured, as in the case of acute abdominal pain, before the diagnosis is established because it effectively removes the protective function of acute pain. It also makes you wonder who decided to put endogenous morphine in our brain so long ago.

Morphine is well absorbed by all routes of administration, but because of the large first-pass effect, its bioavailability is low after ingestion. It is metabolized to morphine-3-glucuronide, with no analgesic properties, and to morphine-6-glucuronide, which produces greater analgesia and less respiratory suppression than the parent compound.[8]

Morphine is an alkaloid from the opium poppy that belongs to the class of phenanthrenes that also includes codeine and thebaine, from which we derive such products as hydromorphone (Dilaudid), hydrocodone (Vicodin), and oxycodone (OxyContin), all prototypic agents of morphine.[9]

## HYDROMORPHONE

Hydromorphone, a semi-synthetic morphine derivative marketed under the trade name Dilaudid, is considered to be a more potent opioid analgesic than morphine and is used to treat more severe pain. It is used mostly by intravenous injection because of its bioavailability by the oral route (8).

## HYDROCODONE

Hydrocodone (Vicodin) is a semi-synthetic derivative of codeine and bears a similar relationship to codeine as hydromorphone has to morphine. It is usually prescribed in combination with acetaminophen for treatment of minor pain. However, its abuse can lead to hepatotoxicity because of the large amount of acetaminophen in the combination prescription.[10]

## OXYCODONE

Oxycodone, a moderately potent semisynthetic opioid analgesic derived from thebaine, is pharmacologically similar to morphine. It is available as a monoproduct in immediate release and sustained release forms but is often combined with acetaminophen and non-steroidal anti-inflammatory medications such as aspirin and ibuprofen. Available in oral forms and prescribed for the treatment of moderate pain, it has been one of the most abused prescription drugs in recent years, especially in the controlled-release formulation, which prior to reformulation in 2014 could be easily crushed and administered intranasally or intravenously for a fast high. To serve as an abuse deterrent, naloxone has been incorporated into some of oxycodone formulations.

## CODEINE

Similar in structure and in clinical effects, codeine is morphine with a methyl substitution on the phenolic hydroxyl group. It is more lipophilic and crosses the blood-brain barrier faster than morphine; its pharmacological effects are due to the morphine produced by its metabolism. It is commonly used in low doses by oral administration for cough suppression and, combined with non-opioid analgesics, to treat mild to moderate pain; the rationale here is that the analgesia is summed, but the side effects are individualized. However, acetaminophen, frequently used in the combination, can cause liver toxicity in high doses.

Although codeine is commonly believed to be less potent—and therefore not as easily abused as morphine—at higher doses it acts much like morphine in both cases.

## MEPERIDINE

Meperidine (Demerol) is the first purely synthetic opioid of the phenylpiperidine class, which also includes fentanyl. It was once perhaps the mostly widely used opioid analgesic in hospital settings. Meperidine use has fallen out of favor in recent years in the United States because of seizures attributable to its metabolite nor-meperidine, and concerns about its drug/drug interaction with the monoamine oxidase inhibitor class of drugs resulting in toxicity—serotonin syndrome—characterized by agitation, and hyperthermia and other neurological manifestations (8).

## PENTAZOCINE

Pentazocine is one of the first "agonist-antagonist" medications; it is a weak antagonist or partial agonist at the mu receptor and also as a partial agonist at the kappa receptor. Pentazocine produces an analgesic "ceiling effect," but abuse of this drug threatened its availability on the market. It was eventually combined with naloxone to mitigate its intravenous abuse since the injection of this combination would precipitate opioid withdrawal in those with opioid dependence.

## HEROIN

Heroin, diacetylmorphine, was created by the English chemist Alder Wright in 1874 by boiling morphine with acetic anhydride in an attempt to find a less addictive form of morphine. It did not attract much interest until it was resynthesized by Felix Hoffmann at the Bayer pharmaceutical company in an attempt to synthesize codeine. Heroin is more potent than morphine because it is less water soluble and enters the brain, where it is converted to morphine more quickly. Bayer marketed it in 1898 as a non-addictive morphine substitute "heroin" and cough suppressant. It was believed then that heroin could be used to treat morphine addiction, which proved not to be the case. The head of Bayer supposedly named it "heroin," from the German *heroisch*, meaning "heroic" on account of the action of the employees who volunteered to test the drug. Today, heroin is the most abused opioid worldwide.[11]

## METHADONE

Synthesized by German scientists during World War II, methadone is a potent synthetic opioid with properties similar to those of morphine and was used extensively for the treatment of pain, especially cancer pain. Certain pharmacological properties make methadone useful in the treating of opioid addiction, including its rapid absorption after oral administration, how quickly it reaches an effective concentration in the body, and how much longer its effects last, continuing for many hours. Unlike heroin, which has to be taken by injection every few hours, methadone can be taken by mouth once daily. Methadone was introduced as a maintenance treatment for heroin addiction in the 1960s and has remained so to this day. More recently there has been a renewed interest in the use of methadone for chronic pain, in part because of its relatively low cost.

Methadone has a complex metabolism in individuals naïve to opioids as well as in those with prior opioid exposures, which alters the individual's sensitivity to methadone. Even in experienced hands methadone must be used with care and caution. The advice to "start low, and go slow" can literally be lifesaving.[12,13]

## LAAM

Levo-alpha-acetylmethadol (LAAM), often referred to as "long-acting methadone" (this is pharmacologically misleading but quite accurate in a clinical sense) by methadone users, is a synthetic congener of methadone. It is metabolized into two active metabolites: nor-LAAM and dinor-LAAM. Together with the parent compound, these combine to produce a prolonged clinical opioid effect lasting 48 hours and even longer, thus making possible a Monday, Wednesday, Friday dosing strategy. It was first studied in the 1970s and approved for treatment of opioid dependence by the US FDA in 1994, with a black-box warning for its potential to prolong QTc intervals that could lead to *torsade de pointes*. LAAM remains approved for clinical use but is not available because the manufacturer has stopped producing it.

## BUPRENORPHINE

Buprenorphine's discovery was the result of a systematic search for a non-addicting opioid to replace morphine. Although the quest to separate the painkilling properties of opioids from their addictive properties has yet to be realized, the availability of buprenorphine is by far the most significant life-changing event for the addicted individual since the introduction of methadone maintenance treatment a half century ago. First synthesized in 1963, buprenorphine is a potent analgesic that has been available worldwide for over forty years in injectable and tablet forms, although only the injectable form was marketed in the United States for use in post-surgical pain. Its use for treatment of opioid addiction has been a recent development.

Dr. Donald Jasinski in the 1970s reasoned that buprenorphine, having properties such as methadone and properties such as naltrexone might be effective in treating heroin addiction. He was right. And it took the entire 1980s and 1990s, and studies involving thousands of patients (plus an act of Congress), to finally make buprenorphine available. In 2002 it became available for patients in the United States suffering with opiate-use disorders.[14]

Buprenorphine's partial agonist properties confers a ceiling effect on respiratory suppression, sedation, and euphoria that makes it much safer than many other opiates. Buprenorphine's tight binding to opiate receptors gives it long duration of action. These properties provide buprenorphine a significant advantage over methadone and makes it possible to be prescribed by a qualified physician in the setting of her office practice, unlike methadone which has to be dispensed out of a highly regulated specially licensed clinic (i.e., opiate treatment program [OTP]).

The antagonist naloxone is incorporated into an additional formulation to help further reduce abuse liability, although it does not eliminate the abuse potential completely. Other recently FDA-approved formulations include a 6-month sustained release implant and novel sublingual delivery mechanisms for opiate dependence, as well as lower dose sublingual preparations and patches for the treatment of pain.

Most importantly, buprenorphine returns to the physician an effective tool to treat opioid addicted patients (like all other patients) in her usual practice environment; it also provides the physician opportunities to educate the community in the proper and humane relief of these patients' suffering.

## NALTREXONE

First synthesized in 1967, naltrexone has properties of a pure opioid antagonist (i.e., rapid onset of action like naloxone but with a long duration of action and oral bioavailability). It has relatively few side effects and was once regarded as an ideal medication for treating heroin addiction. A single 50 mg oral dose blocks the euphoric effect of 25 mg of injected heroin for 24 hours and at a 150 mg dose it can provide blockade for up to 72 hours. It can therefore be given 3 times a week. The rationale for the antagonist approach to treating opioid addiction was that by blocking the euphoric effects of opioids at the opioid receptors, opiate use would become less rewarding and in time, opiate users—animals and humans—would learn to stop.

Unfortunately, naltrexone's favorable pharmacological properties did not translate into clinical success. Unfortunately, medication compliance with naltrexone was so poor that the pharmacologically "perfect drug" was becoming a "victimless cure." Still, there were groups of patients—physicians, nurses, pharmacists, and lawyers who were under threat of losing their professional licenses—who did extremely well with naltrexone. Prisoners on work release and parolees also seemed to be successful. A common thread among these groups includes their having something to lose, the immediacy of the consequences of failure to comply with treatment, and (for the professionals at least) their knowledge that life could be different.

Naltrexone's lack of clinical success was due almost entirely to treatment nonadherence: patients simply were not willing to continue taking the medication. So investigators, policymakers, and funding agencies made concerted efforts to develop a long-acting depot naltrexone, with the first attempts dating back to the 1970s. It took nearly 30 years to get the first US Food and Drug Administration (FDA)—approved form of extended-release naltrexone to the market, with data provided from a study conducted in Russia.[15]

# Epidemiology

Globally, an estimated 69,000 people die from opioid overdoses each year. There are an estimated 15 million people who suffer from opioid use disorders (i.e., addiction to opioids). The majority of people dependent on opioids use illicitly cultivated and manufactured heroin, but an increasing proportion use prescription opioids.

Opiate prescription use disorder has become a problem of epidemic proportions in the United States, with 16,235 overdose deaths from prescription medications in 2013 and another 8,260 from heroin. Although Americans account for less than 5% of the world's population, they consume 80% of the manufactured global opioid supply, 99% of the global hydrocodone supply, and two-thirds of the world's illegal drugs.[16]

## GENETICS

The role of genetics in opiate dependence has been increasingly defined and understood in recent years. As with other substance-use disorders heritability is generally categorized with genetic factors, shared family environmental factors, and random or unique environmental factors. The work of Tsuang et al suggests that compared to other substances of abuse, opiate-use disorder may have a more significant genetic component. Tsuang's group conducted a twin study including 3,372 male twin pairs from the Vietnam Era Twin (VET) Registry, 1,874 of which were monozygotic (MZ) and 1,498 of which were dizygotic (DZ) and found independent models of drug abuse patterns illustrating that marijuana abuse was the only category to be influenced by family environmental factors and that heroin abuse had the largest contribution from specific genetic factors.[17,18]

This group also found heritable factors influencing the transition of users from experimental to occasional, to regular use of opiates. Current evidence suggests that genes related to dopamine, opiate receptors, and neurotrophic factors are most commonly associated with opiate dependence. Opioid dependence appears to be especially influenced by changes in the *DRD2*, *OPRM1*, *OPRD1*, and *BDNF* (19).

At this time no specific genetic testing appears to be the standard of care, but as more large-scale studies are conducted, the ability to identify specific genetic susceptibility may be elucidated.

## DETOXIFICATION AND WITHDRAWAL

While opioids induce a qualitatively unique type of analgesia in acute pain, what the user seeks is the state of euphoria: or that exaggeratedly carefree sense of well-being described as a "rush," or a "high" during acute intoxication. With repeated use, tolerance develops so that steadily increasing amounts of opioid are needed to produce the same euphoric effect. At the same time physical dependence also develops, manifested by the appearance of a specific abstinence syndrome and characterized by manifestations opposite of the acute effects of opioids. This occurs upon cessation of use or when precipitated by administration of an antagonist. Often unappreciated is that the effects sought and obtained by the user when using opioids—the rush and high—are psychological and emotional in nature; however, in abstinence the physical manifestations—nausea, vomiting, cramps, diarrhea—predominate. Acute intoxication can lead to death from acute respiratory depression, but it is the tolerance and dependence from chronic use that bring to medical attention the user. Detoxification is the most common treatment sought and offered in opioid addiction in the United States. Heroin used to be the root cause, but prescription opioids are now the most common.

Withdrawal symptoms appear at the "abrupt termination of opioid administration or administration of competitive opioid receptor antagonists, such as naloxone."

Intense preoccupation with obtaining opioids (craving) develops that often precedes the somatic signs of withdrawal, and this preoccupation is linked not only to stimuli associated with obtaining the drug but also to stimuli associated with withdrawal and internal and external states of stress. This combination of seeking reward, avoiding the aversive stimuli, and changes in cognitive function encourage the user to continue to obtain and use opioids despite sometimes disastrous consequences.

Opioid withdrawal symptoms include yawning, lacrimation, rhinorrhea, perspiration, gooseflesh, tremor, dilated pupils, anorexia, nausea, emesis, diarrhea, restlessness, insomnia, weight loss, dehydration, hyperglycemia, aches, and pains, flulike states, temperature and blood pressure elevations, fluctuations in pulse rate, and a dysphoric state accompanied by depressive and anxiety-like symptoms that do not meet the criteria for a major mental disorder.

Acute opioid withdrawal symptoms can be classified as purposive and nonpurposive symptoms. George Koob defined purposive symptoms as goal oriented, directed at getting more opioids, including complaints, pleas, demands, and manipulations and this type includes cravings or motivational symptoms.[19]

Motivational effects are affected by changes at the level of the ventral tegmental area and nucleus accumbens, where there also occurs a decrease in the firing of dopamine neurons, which may involve the increase of GABA and reduction of the release of glutamate. On the other hand, non-purposive symptoms are described as not goal oriented and are independent of the observer, the patient's will, and the environment; they are outward expressions of the internal reversal of neural adaptation brought about by repeated opioid exposure.

Symptoms of opioid withdrawal change as time increases from the last use. Purposive symptoms are present 6 to 8 hours after last use, peaking at 36 to 72 hours. Non-purposive symptoms become present at 8 to 12 hours are last use, peak at 36 to 48 hours, and continue until 72 hours. If the patient receives no treatment, the physical symptoms last up to 7 to 10 days. A user may also experience what is referred to as "protracted abstinence," which includes "signs of drug abstinence that persist after opioid withdrawal syndrome subsides. Metabolic changes have been reported during an even later stage of protracted abstinence, in which the direction of the changes is *opposite* of the acute signs of abstinence". All of the changes occurring within the body may be contributing to the decrease of the reward system and increase of the stress system activity of opioid dependence and allostatic molecular changes, thus driving craving during protracted abstinence. During abstinence it has been observed that patients struggle with greater sensitivity to pain. Each opioid demonstrates different withdrawal symptoms and time frames depending on its half life, dose, and the duration of exposure.

While the intensity of opioid withdrawal is a progressive syndrome related to the amount of opioids used and the time from the last use, many other things affect the manifestation of withdrawal symptoms. An appreciation of "the set and the setting" of the individual is important in managing patients in withdrawal. The surroundings, treatment settings, and the treating physician's attitude and confidence are all important in determining the intensity of the patient's withdrawal symptoms and ultimately the success of detoxification. Addicts in jails often show little withdrawal symptoms simply from the fear of being found out. An anxious physician is likely to have anxious patients and a calm and confident one likely to have patients who do well. While helpful, medications often play only a minor role. It is often assumed that addicts in withdrawal crave drugs because they cannot find them: this is wrong. Craving happens only when drugs are potentially obtainable. Many addicts in a lock-up facility will stop craving drugs when they discover that no one is smuggling drugs into the place, and drugs are simply unavailable.

## TREATMENT OF OPIATE-USE DISORDERS

The treatment of opiate-use disorders should be comprehensive, individualized, and multimodal. The more customized the combination of biological, psychological, social, spiritual, and nutritional interventions the more likely the treatment is to be successful. The preferences, experiences, and desires of the individual seeking treatment are essential elements in the development of a treatment plan. Treatment plans should be regularly updated and modified to best meet the temporal needs of the patient. Duration of treatment is crucial to successful outcomes in the treatment of opiate use disorders. Addiction *is* a disease characterized by relapse and length and intensity of treatment and should be tailored to meet the needs of each person seeking help.

## MEDICATIONS FOR DETOXIFICATION AND RELAPSE PREVENTION

Detoxification should not be just about quitting drugs; it should help the user stop the recurrence of drug memories that form the basis of the addict's belief system: a system that, in turn, drives the addicted behavior. Detoxification is not complete until the addict no longer thinks and acts like an addict, abstaining from drugs and living without them. Detoxification is rightly called "step one" in the long journey of recovery. A number of medications, including the full opioid agonist methadone, the partial agonist buprenorphine, and the antagonist naltrexone, all can play a role in detoxification and in relapse prevention.

## OPIOID FULL AND PARTIAL AGONISTS

Methadone is used for detoxification and for maintenance in the medication assisted treatment (MAT) of opiate-use disorder (OUD). Its use is regulated and limited to registered clinics. By definition, methadone detoxification means providing methadone in decreasing doses for a period no longer than 21 days. In practice, few patients successfully complete a 21-day detoxification program and remain drug free thereafter. As the doses of methadone decrease, withdrawal symptoms and craving can overwhelm patients within a matter of days leading to treatment drop out and relapse. The real benefit of methadone in treating opioid addiction lies in its use as a maintenance treatment agent. Patients maintained on methadone often decrease or eliminate the use of illicit opioids and achieve significant improvement in many areas of their lives including: enhanced employment status, decreased contraction of HIV and Hep C, and decreased incarceration rates. The main disadvantage of methadone is its highly regulated system of delivery that ties the patient to the clinic. Patients simply cannot get away. There is the general and genuine observation that patients who remain in treatment fare better than those who don't, and methadone treatment's high retention has been commonly cited as proof of methadone's advantage over other medications such as buprenorphine. That may not be so from the patient's perspective if freedom and pursuit of happiness are part of a good life.

Generally speaking, the long-term success of methadone treatment depends on an adequate dose and long duration of treatment. An adequate dose generally means somewhere between 80 mg to 120 mg/day. Lower doses of methadone can prevent emergence of withdrawal symptoms, and at higher doses (80 to 120 mg/d), methadone can produce a tolerance that blocks the opioid effects of exogenously administered opioids such as heroin, hydromorphone, and methadone, hence the term *agonist blockade*. The duration of methadone maintenance treatment should be years rather than weeks and months. Longer-term maintenance provides opportunity for psychosocial stabilization in the context of symptom relief. Common side effects of methadone maintenance treatment include constipation, excess sweating, drowsiness, and decreased sexual interest and performance. Other potential side effects include hypogonadism in men and minor risk of QT prolongation. After several months of methadone stabilization, normalization of stress hormone responses and reproductive functioning can result.

Buprenorphine, a μ-opioid partial agonist and κ-opioid antagonist originally marketed as an analgesic, is used for both detoxification and maintenance. Its major clinical advantage is its high pharmacological safety profile due to its ceiling effect on respiratory depression, sedation, and euphoria and its relatively long duration of action due to its tight receptor binding. It appears to have fewer subjective effects than morphine, a milder withdrawal syndrome, and an ability to block the subjective responses of up to 120 mg doses of morphine. It reduces craving and illicit opioid use, keeping patients in treatment. The sublingual version of buprenorphine is available in two "formulations": one containing only buprenorphine, the other containing buprenorphine and the opioid antagonist naloxone, at a 4:1 ratio. Other formulations are currently under development including 1-week and 1-month injectable forms of the drug as well as a 6-month sub-dermal implant, which was approved in May 2016.[20] Buprenorphine is the only medication available to physicians for use in their usual practice environment to treat opioid addiction that actually activates opiate receptors. Even so there are some specific training and prescribing requirements. As of 2014, there are around 24,000 physicians that can prescribe buprenorphine to treat opioid addiction in an office-based treatment. Each physician must complete an 8-hour continuing medical education course, notify the government of the intention to prescribe buprenorphine for the purposes of treating patients of opioid addiction, have the ability to refer patients for ancillary services, and track the number of patients they treat. Qualified physicians are orginally limited to treating 30 patients, then may seek an increase of their limit to 100 patients after 1 year. Recent legislation allows certain more highly qualified physicians to increase their limit to up to 275 patients (14).[21,22]

Naloxone is a "short-acting, parenterally administered full opioid antagonist medication used to counter the life-threatening depression of the central nervous and respiratory systems caused by opioid overdose". It has an affinity toward u-opioid receptors and antagonism of these receptors causes a reversal of opiate effect and a fast onset of withdrawal symptoms. Naloxone is a first-line therapy of paramedics and EMS providers for obtunded individuals; it has been distributed in "overdose prevention kits" at needle exchanges for more than a decade and has more recently been packaged and marketed for prevention of overdose in patients being prescribed powerful opiates for the treatment of pain. Naloxone is not used in routine opioid detoxification or relapse prevention.

Naltrexone hydrochloride is a competitive opioid antagonist that blocks opioid effects and will induce withdrawal symptoms in those with full opiate agonists on board for up to 24 hours. Naltrexone is long acting and effectively provides a blockade of the u-receptors when taken at least 3 times per week, for a total dose of 350 mg (100, 100, 150 mg). It is used as pharmacological intervention for those who have surpassed withdrawal and are maintaining abstinence. Naltrexone has a variable effect on craving. Some individuals report that cravings are neutralized since they know they "can't get high," but others do not experience this effect. When the drug is discontinued there are no withdrawal effects. Side effects of naltrexone can include gastrointestinal upset, headache, nausea, vomiting, and liver toxicity. An injectable extended release version of naltrexone, Vivitrol™, delivers a steady dose of naltrexone for 4 weeks. Side effects include nausea, vomiting, headache, dizziness, injection site reactions, and hepatic toxicity. After abstinence from opiates or exposure to opiate antagonists, an increased sensitivity of the opioid receptors can lead to an increased risk for potential overdose in the event of reexposure to full opiate agonists (9) (Table 8.1).

## Table 8.1  Withdrawal Effects

| Syndrome (Onset and Duration) | Characteristics |
| --- | --- |
| Anticipatory* (3–4 hrs. after last "fix") | Fear of withdrawal; anxiety; drug-seeking behavior |
| Early (8–10 hrs. after last "fix") | Anxiety; restlessness; yawning; nausea; sweating; nasal stuffiness; rhinorrhea (runny nose); lacrimation (teary eyes); dilated pupils; stomach cramps; drug-seeking behavior |
| Fully Developed (1–3 days after last "fix") | Severe anxiety; tremor; restlessness; piloerection (goosebumps)**; vomiting; diarrhea; muscle spasm***; muscle pain; hypertension(high blood pressure); tachycardia (rapid heartbeat); fever; chills; impulse-driven drug-seeking behavior |
| Protracted abstinence (indefinite duration) | Low blood pressure; bradycardia (slow heartbeat); insomnia; loss of energy; loss of appetite; opiate craving |

## RELAPSE PREVENTION—PSYCHOSOCIAL THERAPIES

Alan Leshner, former head of the National Institute of Drug Abuse, famously said that "addiction is not taking lots of drugs but taking drugs and acting like an addict." There is a huge difference between taking drugs (becoming addicted) and acting like an addict (being an addict). Becoming addicted has to do with what drugs do to the brain; being addicted, and thus acting like an addict, has to do with learning and memory—conditioning. By the same token detoxification should not just be getting rid of the drug effect; successful detox must include detoxing from what makes you act like an addict—that is, remembering drugs and thinking like an addict. You have not finished detox until you stop thinking and behaving like an addict, replacing the drug memories that form the foundation of addicted behavior. Without relapse prevention, detoxification, from hospitalization to incarceration, almost invariably leads to relapse. That is where maintenance pharmacotherapy and non-pharmacological therapies such as cognitive behavioral therapy, acupuncture, mindfulness training, nutrition, and exercise play a role.

Psychological and social therapies for opiate-use disorder are essential to ongoing recovery. All drugs and alcohol, but opiates especially, can be used as psychological "coping mechanisms." Using drugs or alcohol to deal with one's psychological or social problems, is like using a "shredder to deal with a credit card bill. . . your bill is gone, but your balance is just going to go up and up." The last definition in *Merriam-Webster*'s dictionary for opiates is "that which quiets uneasiness." Using opiates to quiet one's "dis-ease," sometimes for decades at a time, can leave psychological skills un- or under-developed. It is essential for individuals in early recovery to enhance their psychological coping skills. This can be accomplished with the forming and maintaining meaningful relationships, individual therapy, group therapy, cognitive behavioral therapy, motivational interviewing, and other forms of therapy. Engaging in the process of coping with all of the unprocessed emotional negativity of those "unpaid credit card bills" and getting used to dealing with new emotional stressors in real time without resorting to opiate or other substance use paves the way to successful recovery.

Group support, whether in the form of AA, Narcotics Anonymous, Heroin Anonymous, Smart Recovery, Rational Recovery, Alanon, Alateen, or Against the Stream can be life saving. People working together on a common goal are more powerful than individuals working alone. Although no one "flavor" of group support is going to be a treatment match for everyone, if individuals can find a suitable peer group in striving toward recovery, they can recieve great benefits. There also appears to be something helpful and protective about the process of going through the 12 steps with a sponsor and then helping someone else through the steps. Individuals can derive an array of different benefits from group support activities including but not limited to: fellowship, identification of non using peers, opportunities to be mentored, opportunities to mentor, opportunities to learn form others' experiences, opportunities to share one's own experiences, service opportunities, and opportunities to enhance a spiritual connection.

Acupuncture has been used as an adjunct treatment for opiate-use disorders. Standard and auricular acupuncture has been investigated for the amelioration of opiate withdrawal with mixed results. Auricular acupressure and self-stimulated auricular acupuncture have also been investigated. Although high-quality trials have yet to yield definitive results, there is basically "no downside" to acupuncture for the individual at any stage of treatment. It remains logical that acupuncture has the potential to benefit patients with opiate use disorder even more so than those in the population at large.

Take, for example, diet and nutrition, we are in the middle of a nutritional crisis; millions of American are overweight and there are almost endless television programs and books and magazines articles on weight loss and proper nutrition. It can be confusing. A lot of programs want to sell you something. Be careful. If something sounds too good to be true, it very likely is. Learn to differentiate facts from fads and fictions. Read up on the positives and negatives of anything pitched enthusiastically. Use common sense and seek advice from someone trustworthy. Believe it or not, you *are* what you eat; there is much truth in "healthy heart, healthy brain." It turns out that the gut has much to do with the brain, so "healthy gut, healthy brain" is true as well. The healthiest diet is the Mediterranean diet or Mediterranean Plus diet, which emphasizes fresh food, fruits, and vegetables.

High on the list of things to eat are olive oil (especially virgin olive oil), fruits, seeds and legumes, non-refined carbohydrates, fish such as wild salmon, milk, and other dairy products (in moderation), eggs, lean meat, and beans; nuts for snacks, 3–4 small cups of coffee per day, and dessert on occasions. Avoid what grandma would not recognize as food.

The discovery of gut bacteria, the microbiomes, informs us that what and how we eat make a difference in recovery because our gut affects our brain by influencing inflammation and the level of free radicals that are unhealthy for the brain. Antioxidants and probiotics can be helpful. Keep a balance with healthy gut, healthy brain, healthy mind, and healthy life. Avoid the metabolic syndrome: high blood pressure, high blood sugar, high triglycerides, unbalanced cholesterol— high LDL and low HDL, and too much fat around your waist. This and other topics are also covered elsewhere in this volume.

Exercise can be an essential element of recovery from opiate dependence. Other than the innumerous physiological benefits of moving one's body, exercise provides a meaningful source of dopamine release. The process of exercising, especially vigorously, can be thought of as the opposite of using drugs. When using, the individual "knows that it is bad for them, but it feels good and does it anyway." When exercising the individual "knows that it is good for them, but it feels bad and does it anyway." This dichotomy is further illustrated by the fact that using drugs produces a net harmful effect while exercise produces a net positive effect for the individual. Exercise may be impossible in the detoxification phase, but patients are encouraged to move their bodies as soon as they are able and to continue to exercise in a way palatable to them on a regular basis as they gain momentum in recovery.

## REFERENCES

1. Jaffe, JH Martin WR. Opiod analgesics and antagonists. In: Gilman, AG, Rall TW, Nies AS, Taylor P, eds. *The Pharmacological Basis of Therapeutics*. 8th ed. New York: Pergamon; 1990:485–521.
2. Ling W, Mooney L, Wu L. Advances in opioid antagonist treatment for opioid addiction. In: Danovitch I, Mariana J., eds. *Addiction. Psychiatric Clinics of North America*. Vol. 35. Philadelphia, PA: Elsevier; 2012:298–308.
3. Rosado J, Walsh SL, Bigelow GE, Strain EC. Sublingual Buprenorphine/Naloxone Precipitated Withdrawal in Subjects Maintained on 100 mg of Daily Methadone. *Drug and Alcohol Dependence*. 2007;90(2–3):261–269.
4. Ling W. A perspective on opioid pharmacotherapy: where we are and how we got here. *Journal of Neuroimmune Pharmacology: The Official Journal of the Society on Neuroimmune Pharmacology*. 2016;11(3):394–400.
5. McNamara, JD. Criminalization of Drug Use. *Psychiatric Times*. 2000;17(9):1–3.

6. Robins LN. *The Vietnam Drug User Returns. Final Report, September 1973: For Sale by Superintendent of Documents*. Washington, DC: US Government Printing Office; 1974.

7. White J. *Addiction Medicine: Science and Practice. Part 8: Opioids: Heroin and Prescription Drugs*. 2nd ed. New York: Springer-Verlag New York; 2010:1029–1048. *Opioids: Heroin and Prescription Drugs and it is in part 8 of the book without a chapter number.*

8. Jaffe JH. *One Bite of the Apple: Establishing the Special Action Office for Drug Abuse Prevention, One Hundred Years of Heroin*. Westport, VA: Auburn House; 2002:43–53.

9. Brands B, Blake J, Sproule B, Gourlay D, Busto U. Prescription Opioid Abuse in Patients Presenting for Methadone Maintenance Treatment. *Drug Alcohol Depend.* 2004;73(2):199–207.

10. Ling W, Rawson RA, Compton, MA. Substitution pharmacotherapies for opioid addiction: From methadone to LAAM and Buprenorphine. *Journal of Psychoactive Drugs.* 1994;26(2):119–128. doi:10.1080/02791072.1994.10472259.

11. Jasinski DR, Pevnick JS, Griffith JD. Human pharmacology and abuse potential of the analgesic buprenorphine: a potential agent for treating narcotic addiction. *Archives of General Psychiatry.* 1978;35(4):501–516.

12. Krupitsky E, Nunes EV, Ling W, Gastfriend, DR, Memisoglu A, Silverman BL. Injectable extended-release naltrexone (XR-NTX) for opioid dependence: Long-term safety and effectiveness. *Addiction.* 2013;108(9):1628–1637. doi:10.1111/add.12208.

13. Nowak BL. America's Pain Points. Web site. http://lab.express-scripts.com/lab/insights/drug-safety-and-abuse/americas-pain-points. Accessed February 14, 2017).

14. Tsuang MT, Lyons MJ, Meyer JM, et al. Co-occurrence of abuse of different drugs in men: the role of drug-specific and shared vulnerabilities. *Archives of General Psychiatry.* 1998;55(11):967–972.

15. Mistry C, Bawor M, Desai D, Marsh D, Samaan Z. Genetics of opioid dependence: A review of the genetic contribution to opioid dependence. *Current Psychiatry Reviews.* 2014;10(2):156–167.

16. Koob G, Arends MA, Moal ML. *Drugs, addiction, and the brain*. San Diego, CA: Academic Press; 2014.

17. *Follow FDA*. Web site http://www.fda.gov/NewsEvents/Newsroom/Press Announcements/ucm503719.htm. Accessed February 14, 2017.

18. 2016 Colleague Letter 275 Limit.

19. Volkow N. *America's Addiction to Opioids: Heroin and Prescription Drug Abuse*. Senate Caucus on International Narcotics Control. 2014. Available at: https://www.drugabuse.gov/about-nida/legislative-activities/testimony-to-congress/2016/fiscal-year-2017-budget-request Accessed February 2, 2017.

20. Stine S, Kosten T. *Addictions. A Comprehensive Guidebook, Opioids*. New York: Oxford University Press; 1999:141–161.

21. Ries RK, Miller SC, Saitz R, Fiellin DA. *The Asam Principles of Addiction Medicine*. 5th ed. Philadelphia: Lippincott Williams and Wilkins; 2014.
22. *2016 Colleague Letter 275 Limit*. https://www.samhsa.gov/sites/default/files/programs_campaigns/medication_assisted/dear_colleague_letters/2016-colleague-letter-275-limit.pdf. Accessed February 14, 2017
23. Ling W. Buprenorphine for opioid dependence. *Expert Review Neurother*. 2009;9(5):609–616

# 9

## Integrative Approach to Nicotine Use Disorder

### DAVID MARTARANO

## Introduction

Tobacco use is an insidious problem and arguably remains the most costly and deadly of addictions.[1] Fortunately, it is also among the most treatable, and treatment is cost effective in comparison to other addictive disorders and medical conditions. In terms of dollars per life saved, the estimated cost is less than $7,000 per life saved. This number is staggeringly inexpensive compared to the widely accepted minimum of $32,000 (in 1998 dollars) per year of life gained that pharmaceutical companies use as a baseline for developing new therapies.[2] Sixty-seven percent of people who wish to quit smoking are interested in alternative medicine as a means to stop.[3]

## Epidemiology

Data from 2013 indicate that 25.5% of the US population aged 12 and older currently use tobacco products, and 21.3% of those smoke cigarettes.[4] E-cigarette data are primarily from industry sources, indicating widespread adoption and significant growth. However, concerning the current statistics, and in terms of continued exposure, overall tobacco use in the United States is down 50% from 50 years ago and continues to decline.

Smoking and tobacco use are frequently comorbid with mental illness. Tobacco use is twice as prevalent in those who have mental illness when compared with the general population. That number doubles again, approaching 80% in persons who have another chemical dependency issue.[4]

Nearly 70% of all smokers report a desire to quit, and over half of those have tried to quit at least once in the past 12 months. Overall, only a small minority succeed, with only 6% of smokers quitting each year. From this data we can infer that 90% of the people who will try to quit smoking in the next 12 months, across all cessation modalities, will fail and revert to regular tobacco use.[4]

In adequately defining a tobacco-use disorder, any exposure to tobacco smoke is detrimental, and there are decades of research so compelling as to causality that the US surgeon general states, "Smoking causes 87 percent of lung cancer deaths, 32 percent of coronary heart disease deaths, and 79 percent of all cases of chronic obstructive pulmonary disease" and "smoking causes diabetes mellitus, rheumatoid arthritis and immune system weakness, increased risk for tuberculosis disease and death, ectopic (tubal) pregnancy and impaired fertility, cleft lip and cleft palates in babies of women who smoke during early pregnancy, erectile dysfunction, and age-related macular degeneration."[5]

From an epidemiological prospective, "Estimated economic costs attributable to smoking and exposure to tobacco smoke continue to increase and now approach $300 billion annually, with direct medical costs of at least $130 billion and productivity losses of more than $150 billion a year."[6]

The statistics on tobacco use are staggering. Twenty million smoking-related deaths in adults since 1964 have been those caused by a history of smoking. Also shocking and sad is that 2.5 million of those deaths have been among nonsmokers who died from diseases caused by exposure to secondhand smoke.

The numbers involving children and infants are sobering; 100,000 babies have died in the last 50 years from Sudden Infant Death Syndrome, complications from prematurity, complications from low birth weight, and other pregnancy problems resulting from parental smoking.[1]

Almost 50 studies have been conducted on SIDS and maternal smoking alone, and every one of them showed an increased risk for the infant of dying from the syndrome. Data suggest that infants of smoking mothers have 5 times the risk of dying from SIDS than infants with non-smoking mothers. When other factors such as bed sharing are introduced, the risk is greater still. It is not only mothers who put their babies at risk, however. Fathers and other household members who smoke near the infant put the baby in danger: although when these case studies adjusted for the mother being a nonsmoker, the risk that others introduce is less than that of the mother herself. Something to note is that it is difficult for any of these studies to distinguish between the risk of SIDS to smoking during pregnancy and the risk of SIDS to maternal smoking postpartum. Most mothers who smoke heavily during gestation do not quit smoking after the baby is born, and it is highly unlikely for a nonsmoking mother to take up smoking with an infant. It is believed that most of the deleterious effects of smoking occur in utero.[1]

1. Mitchell EA, Ford RPK, Stewart AW, et al. Smoking and the Sudden Infant Death Syndrome. *Pediatrics*. 1993;91:893–896.

Of those Americans today who are 18 years of age or younger, 5.6 million are projected to die prematurely from a smoking-related disease.[5] Nicotine has established mutagenic properties, both growth-promoting and anti-apoptotic, directly linking it to carcinogenesis.[7]

## Definition

"Tobacco Use Disorder" is comprehensively defined in *DSM-5*. Like all chemical dependencies, it is a "problematic" pattern of use. Many of the criteria that apply to other substance-use disorders are included in the definition, including interference with work or social function, arguments with family, among others.[8] In real-world practice, most medical professionals and all medical societies that comment on tobacco including the AMA, the APA, and the American Lung Association have published multiple public statements warning of the dangers of tobacco use and smoking. They also now issue cautionary statements about electronic cigarettes.

Nicotine is a tertiary amine found in tobacco and binds stereoselectively to nicotinic cholinergic receptors (nAChRs). When tobacco is ignited, nicotine evaporates and inhaled with smoke particles, where it is absorbed rapidly into the pulmonary venous circulation and quickly moving to the brain where it binds to nAChRs. Nicotine acutely increases activity in the prefrontal cortex, thalamus, and visual system. Stimulation of central nAChRs by nicotine results in the release of a variety of neurotransmitters in the brain, most importantly dopamine. Nicotine causes the release of dopamine in the mesolimbic area, the corpus striatum, and the frontal cortex.[9]

Each of the receptor subunits of nicotine is responsible for a different effect: the $\alpha 4$ is nicotine sensitivity, the $\beta 2$ subunit is reponsible for the behavioral effects of nicotine, the $\alpha 7$ subunit affects learning, and the a $\alpha 3 \beta 4$ subunit primarily dictates cardiovascular response. Nicotine is metabolized to cotinine and other compounds through CYP2A6 and has a 2-hour half-life.[9]

Nicotine addiction is one of the oldest and perhaps most challenging addictions to overcome. What makes nicotine so difficult to quit is the way it acts upon the central nervous system. Smoking tobacco stimulates the prefrontal cortex and nucleus accumbens, which are the reward areas of the brain. The semi-permanent neuroadaptations that occur from chronic use are exactly what make withdrawal symptoms so profound and the cravings so strong. The dip in activity of reward signals in the brain correlates directly to the craving levels during withdrawal.[9] Importantly, smokers manipulate the dose of nicotine in their blood on a puff-by-puff basis. Intake of nicotine during smoking depends on puff volume, depth of inhalation, the extent of dilution with room air, and the rate and intensity of puffing.

Electronic cigarettes, or e-cigarettes as they are called, are the latest trend in the tobacco product world. They have been marketed as definitively safer because they do not burn anything but rather heat up a solution that the user then inhales. This has quickly been proven to be a myth, as researchers are finding that these solutions carry toxic carcinogens, and an even more troubling fact is that there is not much information available as to what the toxins might be from product to product. As of March 2015, there is absolutely no oversight or regulation of e-cigarettes by the Food and Drug Administration. Advertising of these products is unregulated as well, and marketers tend to tout health benefits. One early study found that e-cigarettes (vaping) actually lead to substantially higher plasma levels of nicotine versus smoking. This was attributable to both the nicotine content of the liquid that was vaped and puff duration, which was significantly longer in the vaping group.[10]

As far as the notion that e-cigarettes appear to help a regular smoker transition from cigarettes, the American Lung Association's official website states: "The American Lung Association is troubled about unproven claims that e-cigarettes can be used to help smokers quit. The FDA's Center for Drug Evaluation and Research has not approved any e-cigarette as a safe and effective method to help smokers quit."[11]

In a contemporary review published by the University of California San Francisco's Dr. Stanton Glantz, it was concluded that e-cigarettes deliver large quantities of nanoparticles into the lungs, which can trigger inflammation. Inflammation is a proven link to heart disease, stroke, asthma, and diabetes. According to the American Lung Association, a nationwide study in 2014 found that teenagers' use of electronic cigarettes has now surpassed the use of traditional cigarettes, and the Centers of Disease Control report that the use of e-cigarettes among high schoolers increased 61% in just one year.[11]

Those with mental health and addiction disorders have higher rates of smoking, higher rates of tobacco dependence, and have a lower rate of quitting than the general population.[12] Moreover, "Current smoking rates are about twice as high among those with a current psychiatric disorder as among those with no psychiatric disorder."[13] Lifetime prevalence of tobacco-use disorders approaches 80% in people with another substance-use disorder.[14]

## Genetics

Epidemiological studies strongly suggest that genetic factors operate at all steps of addiction. The most recent studies on smoking and heredity show an unequivocal link between nicotine addiction and genetic predisposition. Proteins on a specific chromosome known to hold genes with nicotinic acetylcholine receptors, undergo biological changes that affect the body's susceptibility to disease. Moreover, variants in several genes, including aldehyde dehydrogenases, *GABRA2*, *ANKK1*, and Neurexins 1 and 3, have been associated with addictions to multiple drugs. Variants of the *CHRNA5–A3–B4* cluster on chromosome 15 were associated with addictions to tobacco, alcohol, and cocaine, as well as lung cancer.[15]

Nicotine dependence has an inverse relationship with metabolism. It is a widely known fact that people of certain genetic makeups struggle to tolerate alcohol because they are lacking the two key alcohol-metabolizing enzymes—alcohol dehydrogenase and aldehyde dehydrogenase. The lack of these enzymes directly influences the risk of alcohol dependence because they mediate the production of acetaldehyde, which is the toxic byproduct of alcohol metabolism that causes the adverse effects of alcohol consumption. What we find with nicotine addiction is that individuals who metabolize nicotine poorly actually have a decreased risk of dependence. With an increased availability of nicotine at the receptor, the overall tobacco usage over the course of a day goes down.

## Detox/Withdrawal

The withdrawal symptoms of nicotine are widely known by now: headaches, irritability, sleep disturbances, nausea, increased appetite, and intense cravings. These particular responses are likely to pass, peaking on day 3, and they disappear altogether within 2 to 3 weeks. However, there is one symptom that is largely overlooked and can have a lasting impact in the long term: depressed mood.

The benefits of smoking cessation begin with a drop in heart rate within 20 minutes of the last puff. The positive impacts of quitting quickly compound and are found to increase for the next 15 years after cessation of smoking. At year 15 the risk of coronary artery disease is equal to a non-smoker's. In that 15-year span a smoker can expect his/her lung cancer risk to drop, as well as the risk of stroke. Lung function will improve remarkably, and the risk of a heart attack is reduced significantly.

## Treatment

Before discussing each of the individual interventions, it seems worthwhile to give an overview of outcome data from one source. West provides such a meta-analysis, with Varenicline providing the best results as monotherapy with a 15% increase in abstinence at the 6- to 12-month intervals and printed self-help materials having the least impact at 2% increased abstinence rates in the same post-cessation attempt intervals.[16]

Level of readiness and motivation to quit provides improved adherence to any intervention and higher rates of abstinence; there is also evidence to support motivational interviewing as preparation for quitting.[13] Not surprisingly, smokers with comorbid mental illness were more likely to quit if they had received treatment in the last year.[17]

Finally, stress itself plays a significant role in abstinence. When both meditation practices and buproprion were studied as smoking cessation aids, decreases in perceived stress were felt to play a crucial role in smoking cessation.[18]

## Pharmacotherapy

Before delving into alternative approaches in supporting smoking cessation, it seems appropriate to review common pharmacotherapeutic options. Keep in mind that approving any patient for alternative medicine must involve reviewing all available options. Textbooks of addiction devote whole chapters to the pharcotherapeutic approach to smoking cessation, and such a review can be found in the American Society of Addiction Medicine's *Principle of Addiction Medicine*, 3rd edition.

Pharmacotherapy of addiction usually involved either substitution/harm reduction (agonists), or antagonism at one or more known receptors. The single most widely studied and used and generally regarded as the safest is nicotine replacement.[19] Although cigarettes contain up to 20 mg of nicotine each, absorption is affected by puff duration[10] but widely estimated at 1–2 mg per cigarette. Nicotine replacement therapy (NRT) is most commonly delivered transdermally in a 6-week taper from a starting dose of 21 mg per day (for 1-pack-per-day smokers) and decreasing at 2-week intervals by 7 mg every other week. Variations of nicotine replacement include oral (gum or lozenge) and inhaled (metered or e-cigarette).[20] There are validated applications of cotinine (a nicotine metabolite) level analysis to determine appropriate daily dosage; however, the additional complexity of this approach versus relying on patient report may only offer the benefit of predicting response to NRT based on pretreatment cotinine levels.[21]

Bupropion stimulates increased activity at dopamine and norepinephrine neurons, simulating the effects of nicotine on these neurotransmitters.[9] Bupropion also antagonizes nicotine receptor-activity, contributing to reduced reinforcement from smoking. Hence, buproprion therapy is initiated 2 weeks in advance of a planned quit date.[22]

Both buproprion and NRT nearly doubled the observed abstinence rate for people attempting to stop smoking; only varenicline is considered superior, achieving cessation rates nearly 50% higher than the other 2 established methods.[23] Varenicline has agonist activity at a wide range of neuronal nicotinic receptors ranging from partial to full agonist activity.[24] Variable activity, specifically partial agonism, is thought to lead to decreased reinforcement versus nicotine via decreased nicotinic-driven dopamine release.[25] However, increased efficacy comes at a price: although varenicline and buproprion were both issued FDA black box warnings in 2011 for neuropsychiatric side effects,[19] varenicline received an updated warning including a potential interaction with alcohol and possible seizure risk.[26]

Clonidine, a high-blood-pressure medication, has demonstrated efficacy in smoking cessation; however, it's probably best reserved for smokers with hypertension, as it has significant side effects including headache and postural hypotension.[27]

Nortriptyline has demonstrated efficacy versus placebo,[28] but a Cochrane review of over 900 patients across 20 studies found that the side effects of tricyclics and safety profile limits their viability in treating tobacco use disorders. Other compounds that have generally failed to demonstrate better results than placebo in the treatment of tobacco-use disorders include selective serotonin reuptake inhibitors.[29]

## Hypnosis

Of all the potential interventions for the management of tobacco-use disorders, none has gained more notoriety than hypnosis. Hypnosis relies on suggestion and is only thought to be effective in treating the highly suggestible portion of the population.[30] For example, Spiegel's method of self-hypnosis instructs patients to focus on the core principles:

1) smoking is a poison to your body;
2) you need your body to live;
3) to the extent that you want to live, you owe your body respect and protection

Uncontrolled studies claim that 45% of smokers were abstinent a year later. Unfortunately, no data exist on whether smokers have a greater probability of being "highly suggestible." The absence of this data and the failure of hypnosis studies to accurately assess this necessary precondition may be the hidden confounder that has resulted in the wild variability of smoking cessation rates in hypnosis studies.[31]

The definitive review of hypnosis in smoking was completed by Green and Lynn in 2000[32] and concluded that there was no appreciable difference in cessation rates through hypnosis versus other behavioral interventions. They attributed the failure to effectively demonstrate hypnosis as superior to 4 main flaws in the 59 studies they reviewed. They were as follows: failure to randomize, non-manualized treatment, small number of participants in individual studies, and poor screening and stratification of study participants.

The Green study limited itself to classic hypnotic interventions. When the search is expanded, more positive results can be found. Spiegel found that proper selection of self-hypnotizable candidates with strong social support (married) led to significantly improved results, a 23% reported abstinence rate at 2 years.[33]

## Acupuncture

Acupuncture has long been used to treat tobacco-use disorders. The efficacy of the treatment has been studied since the 1970s with highly variable outcomes. Almost all studies demonstrate significant, short-term, clinical responses. However, long-term efficacy (continued abstinence at 6 months) has been documented in few studies. At present, acupuncture has yet to gain widespread acceptance as a medical treatment for addiction. Experts believe that the quality of research is improving; but at present, acupuncture is considered to be only "potentially useful" by the most recent National Institute of Health consensus panel.[34]

The theory that acupuncture's role in suppressing the reinforcing effects of abused drugs takes place by modulating mesolimbic dopamine neurons is gaining increased acceptance. This is postulated to be a downstream effect of several afferent inputs including opioid, serotonin, and GABAergic pathways.[35]

Addiction to nicotine is believed to result from increased release of dopamine in the region of nucleus accumbens. Another study out of China reports that acupuncture significantly attenuated expected increase in nicotine-induced locomotor activity in the nucleus accumbens and striatum to subsequent nicotine challenge. Acupuncture is likewise felt to have both negative reinforcing via inhibition of Gabaergic interneurons with subsequent increase in VTA dopaminergic tone while simultaneously positively reinforcing through increased $GABA_b$ and subsequent decreases in nucleus accumbens dopaminergic tone.[36]

One single-blind controlled study found acupuncture to be as effective as nicotine replacement in decreasing smoking and maintaining abstinence at 6 months and included follow-up cotinine levels for validation of self-reported abstinence. However, even this study failed to achieve an acceptable P-value (with a final value of 0.055). Other concerning aspects of this study, as it is the most positive in a group of fairly marginal outcomes, is that it was single blind, and there was 0.0% abstinence rate in the placebo group, which is lower than the anticipated value for people receiving no treatment for smoking cessation.[37] Earlier, open studies compared acupuncture to nicotine replacement and found them to be equivalent.

A meta-analysis of acupuncture as a single modality for treating addiction clearly demonstrated no effect and highlighted poor quality of study design as a key factor.

Acupuncture may be an effective adjunct to an integrated smoking cessation program, but the procedure continues to offer limited promise as monotherapy capable of achieving long-term abstinence. However, compared with pharmaco-therapy, only varenicline is superior to the highest published results in treating tobacco-use disorders.

## Energy Healing

A pub-med review yielded no results for smoking cessation, nor tobacco use in combination with energy healing. A review of websites combining those terms searched through Google indicates that most practitioners of energy healing appear to be using some form of hypnotherapy for smoking cessation at this time.

It is unclear how the practice of energy healing may be beneficial in tobacco-use disorders and the absence of peer-reviewed literature on the practice in general (and more specifically on its efficacy for smoking cessation) may be warranted if practitioners wish to assert that its practice has purported benefits for the management of tobacco-use disorders.

## Yoga

Yoga has been perceived as having established health benefits that have been widely studied. That lens only recently turned toward tobacco cessation and early results are positive. A 2012 randomized, controlled, pilot study demonstrated significant decreases in tobacco use week post-yoga treatment Vinyasa Yoga, when combined with CBT appears to improve cessation rates significantly.[38] The study left many questions that the author hopes to address in the Breath Easy Trial (yoga and smoking cessation trial), which has been underway since 2014.[39]

Yoga is an all-encompassing term that covers a wide variety of practices, each of which would need to be studied individually in relation to determine dose, practice, and efficacy. Practitioners posit that Yoga provides numerous benefits and that specific poses can individually address unique pathologic processes. One of the ongoing challenges to Yoga as a wellness intervention is the heterogeneous nature of its practice. To simply state that the practice of yoga affects tobacco use is far too broad an assumption at this time.

# Diet

There are no studies on nutritional intake as a means to reduce smoking. There is a broad set of literature of varying quality on both the influence of smoking on caloric intake and on how the use of tobacco may alter plasma nutrient levels.

# Herbs and Supplements

Tobacco itself can be classified as an herb; one herb widely studied for its nicotinic activity is *Lobelia inflata*, specifically its alkaloid. Lobeline, a standardized derivative, failed to separate from placebo in clinical trials.[40] At present there appear to be no data to support the use of any herb in the treatment of tobacco-use disorders.

# Vaccination

While only in phase IV clinical trials, nicotine vaccination was thought to be a promising treatment to reduce smoking behaviors and the harmful consequences of nicotine exposure.[9] However, data thus far related to NicVax are not compelling with no separation from controls at 12 months in terms of tobacco consumption. Notably, higher antibody levels were associated with decreased nicotine consumption.[41] Of note, nicotine does reach the brain when it is released from antibody sequestration, but levels are substantially reduced.[42]

# Combined Treatment

Despite an overwhelming number of studies, combined treatment studies have been limited in their impact by their design. Most are naturalistic, have relied on self-reporting, and (if they included psychotherapies) have varied in their applications of psychotherapy complicating effective meta-analysis. However, a 1999 study clearly demonstrated that Wellbutrin, combined with nicotine replacement, was more effective than either of the 2 agents alone, offering greater than 22% abstinence rates at one year.[43]

## REFERENCES

1. Rehm J, Baliunas, D, Brochu, S. *The Costs of Substance Abuse in Canada.* Canadian Centre on Substance Abuse; Ottawa, Ontario: 2006.

2. Owens, DK. Interpretation of cost-effectiveness analyses. *Journal of General Internal Medicine*. 1998;13:716–717.

3. Carim-Todd L, Mitchell SH, Oken BS. Mind-body practices: an alternative, drug-free treatment for smoking cessation? A systematic review of the literature. *Journal of Drug and Alcohol Dependence*. 2004;132;399–410.

4. Substance Abuse and Mental Health Services Administration. *Decline in Tobacco Use Over Fifty Year Period*. Center for Behavioral Health Statistics and Quality; Rockville, Maryland: 2013.

5. States, SGU. The Health Consequences of Smoking—50-years-of-progress: A Report of the Surgeon General. Surgeongeneral.gov. 2012. http://www.surgeongeneral.gov/library/reports/50-years-of-progress/fact-sheet.html. Accessed January 15, 2016.

6. C. f. B. H. S. a. Q. The National Survey on Drug Use and Health Report: Smoking and Mental Illness. 2013. Web site. http://archive.samhsa.gov/data/2k13/NSDUH093/sr093-smoking-mental-illness.htm. Accessed October 12, 2015.

7. Grando SA. *Connections of Nicotine to Cancer*. London: Macmillan. *Nature Reviews*. 2014;(14):419–429.

8. American Psychiatric Association, *DSM-5* Task Force. *Diagnostic and Statistical Manual of Mental Disorders: DSM-5* (5th ed.). Washington, DC: American Psychiatric Association; 2013.

9. Benowitz NL. Pharmacology of nicotine: addiction, smoking-induced disease, and therapeutics. *Annual Revue Pharmacological Toxicology*. 2009;49:57–71.

10. Farsalinos KE, Spyrou A, Tsimopoulou K, Stefopoulos C, Romagna G, Voudris V. Nicotine absorption from electronic cigarette use: comparison between first and new-generation devices. *Scientific Reports*. 2014;4:4133.

11. American Lung Association. Statement on E-Cigarettes. Web site. http://www.lung.org/our-initiatives/tobacco/oversight-and-regulation/statement-on-e-cigarettes.html. Accessed on April 30, 2016.

12. Mackowick KM, Lynch MJ, Weinberger AH, et al. Treatment of tobacco dependence in people with mental health and addictive disorders. *Current Psychiatry Reports*. 2012;14:478–485.

13. Ziedonis D, Hitsman B, Beckham JC, Zvolensky M, et al. Review: Tobacco use and cessation in psychiatric disorders: National Institute of Mental Health report. *Nicotine & Tobacco Research*. 2008;10:1691–1715.

14. Kalman D, Morissette SB, George, TP. Co-morbidity of smoking in patients with psychiatric and substance use disorders. *American Journal on Addictions*. 2005;14:106–123.

15. Li MD, Burmeister M. New insights into the genetics of addiction. *Nature Reviews*. 2009;10:225–231.

16. West R, Raw M, McNeill A, Stead L, et al. Health-care interventions to promote and assist tobacco cessation: a review of efficacy, effectiveness and affordability for use in national guideline development. *Addiction*. 2015;110:1388–1403.

17. Lê Cook B, Wayne GF, Kafali EN, et al. *Trends in Smoking Among Adults With Mental Illness and Association Between Mental Health Treatment and Smoking Cessation*. *JAMA*. 2014 Jan 8;311(2):172–182.

18. Piper M, McCarthy D, Federman EB. Using mediational models to explore the nature of tobacco motivation and tobacco treatment effects. *Journal of Abnormal Psychology.* 2008;117:94–105.

19. FDA. *FDA Drug Safety Communication: Safety review update of Chantix (varenicline) and risk of neuropsychiatric adverse events.* Washington, DC: FDA; 2011.

20. Stead LF, Perera R, Bullen C, Mant D, et al. *Nicotine replacement therapy for smoking cessation.* Hoboken, NJ: John Wiley; 2012.

21. Paoletti P, Fornai E, Maggiorelli F, Puntoni R, et al. Importance of baseline cotinine plasma values in smoking cessation: results from a double blind study with nicotine patch. *European Respiratory Journal.* 1996;(9):643–651.

22. Nicoderm CQ. Physicians Desk Reference Online. *PDR.NET.* Web site. http://www.pdr.net/drug-summary/NicoDerm-CQ-nicotine-1643. Accessed May 15, 2016.

23. Cahill K, Stevens S, Perera R, Lancaster T. *Pharmacological Interventions for Smoking Cessation: An Overview and Network Meta-analysis:* Hoboken, NJ: John Wiley; 2015.

24. Mihalak KB, Carroll FI, Luetje CW. Varenicline is a partial agonist at α4β2 and a full agonist at α7 neuronal nicotinic receptors. *Molecular Pharmacology.* 2009;70:801–805.

25. Elrashidi MY, Ebbert JO. Emerging drugs for the treatment of tobacco dependence: 2014 update. *Expert Opinion on Emerging Drugs.* 2014;19:243–260.

26. FDA. *FDA Drug Safety Communication: FDA Updates Label for Stop Smoking Drug Chantix (Varenicline) to Include Potential Alcohol Interaction, Rare Risk of Seizures, and Studies of Side Effects on Mood, Behavior, or Thinking.* Washington, DC: FDA; 2015.

27. Glassman AH, Stetner F, Walsh BT, Raizman PS, et al. Heavy smokers, smoking cessation, and clonidine. *JAMA.* 1988;259:2863–2866.

28. Prochazka AV, Weaver MJ, Keller RT, Fryer GE, et al. A randomized trial of nortriptyline for smoking cessation. *Achives of Internal Medicine.* 1998;158:2035–2039.

29. Hughes JR, Stead LF, Lancaster T. *Antidepressants for smoking cessation.* Cochrane Database of Systematic Reviews. Hoboken, NJ: Wiley; 2014.

30. Milling LS. Is high hypnotic suggestibility necessary for successful hypnotic pain intervention? *Current Pain Headache Reports.* 2008;12:98–102.

31. Covino NA, Bottari M. Hypnosis, behavioral theory, and smoking cessation. *Journal of Dental Education.* 2001;65:340–347.

32. Green JP, Lynn SJ. Hypnosis and suggestion-based approaches to smoking cessation: an examination of the evidence. *International Journal of Clinical Experimental Hypnosis.* 2000;48:195–224.

33. Spiegel D, Frischholz EJ, Fleiss JL, Spiegel H. Predictors of smoking abstinence following a single-session restructuring intervention with self-hypnosis. *American Journal of Psychiatry.* 1993;150:1090–1097.

34. Sierpina VS, Frenkel MA. Acupuncture: A clinical review. *Southern Medical Journal.* 2005;98:330–337.

35. Yang CH, Lee BH, Sohn, SH. A possible mechanism underlying the effectiveness of acupuncture in the treatment of drug addiction. *Evidence Based Complementary Alternative Medicine.* 2008;5:257–266.

36. Chae Y, Yang CH, Kwon YK, et al. Acupuncture attenuates repeated nicotine-induced behavioral sensitization and c-Fos expression in the nucleus accumbens and striatum of the rat. *Neurosci Letters.* 2004;358:87–90.
37. Waite NR, Clough JB. A single-blind, placebo-controlled trial of a simple acupuncture treatment in the cessation of smoking. *British Journal of General Practice.* 1998;48:1487–1490.
38. Bock BC, Fava JL, Gaskins R, Morrow KM, Williams DM, et al. Yoga as a Complementary Treatment for Smoking Cessation in Women. *Journal of Women's Health.* 2012;21(2):240–248. http://doi.org/10.1089/jwh.2011.2963
39. Bock BC, Rosen RK, Fava JL, Gaskins RB, Jennings, et al. Testing the efficacy of Yoga as a Complementary Therapy for Smoking Cessation: Design and Methods of the *BreathEasy* trial. *Contemporary Clinical Trials.* 2014;38(2):321–332.
40. Glover ED, Rath JM, Sharma E, Glover PN, et al. A multicenter Phase 3 trial of lobeline sulfate for smoking cessation. *American Journal of Health Behavior.* 2010;34:101–109.
41. Hartmann-Boyce J, et al. *Nicotine Vaccines for Smoking Cessation. Cochrane Database of Systematic Reviews.* 2012 Aug 15;(8).
42. Cerny EH, Cerny T. Vaccines against nicotine. *Human Vaccines.* 2009;5:200–205.
43. Jorenby DE, Leischow SJ, Nides MA, Rennard SI, et al. A controlled trial of sustained-release bupropion, a nicotine patch, or both for smoking cessation. *New England Journal of Medicine.* 1999;340:685–691.

# 10

## Integrative Approach to Behavioral Addictions: Internet Gaming Disorder (IGD) and Compulsive Buying Disorder (CBD) and Gambling Disorder

MEREDITH SAGAN AND TIMOTHY FONG

In recent years, there has been a growing awareness and concern regarding "behavioral addictions" defined as the compulsive performance of activities including gambling, sex, use of the Internet and online video games, and shopping. There is much debate over how to classify many of the behavioral addictions (also called "process addictions" or "impulsive-compulsive behaviors"). The *DSM-5* lists the behavioral addictions under the heading "Impulse Control Disorders." This includes illnesses such as pathological gambling and trichotillomania. It does not include compulsive buying disorder, sexual addiction (or "hypersexual disorder"), or Internet/video-game addiction. These disorders have no precise definition in the *DSM-5* and are listed in the broad diagnostic category: impulse control disorder, "not elsewhere classified."

This does not mean, however, that there is not a shared neurobiological mechanism to their underpinning or that the consequences are less severe. The line between behavior as part of normal life and that of addiction can be less concrete in the behavioral addictions. Thus, researchers are trying to collect more data to help identify when a true process addiction has developed without over-diagnosing what is normal behavior. For example, neuro-imaging studies have shown that the act of shopping activates similar brain regions as do drugs of abuse, increasing the signal areas of reward circuitry known as the meso-cortico limbic system and ventral tegmental areas of the brain. This means that the act of shopping leads to increased levels of the brain's pleasure neurotransmitters dopamine, serotonin, and the endorphin system.[1] Additionally, medications that treat Parkinson's and restless leg syndrome and that increase dopamine in the brain have proven to instigate compulsive buying. As with drug users, behavioral addictions also gradually build up a tolerance to their neurochemical response over time, meaning that they have to do the activity more often and/or at a higher level of engagement in order to get the same rush as they did at the beginning. In addition, the dopamine high they get from their behavioral addictions (much like the high people get from using drugs) makes users feel that the rest of their lives are comparatively boring and unstimulating. As a result, behavior addicts tend to lose interest in activities outside of their addictions.

As with any chemical dependence, behavioral addictions can be triggered by cues and memories that help form a habit.[2] Furthermore, if and when they eventually choose to give up the activity, behavioral addicts report suffering from withdrawal symptoms that may be intense and similar to those felt by substance abusers when quitting drugs.

Of course, behaviors such as shopping, online gaming, and spending time on social media sites such as Facebook and Tumblr may be completely innocuous. These activities occur as a normal part of most people's everyday lives. It is only when performing the behavior spirals out of control and begins to negatively impact an individual's life that the activities may be labeled pathological in nature.

Generally speaking, Internet gaming disorder (IGD) and compulsive buying disorder (CBD) are diagnosed as such only when the individuals performing them:[3]

a. Feel they can't control themselves, even in the face of negative consequences to their actions, such as loss of a job, a relationship, or their health.
b. Experience a lack of pleasure in daily activities due to the dopamine insensitivity caused by their behaviors.
c. Show striking, extreme responses to external cues that trigger the behavior, such as an inability to leave the computer for 12 hours at a time despite being hungry, needing to use the bathroom, and loss of sensation in the legs.
d. Demonstrate both cravings for and withdrawals from the behaviors, which are quite similar to the cravings and withdrawals felt with substance addictions.

## Internet Gaming Disorder (IGD)

As recently as 2009, many scientists were still not convinced that people could be addicted to the Internet. Excessive online gaming, they argued, was merely a symptom of depression. The government of China, on the other hand, declared Internet addiction a national epidemic as early as 2004 and began running treatment centers, which thousands of people have since attended.[4]

At the same time, excessive time spent playing video games should not be confused with an actual gaming addiction. Psychologists point out that some people can play games for up to 14 hours a day without exhibiting any of the criteria for diagnosis with a full-blown addiction.[5]

Many experts have argued over the past decade that Internet Gaming Disorder (IGD) should be listed in the *DSM*, the book that highlights psychological disorders and their diagnoses. As of 2013, IGD is included in the *DSM-5* as "a condition warranting more clinical research and experience before it might be considered for inclusion in the main book as a formal disorder."[6]

The following criteria must be met for diagnosis with IGD:[7]

- preoccupation with Internet games
- withdrawal symptoms when Internet gaming is discontinued
- tolerance, the increasing need to spend more time engaged with gaming
- unsuccessful attempts to control Internet gaming
- loss of interest in other hobbies and entertainment
- continued excessive use of Internet games despite knowledge of psychosocial problems
- deception of family, therapists or others regarding Internet gaming
- use of Internet gaming to escape or relieve a negative mood
- loss of significant relationship, career, education or job opportunity due to Internet gaming

In addition to the symptoms listed above, Internet addicts tend to lack interpersonal social skills, having spent a majority of their time socializing online and building many of their closest friendships through chat rooms. They therefore need to learn techniques for dealing with other people face-to-face. Psychologist Larry Rosen has argued that lack of socialization and too much "screen time" among the Internet generation has, in fact, led to increasing rates of personality disorders including antisocialism and narcissism,[8] and others suggest it may be the reason for increasing rates of autism.[9]

The prevalence of IGD is unknown, but several studies suggest that approximately 1 in 10 gamers suffer from the disorder. Out of 7,000 gamers surveyed in the United Kingdom, 12% were found to have an addiction.[10] A US study estimated up to 10–15% of gamers could be addicted.[11] Spekman (2013) found a rate ranging from 9% to 14% based on problematic MAC-R (MacAndrew Alcoholism Scale-Revised) levels.[12] The overwhelming majority of gamers are young men, though women and people of all ages can experience addiction to the Internet.

There are strong similarities between IGD and gambling addiction. Therefore, similar treatment approaches may be used for both disorders.[13] CBT has been used effectively in studies, as well as multimodal counseling, reality therapy, and online self-help.[14] IGD may also be treated with the 12-step method employed originally by AA.

At some Internet gaming treatment programs, patients begin treatment with a technology detox. They are not permitted to use cell phones, computers, tablets, or any device connected to the Internet. They are asked to make phone calls on an old-fashioned payphone and read actual print books. They attend CBT, group sessions, and meditation lessons.[15]

One element that makes treatment of IGD unique is that many of the addicts are young people who have spent so much time in front of computers and other electronic devices growing up that they missed out on learning basic life skills such as doing housework, driving, and cooking. At most treatment programs, all patients must perform daily chores. Furthermore, since most Internet addicts have spent little time outdoors, patients are encouraged to participate in sports and out-door activities such as hiking.

In general, more research into pharmacological as well as alternative treatments of IGD is needed. As far as medical interventions, Bupropion or methylphenidate are medications used to treat IGD among adolescents.[16]

The supplement N-acetylcysteine (NAC), which comes from the amino acid L-cysteine, is an antioxidant sold over the counter in most health food stores. It has shown promise in treating several psychiatric disorders, including substance addiction, and obsessive-compulsive disorder (OCD). In a randomized, placebo-controlled clinical trial of NAC for gambling addiction, 83% of those treated showed significant reductions in their compulsive behavior.[17] This study suggests that NAC may prove a useful treatment for IGD.

Acupuncture may also be an effective intervention for IGD. In a clinical trial of 38 patients in China treated with acupuncture and psychological counseling, 27 were cured, showing an effectiveness rate of over 86%. Results were attributed to the known ability of acupuncture to calm the mind, thereby relieving the anxiety and stress of withdrawal from Internet gaming.[18]

## Compulsive Buying Disorder (CBD)

In an effort to define process addictions, outside researchers are developing valid diagnostic criteria and scales to help identify these patients. McElroy and others have designed criteria for compulsive buying to include:[19]

1. frequent preoccupation with shopping or intrusive, irresistible, "senseless" buying impulses
2. clearly buying more than is needed or can be afforded
3. distress related buying behavior

4. significant interference with work or social functioning
5. not due to hypomania/mania in bipolar disorder

The true costs of this behavior are unknown at this time because longitudinal research to this effect is not available. However, compulsive buyers are often overspending, and this can lead to substantial legal and financial distress, as well as being destructive to personal relationships. Many have credit card debt they cannot afford to pay and must file for bankruptcy or live under tremendous financial strain. Others are spending money on unneeded objects meant for their family's care resulting in chaos and mistrust between the family and the CB. Many times, CB do not even wear or use the clothes/objects they purchased, and the objects/clothes go unused for years, while the CB has a mounting financial burden.

It is important for providers not to confuse the CB sometimes exhibited by people suffering from bipolar disorder during manic or hypomanic episodes with CBD. People may also spend excessively due to the impact of medications, as revenge on ex-spouses, or for a temporary mood boost. These situations do not meet criteria for CBD.

Prevalence by gender is unclear. One study found a 9 to 1 female-to-male ratio, while another found nearly equal levels of CBD across genders (5.5% male to 6.0% female).[20] Currently, there is no evidence that CBD has become more prevalent in the past few decades. The age of onset of CBD appears to be 18 to 30 years old and a greater proportion of these people report incomes under $50,000. There are often psychiatric co-morbid disorders such as substance abuse, eating disorders, and mood disorders. Some studies suggest nearly 60% meet criteria for at least one personality disorder.

There is some evidence that CBD runs in families and that within these families mood, anxiety, and SUDs are excessive. McElroy et al reported that out of 18 individuals with CBD, 17 had 1 or more first-degree relatives (FDRs) with major depression, 11 with an alcohol or drug use disorder, and 3 with an anxiety disorder. Three had relatives with CBD.[21]

Due to its lack of official recognition as a psychological disorder, there are no established treatments for CBD. However, some small studies point to potentially beneficial interventions. CBD is considered similar to OCD and impulse disorders, and impacts the brain's dopamine centers in a manner that is similar to substance addiction. Therefore, treatments for OCD and substance abuse may also prove helpful for compulsive buyers.

The high incidence of comorbidity with mood disorders makes it difficult to discern how effective the pharmacological treatment of CBD might be.[22] There is some evidence that SSRIs may help. Medications for compulsive buying showed that fluvoxamine and citalopram had high placebo response rates that suggest a limited benefit since those receiving the sugar pill also improved.[23] The opiate blocker, naltrexone, was also shown in 4 case reports to help reduce compulsive buying at doses much higher doses than normally used (100–200 mg).

Furthermore, there are no published reports describing psychotherapy-focused interventions for compulsive buying disorder. Preliminary findings suggest that CBT may have promising effects.[24] In a small study with 28 women, those treated with CBT saw improvement, and some did not experience any recurring symptoms of CBD.[25] A team meta-analysis found no results for reducing compulsive buying behavior with psychoanalysis, some improvements with medication, and the most benefits with CBT.[26]

In several small trials, group CBT has reduced CB behavior, with positive results maintained for a period over 6 months.[27] Also, one clinical trial that combined psychotherapy and CBT with motivational interviewing, acceptance and commitment therapy, and mindfulness as a treatment for compulsive buying showed "much promise."[28]

In order to avoid CBD evolving in the first place, psychologists suggest that parents serve as examples of responsible buying behavior for their children. They can reduce emphasis on consumerism by not rewarding their children with "things."[29]

## Gambling Disorder

Gambling can be defined as wagering a valuable item (usually money) on the outcome of an event decided by chance in the hopes of winning a reward or prize. It is a behavior that has been part of the human condition for thousands of years, and evidence of this can be found in mankind's earliest drawings and writings. Today, gambling is widely available in many different formats and has become part of the economic, social, and cultural fabric. Approximately 65% of the general population reported placing a wager, legally or illegally, in the previous 12 months.[30] Since the mid-1990s, legal gambling revenue annually exceeds the combined earnings from all other forms of entertainment combined.

The vast majority of people who gamble regularly do so without incurring long-lasting harm or adverse consequences. For this segment of the population, gambling is social, recreational, no matter the cost or time spent. In comparison, nearly 4% of the general population currently meets criteria for gambling disorder, formerly known as gambling addiction, compulsive gambling, or pathological gambling.[31] Those with gambling disorder are at increased risk to experience financial problems (e.g., bankruptcy, lost job, sizeable debt), legal problems (e.g., crime, arrests), relational problems (e.g., divorce, domestic violence, child abuse), and health problems (e.g., increased stress, sleep disturbances).[32] In addition, these individuals have dramatically higher rates of suicide attempts and completions. One study found that 81% of pathological gamblers in treatment showed some suicidal ideation, and 30% reported one or more suicide attempts in the preceding 12 months.[33] Epidemiological studies, national and locally, have documented that the groups most vulnerable to a gambling disorder are minority groups (African American, Asian American, Hispanic), the disabled, and adolescents and the elderly.[34,35]

Gambling addiction was first recognized as a psychiatric condition in the *DSM-3* and was categorized within the Impulse Control Disorders section under "pathological gambling." Over the ensuing years, research and discussion followed to better characterize this condition as either an addiction, an anxiety disorder, an impulse control disorder, or something in between.[36] In the current *DSM-5*, pathological gambling is categorized as an addictive disorder and places it under a new name: "gambling disorder."[37] This marks a substantial change from previous versions of the *DSM*, cementing gambling disorder as the only recognized behavioral addiction. The 9 *DSM-5* criteria for gambling disorder represent the most common symptoms experienced by those with gambling problems. These symptoms characterize 3 heterogeneous dimensions related to gambling disorder: damage or disruption, loss of control, and dependence. The loss of control over urges and behaviors may be the central component of gambling disorders, and the ability to control gambling may be a component of a progressively worsening process in the life span of some gamblers.

Although there are no substances ingested, the act of gambling has been shown to impact and affect levels of natural neurochemicals, chiefly dopamine, norepinephrine, cortisol, and serotonin.[38] Dopamine is released in the brain, in the same regions as alcohol and drugs of abuse, in response to situations where the prospects of obtaining a reward (increased attention and motivation) and also at earning/winning a reward (experiencing pleasure)[39] are greater. Evidence exists to show that persons with gambling disorder have alterations in functioning in all of these neurotransmitter systems, raising the question of how these changes and alterations occur in the first place. Because there are no objective measures of gambling behaviors, excessive gambling seen in gambling disorder has been termed a truly "hidden addiction" in that the consequences of gambling are felt but cannot be easily detected by observation alone.

## ESTABLISHING THE DIAGNOSIS OF GAMBLING DISORDER

Diagnostic interviews using *DSM-5* criteria allow clinicians to differentiate recreational gambling from gambling disorder. Gambling behavior that arises secondary to dopamine agonists or gambling that occurs during the course of a manic episode must be ruled out, as they are not considered primary gambling disorder. Severity of gambling disorder is established in terms of number of *DSM-5* criteria met: mild gambling disorder is equivalent to having 1 to 3 criteria met (also known as "problem gambling"), moderate gambling disorder is 4 to 5 criteria met, and severe gambling disorder is 6 or more criteria met. During the diagnostic interview and assessment, clinicians should focus on obtaining information about the client's gambling behavior including how often (frequency), how long (duration), and how much (amount) they gamble relative to what they can afford to lose.

## Treatment for Gambling Disorder

Treatment for gambling disorder, like all addictive disorders, is best approached with a biopsychosocial treatment approach with an integrated team creating an individualized treatment plan. Treatment principles for gambling disorder are similar to treatment principles used for SUDs, principally focusing on engaging the client in a lifestyle of recovery and self-care focusing on managing stress, increasing physical activity, raising social capital, maintaining healthy sleep hygiene, and adding structure and purpose.[40]

### BIOLOGICAL TREATMENT APPROACHES

There are no FDA-approved medications for the treatment of gambling disorders. Several medications that are used for other addictive disorders have been examined for gambling disorders. The largest body of evidence supports the use of opioid antagonists (like naltrexone) to reduce the urges, cravings, and preoccupation experienced by those with gambling disorder.[41] Medications from several different classes including antidepressants (SSRIs, bupropion), anticonvulsants (lithium, valproic acid, topiramate), and antipsychotics (olanzapine, quetiapine) have been examined but without establishing a clear signal for efficacy. Additional medications that have been investigated but whose effectiveness have not been established outside of clinical trials include; N-acetyl cysteine, varenicline, injectable naltrexone, quetiapine, tolcapone, and acamprosate.[42]

Several residential gambling treatment programs have employed acupuncture, as a treatment for gambling disorders, over the last 15 years. Although no formal studies have been published, this treatment modality is available because of its availability within treatment programs, acceptability by clients and family, and affordability. Clients with gambling disorders who have benefited from acupuncture describe benefits in reduction of urges, cravings, and preoccupation with gambling. Also, using acupuncture during the first 30 days of gambling cessation may reduce any withdrawal symptoms (such as anxiety, irritability, myalgias) that might occur.

## PSYCHOLOGICAL TREATMENTS

The majority of psychological treatment research studies for gambling disorder have investigated the effectiveness of behavioral, cognitive, cognitive-behavioral, and motivational interviewing therapy.[43] As of 2016, no specific form of psychological treatment has been proven to be superior. Brief, motivational interventions (even a single session) and self-help techniques have been shown to create a significant difference in reducing gambling problems and offer promise as interventions that any health-care provider, therapist, or counselor could support. Research indicates that psychological treatment for gambling disorder not only reduces gambling behavior but can help to reduce comorbid psychiatric symptoms, such as anxiety and depression, improve quality of life, decrease psychological stress, and decrease the likelihood of comorbid psychopathology.[44]

Residential and intensive outpatient programs for gambling disorder are available, but enrollment should be reserved for patients who require significant structure and who are risk for self-injurious behavior or whose continued gambling could cause permanent and severe damage to the family or society.

## SOCIAL TREATMENTS

Gamblers Anonymous (GA) is a mutual self-help group for gambling disorder, patterned after AA and is widely available throughout the world. GA offers support for family members through groups called Gam-Anon. GA has been shown to be most effective when gamblers attend for an extended period of time (more than a year), obtain a sponsor and follow through with a commitment at meetings (such as setting up chairs). Other social treatment modalities include sober companions, life coaches, and personal assistants to help transition patients into a lifestyle of recovery by ensuring compliance with treatment team recommendations, transport to recovery meetings and monitoring of behaviors. No formal studies have examined the utility of these types of social recovery activities but they are currently in use by many gambling treatment programs.

## NOVEL INTEGRATED TREATMENTS APPROACHES

Gambling disorder treatment providers face treatment barriers that are not seen in SUDs and thus require innovative treatment approaches. As an example, there are no urine drug tests or any objective measures to monitor gambling behaviors. Also, relapse to gambling, even for a single gambling session, can create extensive and substantial harm not seen in single sessions of SUDs. Finally, cognitive distortions about gambling exist (e.g., "gambling will solve all of my money problems" or "I'm going to win, it's just a matter of being patient until my luck turns around") that do not persist in SUDs.

Examples of potentially promising integrated treatment approaches include incorporating different forms of physical exercise, virtual reality treatments, mindfulness meditation approaches, and transcranial magnetic stimulation (TMS). Greater use of personal assistants, financial planners, and third-party financial controllers and overseers are also of potential interest in reducing the harm from ongoing gambling.

An example of an emerging integrated treatment approach for gambling would be the use of yoga. Specific benefits of yoga for gambling disorder might include enhanced ability to manage stress, increased ability to let go of urges/craving and desires to gamble, and improved self-control and discipline that will translate to the ability to refrain from gambling. Treatment retention may also improve as clients with gambling disorder have been shown to high frequency of no-show and dropout rates from traditional treatment programs.

In summary, treatment approaches for gambling disorder are similar to SUDs with similar outcomes yet require unique and individualized treatment approaches. Gambling disorder is a behavioral addiction, a non-substance-related disorder characterized by physical, psychological, and social impacts that can be devastating to individuals, families, and society. With a prevalence and incidence rate similar to other major psychiatric illnesses such as schizophrenia or bipolar disorder, gambling disorder is a common disorder that can easily be missed by any health-care or mental health professional. This makes screening tools for gambling disorders all the more useful and important to include in any treatment program for mental health recovery but especially for any program treating SUDs.

## REFERENCES

1. Knutson B, Rick S, Wimmer GE, Prelec D, Loewenstein G. Neural predictors of purchases. *Neuron.* 2007;53:147–156.
2. Karim RCP. Behavioral addictions: an overview. *Journal of Psychoactive Drugs.* 2012;44(1):5–17.
3. Karim RCP. Behavioral addictions: an overview. *Journal of Psychoactive Drugs.* 2012;44(1):5–17`.
4. Brown K. These people are so addicted to the Internet, that they had to go to rehab. 2015. Retrieved from http://fusion.net/story/178702/inside-internet-addiction-treatment/
5. Griffiths MD. The role of context in online gaming excess and addiction: Some case study evidence. *International Journal of Mental Health and Addiction.* 2010;8(1):119–125.

6. American Psychiatric Association. Internet gaming disorder. 2012. Retrieved from http://www.dsm5.org/Documents/Internet%20Gaming%20Disorder%20Fact%20 Sheet.pdf

7. King DL, Delfabbro PH. Internet gaming disorder treatment: A review of definitions of diagnosis and treatment outcome. *Journal of Clinical Psychology.* 2014;70(10): 942–955.

8. Rosen LD, Cheever, NA, Carrier LM. *iDisorder: Understanding our obsession with technology and overcoming its hold on us.* New York: Palgrave Macmillan; 2012.

9. Brown K. These people are so addicted to the internet, that they had to go to rehab. 2015. Retrieved from http://fusion.net/story/178702/inside-internet-addiction-treatment/

10. Karim RCP. Behavioral addictions: An overview. *Journal of Psychoactive Drugs.* 2012;44(1):5–17.

11. Karim RCP. Behavioral addictions: an overview. *Journal of Psychoactive Drugs.* 2012;44(1):5–17.

12. Spekman, MLC, Konijn EA, Roelofsma PHMP, Griffiths MD. Gaming addiction, definition and measurement: A large-scale empirical study. *Computers in Human Behavior.* 2013;29(6):2150–2155.

13. Griffiths MD. The role of context in online gaming excess and addiction: Some case study evidence. *International Journal of Mental Health and Addiction.* 2010;8(1):119–125.

14. King DL, Delfabbro PH. Internet gaming disorder treatment: A review of definitions of diagnosis and treatment outcome. *Journal of Clinical Psychology.* 2014;70(10):942–955.

15. Brown K. These people are so addicted to the internet, that they had to go to rehab. 2015. Retrieved from http://fusion.net/story/178702/inside-internet-addiction-treatment/

16. King, DL, Delfabbro PH. Internet gaming disorder treatment: a review of definitions of diagnosis and treatment outcome. *Journal of Clinical Psychology.* 2014;70(10):942–955.

17. Dean O, Giorlando F, Berk M. N-acetylcysteine in psychiatry: Current therapeutic evidence and potential mechanisms of action. *Journal of Psychiatry & Neuroscience: JPN.* 2011;36(2):78–86.

18. Zheng X-J, Zhang X, Gong X. Mind-regulating needling plus psychological guidance for internet addiction: A report of 38 cases. *Journal of Acupuncture and Tuina Science.* 2012;10(3):160–161.

19. Karim RCP. Behavioral addictions: An overview. *Journal of Psychoactive Drugs.* 2012;44(1):5–17.

20. Karim RCP. Behavioral addictions: An overview. *Journal of Psychoactive Drugs.* 2012;44(1):5–17.

21. Karim RCP. Behavioral addictions: An overview. *Journal of Psychoactive Drugs.* 2012;44(1):5–17.

22. Benson AL, Eisenach DA. Stopping overshopping: An approach to the treatment of compulsive-buying disorder. *Journal of Groups in Addiction & Recovery.* 2013;8(1):3–24.

23. Karim RCP. Behavioral addictions: an overview. *Journal of Psychoactive Drugs.* 2012;44(1):5–17.

24. Karim RCP. Behavioral addictions: an overview. *Journal of Psychoactive Drugs.* 2012;44(1):5–17.

25. Mitchell JE, Burgard M, Faber R, Crosby RD, de Zwaan M. Cognitive behavioral therapy for compulsive buying disorder. *Behaviour Research and Therapy.* 2006;44(12):1859–1865.

26. Lourenço Leite P, Martinho Pereira V, Egidio Nardi A, Cardoso Silva A. Psychotherapy for compulsive buying disorder: A systematic review. *Psychiatry Research.* 2014;219(3).

27. Aboujaoude E. Compulsive buying disorder: a review and update. *Current Pharmaceutical Design.* 2014; 20(25)

28. Benson AL, Eisenach, DA. Stopping overshopping: An approach to the treatment of compulsive-buying disorder. *Journal of Groups in Addiction & Recovery.* 2013;8(1):3–24.

29. Aboujaoude E. Compulsive buying disorder: A review and update. *Current Pharmaceutical Design.* 2014;20(25)

30. Hodgins DC, Stea JN, Grant JE. Gambling disorders. *Lancet.* 2011;378(9806):1874–1884.

31. Lorains FK, Cowlishaw S, Thomas SA. Prevalence of comorbid disorders in problem and pathological gambling: systematic review and meta-analysis of population surveys. *Addiction.* 2011;106(3):490–498.

32. Fong TW, Reid RC, Parhami I. Behavioral addictions: where to draw the lines? *The Psychiatric Clinics of North America.* 2012;35(2):279–296.

33. Ledgerwood DM, Petry NM. Gambling and suicidality in treatment-seeking pathological gamblers. *Journal of Nervous and Mental Disease.* 2004;192(10):711–714.

34. Kessler RC, Hwang I, LaBrie R, et al. DSM-IV pathological gambling in the National Comorbidity Survey Replication. *Psychological Medicine.* 2008;38(9):1351–1360.

35. Petry NM, Stinson FS, Grant BF. Comorbidity of DSM-IV pathological gambling and other psychiatric disorders: results from the National Epidemiologic Survey on Alcohol and Related Conditions. *Journal of Clinical Psychiatry.* 2005;66(5):564–574.

36. Ladouceur R. Gambling: the hidden addiction. *Canadian Journal of Psychiatry.* 2004;49(8):501–503.

37. Petry NM, Blanco C, Auriacombe M, et al. An overview of and rationale for changes proposed for pathological gambling in DSM-5. *Journal of Gambling Studies.* 2014;30(2):493–502.

38. Potenza MN. Neurobiology of gambling behaviors. *Current Opinion in Neurobiology.* 2013;23(4):660–667.

39. Potenza MN. The neurobiology of pathological gambling and drug addiction: an overview and new findings. *Philosophical Transactions of the Royal Society of London Series B-Containing Papers of a Biological Character.* 2008;363(1507):3181–3189.

40. Pulford J, Bellringer M, Abbott M, Clarke D, Hodgins D, Williams J. Reasons for seeking help for a gambling problem: the experiences of gamblers who have sought specialist assistance and the perceptions of those who have not. *Journal of Gambling Studies.* 2009;25(1):19–32.

41. Grant JE, Odlaug BL, Schreiber L. Pharmacological treatments in pathological gambling. *British Journal of Clinical Pharmacology.* 2014;77(2):375–381.

42. Grant JE, Odlaug BL, Schreiber L. Pharmacological treatments in pathological gambling. *British Journal of Clinical Pharmacology.* 2014;77(2):375–381.

43. Fink A, Parhami I, Rosenthal RJ, Campos MD, Siani A, Fong TW. How transparent is behavioral intervention research on pathological gambling and other gambling-related disorders? A systematic literature review. *Addiction.* 2012;107(11):1915–1928.

44. Gooding P, Tarrier N. A systematic review and meta-analysis of cognitive-behavioural interventions to reduce problem gambling: hedging our bets? *Behaviour Research and Therapy.* 2009;47(7):592–607.

# 11

## Hallucinogens: Spiritual and Therapeutic Use, Overuse, and Complications

### CHARLES S. GROB

## Introduction

A fascinating class of psychoactive substances possessing a long and mysterious history of human use are the classic hallucinogens. Forming a vital component of prehistorical and aboriginal culture and belief systems, hallucinogens were ultimately condemned and repressed by evolving civilizations, only to be "rediscovered" in the 20th century. Of compelling interest to anthropologists, ethnobotanists, pharmacologists, medical scientists, and mental health clinicians, their use was diverted to the general culture (particularly youth) during the politically tumultuous 1960s: these drugs were determined to be the cause of a period of cultural upheaval associated with a perceived public health crisis. After decades of quiescence, however, the careful examination of hallucinogens under rigorous and approved research conditions has resumed. This chapter will explore the historical background, risks of adverse events, and discussion of hallucinogenic-use disorder.

### CLASSIC HALLUCINOGENS

The substances under consideration for this chapter are the classic hallucinogens—specifically, mescaline, lysergic acid diethylamide (LSD), psilocybin, and dimethyltryptamine (DMT). These were the compounds of greatest interest to the pioneers of hallucinogen research as well as to modern investigators of hallucinogens. A variety of chemically related compounds, including ketamine, phencyclidine (PCP), salvinorin, ibogaine, 3,4-methylenedioxymethamphetamine (MDMA), and a

184

profusion of recently discovered laboratory phenethylamines and tryptamines have interesting histories, range of effects, relative risks, and in some cases potential therapeutic application. However, the scope of this chapter will be limited to those compounds known as the "classic" hallucinogens.

# Historical Background

## USE OF PLANT HALLUCINOGENS IN PREHISTORY AND BY EARLY CIVILIZATIONS

Hallucinogens, in plant form, have been present since the earliest habitation of the earth and have played a pivotal role in the evolution of human culture. Indeed, recent paleontological investigations have discovered evidence of fossilized grasses covered with ergot, a hallucinogenic fungi (Poinar et al., 2015), and likely a food source for evolving life forms during the primordial epochs of earth's development. This finding may explain the exquisite sensitivity the human central nervous system has to even minute doses of powerful hallucinogens. A case in point is LSD, a compound derived from ergot and active on a microgram level, which is a smaller active dose than virtually all other drugs are known to possess. This recent discovery may explain the remarkable neuro-receptor sensitivity to LSD and provide a possible biological explanation to the question of why the human species appears to be "wired" to be receptive to such remarkably low doses of these powerful psychoactive compounds.

## Hallucinogens and Shamanism

It is by now well established that indigenous tribal groups around the world have, since time began, used plant hallucinogens to catalyze shamanic ceremonies designed to facilitate individual and group healing as well as cultural cohesion (Dobkin de Rios, 1984). Individual and collective experiences with these mind-altering plants and fungi established the psychospiritual bedrock out of which emerged the great world religions and civilizations. Archeological finds have identified evidence of early ceremonial plant hallucinogen use dating back many thousands of years. This evidence includes pre-Neolithic rock paintings on the Tassili Plain in southeast Algeria believed to have been created in the range of 7,000 to 9,000 years ago, depicting tribal shamans wearing masks adorned with symbolic representations of hallucinogenic mushrooms (Samorini, 1992). In plant form, hallucinogens were employed by many prehistoric and early civilizations as integral components of their religious, healing, and initiation rituals. More than

100 species of plant hallucinogens have been cataloged, the majority in the western hemisphere, and identified as possessing a history of use within indigenous cere-monial practice (Schultes & Hofmann, 1992).

## NEUROPHARMACOLOGY, PHENOMENOLOGY, AND PHYSIOLOGY

Through the years of repression and taboo, most mainstream health and mental health professionals were not aware of the vital role hallucinogens played in the early discovery and elucidation of the serotoninergic neurotransmitter system, which has wide-ranging effects on mood, anxiety, social behavior, memory, sleep, appetite, and sexuality. Serotonin was discovered in 1953. The chemical structure of serotonin (Twarog & Page, 1953), was found to be very similar to the prototype hallucinogen, LSD (discovered 10 years earlier), and later to the tryptamines psilocybin and DMT, all of which contain an indole nucleus. Indeed, it was through preclinical research studies in the late 1950s, some led by Daniel X. Freedman at the University of Chicago, that it was discovered where in the brain serotonin was located in highest quantities by radioligand tagging LSD and injecting them into non-human primates. The hallucinogens (and par-ticularly LSD's) contribution to the early evolution of neuroscience is rarely ap-preciated (Freedman, 1961).

Hallucinogens may be regarded as potent "non-specific amplifiers of the un-conscious," according to Stanislav Grof, a pioneer of the field who over the course of his extensive career as a psychiatric researcher of hallucinogens starting in the early 1950s in Prague, Czechoslovakia, until the closure of investigations by the early 1970s, personally treated more clinical research subjects with a halluci-nogen in an approved setting than any other investigator of that era (Grof, 1980; Grof, 2005).

While the previous, progenitor generation of researchers were primarily focused on the intra-subjective process, later investigators identified the neurobiologic mechanism involving stimulation of the serotonin 5-HT2A receptor. Investigators have demonstrated that hallucinogens are 5-HT2A agonists or partial agonists, whose action can be blocked by the selective 5-HT2A antagonist ketanserin (Vollenweider et al., 1998). Hallucinogens also have additional effects on other neurotransmitter systems, with particular interest recently being directed at the glutamergic system, and the potential of classic hallucinogens to facilitate increased glutamate production and glutamate-dependent neuroplastic adaptation—a mechanism suggested as the potential basis for therapeutic outcomes (Ross, 2012).

The classic hallucinogens produce an altered state of consciousness that is characterized by changes in perception, mood, and cognition in the presence of an otherwise clear sensorium, along with visual illusions and internal visionary experiences (though rarely frank hallucinations), states of ecstasy, dissolution of ego boundaries, and the experience of union with others and with the natural world. Set (mental expectation) and setting (environment) are critical factors for determining subjective experiences under the influence of hallucinogens. In a recent study of the acute effects of LSD in normal volunteers, investigators observed sustained (up to 12 hours) alterations in waking consciousness, including visual hallucinogens, audio-visual synesthesia, and positively experienced depersonalization and derealization. Compared to subjects receiving placebo, the hallucinogen facilitated enhanced feelings of well-being, improved mood, rapport with others, openness, and trust. Safe physiological parameters were maintained, with no serious acute adverse effects reported (Schmid et al., 2015).

Pharmacologically, tolerance and cross-tolerance to other hallucinogens has been developed in both animal and human models. Repeated administration of hallucinogens leads to rapid development of tolerance and downregulation of the 5-HT2A receptor (Nichols, 2016). This has been demonstrated in the laboratory setting, with experimental animals but also is a phenomenon well known to aficionados of hallucinogen use, who have collectively long understood that the drugs cannot be administered on a frequent basis owing to the rapid attenuation of positive effects with repeated dosing. Hallucinogens would then appear to possess an innate deterrent mechanism for overuse and abuse. Medically, hallucinogens are generally considered to be safe within particular dosage ranges, careful subject selection, and optimal treatment structures. They do not cause physiological addiction, although psychological dependence can occur. Particularly when taken in unmonitored settings, and by individuals with serious underlying vulnerabilities, disturbance of psychological function can occur. They are generally well-tolerated physiologically, although individuals with underlying organ system vulnerabilities may be at some risk. A case in point is a recent report in the medical literature of a fatal ingestion of hallucinogenic mushrooms by a young woman who had received a heart transplant ten years previously for end-stage rheumatic heart disease (Lim et al., 2012). Nevertheless, such cases of either acute medical crises or chronic physical disability caused by the classic hallucinogens, when taken under optimal conditions, are remarkably rare.

## EPIDEMOLOGY OF HALLUCINOGEN USE

Until the 1960s the use of hallucinogens in Western society was virtually unheard of. But within the context of the social and political upheaval of a half-century ago, these drugs, and LSD in particular, became widely popular, particularly among youth. While formal data collection was minimal during that time, observers in

North America and across Europe and elsewhere noted radical shifts in youth culture believed to be associated with the emergence of information (albeit limited) and supplies (often plentiful and at high dosages) of LSD suddenly available to large populations of young people. Curiously, the popularity of the "psychedelics," as they were commonly known, was mainly identified with middle- to upper-level socioeconomic classes of Caucasian youth. These powerful mind-altering substances that heightened awareness of one's surroundings and raised questions of ontological security were evidently far less popular among disenfranchised segments of the population, including those from lower socioeconomic strata and ethnic minority groups who were primarily focused on day-to-day survival within a larger and historically hostile culture.

Establishing precise estimates of current use of classic hallucinogens remains difficult, partly because of the frequent lumping together for the purpose of data collection of various drugs, including the dissociative hallucinogen, PCP, as well as the popular Ecstasy (or Molly), along with the compounds of primary interest to this chapter, LSD, mescaline, psilocybin, and DMT. Nevertheless, from the available data, coupled with reports from health providers and others aware of cultural trends, it is evident that there is far less general use of classic hallucinogens currently than during the era of the youth counterculture activism during the late 1960s and 1970s. According to the government-sponsored SAMHSA, the best data source for behavioral trends in the United States found fairly consistent hallucinogen-use patterns from the early 2000s up to 2014. In 2014, 1.2 million individuals aged 12 and older reported use of hallucinogens in the previous month, representing approximately 0.4% of the population (SAMHSA, 2014). According to the National Survey on Drug Use and Health the number of first-time users of hallucinogens has remained fairly stable. In 2014 slightly less than 1 million people in the United States were reported to have tried a hallucinogen for the first time. Almost twice as many males as females have taken a hallucinogen. Recent data for 2015 from the National Survey on Drug Abuse and Health revealed that 4.3% of high school seniors reported having taken LSD while similar data from the year before, 2014, reported a past year prevalence of LSD use histories of 10.9% among adults aged 26 and older. Examining the US population as a whole, a 2008 NSDUH (National Survey on Drug Use and Health) survey reported 23.5 million US citizens aged 12 or older have used LSD in their lifetime representing 9.4% of the overall population (SAMHSA, 2008). Epidemiologists have also found that the earlier the onset of hallucinogen use, the more likely individuals will develop a polysubstance pattern of use (Rickert et al., 2003; Wu et al., 2006). Those individuals with an identified preference for hallucinogens over other available drugs are more likely to have deferred initiating drug experimentation until after their high school years.

# Suboptimal Use and Adverse Events

## HALLUCINOGEN-USE DISORDER

According to the *DSM-5*, problematic use of hallucinogens is considered to be a sign of psychological disturbance if the drug use causes clinically significant functional impairment that may manifest at work, school, or home settings. Evidence of a disturbance is also exhibited in impaired social judgment; interference with social, work, and school obligations; failure to control use when attempted; increased tolerance and use of larger quantities of the drug over time; persistence of use despite harmful consequences; and engaging in high-risk activities associated with drug use (SAMHSA, 2015).

## COMPLICATIONS OF HALLUCINOGEN USE

Transient anxiety reactions also known as a "bad" trip can occur during the course of hallucinogen use and are common. Indeed, there may be a neurobiologic basis for this phenomenon, as the prominent preclinical hallucinogen researcher, David Nichols, formerly of Purdue University (and more recently at the University of North Carolina), as well as founding president of the Heffter Research Institute, has suggested that 13 hydroxy-LSD, a metabolite of LSD generated several hours after ingestion and a highly potent dopamine agonist, may be responsible for some of the anxiety observed clinically (Nichols, 2016). The degree and duration of the anxiety response are influenced by dose, setting, underlying psychological stability, and experience of the user with altered states of consciousness. During the 1960s, when there was limited familiarity with the range of effects of hallucinogens individuals experiencing high levels of anxiety, particularly after taking LSD, were often taken to local hospital emergency rooms for treatment and monitoring. It was quickly realized, however, that the intensity and sensory overloading of an ER setting was not conducive to rapid recovery from anxiety responses caused by hallucinogens and in fact often exacerbated the presenting condition. Furthermore, the convention of administering strong antipsychotic medications to sedate recreational "trippers" who had unexpectedly found themselves to be experiencing high levels of fear and apprehension that they were "losing their mind" was found to be contraindicated, as the antipsychotics often appeared to intensify the depressed mood and compound the growing sense of demoralization over time.

Rather than relying on traditional psychiatric emergency services, the counterculture communities of individuals drawn to collectively participate in what was a new and poorly understood drug trend at that time, took a gentler and more supportive approach in settings that were without excessive sensory stimulation.

In such quiet and contained environments it was often possible to facilitate the rapid reorientation of the individual, along with attenuation of presenting anxiety and return to baseline status. Usually, establishing rapport and providing reassuring statements that the individual will return to normal is sufficient, allowing what is often the most salient fear—that sanity and "normality" will never be reestablished—to dissipate. If any medication is indicated, a low dose of an anti-anxiety benzodiazepine is often found to be sufficient and without the lingering sense of an "incomplete process" that individuals on hallucinogens treated with antipsychotic medications often report. In contemporary settings where large groups of people collectively take hallucinogens, those communities have established their own interventions, modeled on the knowledge accrued by earlier generations who learned by trial and error how to successfully contain most anxiety reactions incurred during social hallucinogen use. An effective example of current efforts to provide the quiet space and gentle "talking down" that "bad trips" require are the Green Dot Rangers who are active in many festivals, including the annual end-of-summer Burning Man gathering in the Nevada desert, organizing psychological first aid interventions for "trippers" experiencing disturbing levels of anxiety and disorientation.

## SUSTAINED PSYCHOTIC REACTIONS

In individuals with severe vulnerability for underlying psychopathology and for those taking hallucinogens under adverse conditions, there is a risk for serious mental health deterioration. Risk of long-term psychological damage is relatively rare, and much less frequent than in the 1960s, when less was known about hallucinogens and higher dosages (particularly of LSD) were routinely employed. But there still remains a real risk for sustained psychotic reaction following hallucinogen use, often when excessive frequency of administration and higher dosing occur. Individuals who deteriorate following hallucinogen use often have strong biological family histories for major mental illness and are thus genetically at risk. They may also have suffered from relative degrees of instability in their lives, involving family, and relationships as well as school and work. Furthermore, there may be histories of chronic, untreated PTSD. With some hallucinogens, such as psilocybin containing mushrooms, if the user consumes them at too frequent an interval, there is a tendency to become "lost" in alternate perceptual experiences and belief systems that obstruct the individual from effectively engaging in consensus reality. Other hallucinogens, such as ayahuasca, appear to be better tolerated if taken regularly for a limited period of time, as can be observed with the Brazilian syncretic ayahuasca churches. However, the rapidly growing awareness and interest in the ayahuasca experience has led to an increasing number of North Americans and Europeans traveling to South America in search of the legendary plant brew and, consequently, more problematic outcomes. The problem with quality control regarding the ayahuasca experience is an important consideration, both with regard to the integrity and expertise of the facilitator of the ayahuasca experience as well as the actual quality and constituents of the brew employed. Sometimes ayahuasceros add powerful admixture plants to increase the potency and range of effects of the brew, including the leaves of *Brugmansia*, which is a powerful cholinergic hallucinogen, and may significantly increase the potency and duration of the ayahausca ceremony. It may be that the added *Brugmansia*, its powerful psychoactive effects amplified by the monoamine oxidase inhibitoractivity of the harmala alkaloids from the *Banisteriopsis* vine in ayahuasca, is responsible for many of the psychotic events observed with the growing number of Westerners drawn to the Amazon.

The increasing knowledge and interest in ayuahuasca seen over the past decade has led to a rapid increase in what has been called "ayahuasca tourism" to the Amazon, and particularly to Peru, where cases have emerged, often involving young men and women. After a long and exhausting trip to South America from North American and Europe, these people participated in multiple ayahuasca sessions spaced at brief intervals (often only a day or two), deteriorated into a disoriented state along with disturbed reality testing, impaired judgment, and disturbances of relatedness. While the majority of such ayahuasca initiates tolerate the experience without evident adverse effect, there is that small yet appreciable number who return home with relative degrees of psychological impairment. These cases have also often proved to be poorly responsive to conventional psychiatric treatment, though with a supportive environment and gentle reassurance over time some improvements have been noted. Nevertheless, these challenging and difficult-to-treat cases represent a call to develop alternative models of intervention. Given the limited efficacy often observed with conventional treatments for continued perceptual disturbance and anxiety—it has become increasingly evident that novel treatment interventions will need to be developed that mirror the unique experience encountered in a hallucinogen-induced altered state of consciousness. It has even been suggested that the judicious use of a hallucinogen administered under optimal conditions may facilitate the resolution of the psychotic experience. While anecdotal accounts support this model, that "the best treatment for a bad trip is a good trip," because of the lack of research in the field the efficacy and safety of such a novel treatment remain unknown. Nevertheless, it should also be noted that repeat use of hallucinogens, particularly in unwise settings and at inopportune times may not ameliorate the underlying disturbance and may instead lead to exacerbation of the impaired state.

During the 1960s and 1970s many young people who experimented with hallucinogens encountered various degrees of anxiety, often of an existential nature. At that time the growing cultural interest in Asia stimulated an increasing fascination with previously obscure and remote Eastern religions and philosophical systems. Of particular appeal to many young people who had participated in the social events of that era were the various forms of Buddhist meditation. The discipline involved with meditation, along with the systemized restructuring of thought patterns, worked to establish a more grounded perspective and capacity to effectively contain and work through the residual anxiety of their early hallucinogen experimentation. The capacity for trained meditators to improve their internal self-regulation of anxiety and mood appears to be a critical component in the efficacy of meditation as an adjunct to treatment (Shapiro & Giber, 1978). Another novel approach that may potentially ameliorate the persistent anxiety and psychological disturbance that sometimes follows difficult and unprocessed hallucinogen experiences is holotropic breathwork therapy, developed by the veteran researcher Stanislav Grof, after hallucinogen research was shut down in the late 1960s and early 1970s. Grof, along with his wife Christina, developed a non-drug technique, including control of breathing, that he believed replicated the hallucinogen-induced altered state of consciousness. While not the initial focus in the development of the holotropic therapy technique, cases did emerge of successful amelioration of residual anxiety, some quite distant in time, that had been initially catalyzed by past hallucinogen use. This method may offer another alternative non-drug treatment approach that merits investigation (Grof & Grof, 2010).

## POSTTRAUMATIC RESPONSE

Often-overlooked adverse phenomena are the responses to traumatic experience, which may occur after having taken a hallucinogen. This can be the result of having experienced overwhelming intrapsychic conflict while under the influence or from sequelae of having incurred actual mental or physical trauma while in a vulnerable altered state. As amplifiers of experience, the hallucinogen state response to a normally frightening encounter becomes strongly accentuated. This resultant impairment from persistent posttraumatic stress catalyzed during the amplified hallucinogen-induced state often has a strong impact on subsequent function. Both in the world of the social hallucinogen experimenter as well as that of the psychospiritual seeker working with a presumably trained facilitator, there is a heightened degree of vulnerability that can potentially be preyed upon by someone in a position of power who possesses inappropriate motives. Such unfortunate events of course occur in other contexts as well, including spiritual retreats, but the drug-altered condition of the victim can intensify the subsequent traumatized psychological reaction and provide additional treatment challenges.

Difficult experiences with hallucinogens may also lead to another form of sustained and posttraumatic stress, as the individual's efforts to work through conflicts, disruptions in sense of self, and disturbed affect are fruitless, leading to a reinforced states of despair and inadequacy. Disturbing images along with intrusive thoughts from the hellish experience may persist over time. Such adverse experiences with hallucinogens are particularly likely to occur in uncontrolled settings with over-stimulating environments and often in the context of alcohol and polydrug use. This severe psychological distress and despair often responds inadequately to con-ventional treatments, although it should always be remembered that many cases over the course of time do experience gradual healing, sometimes with valuable insights. A famous historical example from the 1930s of a catastrophic intrapsy-chic experience leading to a peculiar enlightenment revealing truths previously obscured, was the terrifying experience induced by the hallucinogen mescaline that precipitated the existential crisis of French philosopher Jean-Paul Sartre, who emerged from his staggering encounter with the void to develop the philosophical movement of Existentialism (Sartre, 1938; Riedlinger, 2002).

## HPPD (HALLUCINOGEN PERSISTING PERCEPTION DISORDER)

Though only a relatively small number of cases have been reported, a serious concern in recent years has been the risk of a condition involving sensory disturbances (primarily visual) and similar to those sometimes acutely gener-ated by hallucinogens but sustained long after hallucinogens were last taken and long after perceptual effects should have faded away. This is known as halluci-nogen persisting perception disorder (HPPD). Often occurring in individuals with a substantial history of taking hallucinogens as well as other drugs, HPPD can be a debilitating condition. Typical symptoms include visually perceived auras surrounding objects, trails following objects in motion, distortion of dimensions, and other visual aberrations, often including persistent floaters. HPPD was first identified and defined in the 1990s by psychiatrist Henry David Abraham of Rhode Island. In previous years, during the tumultuous events of the psychedelic 1960s, these after-effects, were generally referred to as "flashbacks." Flashbacks, as commonly understood, were relatively transient, while HPPD is notable for its persistence of symptoms, which over time may be unnerving for those with the condition. Comorbidity with depressive and anxiety disorders are often a persist-ent concern with HPPD, as demoralization and a growing sense of despair often aggravate the condition. While relatively uncommon in frequency, they often present clinically as serious treatment challenges. Given these seeming organic symptoms, in the absence of ophthalmologic findings, pharmacotherapy has often been used. Unfortunately, most conventional psychopharmacology treatments have not helped much, and the atypical neuroleptic risperidone in particular has been documented to exacerbate underlying HPPD (Abraham & Mamen,

1996). However, a positive report was recently published on the successful use of the mood stabilizer lamotrigine to treat HPPD (Hermle et al., 2012). Whether or not lamotrigine as a treatment model holds up over time, the identification and treatment of HPPD is a neglected clinical area that is in desperate need of rigorous study.

A rarely asked question has been whether the risk of HPPD is increasing. If indeed HPPD is distinct from flashbacks, because of its long duration, why are there more cases of persistent visual anomalies now than during the 1960s? One reason for this may be purity of product, as years ago during the apex of the psychedelic movement a small number of highly skilled chemists (and as it turned out, often ethically attuned) were responsible for manufacturing most of the relatively high-quality LSD consumed by that generation. Since the 1990s, however, a new phenomenon has often been observed: drug substitution. Many sufferers of HPPD have not only taken LSD or other classic hallucinogens, they also have histories of taking non-classic hallucinogens, particularly MDMA—and have often done so in large quantities. Surveys since the 1990s have demonstrated that an alarming proportion of drugs sold for MDMA as Ecstasy and later Molly, were in fact adulterated with other drugs, with or without MDMA present. In recent years newly designed synthetic phenethylamines and tryptamines have been widely distributed, with much of it manufactured abroad; in fact, China is the chief exporter of untested and only recently discovered drugs that have never been rigorously studied, are not known to be safe, and are manufactured under conditions of poor quality control. Consequently, the role of polysubstance use, toxic adulterants, and excessive-use histories cannot be disregarded when examining for possible contributors to the increasing reports of HPPD.

An additional concern that may be related to the suspected increased occurrence of HHPD is that young people over the past few decades have been exposed to far greater degrees of treatment with conventional psychotropic medication than their predecessors were. While the generation that experimented with hallucinogens in the 1960s was much less likely to have a history of past or current psychiatric medication use, young people nowadays are increasingly likely to have been prescribed—and often over prolonged periods of time—various antidepressants, mood stabilizers, anxiolytics, antipsychotics, stimulants, and other pharmaceutical products. Consequently, between relative frequent use of recreational phenethylamines (most prominently MDMA/Ecstasy) and likely occurrence of prior (or current) use of prescription psychotropic medications, it is quite probable that the brain substrate of today's youth is fundamentally different than in preceding generations, leading to a variety of potential consequences: including the acquisition of particular neuropsychiatric vulnerabilities, which leads to a heightened risk of developing HPPD after exposure to hallucinogens.

## POLYSUBSTANCE ABUSE

A common cause of acute psychological decompensation is when alcohol and other drugs are taken concomitantly with use of a hallucinogen. The behavioral disinhibition, along with the affective and aggressive dysregulation effects of alcohol and some stimulant drugs such as cocaine and methamphetamine, can create a toxic combination with a hallucinogen, capable of provoking severe confusional states that heighten the risk of engaging in self-harm or acts of harm to others. This may occur knowingly in recreational drug-use settings, or unwittingly in the context of surreptitious administration of a hallucinogen (for instance, mixed in with an alcoholic beverage at a social gathering). There is also the risk of ill-advised alcohol and drug combinations with hallucinogens causing sustained adverse impact on mood, anxiety, and reality testing. While the deleterious impact of mixing alcohol and many drugs with hallucinogens are unquestioned, there is some divergence of views in the case of cannabis. Cannabis is not likely to precipitate psychotic or dangerous reactions, and some experienced users report taking it, with no ill-effects, to ameliorate anxiety or to aid with problems with fatigue and muscular tension at the later stages of a hallucinogen experience. However, cannabis in certain hallucinogen-use settings is explicitly prohibited. This is particularly evident in the Amazon region of South America, where commonly mestizo healers in Peru view cannabis to be contraindicated before or during ayahuasca ceremonies. Similarly, in Brazil the syncretic ayahuasca religion Uniao do Vegetal (UDV) has a strong proscription against using cannabis at their religious meetings, and believe the effects of cannabis taken along with ayahuasca impair the capacity of participants to clearly focus on the spiritual process the religious community is engaged in. Nevertheless, some branches of the other (and less hierarchical) main Brazilian ayahuasca church, the Santo Daime, encourage the use of cannabis (referred to as "Santa Maria") during their ceremonies and consider it an adjunct to spiritual attainment.

# Optimal Use, Cultural Resistance, and Therapeutic Application

## SHAMANIC CONTEXT

The use of hallucinogens in ceremonial contexts dates back to prehistory and the earliest civilizations, where plant-based hallucinogens were deemed to be powerful psychoactive substances imbued with sacred qualities that allowed the user to access the celestial realms for the purpose of healing, divination, or obtaining knowledge necessary for the well-being of the tribal group. Hallucinogens were never profaned for purposes of recreational or hedonic use and never consumed with alcoholic beverages or other psychotropic plants. Strict purification practices were often employed prior to participating in a hallucinogen activated ceremony, including prolonged fasting, sexual abstinence, and isolation. Such preparation was designed to protect the individual from malevolent spirits or influences during the hallucinogen experience and to assist him or her to maintain focus on the serious purpose that the hallucinogen ceremony was designed to address (Grob & Dobkin de Rios, 1992).

As modern culture and science begin to carefully reevaluate the potential use of hallucinogens for purposes of healing, it would be instructive to examine some of the extra-pharmacological structures utilized by shamanic practitioners from remote indigenous groups. While much of the knowledge accrued by ancient cultures has been lost to history, available anthropological records have provided a roadmap for altered states of consciousness exploration that optimizes safe and efficacious outcome. These involve careful preparation of the session, including the establishment of a strong rapport between the healer and the patient. This process often involves discussing the goals, or intentions, of the treatment, imparting information about the treatment and addressing any concerns or fears the patient may have. Instructions are provided regarding fasting and other dietary restrictions, abstinence from sex and other intoxicants and the use of particular techniques designed to quiet the mind, such as meditation or prayer (Bravo & Grob, 1989). Shamanic practitioners are often adept at establishing powerful expectation effects directed toward predetermined therapeutic goals. Indeed, hallucinogens are understood to possess powerful hyper-suggestible effects, and depending upon the mindset of the user and the explicit as well as implicit messages conveyed by the practitioner and the general setting, there may be a strong impact upon the content and outcome of the session (Dobkin de Rios & Grob, 1994). The need to develop an effective set and setting for the experience in order to increase the likelihood of optimal outcome can be seen in the structures employed by the ancient practitioners of the shamanic arts. These structures are instructive to contemporary efforts designed to reopen this field of study while maintaining strong safety parameters and facilitating a salutary therapeutic outcome for the patient.

## MEDICAL USE REFRACTORY PSYCHIATRIC CONDITIONS

Clinical investigators working with hallucinogens in the 1950s and 1960s were highly impressed with the results of treatment, often with patients who had not responded to conventional treatments. While the cultural reaction of the 1960s and the relative immaturity of the field led to a lengthy hiatus in approved use of these novel treatment models, we are once again being allowed the opportunity to carefully study the range of effects of hallucinogens, including their potential utility in treatment, provided we can demonstrate that these compounds can be used safely and without disruptive public fanfare. It is time to approach this class of psychoactive substances with respect for its ancient lineage and regard for its potential to heal when applied under ideal conditions. Since the collapse of the early generation of hallucinogen research in the 1960s, modern psychiatry has shifted strongly toward pharmaceutical treatment models, largely abandoning the more introspective, insight-oriented psychotherapies that previously dominated the field. Prevailing mainstream drug treatment models, while having some success ameliorating presenting symptoms, often fall short with particular refractory conditions, including some that were demonstrated to respond to hallucinogen treatment years ago, such as obsessive-compulsive disorder, existential anxiety associated with terminal medical illness, chronic posttraumatic stress disorder, refractory mood and anxiety disorders, and character pathologies. There is an urgency now to establish new treatment investigations designed to gauge the safety and effectiveness of the hallucinogen treatment model, given the high rate of conventional treatment failures. Finally, we have reached a critical point in time, with a new opportunity to develop prospective investigations conducted under optimal conditions of the use of the hallucinogen treatment model, particularly with patient populations that are widely considered the most difficult to treat clinical cases (Mithoefer et al., 2016).

## ADDICTION MEDICINE

Some of the more impressive treatment responses to hallucinogen treatment in the 1950s and 1960s were with severe alcoholics and drug addicts. Humphrey Osmond reported from Saskatchewan, in northwest Canada, the impressive responses to mescaline treatment of a large series of chronic alcoholic patients who demonstrated sustained sobriety far surpassing responses to standard treatments (Osmond, 1957). Even Bill Wilson, the founder of AA, after volunteering to be a subject in UCLA research Sidney Cohen's LSD studies in the late 1950s, spoke passionately about the potentials of hallucinogen treatment to aid the treatment of alcoholism (Lattin, 2012). However, his recommendations were rejected by the Board of Trustees of AA, who by the early 1960s had become alarmed over the controversies at Harvard involving Timothy Leary and Richard Alpert's exuberant endorsement of hallucinogen experimentation.

While highly impressive outcomes in alcohol abuse treatment studies were observed in investigations utilizing optimal structures designed to facilitate positive therapeutic outcomes in the 1950s and early to mid 1960s (Chwelos et al., 1959; Maclean et al., 1961; Van Dusen et al., 1967), by the late 1960s a clear shift in research strategy had occurred. Investigators were under increasing pressure to invalidate the hallucinogen treatment model, which they gradually did, by dismissing the standard rules of set and setting, and utilizing suboptimal, as well as (by today's standards) unethical treatment structures, including little or no preparation, minimal monitoring or support during the experience and minimal integration afterward. Investigators who demonstrated positive therapeutic outcomes with hallucinogens were increasingly disregarded and marginalized by their peers. However, those whose findings corroborated the need to demonstrate that the earlier claims of therapeutic success with the treatment model had been exaggerated, and that hallucinogens were more dangerous than had been acknowledged, found themselves rewarded with generous new research grants and professional honors, including in 1970 the prestigious American Psychiatric Association Lester N. Hofheimer Prize for Research (Ludwig et al., 1970). Years later, Stanislav Grof, veteran hallucinogen researcher from the early 1950s to the early 1970s, described the group so honored: "At a time when LSD was popular, (they) had reported positive results . . . When LSD fell out of favor and the positive results became politically unwise, they obtained negative results. Unconsciously or consciously they built into their study a number of anti-therapeutic elements that guaranteed a therapeutic failure" (Grof, 1980).

One rather unusual psychological mechanism that may account for the effectiveness of the hallucinogen treatment model is the emergence of a powerful psychospiritual epiphany during the course of the optimally controlled hallucinogen augmented therapy session. While all churches likely have their members who had at one time suffered from alcohol- or drug-use disorders and subsequently had established sobriety, an intriguing phenomenon is presented by the use of particular plant hallucinogens as ceremonial sacrament in particular religions that have become established over the last 140 years. Beginning in the1870s and 1880s Native American Indians in the southwestern United States began to develop religious ceremonies using the psychoactive cactus, peyote, which contains the hallucinogen alkaloid mescaline. Eventually incorporated in the United States as the Native American Church (NAC), peyote ceremonies are now permissible under the law for individuals who can demonstrate at least 25% native ethnicity. The impact of the NAC ceremonies on the surviving indigenous people of North America has been impressive, particularly with regard to its evident capacity to actively facilitate recovery from alcohol abuse, a condition endemic to native people. Indeed, Karl Menninger, a revered figure in the development of American psychiatry in the mid-20th century, during a period of controversy and threat to terminate the rights of native people stated, "Peyote is not harmful to these people; it is beneficial, comforting, inspiring, and appears to be spiritually nourishing. It is a better antidote to alcohol than anything the missionaries, the white man, the American Medical Association, and the public health services have come up with" (Bergman, 1971).

Another contemporary example of the spiritual and legal use of a ceremonial plant hallucinogen is the ayahuasca churches of Brazil. Since the late 1980s ayahuasca has been legal in Brazil when used in religious context. An investigation of the acute and long-term effects of ayahuasca on long-term members of the Uniao do Vegetal (UDV) in the early 1990s identified a number of individuals there whose establishment and maintenance of sobriety they attributed to their experiences with ceremonial administered ayahuasca within the context of the UDV church structure (Grob et al., 1996; Grob, 1999). In addition to the strong community support provided by the UDV, participants in ayahuasca ceremonies often report experiencing profound psychospiritual epiphanies, which are understood and integrated according to their religious belief system. Hallucinogens are known to facilitate psychological states of hyper-suggestibility. In addition to reflections on the beauties of nature and the divine value of life, UDV ceremonies are also structured to provide sermons by church leaders, along with commentary by congregants, that are instructive lessons on the importance of conducting ethical and moral lives. Hearing these positive messages while under the influence of ayahuasca at a UDV ceremony, individuals receive powerful psychological suggestions to mend their ways and transform their lives for the better. Consequently, it is evident that under optimal conditions these powerful substances have the innate capacity to facilitate a radical restructuring of the sense of self with the result that chronic maladaptive and unhealthy behaviors, including chronic alcoholism, often cease. These contemporary examples of state sanctioned religious ceremonial use of classic hallucinogens, in plant form, including the Native American peyote church in North America and the UDV ayahuasca religion in Brazil, provide a unique opportunity to carefully examine the range of their potential therapeutic applications, including the extinction of alcohol and drug abuse.

## Conclusions and Implications for the Future

After decades of repression, both during the modern era and throughout much of our history, hallucinogens have resurfaced once again, though now as respectable and potentially valuable objects of formal scientific research. No longer the objects of derision or repression, hallucinogens are being seriously examined at academic research settings around the world as potential tools for learning and healing. Indeed, the time may have come in which the optimal use of hallucinogens can be thoroughly explored and understood, under legally sanctioned and culturally supported conditions. It will be essential, nevertheless, to learn from the lessons of the past and optimize conditions under which these compounds are administered. The greatest attention must be consistently given to establishing and maintaining strong safety parameters and to that end ensure that investigator-therapists employ the highest ethical standards in their work. The nascent field must also guard against pathologic narcissism and hubris. Adhering to proper standards of conduct and respecting personal boundaries will ultimately support the safe passage of the normal volunteer research subject and the healing of the patient seeking relief from suffering. It will also serve to protect the field from further obstructions to achieving its long-hoped-for but unrealized potential.

Moving forward, the greatest attention needs to be directed at minimizing adverse outcomes. The lessons learned, not only by a prior generation of modern researchers but also from the shamanic traditions, will be of great value to current research efforts as well as to future practitioners. For those who have fully understood the value of these highly unusual compounds, they are never taken for recreational or hedonic purposes. Intention is a key factor and will likely frame the content of the experience. Serious purposes for embarking on the hallucinogen experience, including healing and spiritual, provide a structure that provides protection and the optimal conditions under which to heal, to learn, and to grow. Attention to set and setting, as was fully understood by our predecessors, from those in the recent past back to the ancients, will optimize the likelihoods of safe and efficacious outcomes.

There is growing recognition that the judicious use of the hallucinogen treatment model, when administered under optimal conditions, may achieve successful therapeutic outcomes even in patients refractory to conventional treatments. The implications to the future of psychiatry and even other fields in medicine, are compelling. An integrative approach will need to be taken, incorporating all that has been learned from those who have explored this inner terrain from other times and other cultures, as well as from our predecessors from a half-century ago. In the 21st century, we also have access to an extraordinary neuroscience and medical technology that allows us to comprehensively examine the range of effects of hallucinogens: its mechanisms of action and putative models for healing. Recent interest in microdosing regimens, where a classic hallucinogen may only be administered sporadically, at supposed subthreshold dosages, raise new questions that await answers. Future research into mechanisms of action, as well as the potential medical and psychiatric uses of the hallucinogen treatment model, may over time achieve a significant impact on how we facilitate health and healing, on both individual and collective levels.

## REFERENCES

Abraham HD, Mamon A. LSD-like panic from risperidone in post-LSD visual disorder. *Journal Clinical Psychiatry*. 1996;16:238–241.

Bergman RL. Navajo peyote use: its apparent safety. *American Journal Psychiatry*. 1971;128:695–699.

Bravo G, Grob, CS. Shamans, sacraments and psychiatrists. *Journal Psychoactive Drugs.* 1989;21:123–128.

Chwelos N, Blewett DB, Smith CM, Hoffer, A. Use of d-lysergic acid diethylamide in the treatment of alcoholism. *Quarterly Journal Studies Alcohol.* 1959;20:577–590.

Dobkin de Rios M. *Hallucinogens: Cross-Cultural Perspective.* Albuquerque: University of New Mexico Press; 1984.

Dobkin de Rios M, Grob CS. Hallucinogens, suggestibility and adolescence in cross-cultural perspective. *Yearbook Ethnomedicine Study Consciousness.* 1994;3:113–132.

Grob CS. The psychology of ayahuasca. In: Metzner, R. ed., *Ayahuasca: Hallucinogens, Consciousness and the Spirit of Nature.* New York: Thunder's Mouth; 1999:214–249.

Grob CS, Dobkin de Rios M. Adolescent drug use in cross-cultural perspective. *Journal Drug Issues.* 1992;22:121–138.

Lattin D. *Distilled Spirits.* Oakland: University of California Press; 2012.

Lim TH, Wasywich CA, Ruygrok PH. A fatal case of magic mushroom ingestion in a heart transplant recipient. *Internal Medicine Journal.* 2012;42:1268–1269.

Ludwig AM, Levine J, Stark LH. *LSD and Alcoholism: A Clinical Study of Treatment Efficacy.* Springfield, IL: Charles C. Thomas; 1970.

MacLean JR, MacDonald DC, Byrne UP, Hubbard AM. LSD in treatment of alcoholism and other psychiatric problems. *Quarterly Journal Studies Alcoholism.* 1961;22:34–45.

Mithoefer MC, Grob CS, Brewerton TD. Novel psychopharmacological therapies for psychiatric disorders: psilocybin and MDMA. *Lancet Psychiatry.* 2016;3(5):481–488.

Poinar G, Alderman S, Wunderlich J. One hundred million year old ergot: psychotropic compounds in the Cretaceous. *Palaeodiversity.* 2015;8:13–19.

Samorini G. The oldest representation of hallucinogenic mushrooms in the world (Sahara Desert, 9000–7000 BC). *Integration.* 1992;2:69–78.

Van Dusen W, Wilson W, Miners W, Hook H. Treatment of alcoholism with lysergide. *Quarterly Journal Studies Alcoholism.* 1967;28:295–304.

# SECTION III

## The Tools

# 12

## Psychiatric Assessment and Co-Occurring Disorders

### SHAHLA J. MODIR AND JOHN TSUANG

People with substance-use disorders are more likely to suffer from a psychiatric diagnosis. In the last few decades, major studies have determined the prevalence of drug- and alcohol-use disorders and concurrent psychiatric disorders among the general population in the United States. Some of these studies include: the Epidemiologic Catchment Area (ECA) Study, the National Comorbidity Survey (NCS), National Epidemiologic Survey on Alcohol and Related Conditions (NESARC), and National Survey on Drug Use and Health (NSDUH).[1-4] Results from these studies show that the presence of alcohol and/or drug dependence increases the risk of having some type of mental disorder.

Drug- and alcohol-use data in 2013 showed that 24.6 million Americans (or 9.4% of the population age 12 and older) used an illicit drug within the last month, and 2.6% had a lifetime diagnosis of drug dependence.[4] In the same study, 8.2% of population met *DSM-IVTR* criteria for substance-use disorder (either abuse or dependence), and this rate has been stable for the last 10 years. In 2013 of the 20.3 million adults 18 years and older who have a past-year substance-use disorder, 37.8% have a co-occurring mental illness. In contrast, among adults without a past-year substance-use disorder, 16.7% had mental illness in the past year.[5] Thus, from this recent data, it has been determined that having a substance-use disorder in the past year increases the risk of having a co-occurring mental illness by 2.2 times.

According to NSDUH 2013, 52.2% of Americans are current alcohol drinkers, 22.9% participated in binge drinking (5 or more drinks per occasion), and 6.3% report heavy drinking (binge drinking 5 days in the past 30 days). Twelve-month and lifetime prevalence of alcohol-use disorder (AUD) were 13.9% and 29.9%.[5] Many significant associations were found between AUD and other substance use disorders (OR = 4.1), bipolar I disorder (OR = 2.0), major depression (OR = 1.3), antisocial personality disorder (OR = 1.9), borderline personality disorder (OR = 2.0). Additional associations were found between AUD and anxiety disorders (OR = 1.3), such as panic (OR = 1.3), specific phobia disorder (OR = 1.2), and generalized anxiety disorder (OR = 1.2). Furthermore, AUD also increased the risk of PTSD and schizotypal PD.[5] These higher odd ratios mean that those with AUD were at higher risk for developing a specific mental disorder as compared to those without AUD. For those with any substance-use disorder in the past year, researchers found that patients have higher rates of independent mood and anxiety disorders, including 19.67% for any mood disorder, 17.71% for any anxiety disorder. When looking at each anxiety disorder, specific phobia has the highest rate of 10.54%, social phobia at 4.72%, generalized anxiety disorder 4.2%, and panic disorder without agoraphobia at 2.86%.[3]

Another area of major concern is the high prevalence of smoking among people with psychiatric disorders, as well as co-occurrence of ADHD with psychoactive drug use among adults[6]. Studies showed that 50% to 90% of individuals with addiction or mental illness are tobacco dependent. Forty-four percent of cigarettes smoked in the United States are by individuals with either psychiatric diagnosis and/or drug addiction.[7] Other studies reported that the dual diagnosis population is 2 to 3 times more likely to be dependent on tobacco than the general population.[8,9] Rates of cigarette smoking by psychiatric patients vary according to their psychiatric diagnoses, with substance dependence and psychotic disorders having the highest use.[6]

The lifelong prevalence of ADHD in the general population is 1% to 5%. In patients with substance-use disorder, the ADHD prevalence rates are overly represented at rates ranging from 14% to 23% (Van Emmerik-van Oottmerssen, 2012; Vanden Glind et al., 2013).[10,11] These results come from a recent meta-analysis completed in both the United States and Europe, and both reflect the higher rates of ADHD in the substance-use disorder population. In addition to having ADHD, studies have shown that 65% to 89% of all adults with ADHD suffer from one or more additional psychiatric disorders, with a strong connection between ADHD, drug abuse, and alcoholism. ADHD is 5 to 10 times more common among adult alcoholics than in people without the alcohol problem. Among adults being treated for alcohol and substance abuse, the rate of ADHD is about 25%.[12]

## Differential Diagnosis

When patients with concurrent substance-use disorder and psychiatric symptoms, also called dual diagnosis patients (DDX), present for help, there can be a great deal of confusion in making accurate diagnoses and establishing a treatment plan. Diagnosis in this population can be difficult because substances of abuse can cause a wide range of psychological symptoms. In order to make an accurate diagnosis in the presence of substance abuse, one must determine what role substances played in the initiation and maintenance of these psychological symptoms. Clinicians must not only know what substances an individual is using but also the amount and duration of use, time of last use, and whether there are contaminants by other drugs. For the average dually diagnosed patient, this information is often missing or concealed, and its impact on patients' psychiatric symptoms is unclear. Even if clinicians perform a urine toxicology exam, results are often unhelpful because the window of detection has passed, or the test failed to pick up the specific drugs of abuse. Thus, the clinicians are often faced with the difficult dilemma of being unable to make an accurate diagnosis in this patient population.

There are multitudes of diagnostic possibilities when patients are abusing substances and suffer from psychiatric symptoms simultaneously. First, some psychiatric symptoms are consequences of intoxication and/or withdrawal from substances of abuse and they are temporary in nature and usually resolved when substances uses are discontinued or withdrawal symptoms are complete. This is defined as substance-induced mental disorders.[12] People suffering from these substance-induced psychiatric symptoms are indistinguishable from those with functional psychiatric disorders. There are many examples of substance-induced depression, anxiety, and psychosis. Repeated heavy drinking of alcohol can be associated with a temporary depressive episodes, severe anxiety, and/ or insomnia. Acute withdrawal and chronic withdrawal from alcohol can lead to transient psychosis with auditory and visual hallucinations and autonomic instability. Acute intoxication of stimulants can produce psychosis and manic-like symptoms, while withdrawal from stimulants can present with depressive symptoms. Chronic marijuana use can cause depressive and anxiety symptoms, while less likely, its use also are associated with psychosis. However, if these symptoms are purely substance induced, they are likely to improve within 2 to 4 weeks of abstinence.[13,14]

Another possibility is that the secondary diagnosis might develop due to an attempt to reduce problems associated with the first diagnosis. For example, some individual might escalate their alcohol use to reduce symptoms of depression and insomnia. Thus they developed a secondary alcohol-related problem in an attempt to resolve the primary depression. Another possibility is that this co-occurrence might be represented by two independent conditions: each disorder occurring independently of each other, and this combination could occur by chance alone or caused by similar predisposing factors shared by both conditions. These factors might be a high stress level, a predisposing personality traits, childhood impact, and/or genetic impact.[15] Finally, the first disorder can cause the development of the second disorder, which then becomes an independent disorder by itself. A perfect example of this is methamphetamine-induced psychosis in people with some predisposition resulting in chronic psychosis resembling schizophrenia.[16]

## Diagnosing Comorbidity

Clinicians have tried different methods to make an accurate diagnosis in DDX patients. One common way is the using of the primary and secondary diagnosis distinction, where the first condition to develop is the primary diagnosis and the second condition to occur is the secondary diagnosis.[17-19] This method is based purely on age of onset of each condition and not focused on cause and effect. Another method is to emphasize the distinction between substance-induced disorders versus the independent mental disorders. One needs to determine if psychiatric syndrome is present while someone is sober for a period of time. Thus, a psychiatric disorder can only be diagnosed during a period of abstinence. It is imperative for patients to have a period of sobriety to utilize this method of diagnosis. Finally, some clinicians accept the difficulty of making a diagnosis among active using patients and endorse the strategy of classifying DDX patients into four categories: category I is the less severe mental disorder/less severe substance abuse disorder, category II is the more severe mental disorder/less severe substance abuse disorder, category III is the less severe mental disorder/more severe substance abuse disorder, category IV is the more severe mental disorder/more severe substance abuse disorder.[20] Thus, their treatment will be dictated according to which category patients fit into. It is recommended to have serial longitudinal assessments to further improve diagnostic certainty, especially in the first 3 months of sobriety where the brain is in a recovery state.

## Medication Strategy

Medication strategies for the treatment of DDX patients are complicated. First, one needs to determine if medications are necessary for management of withdrawal symptoms. Second, clinicians must think about how to treat psychiatric symptoms occurred in the midst of withdrawal. Third, doctors must decide when to treat psychiatric symptoms that persist after the withdrawal state. Finally, physicians must figure out the role of substance reducing medications for treatment of substance abuse disorders in their practice. In the beginning, regardless of their diagnosis, patients suffering from severe withdrawal symptoms from alcohol, benzodiazepines, and opiates will need medical treatment. We must safely detoxify patients to prevent any life threatening consequences from happening. Furthermore, one needs to keep in mind the possibility that patients might be abusing multiple substances simultaneously, such as drinking alcohol and abusing benzodiazepines at the same time. Thus, careful assessment to determine potential multiple substances of abuse and the need of using medications to treat withdrawal symptoms is essential. Next, during substances withdrawal, it is not uncommon for patients to suffer from debilitating psychiatric symptoms such as psychosis, mania, and agitation, despite receiving proper withdrawal medications. Clinicians must decide whether to increase medications for treatment of withdrawal symptoms, or add additional psychiatric medications to treat them appropriately. Sometimes, we might need to add an antipsychotic medication or a mood stabilizer to manage a complicate withdrawal state. If these additional psychiatric symptoms are ignored, patients might be at higher risk for relapse or have a complicated and prolonged withdrawal period. During the withdrawal state, neuroadaptive changes can occur in the brain, which can increase the risk of seizure and worsen the severity of future withdrawal symptoms. Often, the most commonly asked question after withdrawal is: how long does a patient needs to be sober before a clinician should initiate psychiatric medications for treatment of depression or anxiety state? According to *DSM-5*, substance-induced mental disorder should not last longer than a month. Thus, most clinicians will abide by this strategy and start treatment only when patients have been sober for a month or longer. However others disagree with this strategy and advocate for initiating medication treatment dependent on the severity of psychiatric symptoms rather than waiting for the 1-month sober period. One common strategy is the treatment of severe, life-threatening psychiatric symptoms such as psychosis, mania, suicidal depression—regardless of the duration of the sober period. In the case of other psychiatric symptoms that are non-life threatening, such as depression or anxiety, one might wait for a period of time before treatment. Some anti-depressants can cause significant agitation and anxiety during detoxification. It is advisable to wait until the detoxification is complete to start on anti-depressants. Most clinicians will choose safety first, carefully weighing the benefit of treatment versus the risks of prescribing medications that have overdose potential or can produce significant side effects. Clinicians also need to be careful when prescribing medications that can be abused or worsen the addiction process (e.g., benzodiazpines and psychostimulants). Some of these medications might even be diverted because of their street value; thus one needs to choose medications that are longer acting in nature and that tend to have less abuse liability. Additionally, non-medication intervention such as neurofeedback and mindfulness can be tremendously helpful and while not increasing the risk of relapse.

## Pharmacological Treatments for Co-Occurring Substance Abuse and Psychiatric Conditions

Anti-depressants are common pharmaceutical treatments for depressive disorders co-occurring with alcoholism and other substance-use disorders. Two major meta-analytic studies found a similar outcome that anti-depressant medication is more effective than placebo for AUD patients with co-occurring depression.[21-22] The outcome for cocaine and opiate-use disorder patients with comorbid depression was less clear. The effect size for using anti-depressants for the treatment of depression with substance abuse was reviewed in a major *JAMA* article from 2004 by Nunes, and it looked at 14 placebo-controlled studies encompassing 800 carefully selected patients who had co-occurring alcohol-, cocaine-, and opiate-use disorders. The researchers found an elevated placebo response rate with the effect size for the treatment of depression using medication of 0.38, similar to outpatient medication trials for treatment of depression without substance abuse. The studies with best outcome results for treatment of depression were ones where the patients were abstinent at least 1 week before any diagnosis or treatment with medication was initiated.[23,24] Where criteria for a depression disorder from the *DSM-4* were not met, anti-depressants were not effective. All 5 studies using SSRIs showed no benefit in reducing depression, but the 2 studies that controlled for placebo response did show a positive effect for reduction of depressive symptoms.[25] The high placebo rates in most substance abuse studies demonstrated that substance related depression often remits within days to weeks after quitting substances such as alcohol.[26,27] In the Nunes study, if there was a benefit in using anti-depressants for co-occurring depression, there was a commiserate level of improvement in self reported substance use.[28] In all studies, however, improving depression did not correlate with improved substance use outcomes, and it is clear that both substance abuse problems as well as mental health issues need to be treated for both to improve.

Additionally, there is a subgroup of alcoholics who have increased relapse rates under the influence of SSRI treatment.[29,30,33] Studies showed that when using SSRI for treatment of Type B alcoholics (those individuals characterized as having an early onset of alcohol use, weak environmental influences, more severe dependence, and a higher frequency of antisocial and impulsive traits), they had worse drinking outcomes as compared to those receiving placebo.[31] This result was replicated in a study of patients suffering from PTSD and alcoholism whereby sertraline treatment provided increased relapse rates for Type B alcoholics.[32] By contrast, Type A alcoholics (those having a later onset of alcohol use, a lower rate of comorbidities, and less severe alcohol use), they responded well to treatment with sertraline for their depression as well as to treatment for PTSD in a separate trial.[32,33]

While SSRIs might have questionable effectiveness for treatment of alcohol dependence and depression, the combination of naltrexone with SSRIs may be useful for reducing alcohol consumption and depression. One double-blind, placebo-controlled trial tested the effectiveness of combining sertraline with naltrexone as treatment for both depression and alcohol dependence in 170 individuals. Results showed that the combination of naltrexone with sertraline yielded a significantly higher abstinence rate (53.7%) than sertraline alone (27.5%), naltrexone alone (21.3%), and placebo (23.1%).[34] The group treated with both naltrexone and sertraline also showed fewer adverse effects and less depressive symptoms at the end of the trial.

Research on the management of bipolar disorder with substance misuse is less robust. There is a high prevalence of substance abuse among bipolar patients. Studies showed that the course of mania is more severe, and they have worse prognosis in comorbid substance abusing bipolar patients.[35] Additionally, findings showed that these patients are more likely to be hospitalized, less responsive to treatment, and have a higher risk for suicide.[36,37] Unfortunately, there is not an optimized treatment approach for care of this population, but research suggested that integrating treatment of substance abuse and mental health is critically important in the treatment of bipolar patients with substance abuse problems. Integrated group therapy (IGT) is a type of group therapy that was designed to address patients suffering from bipolar disorder and substance use disorder. IGT has been shown to have beneficial effects in comorbid management.[38,39] As far as pharmacological options, open label trials have been completed using gabapentin, lamictal, and depakote. The results showed that all three medications showed some beneficial effects for this population.[40–43] An open label study on the use of quetiapine in bipolar patients with cocaine use disorder showed some improvement for cocaine use.[44] Another open label trial using quetiapine for bipolar patients with alcohol dependence showed bipolar depression improved, but it had no effect on alcohol use.[45]

Unfortunately, double-blind placebo-controlled studies examining medication treatment of bipolar patients and co-occurring substance use disorder are lacking. One study suggested that using depakote plus lithium was more effective than using lithium alone in reducing the number of heavy drinking days in patients with alcoholism and bipolar disorder.[46] In another study, utilizing lithium alone, adolescents with bipolar disorder, and substance-use disorder had positive results with improved mood and reduced substance use.[47]

With respect to anxiety disorders and substance-use disorders, there is a paucity of trials looking at treating the comorbid conditions. There have been 2 studies done using the SSRI paroxetine to treat anxiety in alcoholics, and the results showed a reduction in anxiety and social anxiety without changes in alcohol consumption.[48,49] There were 4 double-blind trials using buspirone, a partial 5 HT1A agonist, for treatment of anxiety in alcoholic patients. Bruno and Tollefson both found that buspirone treated patients stayed in treatment longer, and had decreased alcohol craving, as well as reduction in their anxiety and depression.[50,51] In another study by Kranzler, buspirone was more effective than placebo at reducing anxiety in alcoholics but also in delaying relapse to heavy drinking and had lower number of drinking during follow-up.[52] Buspirone had the greatest effect for those patients with the highest baseline anxiety. However, another study showed that buspirone was not effective at reducing anxiety or alcohol use among severe alcoholics.[53]

The management of psychosis in substance-use disorder patients has been studied under many different circumstances. There are various associations between psychosis and substances of abuse. There are drugs that can cause acute psychosis, such as cocaine, amphetamines/methamphetamine, marijuana, alcohol, and club drugs. Psychosis can also occur as part of withdrawal symptom from alcohol and other substances. Marijuana or methamphetamine use may lead to chronic psychosis or the development of schizophrenia-like syndrome. Patients with schizophrenia can use drugs that precipitate psychosis independent of their schizophrenia pathology. It is also true that chronic drug use can lower the threshold of developing psychosis.[54] It is important to treat psychotic symptoms with anti-psychotic medication whether it is a temporary or more prolonged state in order to retain patients in treatment and improve their outcomes. In studying the treatment of schizophrenia with substance use, there is some evidence that reward dysfunction in schizophrenia predisposes these patients to higher rates of substance abuse, and clozapine has proven to be more effective than others in reducing psychosis and drug use in some trials.[55] Clozapine has shown some promise in reducing smoking, cannabis, and alcohol use among schizophrenic patients. In a posteriori study of 151 patients with schizophrenia or schizoaffective disorder and co-occurring substance-use disorder, 36 patients received clozapine for treatment of their psychotic disorder. The participants were assessed prospectively at baseline and every 6 months over 3 years for psychiatric symptoms and substance use. Results of the study showed that alcohol-abusing patients taking clozapine experienced significant reductions in severity of alcohol abuse and days of alcohol use while on clozapine and improved more than patients who did not receive clozapine. Seventy-nine percent of the patients on clozapine were in remission from AUD for 6 months or longer at the end of the study, while only 33.7% of those not taking clozapine were remitted.[56] Side effects are a major consideration before deciding to use this medication, since weight gain, hyperlipidemia, diabetes mellitus, and agranulocytosis are possible. Additionally, a study that evaluated adding naltrexone to antipsychotic medication for the treatment of schizophrenia and AUD found reduced heavy drinking days and number of drinking days.[57] In general, however, problems such as medication noncompliance, unemployment, legal problems, homelessness, and cognitive impairment are common in the schizophrenic population, and outcomes for substance abuse are much less successful. It is clear that integrating treatment of both disorders is the only way to achieve any success.

For the treatment of comorbid ADHD and substance-use disorder here have been 13 double-blind placebo-controlled trials looking at pharmacotherapy. Twelve of these were outpatient studies and looked at a variety of different substances of misuse. Only 4 studies of ADHD with comorbid substance-use disorder including 2 with nicotine-use disorder, one with amphetamine misuse, and one with alcoholism showed efficacy when using stimulants or atmoxetine for the treatment of ADHD.[58,59,60] One of the positive studies examined atomoxetine in adults with comorbid AUD and ADHD. This study did find that atomoxetine did improve ADHD symptoms but did not improve alcohol use. However, there was a reduction in the number of heavy drinking days in the active versus placebo group.[61] Each of the other studies were mixed in their results in eliciting any major benefit of using medication to treat ADHD with comorbid substance use.[62–69] Several trials have looked at cocaine addiction and ADHD with use of long acting methylphenidate.[70,71] They found no increased risk of diversion and that the subjective high of cocaine was reduced in the methylphenidate groups. Results were mixed, however, in the treatment of ADHD, and there was not an improvement detected for cocaine use. In one of the studies, there was an initial efficacy in favor of methylphenidate for ADHD and comorbid cocaine use.[71] However, by the end of the trial at week 12, the differences in response rates between drug and placebo became nearly equal for methylphenidate 50% versus placebo 56%. There was no effect on cocaine use, and methylphenidate did not improve or worsen the cocaine use in the treated patients versus placebo. Additionally, in only 1 out of these 12 outpatient studies was there a tendency toward positive effects on the substance abuse when treating comorbid ADHD with medication.[72] In all these studies the patients received additional psychosocial therapy.

It is clear that the treatment of comorbid ADHD and substance abuse is essential for recovery, but the current model does not have favorable outcomes. In general, we recommend waiting periods of at least 1 week to 1 month before making a firm diagnosis and remembering that the symptoms need to be present in more than one setting, are clinically impairing, and ensuring that there are not other psychiatric disorders such as bipolar disorder, PTSD, or anxiety that may account for attentional symptoms. We also recommend favoring nonabusable medications such as strattera, guanfacine er, clonidine er, modafinil, and wellbutrin over stimulants. If stimulants are necessary, we recommend the long acting preparations over short acting and monitoring closely for signs of diversion/misuse.

## Summary of Integrative Treatments

In the management of complex co-occurring disorder patients, medications are not the only solution: using complementary tools can be of great benefit. In the treatment of comorbid depression, adding fish oil, folic acid, or SAM-E is recommended where appropriate as an augmentation to pharmacotherapy of depression.[73–81] Avoid using St. John's Wort for depression except in mild cases due to several drug/drug interactions.[82] Exercise, neurofeedback, and mindfulness are other useful tools that can reduce drug craving and depression.[83–89] These effects are discussed more extensively in Dr. Weil's book *Integrative Psychiatry*.

In the management of bipolar disorder comorbid with substance use, we recommend adding N-acetyl cysteine and fish oil.[90,91,96] In the case of cocaine and marijuana use with bipolar patients, N-acetyl cysteind and citicholine might be helpful to reduce craving and improve cognition.[92-95] Social rhythm therapy, exercise, neurofeedback, and meditation are also useful adjuncts to neutralize circadian rhythm and improve outcomes in bipolar disorder.[96-99]

With respect to anxiety, we recommend both yoga and exercise as beneficial tools in reducing worrying and physical anxiety symptoms.[100-102] Meditation/MBSR has also been shown to reduce anxiety.[103] We recommend a high potency B complex vitamin for anxiety patients along with magnesium and calcium to help create relaxing sleep and aide in reducing muscle tension.[101,104] Additionally, we often use passionflower, L-theanine and inositol in cases where patients have poor tolerance to medications but are in need of relief.[101]

In cases of ADD/ADHD, neurofeedback has been shown to improve cognitive function and executive function.[105,106] We also recommend fish oil as evidence based supplement for the management of ADD/ADHD and phosphadtidylserine serine also shown to be helpful for treatment of attention symptoms.[107-109] Exercise and meditation can both improve executive functions and reduce brain stress to help patients who suffer from attention disorders.[110-113]

For psychotic disorders, N-Acetyl Cysteine has been shown to improve psychotic symptoms in treatment resistant cases and is well tolerated with few side effects.[114,115] We also recommend neurofeedback and exercise as reasonable tools for patients suffering from schizophrenia.[116-120]

In summary, psychiatric comorbities are frequent in the substance-abusing population. The presence of a dual diagnosis should be properly evaluated by using a waiting period and ensuring treatment of symptoms during the withdrawal period. Over- and under-diagnosis is common in this population, and a waiting period of at least 1 week to 1 month can be helpful to assist in diagnostic accuracy and treatment outcomes. While we briefly addressed the integrative treatment of specific psychiatric comorbities in limited matter, other chapters in this book will address this in a warranted level of complexity. It is clear that self-medication is frequently occurring in the substance-abusing population; however, treating only the psychiatric symptoms does not always improve the substance abuse outcome. It is evident that both disorders have to be addressed in an integrative way to be optimal. The question of using anti-depressants for both the treatment of addiction and related psychiatric disorders was mentioned to ensure the reader understands that they don't always help as we previously thought. Further, they may actually worsen addiction and increased relapse rates when they are used in particular sub-populations. The possibility of using an integrative approach, in addition to the use of medications, is essential in the treatment of these co-occurring patients. Using a more holistic approach as the one described throughout this book and in the Dr. Weil textbook *Integrative Psychiatry* can be beneficial for treatment of this population.[121]

# REFERENCES

1. Regier DA, Farmer ME, Rae, DS, et al. Comorbidity of mental disorders with alcohol and other drug abuse: Results from the Epidemiologic Catchment Area (ECA) Study. *Journal of the American Medical Association.* 1990;21:2511–2518.
2. Kessler RC, Berglund P, Demler O, Jin R, Merikangas KR, Walters EE. Lifetime prevalence and age-of-onset distributions of *DSM-4* disorders in the National Comorbidity Survey Replication. *Archives of General Psychiatry.* 2005;62:593–602.
3. Grant BF, Stinson FS, Dawson DA, et al. Prevalence and co-occurrence of substance use disorders and independent mood and anxiety disorders. *Archives of General Psychiatry.* 2006;29:107–120.
4. SAMHSA. Results from the 2013 National Survey on Drug Use and Health: Summary of National Findings, NSDUH Series H-48, HHS Publication No. (SMA) 14-4863. Rockville, MD: Substance Abuse and Mental Health Services Administration; 2014.
5. Grant BF, Goldstein RB, Saha TD, et al. Epidemiology of *DSM-5* Alcohol use disorder: Results from the National Epidemiologic Survey on Alcohol and Related Conditions III. *Journal of the American Medical Association.* 2015;72:757–66.
6. Williams JM, Ziedonis D. Addressing tobacco among individuals with a mental illness or an addiction. *Addictive Behaviors.* 2004;29:1067–1083.
7. Lasser K, Boyd W, Woolhandler S, Himmelstein DU, McCormik D, Bor DH. Smoking and mental illness: A population-based prevalence study. *Journal of the American Medical Association.* 2000;284:2606–2610.
8. Lohr JB, Flynn K. Smoking and schizophrenia. *Schizophrenia Research.* 1992;8:93–102.
9. World Health Report. *Mental Health: New Understanding, New Hope.* Geneva, Switzerland: World Health Organization; 2001.
10. Van de Glind G, Konstenius M, Koeter MWJ, van Emmerik-van Oortmerssen K, Carpentier PJ, Kaye S. IASP Research Group: Variability in the prevalence of adult ADHD in treatment seeking substance use disorder patients: Results from an international multi-center study exploring *DSM-4* and *DSM-5* criteria. *Drug and Alcohol Dependence.* 2014;134:158–166.
11. van Emmerik-van Oortmerssen K, van de Glind G, Koeter MW, et al. Psychiatric comorbidity in treatment-seeking substance use disorder patients with and without attention deficit hyperactivity disorder: results of the IASP study. *Addiction.* 2014;109(2):262–272.
12. Sobanski E. Psychiatric comorbidity in adults with attention-deficit/hyperactivity disorder (ADHD). *European Archives of Psychiatry and Clinical Neuroscience.* 2006;256:1–27.
13. American Psychiatric Association. Diagnostic and Statistical Manual of Mental Disorders: *DSM-5.* Washington, DC: American Psychiatric Association; 2013.
14. Shuckit MA. Comorbidity between substance use disorders and psychiatric conditions. *American Psychiatric Association.* 2006;101:76–88.
15. Lukasiewics M, Blecha L, Falissard B, et al. Dual diagnosis: Prevalence, risk factors, and relationship with suicide risk in a nationwide sample of French prisoners. *Alcoholism: Clinical & Experimental Research.* 2008;33:160–168.

16. Zorick TS, Rad D, Rim C, Tsuang J. An overview of methamphetamine-induced psychotic syndromes. *Addictive Disorders and Their Treatment.* 2008;7:143–156.

17. Lehman AF, Myers CP, Corty E, Thompson JW. Prevalence and patterns of 'dual diagnosis' among psychiatric inpatients. *Comprehensive Psychiatry.* 1994;35:106–112.

18. Shuckit MA. The clinical implications of primary diagnostic groups among alcoholics. *Archives of General Psychiatry.* 1985;42:1043–1049.

19. Shuckit MA. Genetic and clinical implications of alcoholism and affective disorder. *American Journal of Psychiatry.* 1986;143:140–147.

20. Ries RK. The dually diagnosed patient with psychotic symptoms. *Journal of Addictive Disorders.* 1993;12:103–122.

21. Nunes EV, Levin FR. Treatment of depression in patients with alcohol or other drug dependence: a meta-analysis. *Journal of the American Medical Association.* 2004;291(15):1887–1896.

22. Walsh BT, Seidman SN, Sysko R, Gould M. Placebo response in studies of major depression: variable, substantial, and growing. *Journal of the American Medical Association.* 2002;287(14):1840–1847.

23. Altamura AC, Mauri MC, Girardi T, Panetta B. Alcoholism and depression: a placebo controlled study with viloxazine. *International Journal of Clinical Pharmacology Research.* 1990;10(5):293–298.

24. Cornelius JR, Salloum IM, Ehler JG, et al. Fluoxetine in depressed alcoholics: a double-blind, placebo-controlled trial. *Archives of General Psychiatry.* 1997;54(8):700–705.

25. Nunes EV, Levin FR. Treatment of depression in patients with alcohol or other drug dependence: a meta-analysis. *Journal of the American Medical Association.* 2004;291(15):1887–1896.

26. Brown SA, Schuckit MA. Changes in depression among abstinent alcoholics. *Journal of Studies on Alcohol.* 1988;49(5):412–417.

27. Schuckit MA, Smith TL, Danko GP, et al. A comparison of factors associated with substance-induced versus independent depressions. *Journal of Studies on Alcohol and Drugs.* 2007;68(6):805–812.

28. Nunes EV, Levin FR. Treatment of depression in patients with alcohol or other drug dependence: a meta-analysis. *Journal of the American Medical Association.* 2004;291(15):1887–1896.

29. Pettinati HM, Volpicelli JR, Kranzler HR, Luck G, Rukstalis MR, Cnaan A. Sertraline treatment for alcohol dependence: interactive effects of medication and alcoholic subtype. *Alcoholism, Clinical and Experimental Research.* 2000;24(7):1041–1049.

30. Pettinati H, Oslin D, Decker K. Role of serotonin and serotonin-selective pharmacotherapy in alcohol dependence. *CNS Spectrums.* 2000;5(2):33–46.

31. Kranzler H, Burleson J, Brown J, Thomas F. Fluoxetine treatment seems to reduce the beneficial effects of cognitive-behavioral therapy in Type B alcoholics. *Alcoholism: Clinical and Experimental Research.* 1996;20(9):1534–1541.

32. Brady KT, Sonne S, Anton RF, Randall CL, Back SE, Simpson K. Sertraline in the treatment of co-occurring alcohol dependence and posttraumatic stress disorder. *Alcoholism: Clinical and Experimental Research.* 2005;29(3):395–401.

33. Kranzler H, Armeli S, Tennen H, et al. A double-blind, randomized trial of sertraline for alcohol-dependence: moderation by age of onset and 5-HTTLPR genotype. *Journal of Clinical Psychoparmacology.* 2011;31(1):22–30.
34. Pettinati H, Oslin D, Kampman K, et al. A double-blind, placebo-controlled trial combining sertraline and naltrexone for treating co-occuring depression and alcohol dependence. *American Journal of Psychiatry.* 2010;167(6):668–675.
35. Salloum IM, Cornelius JR, Mezzich JE, Kirisci L. Impact of concurrent alcohol misuse on symptom presentation of acute mania at initial evaluation. *Bipolar Disorders.* 2002;4(6):418–421.
36. Cassidy F, Ahearn EP, Carroll BJ. Substance abuse in bipolar disorder. *Bipolar Disorders.* 2001;3(4):181–188.
37. Dalton EJ, Cate-Carter TD, Mundo E, Parikh SV, Kennedy JL. Suicide risk in bipolar patients: the role of co-morbid substance use disorders. *Bipolar Disorders.* 2003;5(1):58–61.
38. Weiss RD. Treating patients with bipolar disorder and substance dependence: lessons learned. *Journal of Substance Abuse Treatment.* 2004;27(4):307–312.
39. Weiss RD, Griffin ML, Kolodziej ME, et al. A randomized trial of integrated group therapy versus group drug counseling for patients with bipolar disorder and substance dependence. *American Journal of Psychiatry.* 2007;164(1):100–107.
40. Rubio G, López-Muñoz F, Alamo C. Effects of lamotrigine in patients with bipolar disorder and alcohol dependence. *Bipolar Disorders.* 2006;8(3):289–293.
41. Brady KT, Sonne SC, Anton R, Ballenger JC. Valproate in the treatment of acute bipolar affective episodes complicated by substance abuse: a pilot study. *Journal of Clinical Psychiatry.* 1995;56(3):118–121.
42. Salloum IM, Cornelius JR, Daley DC, Kirisci L, Himmelhoch JM, Thase ME. Efficacy of valproate maintenance in patients with bipolar disorder and alcoholism: a double-blind placebo-controlled study. *Archives of General Psychiatry.* 2005;62(1):37–45.
43. Perugi G, Toni C, Frare F, Ruffolo G, Moretti L, Torti C, Akiskal HS. Effectiveness of adjunctive gabapentin in resistant bipolar disorder: is it due to anxious-alcohol abuse comorbidity? *Journal of Clinical Psychopharmacology.* 2002;22(6):584–591.
44. Brown ES, Nejtek VA, Perantie DC, Bobadilla L. Quetiapine in bipolar disorder and cocaine dependence. *Bipolar Disorders.* 2002;4(6):406–411.
45. Brown ES, Garza M, Carmody TJ. A randomized, double-blind, placebo-controlled add-on trial of quetiapine in outpatients with bipolar disorder and alcohol use disorders. *Journal of Clinical Psychiatry.* 2008;69(5):701–705.
46. Salloum IM, Cornelius JR, Daley DC, Kirisci L, Himmelhoch JM, Thase ME. Efficacy of valproate maintenance in patients with bipolar disorder and alcoholism: a double-blind placebo-controlled study. *Archives of General Psychiatry.* 2005;62(1):37–45.
47. Geller B, Cooper TB, Sun K, Zimerman B, Frazier J, Williams M, Heath J. Double-blind and placebo-controlled study of lithium for adolescent bipolar disorders with secondary substance dependency. *Journal of the American Academy of Child and Adolescent Psychiatry.* 1998;37(2):171–178.

48. Book SW, Thomas SE, Randall PK, Randall CL. Paroxetine reduces social anxiety in individuals with a co-occurring alcohol use disorder. *Journal of Anxiety Disorders.* 2008;22(2):310–318.

49. Thomas SE, Randall PK, Book SW, Randall CL. A complex relationship between co-occurring social anxiety and alcohol use disorders: what effect does treating social anxiety have on drinking? *Alcoholism, Clinical and Experimental Research.* 2008;32(1):77–84.

50. Bruno F. Buspirone in the treatment of alcoholic patients. *Psychopathology.* 1989;22(Suppl 1):49–59.

51. Tollefson GD, Montague-Clouse J, Tollefson SL. Treatment of comorbid generalized anxiety in a recently detoxified alcoholic population with a selective serotonergic drug (buspirone). *Journal of Clinical Psychopharmacology.* 1992;12(1):19–26.

52. Kranzler HR, Burleson JA, Del Boca FK, et al. Buspirone treatment of anxious alcoholics. A placebo-controlled trial. *Archives of General Psychiatry.* 1994;51(9):720–731.

53. Malcolm R, Anton RF, Randall CL, Johnston A, Brady K, Thevos A. A placebo-controlled trial of buspirone in anxious inpatient alcoholics. *Alcoholism, Clinical and Experimental Research.* 1992;16(6):1007–1013.

54. Brady KT, Lydiard RB, Malcolm R, Ballenger JC. Cocaine-induced psychosis. *Journal of Clinical Psychiatry.* 1991;52(12):509–512.

55. Green AI. Pharmacotherapy for schizophrenia and co-occurring substance use disorders. *Neurotoxicity Research.* 2007;11(1):33–40.

56. Drake RE, Xie H, McHugo GJ, Green AI. The effects of clozapine on alcohol and drug use disorders among patients with schizophrenia. *Schizophrenia Bulletin.* 2000;26(2):441–449.

57. Petrakis IL, O'Malley S, Rounsaville B, Poling J, McHugh-Strong C, Krystal JH. VA Naltrexone Study Collaboration Group: Naltrexone augmentation of neuroleptic treatment in alcohol abusing patients with schizophrenia. *Psychopharmacology (Berl).* 2004;172(3):291–297.

58. Kollins SH, English JS, Itchon-Ramos N. A pilot study of lis-dexamfetamine dimesylate (LDX/SPD489) to facilitate smoking cessation in nicotine-dependent adults with ADHD. *Journal of Attention Disorders.* 2014;18(2):158–168.

59. Konstenius M, Jayaram-Lindström N, Guterstam J, Beck O, Philips B, Franck J. Methylphenidate for attention deficit hyperactivity disorder and drug relapse in criminal offenders with substance dependence: a 24-week randomized placebo-controlled trial. *Addiction.* 2014;109(3):440–449.

60. Winhusen TM, Somoza EC, Brigham GS, et al. Impact of attention-deficit/hyperactivity disorder (ADHD) treatment on smoking cessation intervention in ADHD smokers: a randomized, double-blind, placebo-controlled trial. *Journal of Clinical Psychiatry.* 2010;71(12):1680–1688.

61. Wilens TE, Adler LA, Weiss MD. Atomoxetine ADHD/SUD Study Group. Atomoxetine treatment of adults with ADHD and comorbid alcohol use disorders. *Drug Alcohol Depend.* 2008;96(1–2):145–154.

62. Schubiner H, Saules KK, Arfken CL, et al. Double-blind placebo-controlled trial of methylphenidate in the treatment of adult ADHD patients with comorbid cocaine dependence. *Experimental and Clinical Psychopharmacology.* 2002;10(3):286–294.

63. Riggs PD, Winhusen T, Davies RD, et al. Randomized controlled trial of osmotic-release methylphenidate with cognitive-behavioral therapy in adolescents with attention-deficit/hyperactivity disorder and substance use disorders. *Journal of the American Academy of Child and Adolescent Psychiatry.* 2011;50(9):903–914.

64. Levin FR, Evans SM, Brooks DJ, Kalbag AS, Garawi F, Nunes EV. Treatment of methadone-maintained patients with adult ADHD: double-blind comparison of methylphenidate, bupropion and placebo. *Drug Alcohol Depend.* 2006;81(2):137–148.

65. Levin FR, Evans SM, Brooks DJ, Garawi F. Treatment of cocaine dependent treatment seekers with adult ADHD: double-blind comparison of methylphenidate and placebo. *Drug Alcohol Depend.* 2007;87(1):20–29.

66. Konstenius M, Jayaram-Lindström N, Beck O, Franck J. Sustained release methylphenidate for the treatment of ADHD in amphetamine abusers: a pilot study. *Drug Alcohol Depend.* 2010;108(1–2):130–133.

67. McRae-Clark AL, Carter RE, Killeen TK, Carpenter MJ, White KG, Brady KT. A placebo-controlled trial of atomoxetine in marijuana-dependent individuals with attention deficit hyperactivity disorder. *American Journal on Addictions.* 2010;19(6):481–489.

68. Thurstone C, Riggs PD, Salomonsen-Sautel S, Mikulich-Gilbertson SK. Randomized, controlled trial of atomoxetine for attention-deficit/hyperactivity disorder in adolescents with substance use disorder. *Journal of the American Academy of Child and Adolescent Psychiatry.* 2010;49(6):573–582.

69. Riggs PD, Hall SK, Mikulich-Gilbertson SK, Lohman M, Kayser A. A randomized controlled trial of pemoline for attention-deficit/hyperactivity disorder in substance-abusing adolescents. *Journal of the American Academy of Child and Adolescent Psychiatry.* 2004;43(4):420–429.

70. Levin FR, Evans SM, Brooks DJ, Garawi F. Treatment of cocaine dependent treatment seekers with adult ADHD: double-blind comparison of methylphenidate and placebo. *Drug Alcohol Depend.* 2007;87(1):20–29.

71. Schubiner H, Saules KK, Arfken CL, et al. Double-blind placebo-controlled trial of methylphenidate in the treatment of adult ADHD patients with comorbid cocaine dependence. *Experimental and Clinical Psychopharmacology.* 2002;10(3):286–294.

72. Konstenius M, Jayaram-Lindström N, Guterstam J, Beck O, Philips B, Franck J. Methylphenidate for attention deficit hyperactivity disorder and drug relapse in criminal offenders with substance dependence: a 24-week randomized placebo-controlled trial. *Addiction.* 2014;109(3):440–449.

73. Appleton KM, Sallis HM, Perry R, Ness AR, Churchill R. Omega-3 fatty acids for depression in adults. *Cochrane Database System Review.* 2015;11:CD004692.

74. Grosso G, Pajak A, Marventano S, et al. Role of omega-3 fatty acids in the treatment of depressive disorders: a comprehensive meta-analysis of randomized clinical trials. *PLoS One.* 2014;9(5):e96905.

75. Bloch MH, Hannestad J. Omega-3 fatty acids for the treatment of depression: systematic review and meta-analysis. *Molecular Psychiatry*. 2012;17(12):1272–1282.
76. Sublette ME, Ellis SP, Geant AL, Mann JJ. Meta-analysis of the effects of eicosapentaenoic acid (EPA) in clinical trials in depression. *Journal of Clinical Psychiatry*. 2011;72(12):1577–1584.
77. Morris DW, Trivedi MH, Rush AJ. Folate and unipolar depression. *Journal of Alternative and Complementary Medicine*. 2008;14(3):277–285.
78. Fava M, Mischoulon D. Evidence for folate in combination with antidepressants at initiation of therapy. *Journal of Clinical Psychiatry*. 2010;71(11):e31
79. Papakostas GI. Evidence for S-adenosyl-L-methionine (SAM-e) for the treatment of major depressive disorder. *Journal of Clinical Psychiatry*. 2009;70(Suppl 5):18–22.
80. Papakostas GI, Cassiello CF, Iovieno N. Folates and S-adenosylmethionine for major depressive disorder. *Canadian Journal of Psychiatry*. 2012;57(7):406–413.
81. Owen RT. Folate augmentation of antidepressant response. *Drugs Today (Barc)*. 2013;49(12):791–798.
82. Russo E, Scicchitano F, Whalley BJ, et al. Hypericum perforatum: pharmacokinetic, mechanism of action, tolerability, and clinical drug-drug interactions. *Phytotherapy Research*. 2014;28(5):643–655.
83. Krogh J, Nordentoft M, Sterne JA, Lawlor DA. The effect of exercise in clinically depressed adults: systematic review and meta-analysis of randomized controlled trials. *Journal of Clinical Psychiatry*. 2011;72(4):529–38.
84. Mead GE, Morley W, Campbell P, Greig CA, McMurdo M, Lawlor DA. Exercise for depression. *Cochrane Database of Systematic Reviews*. 2009 Jul 8;(3):CD004366. doi:10.1002/14651858.CD004366.pub4
85. Carek PJ, Laibstain SE, Carek SM. Exercise for the treatment of depression and anxiety. *International Journal of Psychiatry in Medicine*. 2011;41:15–28.
86. Robertson R, Robertson A, Jepson R, Maxwell M. Walking for depression or depressive symptoms: a systematic review and meta-analysis. *Mental Health and Physical Activity*. 2012;5(1):66–75.
87. Strauss C, Cavanagh K, Oliver A, Pettman, D. Mindfulness-based interventions for people diagnosed with a current episode of an anxiety or depressive disorder: A meta-analysis of randomised controlled trials. *PLoS One*. 2014;9(4):e96110.
88. Segal ZV, Walsh KM. Mindfulness-based cognitive therapy for residual depressive symptoms and relapse prophylaxis. *Current Opinion in Psychiatry*. 2016;29(1):7–12.
89. Cheon EJ, Koo BH, Choi JH. The efficacy of neurofeedback in patients with major depressive disorder: An open labeled prospective study. *Applied Psychophysiology and Biofeedback*. 2016;41(1):103–110.
90. Berk M, Dean OM, Cotton SM, et al. Maintenance N-acetyl cysteine treatment for bipolar disorder: A double-blind randomized placebo controlled trial. *BMC Medicine*. 2012;10: 91.
91. Berk M, Dean O, Cotton SM, et al. The efficacy of N-acetylcysteine as an adjunctive treatment in bipolar depression: an open label trial. *Journal of Affective Disorders*. 2011;135(1–3):389–394.

92. Wignall ND, Brown ES. Citicoline in addictive disorders: a review of the literature. *American Journal of Drug and Alcohol Abuse.* 2014;40(4):262–268.

93. Deepmala J, Slattery J, Kumar N, et al. Clinical trials of N-acetylcysteine in psychiatry and neurology: A systematic review. *Neuroscience and Biobehavioral Reviews.* 2015;55:294–321.

94. Moussawi K, Pacchioni A, Moran M, et al. N-Acetylcysteine reverses cocaine-induced metaplasticity. *Nature Neuroscience.* 2009;12(2):182–189.

95. Mardikian PN, LaRowe SD, Hedden S, Kalivas PW, Malcolm RJ. An open-label trial of N-acetylcysteine for the treatment of cocaine dependence: a pilot study. *Progress in Neuro-Psychopharmacology and Biological Psychiatry.* 2007;31(2):389–394.

96. Bauer IE, Gálvez JF, Hamilton JE, et al. Lifestyle interventions targeting dietary habits and exercise in bipolar disorder: A systematic review. *Journal of Psychiatric Research.* 2016;74:1–7.

97. Crowe M, Beaglehole B, Inder M. Social rhythm interventions for bipolar disorder: a systematic review and rationale for practice. *Journal of Psychiatric and Mental Health Nursing.* 2016;23(1):3–11.

98. De Sa Filho AS, de Souza Moura AM, Lamego MK, et al. Potential therapeutic effects of physical exercise for bipolar disorder. *CNS and Neurological Disorders Drug Targets.* 2015;14(10):1255–1259.

99. Ives-Deliperi VL, Howells F, Stein DJ, Meintjes EM, Horn N. The effects of mindfulness-based cognitive therapy in patients with bipolar disorder: a controlled functional MRI investigation. *Journal of Affective Disorders.* 2013;150(3):1152–1157.

100. Li AW, Goldsmith CA. The effects of yoga on anxiety and stress. *Alternative Medicine Review.* 2012;17(1):21–35.

101. Lakhan SE, Vieira, KF. Nutritional and herbal supplements for anxiety and anxiety-related disorders: systematic review. *Nutrition Journal.* 2010;9:42.

102. Carek PJ, Laibstain SE, Carek SM. Exercise for the treatment of depression and anxiety. *International Journal of Psychiatry in Medicine.* 2011;41(1):15–28.

103. Fjorback LO, Arendt M, Ornbøl E, Fink P, Walach H. Mindfulness-based stress reduction and mindfulness-based cognitive therapy: a systematic review of randomized controlled trials. *Acta Psychiatrica Scandinavica.* 2011;124(2):102–119.

104. Lewis JE, Tiozzo E, Melillo AB. The effect of methylated vitamin B complex on depressive and anxiety symptoms and quality of life in adults with depression. *ISRN Psychiatry.* 2013:1–7.

105. Ryoo M, Son C. Effects of Neurofeedback training on EEG, Continuous Performance Task (CPT), and ADHD Symptoms in ADHD-prone college students. *Journal of Korean Academy of Nursing.* 2015;45(6):928–938.

106. Moriyama TS, Polanczyk G, Caye A, Banaschewski T, Brandeis D, Rohde LA. Evidence-based information on the clinical use of neurofeedback for ADHD. *Neurotherapeutics.* 2012;9(3):588–598.

107. Bloch MH, Qawasmi A. Omega-3 fatty acid supplementation for the treatment of children with attention-deficit/hyperactivity disorder symptomatology: systematic review and meta-analysis. *Journal of the American Academy of Child and Adolescent Psychiatry*. 2011;50(10):991–1000.

108. Manor I, Magen A, Keidar D, et al. The effect of phosphatidylserine containing Omega3 fatty-acids on attention-deficit hyperactivity disorder symptoms in children: a double-blind placebo-controlled trial, followed by an open-label extension. *European Psychiatry*. 2012;27(5):335–342.

109. Hirayama S, Terasawa K, Rabeler R, et al. The effect of phosphatidylserine administration on memory and symptoms of attention-deficit hyperactivity disorder: a randomised, double-blind, placebo-controlled clinical trial. *Journal of Human Nutrition and Dietetics*. 2014;27(Suppl 2):284–291.

110. Vysniauske R, Verburgh L, Oosterlaan J, Molendijk ML. The effects of physical exercise on functional outcomes in the treatment of ADHD: A meta-analysis. *Journal of Attention Disorders*. 2016;9.

111. Zylowska L, Ackerman DL, Yang MH, et al. Mindfulness meditation training in adults and adolescents with ADHD: a feasibility study. *Journal of Attention Disorders*. 2008;11(6):737–746.

112. Mitchell JT, Zylowska L, Kollins SH. Mindfulness meditation training for attention-deficit/hyperactivity disorder in adulthood: Current empirical support, treatment overview, and future directions. *Cognitive and Behavioral Practice*. 2015;22(2):172–191.

113. Mitchell JT, McIntyre EM, English JS, Dennis MF, Beckham JC, Kollins SH. A pilot trial of mindfulness meditation training for ADHD in adulthood: Impact on core symptoms, executive functioning, and emotion dysregulation. *Journal of Attention Disorders*. 2013;21(13):1105–1120.

114. Berk M, Copolov D, Dean O, et al. N-acetyl cysteine as a glutathione precursor for schizophrenia--a double-blind, randomized, placebo-controlled trial. *Biological Psychiatry*. 2008;64(5):361–368.

115. Farokhnia M, Azarkolah A, Adinehfar F, et al. N-acetylcysteine as an adjunct to risperidone for treatment of negative symptoms in patients with chronic schizophrenia: a randomized, double-blind, placebo-controlled study. *Clinical Neuropharmacology*. 2013;36(6):185–192.

116. Gorczynski P, Faulkner G. Exercise therapy for schizophrenia. *Cochrane Database of Systematic Reviews*. 2010;5:CD004412.

117. Gruzelier J, Hardman E, Wild J, Zaman R. Learned control of slow potential interhemispheric asymmetry in schizophrenia. *International Journal of Psychophysiology*. 1999;34:341–348.

118. Bolea AS. Neurofeedback treatment of chronic inpatient schizophrenia. *Journal of Neurotherapy*. 2010;14:47–54.

119. Surmeli T, Ertem A, Eralp E, Kos IH. Schizophrenia and the efficacy of qEEG-guided neurofeedback treatment: a clinical case series. *Neuroscience Letters.* 2011;500S:e16.

120. Ruiz S, Lee S, Soekadar S, et al. Acquired self-control of insula cortex modulates emotion recognition and brain network connectivity in schizophrenia. *Human Brain Mapping.* 2013 Jan;34(1):200–212.

121. Monti DA, Beitman, BD. *Integrative Psychiatry.* Oxford: Oxford University Press; 2010.

# 13

# Psychosocial Treatment Approaches
# for Substance Use

## LYNN MCFARR, JULIE SNYDER, LISA BENSON, AND RACHEL HIGIER

Multiple psychosocial treatments for substance-use disorders have been studied for efficacy. A recent meta-analysis indicates that psychosocial interventions are effective across multiple types of substances used. In the case of opiates, psychosocial interventions combined with medication appear to be the most effective.[1] Many studies further agree that psychosocial interventions are an integral and necessary part of treating substance-use disorders.

Although theoretical orientations may differ across psychosocial treatments, they have several principles and practices in common. All involve talk therapy or talk in communities as a way to clarify triggers, build commitment, and improve accountability. Many also target addiction behaviors and work to develop alternative contingencies to reduce or eliminate use. Finally, as in all good cognitive and behavioral treatments, targeting repeated performance (or building "chains of committed behavior") decreases the likelihood of relapse. This chapter discusses the most frequently studied and employed psychosocial treatments for substance use, including CBT, motivational interviewing, contingency management, mindfulness, and community-based programs.

## Cognitive Behavioral Therapy for
## Substance-use Disorders

CBT incorporates a variety of interventions: cognitive, conditioning based, and skills building.[2] The contingency management procedures discussed elsewhere in this chapter also have their foundation in basic behavioral principles but differ in their emphasis on altering the structure of the environment. CBT emphasizes changing the cognitions and the behaviors of the individual.

The defining feature of CBT is functional analysis of the antecedents (cognitive and behavioral) and consequences of the individual's drug or alcohol use,[3] followed by training the individual in skills for avoiding these antecedents and preventing use. Because of this emphasis on individualized case conceptualization, CBT is a highly flexible approach that can be delivered in multiple modalities: individual or group, inpatient or outpatient. Using the conceptualization also facilitates combination of CBT for substance-use disorders with CBT for comorbid conditions such as mood and anxiety disorders. The principles of CBT for substance-use disorders can also inform adjunctive treatments such as couple's and family therapy.

## COMPONENTS OF CBT FOR SUBSTANCE-USE DISORDERS

Treatment proceeds in 4 major stages: building a collaborative relationship, psychoeducation, functional analysis of the patient, and skills training.[4] In the early stages of treatment, it is critical to build a collaborative therapeutic relationship between the therapist and patient. Like the motivational interviewing practitioner, CBT clinicians do not argue with patients or attempt to convince them not to engage in drug or alcohol use. Instead, they will use CBT techniques to help patients evaluate the evidence for whether their beliefs are helpful, as well as the pros and cons of their behaviors.

Psychoeducation about the CBT model of substance-use disorders includes explanation of the differences between situations, cognitions, emotions, and behaviors. Patients are introduced to an example of a CBT model of a craving, one in which an individual is in circumstances he or she has associated with drug use. Also in this example, the individual has aversive internal experiences such as boredom, underlying core beliefs such as "I'm a failure," use-congruent intermediate beliefs such as "my life is already terrible so it doesn't matter if I use," an automatic thought such as "I'm going to go for it," and chooses to engage in drug-use behavior. The individual then experiences short-term relief from the aversive state—together with unwanted long-term consequences such as losing a job. Emphasizing the power of core and intermediate beliefs in influencing behavior is critical for both helping the patient understand how to change their behavior patterns and also validating the patient in a way likely to build rapport: the same also goes for the impact of relief from aversive states (a negative reinforcement paradigm) on increasing the likelihood of that behavior in the future.

The patient and therapist then collaboratively develop a functional analysis specific to this patient. The analysis should include all major controlling variables: environmental factors or internal experiences that seem to be particularly influential over whether a patient engages in substance use. These variables are likely to include aversive internal experiences such as anxiety and boredom; people, places, and things associated with substance use; permission-giving beliefs about substance use, expectancies about substance use, and experiences of pleasure during substance use.

Once the patient and therapist have developed a working version of the conceptualization, the therapist can identify which skills will be most helpful to the patient for ceasing substance use-related behaviors and developing new behavioral patterns. It is preferable for the interventions to be driven by the conceptualization rather than the same ones being provided to all patients. For example, for a patient with strong permission-giving beliefs, learning to remediate these cognitions and develop new coping thoughts would be crucial. For people, places, and things associated with substance use, planning ahead to avoid contact with these triggers as much as possible ("stimulus control") is necessary. For avoidance of aversive experiences such as anxiety, several strategies are likely to be helpful: (1) planned exposure to these experiences so patients learn they can tolerate them without substance use, and (2) learning coping skills such as distraction or muscle relaxation. For patients for whom it is salient that substance use results in current pleasure (or is associated with past pleasure), it is particularly important to help them develop alternative sources of reinforcement by scheduling enjoyable activities throughout the week and teaching interpersonal skills for developing more satisfying relationships.

As treatment progresses, the therapist and patient may find new controlling variables and are encouraged to update the functional analysis and treatment plan to reflect these new data. For example, a patient may initially focus on decreasing marijuana use primarily through stimulus control (not going near dispensaries or friends who use) but find that his or her cravings increase dramatically in association with an increase in anxiety; exposure to anxiety and coping strategies for tolerating it would then be indicated.

## EMPIRICAL FINDINGS ON CBT FOR SUBSTANCE-USE DISORDERS

The literature on CBT for substance-use disorders generally supports the view that it is efficacious. DeRubeis and Crits-Christoph[5] reviewed the literature at that time on manualized treatments for alcohol and substance-use disorders to classify treatments as "efficacious and specific," "efficacious," and "possibly efficacious." They found cue exposure therapy, cue exposure therapy plus coping skills training, and social skills training to be possibly efficacious treatments for alcohol dependence. Cognitive therapy with drug counseling was found to be a possibly efficacious treatment for opiate dependence.[5] Chambless and Ollendick[6] then summarized the efforts of several workgroups to classify treatments as "well established," "probably efficacious," or "promising." They found that all groups classified cue exposure therapy for alcohol abuse and dependence, CBT for benzodiazepine withdrawal, behavior therapy and CBT relapse prevention for cocaine abuse, and cognitive therapy for opiate dependence as "probably efficacious."

A more recent meta-analysis of 53 studies found a large effect size for CBT as compared to no treatment, Hedges's $g = 0.796$ across substance-use disorders.[7] The effect size for CBT as compared to other active treatments was small ($g = 0.154$) but statistically significant. This effect size diminished to 0.096 at 12-month follow-up. As Carroll and Onken[3] note, a limitation of CBT for substance-use disorders is that training clinicians in conceptualization-based intervention may be relatively more difficult than some other treatments. Additional training and supervision might result in the effect sizes for CBT comparing even more favorably.

## Motivational Interviewing and Motivational Enhancement Therapy

Not only is cognitive behavioral therapy applicable to the treatment of substance-use disorders, more specific, brief, time-limited behavioral interventions are often utilized in substance-use disorder treatment as well. Two well-known interventions are Miller and Rollnick's[8–10] motivational interviewing and a variation known as "motivational enhancement therapy."[5]

### MOTIVATIONAL INTERVIEWING

Motivational interviewing (MI) is a therapeutic stance designed to facilitate individuals looking at and ultimately resolving ambivalence around changing a behavior, through an assortment of therapeutic components.[8–11] MI views the therapy relationship as collaborative and democratic, with the therapist taking a directive stance in the session to elicit motivational statements and behavioral change in the patient[11] with the balance of acceptance and meeting the patient where they are, in the present moment.

Patients in treatment are often at varying levels of readiness for behavioral change.[12] Motivational interviewing utilizes the stages of change model outlined by Prochaska and DiClemente,[13] recognizing that some patients may be in treatment for the first time, only really thinking about the idea of change and not yet engaged in any behavioral changes. Some patients, meanwhile, may have been in an active stance of behavioral change for many years. A motivational interviewing stance utilizes therapeutic interventions based on where the patient is at in terms of readiness for change.[8]

Miller and Rollnick[10] explain that motivational interviewing is pragmatic and compassionate, where the therapist utilizes a clear set of strategies for increasing intrinsic motivation, eliciting change talk and commitment while balancing acceptance. There are 5 main strategies in MI: (1) express empathy; (2) develop discrepancy; (3) avoid argument; (4) roll with resistance; (5) support self-efficacy, and these components are further detailed below.

## COMPONENTS OF MOTIVATIONAL INTERVIEWING

Miller and Rollnick[8] discuss the 5 components of motivational interviewing in detail. To start, expressing empathy in counseling individuals with substance-use disorders utilizes reflective listening as the main conduit to being able to communicate a sense of understanding and acceptance of the patient's situation. Developing discrepancy is where the therapist helps the patient to highlight the difference between the patient's current substance using behaviors and their valued or desired behaviors. The perception of discrepancy between actual and ideal behavior enhances patient's motivation to change a problematic behavior. Here, the patient should present the case for change. Subsequently, avoiding argument is key because arguing with a patient around a behavior pulls for defensiveness and is counterproductive in eliciting acceptance and change. In order to avoid argument, rolling with resistance focuses on providing validation and an imparting a sense of understanding where the patient may be pulled to become more willful or grounded in previous ways of thinking. Finally, supporting self-efficacy helps to instill a sense of hopefulness that change is possible. Oftentimes, individuals with substance-use disorders have less confidence that they can create long-term change. In motivational interviewing, the therapist can support self-efficacy by eliciting and reinforcing hope as well as recognizing and calling attention to patient's strengths.

## MOTIVATIONAL ENHANCEMENT THERAPY

Arising from motivational interviewing, motivational enhancement therapy (MET) is a 4-session treatment outlined by Miller, Zweben, DiClemente, and Rychtarik[14,15] for a Project MATCH treatment manual series. Before MET starts, the patient is asked to complete several assessments that are discussed in session. The patient is also asked to bring a significant other to treatment sessions 1 and 2 in service of support. Finally, MET stipulates that the patient must attend the first session sober, and a breathalyzer is administered as a way of ensuring sobriety. If the patient is not sober for the first session, it is rescheduled. The first 2 sessions are structured to explore and identify motivating factors as well as readiness for change, providing the patient with information from assessments as well as moving toward commitment and change. The latter 2 sessions are focused on situations where the patient sustained or did not sustain behavioral change, and renewed commitment to new behaviors takes place. This component of discussing obstacles that arose in the face of commitment to change and problem feedback is an enhancement that MET offers as compared to MI.[16]

## DIFFERENCES ACROSS TREATMENTS

Further differences can be extrapolated from MET and other treatments. MET differs from CBT in that MET does not teach direct skills or modify problematic thoughts but utilizes the above MI principles to build patient motivation and elicit change strategies intrinsically. In MET, the responsibility for change is left with the patient, whereas in CBT there is direct instruction and practice with feedback from the therapist.[16]

When MET is compared to other treatments, MET produced results equal to CBT and 12-step programs in less time.[17] As it is more structured, it also may be easier for therapists to learn when compared to MI alone. However, if combining MI with another treatment, then MI is sufficient and the preferred mode.[16] Therefore, if being used as a standalone treatment, or if time is of the essence, MET may serve to enhance motivation and commitment to change in an individual with a substance-use disorder in a shorter treatment timeline. However, if one wants to combine MI with another treatment, such as CBT, there may be more opportunity and occasion to utilize MI principles with direct practice, skills training, and cognitive modification.

## EMPIRICAL SUPPORT

There has been a wealth of support for utilization of both MI and MET interventions with not only individuals with substance-use disorders but also a growing body of support for other problems as well, highlighting the efficacy of this therapeutic stance.

Project MATCH[17] conducted a large (N = 1726) multisite clinical trial that tested treatment of alcohol-use disorder across 3 treatments: twelve-step facilitation therapy (TSF); MET, and CBT. This study found that these treatments were all efficacious in reducing alcohol use as well as related measures (e.g., depression, social functioning, liver function). It is notable that when compared to TSF or CBT, MET was less likely to have reduction in alcohol consumption and alcohol-related consequences during the treatment phase. But this was not the case following the completion of treatment, where differences among treatment modalities were not significant. This extensive study highlights the efficacy of MET, especially post-intervention.

Sellman and colleagues[18] compared MET with non-directive reflective listening (NDRL) and no further counseling (NFC) in a randomized clinical trial (N = 122). It was found that MET was more effective in reducing heavy drinking than either a feedback or education session as well as more effective than NDRL. The authors suggest that MET is a "value-added" intervention when compared to other treatments.

Looking forward, empirical studies provide support for the efficacy of MI and MET extending to more than just substance-use disorders. For example, MET intervention was supported in the treatment of obesity[19] and binge eating disorder,[20] both in enhancing motivation to change. Additionally, MET has been found to be useful in increasing motivation for engagement in CBT in generalized anxiety disorder,[21,22] obsessive-compulsive disorder,[23] as well as anxiety sensitivity, which is a risk factor for development of anxiety disorders.[24] Not only are MI and MET efficacious in the treatment of substance-use disorders, their efficacy can also be seen across multiple clinical problems, thus enhancing treatment outcomes.

# Contingency Management

Contingency management sees substance use as being operantly conditioned; that is, substance use is shaped by consequences, where substances serve as unconditioned positive reinforcers.[25] Utilizing the underpinnings of behavioral theory, substance use therefore will be mediated by the context and amount of reinforcers available, utilizing high rates of positive reinforcement and some use of negative punishment.[26] For example, non-substance reinforcers should decrease substance use if they are available at a sizeable scale and on a behavioral schedule that does not align with substance use or substance-use behaviors.[27] From this behavioral foundation, contingency management (CM) is a behaviorally based treatment that has been used successfully with individuals with substance-use disorders, where the treatment provides a reinforcer upon objective evidence of abstinence.[28]

## DIFFERENT TYPES OF CONTINGENCY MANAGEMENT

Stemming from various studies, several different types of contingency management have been developed. One frequently used type of contingency management is known as voucher-based reinforcement therapy (VBRT).[29] VBRT was initially developed as a way to help outpatient treatment retention and abstinence for individuals dependent on cocaine.[30] In VBRT, patients receive "vouchers" that have designated monetary values in exchange for providing substance toxicology screens (e.g., urine test) that are negative for substances screened (positive reinforcement). Conversely, if a toxicology screen is positive for substances, the voucher is not provided (negative punishment). Once the patient has started earning vouchers, these can be traded for products that are incompatible with a drug-free lifestyle.

An example of VBRT is commonly utilized at methadone maintenance clinics. At these clinics, patients who have been struggling with opioid-use disorder come into the clinic daily to receive a dose of methadone to help manage cravings and counteract withdrawal symptoms. Coming to the clinic daily, including weekends and holidays, can be cumbersome and demanding schedule and resource wise. To reinforce and promote abstinence, it is common for a patient to be able to earn "take-home" doses of medication, where a patient can pick-up doses of medication to administer at home, increasing freedom around the ability to travel at distances from the clinic as well as time available to engage in other pursuits, such as work or family activities.

In VBRT, there are countless variations on reinforcement schedules. It is also important to note that most schedules increase the value of the voucher with increase abstinence time, so that with each successive negative toxicology screen, the value of the voucher would substantially increase. Additionally, the voucher is reset to a lower value following a positive toxicology screen, or a bonus is provided after a certain number of negative screens.[31]

Using the above example of "take-home" doses, a possible reinforcement schedule could be established where patients would have the ability to earn one dose on a weekend day after 4 negative toxicology screens. Further contingencies might stipulate that these doses are available after dosing daily for a 30-day period and attending all scheduled clinic appointments within the 30-day period. After the patient has earned one "take-home" dose and maintained abstinence with the behavioral indicator of continued negative toxicology screens, the ability to earn another dose is given after another month of continued adherence to the behavioral stipulations. The increase in the voucher in this case would be a free weekend of not traveling to the clinic. The schedule to earn more doses may shorten as time of abstinence (and earning negative toxicology screens as vouchers) increase (e.g., 14 days versus 30 days). Similarly, if the patient provides a toxicology screen that is positive for illicit substances, the take-home doses could be decreased in frequency or suspended all together as stipulated in the schedule.

Another type of contingency management is known as variable magnitude of reinforcement and was developed by Petry and colleagues.[32,33] In this setup, participants do not receive vouchers directly as in VBRT but instead earn a chance to draw a slip of paper kept in a bowl. Each draw has the possibility of winning a prize, but not every draw wins a prize. And some draws earn a small prize, while even fewer draws earn a large prize—similar to a state lottery. This approach continues to reinforce the increase in reinforcers with sustained behavior (e.g., more draws with continued negative screens), although is substantially less costly for clinics. In addition to negative toxicology screens as a means to earn chances, behavioral goals have also been studied as a way of earning further reinforcers or draws. For example, attending a job interview or a parenting class may earn a patient additional draws. Petry and colleagues have found that the variable magnitude of reinforcement helps with treatment retention, increasing length of treatment time—and with it, often successful outcomes.[34]

## EMPIRICAL SUPPORT

Of the psychosocial treatments for substance-use disorders, contingency management (CM) is the intervention with the most efficacy in abstinence when compared to relapse prevention and CBT in several meta-analysis.[28,35,36] Prendergast and colleagues[28] also found that CM was more effective in treating specific kinds of substance use (namely, opiate, and cocaine) when compared to other drugs (e.g., nicotine and polysubstance use).

Lussier and colleagues[37] further replicated the above findings more specifically in a meta-analysis of VBRT. The analysis found that VBRT significantly improved treatment outcomes compared to control conditions. Therefore, the results provide further evidence supporting the efficacy of voucher-based reinforcement for treatment of substance-use disorders.[37]

McPherson and colleagues[38] looked at 2 parallel randomized clinical trials, investigating the impact of contingency management on both longitudinal stimulant use and on treatment attendance. Results indicated that CM had a significant impact on decreased overall simulant use and treatment attendance, and also highlighted the distinctive nature of each treatment outcome. The authors also highlight that treatment attendance does also not necessarily equate to efficacious treatment, and more research would be beneficial.

Although highly effective in improving substance-use outcomes, CM does include a con of adding direct costs as well as staff time and energy, and this expenditure of resources may not be essential for all patients in treatment for substance-use disorders.[33,34] In consideration of this drawback, identifying subgroups who respond well to this enhanced intervention could help modulate resource output.[37]

Identification of subgroups who will respond to CM will help fine tune applicability of CM across populations. One example of this subgroup identification was conducted in a large study ($N = 1,013$) examining the impact of contingency management in individuals with substance-use disorders and physical disability status, the authors found patients who were receiving physical disability payments,

CM improved all substance use outcomes (treatment retention, percent negative screening samples, and longest duration of abstinence).[39]

In summary, contingency management is a widely utilized and studied treatment intervention for substance-use disorders. It has significant pros in that it is effective and helps to increase the likelihood of abstinence over time as well as treatment retention. Cons include cost in both incentives in addition to staff time and resources to administer.

## Mindfulness-based Treatments

Attention has gradually shifted toward mindfulness-based interventions for substance-use disorders. Mindfulness tends to be considered part of third-wave cognitive behavioral therapies and has been described as "paying attention in a particular way: on purpose, in the present moment, and non-judgmentally."[40] This approach is generally based on the acceptance of thoughts, emotions, and sensations rather than on attempts to manage or control them. Recent evidence indicates an important role of mindfulness in the treatment of substance abuse, with several clinical trials supporting the efficacy of mindfulness techniques and practices.[41,42] This section aims to briefly describe mindfulness-based approaches and their theoretical underpinnings in the treatment of substance use.

Perhaps the primary function of mindfulness, in conjunction with traditional cognitive behavioral therapy approaches, is to prevent the escalation of thought and behavior patterns that may lead to relapse. Mindfulness techniques aim to increase the patient's awareness of cravings and their associated experiences as well as urges to use substances, thereby attempting to interrupt the previous cycle of automatic substance-use behavior.[43] That is, mindfulness training works to help patients observe and describe challenging emotional or craving states without routinely reacting and engaging in substance use behaviors—a technique sometimes known as "urge surfing." This technique is used to improve patients' ability to tolerate difficult urges and inner experiences without engaging in a prepotent response (e.g., using substances to alleviate cravings).[44,45] Moreover, the practice of increasing acceptance and tolerance of positive and negative physical, emotional, and cognitive states associated with craving is thought to decrease the overarching need to ameliorate associated discomfort by engaging in substance use. In fact, research on urge states suggests the duration of urges decreases with increased abstinence time.[46] Importantly, an urge-surfing approach circumvents the often-harmful effects of suppression or avoidance of cognitive and affective internal responses.[47,48,49] Instead, it promotes increased awareness and acceptance of these internal states, which is thought to help individuals approach discomfort from a nonjudgmental and nonreactive stance. Through repeated exposure to cravings without behavioral response, patients are taught to tolerate unpleasant experiences and build a behavioral repertoire of alternative responses.

Additionally, mindfulness may enhance the ability to cope with potential relapse cues and triggers. Mindfulness-based interventions encourage increased awareness and tolerance of potential precipitants to relapse. That is, patients are taught to recognize internal (i.e., thoughts, emotions, sensations) and external (i.e., situations) cues previously associated with substance-use behaviors. The practice of increasing awareness of triggers helps patients to monitor their internal reactions and develop more skillful behavioral choices aligned with their overall goals. The emphasis is on helping patients shift from habitual reactions to cues and triggers towards more skillful and effective behavioral responses. Furthermore, increased awareness helps patients identify critical cues and triggers, which may later lead to the practice of stimulus control. This is where patients remove stimuli from the environment that may trigger craving experiences and thereby increase the likelihood of success.

Some authors encourage a dialectical approach to recovery and suggest utilizing mindfulness around substance-use behaviors themselves. Linehan and colleagues coined the term "dialectical abstinence" to describe how patients may work toward abstinence even in the presence of cravings and urges to use.[45,50] In fact, it could be argued that cravings and urges are expected to emerge throughout the course of treatment, and mindfulness provides a frame in which approach such discomfort. The expectation of cravings may reduce risk of relapse and improve the likelihood of recovery. Terms such as "clean mind" versus "addict mind" are labels aimed to help patients increase awareness of their current state of mind and the associated inner experiences. In the event of relapse, the awareness and acceptance fostered by mindfulness may help to reduce the guilt and negative thinking that often serves to increase the risk of relapse.[51] Still others have supported a harm-reduction approach, which emphasizes reducing the harmful consequences associated with substance-use behaviors.[52,53] This approach also necessitates some level of mindful awareness in order to first identify and then minimize risk associated with substance use.

While a review of the neurobiological changes association with addiction and meditation is beyond the scope of this chapter[54] several studies have examined the neural mechanisms subserving mindfulness training in the context of substance use. Disruptions in dopaminergic fronto-striatal circuitry appear to underlie reward processing as well as emotional control and executive decision making that contribute to addictive behaviors.[55,56] Two candidate neural pathways have been proposed as mechanisms of action.[57] First, top-down pathways supporting prefrontal cognitive control over craving sensations may operate in an inhibitory manner on lower subcortical processing. Second, bottom-up pathways may serve to modulate craving-related activation in brain regions involved in subcortical limbic processing. That is, mindfulness training may strengthen the inhibitory pathways of prefrontal executive function over affective neural responsivity or directly enhance affective modulation of subcortical regions, respectively, or both.

In conclusion, there is a growing literature of clinical trials for mindfulness in the treatment of substance use.[58] Mindfulness Based Relapse Prevention (MBRP),[59] which utilizes mindfulness techniques to target experiences of craving and negative affect, has garnered perhaps the most empirical support to date.[59,60] Several outcome studies of MBRP have demonstrated reductions in substance-use or related experiences, such as cravings or reactivity to substance-use cues.[41,61,62,63,64] Other treatments, such as acceptance and commitment therapy[65] (ACT) and dialectical behavior therapy[45,51] (DBT) incorporate mindfulness practice as a core component of treatment. While initial reports support the role of mindfulness meditation in the treatment of substance-use disorders, larger systematic clinical trials are needed. Future research may evaluate mindfulness-based interventions as a standalone treatment of substance-use disorders versus in conjunction with other cognitive behavioral therapies. Moreover, brain-behavior studies are necessary to fully elucidate the mechanisms of change in mindfulness-based treatments.

## Community Interventions

### TWELVE-STEP PROGRAMS

AA started in 1935 and is a well-established support base for individuals with substance-use disorders.[66] Individuals can attend meetings anonymously and for free often wherever they are in the world. Because they are "anonymous" there are inherent complications in conducting research with 12-step programs as a treatment intervention. As AA has been around the longest, when compared to other 12-step programs such as NA (Narcotics Anonymous) or CA (Cocaine Anonymous), the research often focuses on AA.

Although there are complications with data collection, nevertheless there is a wealth of data. For example, better treatment outcomes have been associated with AA affiliation, including increased abstinence from alcohol[67] and sustained recovery.[68] Further, treatment costs for individuals engaged in AA were shown to be 45% lower than for individuals who engaged in outpatient treatment, with similar outcome results after 3 years.[69]

Originally, attendance at AA meetings was the operationalized variable in treatment studies of AA and treatment outcomes, but more recent studies have shown that greater involvement in AA (versus just simple attendance) is associated with more favorable treatment outcomes.[70] Involvement could include attendfance as well as engagement with a sponsor and/or sponsees, being of service (such as setting up chairs for the meeting), reading 12-step materials, speaking at the meeting, and connecting with other attendees.

Project MATCH (Matching Alcoholism Treatments to Client Heterogeneity)[71] investigated efficacy of treatment options for individuals diagnosed with alcohol dependence. This study compared 12-step treatment, cognitive-behavioral skills therapy, and motivational enhancement treatment randomly assigned 774 individuals coming from inpatient treatment and 952 individuals who had only received outpatient services (total N = 1,726). The authors found that individuals without significant mental health issues assigned to the 12-step treatment achieved significantly greater abstinence rates than those assigned to the cognitive behavioral treatment option. This highlights the efficacy of AA as a community-based intervention.

Morgenstern and colleagues[72] illustrate that affiliation with AA was significantly associated with commitment to abstinence and active coping efforts to manage relapse, in addition to increased self-efficacy. Similarly, Sheeren[73] found that AA involvement was not only correlated with lower rates of relapse for individuals with alcohol dependence, but AA involvement, specifically with reaching out to other AA members and the use of a sponsor, had the strongest correlation with maintenance of abstinence.

## ASSERTIVE COMMUNITY TREATMENT

The move from hospital-based treatment to community-based treatment started in the 1950s in an effort to "deinstitutionalize" psychiatric care.[74] As care moved into the community, it became increasingly fragmented due to the number of providers and supports, such as psychiatric care, medical care, housing and employment services, and substance-use treatment. The number of individuals involved with the patient's care increased, and often it was difficult for individuals to coordinate care. To address this difficulty, Stein and Test[75] developed what came to be known as assertive community treatment (ACT), which was developed as creating a multidisciplinary and holistic team, including case managers, psychiatrists, nurses, social workers, and vocational rehabilitation counselors to help individuals with serious mental illness integrate services in the community.

As outlined by the developers, ACT's focus was helping the individual remain in the community, focusing on physical and mental health treatment, including treatment of substance-use disorders. ACT also focused on practical challenges, including housing, finances, and transportation to promote recovery.[76] In ACT, the team provides services directly rather than referring to other providers, and originally services were available 24 hours a day, 7 days a week and were "unlimited" in longitudinal duration. Due to considerable budgeting and time constraints, this approach was later modified, limiting hours and with a goal of graduation.[76]

The ACT approach is tailored to the patient's needs and goals, and has been proven effective with a variety of mental health issues and problems, including individuals struggling with homelessness and problems related to dual diagnosis.[77] ACT has also been shown to be efficacious in reducing hospitalizations,[78] and challenges and recommendations have been identified for individuals transitioning care.[79]

Additionally, Drake and colleagues[80] compared the effectiveness of ACT with standard case management for 203 patients who met criteria for both mental health and substance-use disorders for over 3 years. The individuals receiving ACT showed greater improvements on some measures of substance abuse and quality of life. However, the groups did not exhibit significant differences in several areas, including stable community days, hospital days, psychiatric symptoms, and remission of substance-use disorder symptoms.

## Conclusion

CBT, MI, CM, mindfulness, and community-based interventions represent the current most studied psychosocial interventions for substance-use problems. There is empirical support for each showing effectiveness, and in general, any psychosocial treatment is better than no treatment. However, despite multiple studies, there is no clear winner. Efforts to match patients to specific treatments based on substance of choice, demographic data, or severity of problem usage have yielded promising but not definitive findings.

What seems clear is that several principles are common throughout the approaches and may, in part, underlie the effectiveness of these treatments. Heightened awareness of beliefs, contingencies, goals, emotions, thoughts, and sensations associated with using may help patients develop insight, increase motivation, and promote problem solving and skill application when an individual is faced with urges to use. Likewise, accountability to a community, case manager, or therapist may also accelerate recovery. Rewards (either interpersonal, as in community support, or objective as in "take home doses" of methadone) are also effective in curbing use. Finally, an emphasis on practicing skills repeatedly (mindfulness, urge surfing, etc.) to respond to urges to use may also contribute the positive effects across these psychosocial treatments.

### REFERENCES

1. Jhanjee S. Evidence based psychosocial interventions in substance use. *Indian Journal of Psychological Medicine.* 2014;36(2):112–118. http://doi.org/10.4103/0253-7176.130960
2. McHugh RK, Hearon BA, Otto MW. Cognitive-behavioral therapy for substance-use disorders. *Psychiatric Clinics of North America.* 2010;33(3):511–525.

3. Carroll KM, Onken LS. Behavioral therapies for drug abuse. *American Journal of Psychiatry.* 2005;162(8):1452–1460.
4. Beck AT, Wright FD, Newman CF, Liese BS. Cognitive therapy of substance abuse. New York: Guilford; 1993.
5. DeRubeis RJ, Crits-Christoph P. Empirically supported individual and group psychological treatments for adult mental disorders. *Journal of Consulting and Clinical Psychology.* 1998;6(1):37–52.
6. Chambless DL, Ollendick TH. Empirically supported psychological interventions: controversies and evidence. *Annual Review of Psychology.* 2001;52:685–716.
7. Magill M, Ray LA. Cognitive-behavioral treatment with adult alcohol and illicit drug users: a meta-analysis of randomized controlled trials. *Journal of Studies on Alcohol and Drugs.* 2009; 70(4):516–527.
8. Miller WR, Rollnick S. *Motivational Interviewing: Preparing People to Change.* 3rd ed. New York: Guilford; 2012.
9. Miller WR, Rollnick S. *Motivational Interviewing: Preparing People to Change,* 2nd ed. New York: Guilford; 2002.
10. Miller WR, Rollnick S. *Motivational Interviewing: Preparing People to Change Addictive Behavior.* New York: Guilford; 1991.
11. Rollnick, S., Miller, W.R., Butler, C.C. *Motivational Interviewing in Health Care: Helping Patients Change Behavior.* New York: Guilford; 2008.
12. Center for Substance Abuse Treatment. *Enhancing Motivation for Change in Substance Abuse Treatment.* Treatment Improvement Protocol (TIP) Series, No. 35. HHS Publication No. (SMA) 12-4212. Rockville, MD: Substance Abuse and Mental Health Services Administration; 1999.
13. Prochaska JO, DiClemente CC. Stages of change in the modification of problematic behaviors. In: Herson M, Eisler RM, Miller PM, eds. *Progress in Behavior Modification.* Sycamore, IL: Sycamore; 1992:184–214.
14. Miller WR, Zweben A, DiClemente CC, Rychtarik RG. *Motivational Enhancement Therapy Manual.* Washington, DC: National Institute on Alcohol Abuse and Alcoholism; 1992.
15. Miller WR, Zweben A, DiClemente CC, Rychtarik RG. Motivational Enhancement Therapy Manual: A Clinical Research Guide for Therapists Treating Individual With Alcohol Abuse and Dependence. Project MATCH Monograph Series 2. NIH Pub. No. 94-3723. Rockville, MD: National Institute on Alcohol Abuse and Alcoholism; 1995.
16. Lundahl BW, Kunz C, Brownell C, Tollefson D, Burke BL. A meta-analysis of motivational interviewing: Twenty-five years of empirical studies. *Research on Social Work Practice.* 2010;20(2):137–160. doi: 10.1177/1049731509934785.
17. Project MATCH Research Group. Matching patients with alcohol disorders to treatments: Clinical implications from Project MATCH. *Journal of Mental Health.* 1998;7(6):589–602. doi:10.1080/09638239817743.
18. Sellman JD, Sullivan PF, Dore GM, Adamson SJ, MacEwan I. A randomized controlled trial of motivational enhancement therapy (MET) for mild to moderate

alcohol dependence. *Journal of Studies on Alcohol.* 2001;62(3):389–396. http://dx.doi.org/10.15288/jsa.2001.62.389

19. Fioravanti G, Rotella F, Cresci B, Pala L, DeVita G, Mannucci E, Rotella CM, Motivational enhancement therapy in obese patients: A promising application. *Obesity Research and Clinical Practice.* 2015. doi:10.1016/j.orcp.2015.06.003

20. Vella-Zarb RA, Mills JS, Westra HA, Carter JC, Keating L. A randomized controlled trial of motivational interviewing + self-help versus psychoeducation + self-help for binge eating. *International Journal of Eating Disorders.* 2015;48:328–332. doi: 10.1002/eat.22242

21. Westra HA, Arkowitz H, Dozois DJA. Adding motivational interviewing pretreatment to cognitive behavioral therapy for generalized anxiety disorder: A preliminary randomized controlled trial. *Journal of Anxiety Disorders.* 2009;23:1106–1117.

22. Button ML, Westra HA, Hara KM, Aviram A. Disentangling the impact of resistance and ambivalence on therapy outcomes in cognitive behavioural therapy for generalized anxiety disorder. *Cognitive Behaviour Therapy.* 2015;44(1): 44–53. doi:10.1080/16506073.2014.959038

23. Maltby N, Tolin D. A brief motivational intervention for treatment-refusing OCD patients. *Cognitive Behavioral Therapy.*2005;34:176–184.

24. Korte KJ, Schmidt NB. The use of motivational enhancement therapy to increase utilization of a preventative intervention for anxiety sensitivity. *Cognitive Therapy and Research.* 2015;39(4):520–530, 2015. doi 10.1007/s10608-014-9668-y

25. Deneau G,Yanagita T, Seevers, MH. Self-administration of psychoactive substances by the monkey. *Psychopharmacologia.* 1969;16(1):30–48.

26. Bigelow G, Silverman K. Theoretical and empirical foundations of contingency management treatments for drug abuse. In: Higgins ST, Silverman K, eds. *Motivating Behavior Change Among Illicit Drug Abusers: Research on Contingency Management Interventions.* Washington, DC: American Psychological Association; 1999:15–31.

27. Roll JM, Higgins ST. A within-subject comparison of three different schedules of reinforcement of drug absti- nence using cigarette smoking as an exemplar. *Drug Alcohol Depend.* 2000;58:103–109.

28. Prendergast M, Podus D, Finney J, Greenwell L, Roll J. Contingency management for treatment of substance-use disorders: A meta-analysis. *Addiction.* 2006;101(11): 1546–1560.

29. Higgins ST, Alessi SM, Dantona RL. Voucher-based incentives: a substance abuse treatment innovation. *Addictive Behaviors.* 2002;27:887–910.

30. Higgins ST, Delaney DD, Budney AJ, et al. A behavioral approach to achieving initial cocaine abstinence. *American Journal of Psychiatry.* 1991;148:1218–1224.

31. Silverman, K, Chutuape MA, Bigelow GE, Stitzer ML. Voucher-based reinforcement of cocaine abstinence in treatment-resistant methadone patients: Effects of reinforcement magnitude. *Psychopharmacology.* 1999;146(2):128–138. Voucher-based reinforcement of cocaine abstinence in treatment-resistant methadone patients: Effects of reinforcement magnitude. *Psychopharmacology.* 1999;146(2):128–138.

32. Petry NM, Martin B, Cooney JL, Kranzler HR. Give them prizes, and they will come: contingency manage- ment for treatment of alcohol dependence. *Journal of Consulting and Clinical Psychology.* 2000;68:250–257.
33. Petry NM, Martin B. Low-cost contingency management for treating cocaine- and opioid-abusing methadone patients. *Journal of Consulting and Clinical Psychology.* 2002;70:398–405.
34. Petry NM, Peirce JM, Stitzer M, et al. Prize-based incentives increase retention in outpatient psychosocial treatment programs: results of the national drug abuse treatment clinical trials network study. *Archives of General Psychiatry.* 2005;62:1148–1156.
35. Dutra L, Stathopoulou G, Basden SL, Leyro TM, Powers, MB, Otto MW. A meta-analytic review of psychosocial interventions for substance-use disorders. *American Journal of Psychiatry.* 2008;165(2):179–187.
36. Griffith JD, Rowan-Szal GA, Roark RR, Simpson, DD. Contingency management in outpatient methadone treatment: a meta-analysis. *Drug and Alcohol Dependence.* 2000;58(1):55–66.
37. Lussier JP, Heil SH, Mongeon JA, Badger GJ, Higgins ST. A meta-analysis of voucher-based reinforcement therapy for substance-use disorders. *Addiction,* 2006;101(2):192–203.
38. McPherson S, Brooks O, Barbosa-Leiker C, et al. Examining longitudinal stimulant use and treatment attendance as parallel outcomes in two contingency management randomized clinical trials. *Journal of Substance Abuse Treatment.* 2015(61):18–25.
39. Burch AE, Morasco BJ, Petry NM. Patients undergoing substance abuse treatment and receiving financial assistance for a physical disability respond well to contingency management treatment. *Journal of Substance Abuse Treatment.* 2015;(58):67–71.
40. Kabat-Zinn J. *Wherever You Go, There You Are: Mindfulness Meditation in Everyday Life.* New York: Hyperion; 1994.
41. Bowen S, Chawia N, Collins SE, et al. Mindfulness-based relapse prevention for substance-use disorders: A pilot efficacy trial. *Substance Abuse.* 2009;30:295–305.
42. Alterman AI, Koppenhaver JM, Mulholland E, Ladden LJ, Baime MJ. Pilot trial of effectiveness of mindfulness meditation for substance abuse patients. *Journal of Substance Use.* 2004;9:259–268.
43. Marlatt GA. Buddhist philosophy and the treatment of addictive behavior. *Cognitive and Behavioral Practice.* 2002;9:44–49.
44. Marlatt GA, Gordon JR, eds. *Relapse Prevention: Maintenance Strategies in the Treatment of Addictive Behaviors.* New York: Guilford; 1985.
45. Dimeff LA, Linehan MM. Dialectical behavior therapy for substance abusers. *Addiction Science and Clinical Practice.* 2008;4:39–47.
46. Bohn MJ, Krahn DD, Staehler BA. Development and initial validation of a measure of drinking urges in abstinent alcoholics. *Alcoholism, Clinical and Experimental Research.* 1995;19:600–606.
47. Clark DM, Ball S, Pape D. An experimental investigation of thought suppression. *Behaviour Research and Therapy.* 1991;29:253–257.

48. Wegner DM, Schneider DJ, Carter SR, White TL. Paradoxical effects of thought suppression. *Journal of Personality and Social Psychology.* 2003;85:348–362.

49. Bowen S, Witkiewitz K, Dillworth TM, Marlatt GA. The role of thought suppression in the relationship between mindfulness meditation and alcohol use. *Addictive Behaviors.* 2007;32:2324–2328.

50. Linehan MM. *Cognitive-Behavioral Therapy of Borderline Personality Disorder.* New York: Guilford; 1993.

51. Breslin FC, Zach M, McMain S. An information-processing analysis of mindfulness: Implications for relapse prevention in the treatment of substance abuse. *Clinical Psychology: Science and Practice.* 2002;9:275–299.

52. Carey KB. Substance use reduction in the context of outpatient psychiatric treatment: A collaborative, motivational, harm reduction approach. *Community Mental Health Journal.* 1996;32:291–306.

53. Marlatt GA, Larimer ME, Witkiewitz K, eds. *Harm Reduction: Pragmatic Strategies for Managing High-Risk Behaviors.* New York: Guilford; 1996.

54. Witkiewitz K, Lustyk KB, Bowen S. Re-training the addicted brain: A review of hypothesized neurobiological mechanisms of mindfulness-based relapse prevention. *Psychology of Addictive Behaviors.* 2013;27:351–365.

55. Volkow N, Wang G-J, Fowler JS, Tomasi D, Telang F. Addiction: beyond dopamine reward circuitry. *Proceedings of the National Academy of Sciences of the United States.* 2010;108:15037–15042.

56. Kalivas PW, Volkow ND. The neural basis of addiction: A pathology of motivation and choice. *American Journal of Psychiatry.* 2005;162:1403–1413.

57. Westbrook C, Creswell JD, Tabibnia G, Julson E, Kober H, Tindle HA. Mindful attention reduces neural and self-reported cue-induced craving in smokers. *Social Cognitive and Affective Neuroscience.* 2013 Jan;8(1):73–84.

58. Zgierska A, Rabago D, Chawla N, Kushner K, Koehler R, Marlatt A. Mindfulness meditation for substance-use disorders: A systematic review. *Substance Abuse.* 2009;30:266–294.

59. Bowen S, Chawla N, Marlatt GA. *Mindfulness-Based Relapse Prevention for the Treatment of Substance Use Disorders: A Clinician's Guide.* New York: Guilford; 2010.

60. Bowen S, Witkiewitz K, Clifasefi SL et al. Relative efficacy of mindfulness-based relapse prevention, standard relapse prevention, and treatment as usual for substance-use disorders: A randomized clinical trial. *Journal of the American Medical Association Psychiatry.* 2014;71:547–556.

61. Brewer JA, Sinha R, Chen JA, et al. Mindfulness training and stress reactivity in substance abuse: Results from a randomized, controlled stage I pilot study. *Substance Abuse.* 2009;30:306–317.

62. Vieten C, Astin JA, Buscemi R, Galloway GP. Development of an acceptance-based coping intervention for alcohol dependence relapse prevention. *Substance Abuse.* 2010;31:108–116.

63. Zgierska A, Rabago D, Zuelsdorff M, Miller M, Coe C, Fleming MF. Mindfulness meditation for relapse prevention in alcohol dependence: A feasibility pilot study. *Journal of Addiction Medicine.* 2008;2:165–173.

64. Bowen S, Witkiewitz K, Chawla N, Grow J. Integrating mindfulness and cognitive behavioral traditions for the long-term treatment of addictive behaviors. *Journal of Clinical Outcomes Management Journal.* 2011;18:473–479.
65. Hayes SC, Strosahl KD, Wilson KG. *Acceptance and Commitment Therapy: An Experiential Approach to Behavior Change.* New York: Guilford; 1999.
66. Humphreys K. Alcoholics Anonymous and 12-step alcoholism treatment programs. *Recent Developments in Alcoholism.* 2003;16:149–164. doi: 10.1007/0-306-47939-7_12
67. Moos RH, Moos BS. Long-term influence of duration and frequency of participation in alcoholics anonymous on individuals with alcohol use disorders. *Journal of Consulting and Clinical Psychology.* 2004;72(1): 81.
68. Fiorentine R. After drug treatment: are 12-step programs effective in maintaining abstinence?. *The American Journal of Drug and Alcohol Abuse.* 1999;25(1):93–116.
69. Humphreys K, Moos RH. Reduced substance-abuse-related health care costs among voluntary participants in Alcoholics Anonymous. *Psychiatric Services.* 1996;47(7):709–713.
70. Tonigan JS, Miller WR, Connors, GJ. Project MATCH client impressions about Alcoholics Anonymous: Measurement issues and relationship to treatment outcome. *Alcoholism Treatment Quarterly.* 2000;18(1):25–41.
71. Project MATCH Research Group. Matching alcoholism treatments to client heterogeneity: Project MATCH posttreatment drinking outcomes. *Journal of Studies on Alcohol.* 1997;(58):7–29.
72. Morgenstern J, Labouvie E, McCrady BS, Kahler CW, Frey RM. Affiliation with Alcoholics Anonymous after treatment: A study of its therapeutic effects and mechanisms of action. *Journal of Consulting and Clinical Psychology.* 1997;65(5):768.
73. Sheeren M. The relationship between relapse and involvement in alcoholics anonymous. *Journal of Studies on Alcohol.* 1988;49(1):104–106.
74. Drake RE. Brief history, current status, and future place of assertive community treatment. *American Journal of Orthopsychiatry.* 1998;68(2):172–175. http://dx.doi.org/10.1037/h0085086
75. Stein LI., Test, MA. Alternative to mental hospital treatment: I. Conceptual model, treatment program, and clinical evaluation. *Archives of General Psychiatry.* 1980;37(4): 392–397.
76. Bond GR, Drake RE. The critical ingredients of assertive community treatment. *World Psychiatry.* 2015;14(2). doi: 10.1002/wps.20234
77. Tsemberis S, Gulcur L, Nakae M. Housing First, consumer choice, and harm reduction for homeless individuals with a dual diagnosis. *American Journal of Public Health.* 2004;94:651–656.
78. Bond GR, Drake RE, Mueser KT, Latimer E. Assertive community treatment for people with severe mental illness. *Disease Management and Health Outcomes.* 2001;9(3):141–159.

79. Finnerty MT, Manuel JI, Tochterman AZ, et al. Clinicians' perceptions of challenges and strategies of transition from assertive community treatment to less intensive services. *Community Mental Health Journal.* 2015;51:85–95. doi:10.1007/s10597-014-9706-y

80. Drake RE, McHugo GJ, Clark RE, Teague GB, Xie Haiyi, Miles K, Ackerson TH. Assertive community treatment for patients with co-occurring severe mental illness and substance use disorder: a clinical trial. *American Journal of Orthopsychiatry.* 1998;68(2):201–215. http://dx.doi.org/10.1037/h0080330

# 14

## Homeopathic Approach to Addiction

### AVGHI CONSTANTINIDES AND SHAHLA J. MODIR

Integrative approaches to the treatment of addiction have expanded over the last 10 years. As a chronic disease, the treatment and management of addiction is complex and has left many patients searching for different methods to seek relief. In this chapter, we explore how homeopathy works and canbe helpful in the treatment of addiction.

## Introduction to Homeopathy and History

The founder of homeopathy was a German physician, Samuel Hahnemann, who became a medical doctor on August 10, 1779, in Leipzig, Germany. At that time, popular methods of orthodox treatment included bloodletting, cupping, using leeches, and ingesting large doses of chemical agents such as mercury or arsenic. Hahnemann was disappointed with these methods since they often harmed his patients rather than helped them. He decided to relinquish Western medicine, and after much research created an alternative system of medicine he called homeopathy.

When Hahnemann first quit his practice, he needed to make money. He spoke many languages and started translating medical texts. While translating a book on the herb Cinchona bark, (the basis for quinine) the symptoms he read about sounded similar to the symptoms of malaria. He decided to experiment with the Cinchona bark; but instead of taking the substance raw, he ground it up and diluted it. The symptoms that he experienced were similar to malaria. He hypothesized that if he were to dilute this herb and give it to patients who have malaria, it may cure them. He found that by diluting the substance and succussing/shaking it, the herb became more powerful medicinally. The Cinchona bark became the first homeopathic remedy and has helped cure many cases of malaria over the past 200 years.

## QUOTES FROM HAHNEMANN IN HIS *MATERIA MEDICA PURA*

Hahnemann was quoted as saying the following:

> A very small dose of China officinalis (Cinchona bark) acts for but a short time, hardly a couple of days, but a large dose, such as is employed in the practice of every day, often acts for several weeks if it be not got rid of by vomiting or diarrhea, and thus ejected from the organism. From this we may judge how excellent the ordinary practice is of giving every day several and moreover large doses of bark!
>
> If the Homeopathic law be right, as it incontestably is right without any exception, and is derived from a pure observation of nature, that medicines can easily, rapidly, and permanently cure cases of disease only when the latter are made up of symptoms *similar* to the medicinal symptoms observed from the administration of the former to healthy persons; then we find, on a consideration of the symptoms of China, that this medicine is adapted for but few diseases, but that where it is accurately indicated, owing to the immense power of its action, one single very small dose will often effect a marvelous cure.
>
> I say cure, and by this I mean a 'recovery undisturbed by after-sufferings.' Or have practitioners of the ordinary stamp another, to me unknown, idea of what constitutes a cure?

In Hahnemann's clinical practice, he gave remedies to patients and recorded observations of their symptoms and any cure. Through this method, Hahnemann went on to successfully test over 60 substances for efficacy between 1820 and 1827, culling his remedies from a variety of sources including the mineral, animal, and plant kingdoms. One of main texts used in homeopathy (the *Materia Medica Pura*) was developed from these observations and published by Hahnemann.[6] It is a collective reference compendium of the substances and the associated symptoms found in remedy "provings." To date, the text now has over 200 years of scientific backing on how these remedies work along with thousands of case studies. The case logs are used to help correlate symptoms with remedies to improve accuracy in treatment. Based on these findings, homeopaths select a remedy and then decide on the dilution based on their assessment of the patient. Today, tests "provings" continue to be conducted on healthy, individual volunteers in double-blind studies.

Homeopathic remedies have been FDA regulated in the United States since 1938 and do not have any major side effects or addictive characteristics. They are safe medicines to use when treating addiction and will not harm the patient. Additionally, they are safe for pregnant women, infants, and children.

## How Does Homeopathy Work?

"It is vital to have a clear understanding of the laws and principles of Homeopathy in order to have an appreciation of the complexity in its curative powers."

—*Hahnemann*

*Similia similibus curentur* means "like cures like," and this is the foundation of homeopathy. Paracelsus, from the 16th century, was the first physician to come up with this idea, but Paracelsus did not pursue the idea at that time. It was not until Hahnemann's efforts in the early 1800s that this principle finally became a hypothesis to be tested and evaluated.

Hahnemann emphasizes the law of similars and how it can lead to actually curing disease and not just the alleviation of symptoms. The term homeopathy, first published in 1810, denotes this in its linguistics. The first part "homeo" means *similar*, not the same. While the second part of the word, "pathos," in Greek means *suffering*.

In contrast, the word "allopathy" is a word coined by Hahnemann in 1842 to describe conventional medical treatment of symptoms. Allopathic treatment of disease symptoms uses substances or techniques to oppose or suppress the symptoms. The breakdown of the word "allopathy" goes as follows: "allo" means "oppose" or "opposite," and "pathos" means suffering. In this way, the juxtaposition between the two systems can be identified through the terms used to describe them.

Many fields now acknowledge that the mind and body are interlinked. Hahnemann recognized this principle long ago and stressed that physical and mental symptoms are to be taken together to form a portrait of disease. The main principle of treatment is that homeopathic remedies restore the body's homeostasis by giving a remedy that is similar to the patients' symptoms. A homeopath will choose a remedy according to homeopathic principals and through this the remedy stimulates the body, the mind, the vital force, and the immune system.

Homeopathy is a tried-and-true method of healing people who experience a wide range of acute, chronic, and even hereditary ailments.

## Homeopathic Remedies and Symptoms

Upon administration of a remedy to a healthy individual, that individual will exhibit symptoms unique to that remedy without experiencing illness. However, the same remedy given to an individual who is ill with those same symptoms will prove to be curative.

Think of a common red onion. What happens to you when you cut an onion? You may experience watery eyes with a burning sensation. A clear, watery discharge may come from your nose, and as it drops out of your nose the fluid burns. There can be an itchy and burning sensation in the throat. These symptoms are similar to hay fever or allergies. So by giving a diluted version of the common red onion (*Allium cepa*) it will be curative in the person suffering from hay fever.

## LAWS OF HOMEOPATHY

- **Law of Similars**. *Similia similibus curentur*, which means "like cures like." Finding the right remedy for each individual. It is the remedy that is most similar, as if it were tailor-made for each individual.
- **Vital Force**. Acupuncturists call this *Chi*, Ayurvedics call it *Prana*, and homeopaths call it "vital force." We are all speaking of the life force. It is the energy that starts when the sperm enters the egg and starts to grow. That same energy is with us our whole lives and leaves us when we die. Homeopathic medicines are treating and stimulating the vital/life force.
- **Minimum dose**. Giving small amounts of a substance that is similar to the patient. By giving the minimum dose, this stimulates the vital force back into homeostasis.

This means a medicine capable of producing certain effects when taken by a healthy human being is capable of curing any illness that displays similar effects.

- **Treating the whole person.** A fundamental principle of homeopathy is that it treats the person as an individual. Truly looking at the mental, emotional, and physical states of a person is where homeopathy goes deep. It is less common in the Western allopathic approach that someone will ask a patient about their bowel movements and dreams in the same appointment.

Where homeopaths depart from the Western medicine model of diagnosis is seen in the homeopathic patient consultation. Patients often come in with a diagnosis, which may be helpful; however, this is only part of the entire scope of the person. What sets the homeopathic consultation apart is the level of depth and collecting all of the details of a patient's routine, personality, and symptoms. These are seen as relevant to each person's case and create the basis for selecting remedy.

For example, if a person comes in with a diagnosis of migraine headaches, the homeopath knows that the headaches are severe but not the details of how the person experiences them. Knowing how long the patient has had them and what life events caused them is important to understand. In addition, the homeopath will want to know the type of pain the migraine is causing, what makes it better or worse, and what causes it. In other words, every characteristic of the migraine is considered essential knowledge. Along with physical symptoms, knowing a person's mental and emotional state completes the whole picture.

The remedy is in understanding those details; this then enables the homeopath to easily match the patient with the ideal remedy. Whether treating a migraine headache or a dangerous addiction, the homeopath is looking to understand the "why" behind the person's state. By learning the whole history of the person from birth to the present moment (including any traumatic experiences that may have impacted their lives), the homeopath sees a complete picture and can grasp the underlying nature of that person and why they were affected so deeply. In the case of addiction, underneath the façade of the substance-use habit is a deep sense of fear and often anxiety that can lead to mental suffering. Understanding this underlying state helps the homeopath immensely in finding the correct remedy. With the right remedy, the chances of relapse become progressively less likely.

As a result of the basis for homeopathy, it has been difficult to develop research paradigms that actually represent the fair use of the model for a particular illness. The holistic model of homeopathy focuses on individual treatment, and research design is based on a standard treatment of all subjects against a placebo. This has made finding any meaningful research on homeopathy for addiction treatment a challenge. Modern homeopathy attempts to use its collective databases to guide treatments. Reference Works is a homeopathic computer program widely used by homeopaths around the world. It is a library of over 900 reference books of *Materia Medicas*, repertories, journals, and case studies. For example, in looking up the word "addiction," the program pulls up "974" references and "275" remedies. In adding in the word "alcoholism" it pulls up "2952" references and "436" remedies. One can see that there is a tremendous amount of data to use along with the patient's clinical picture to determine the best remedy.

The following case examples show many different types of addiction, and emphasized here are not only physical characteristics but also archetypal personalities relating to each remedy. In homeopathy, finding constitutional remedies is done in part by matching the patient's symptoms to the cases that have the associated remedy attached. Below are a list of remedies commonly used in the treatment of addictions and their associated constitutional archetypes and symptoms.

# Case A

**Remedy**: *Nux Vomica*

**Addiction and/or related symptoms:** alcohol or stimulants/gastrointestinal complaints/insomnia

**Personality:** Type "A" personality and very competitive.

This person might be a high-functioning vice president of a company, or an ambitious climber of the corporate ladder. These personality types can often be irritable and lack the patience to deal with lower-level people. As you will see, their irritability often stems from uncomfortable physical ailments. They are ambitious and will do anything to get ahead and beat out another person for the same position. As workaholics, they know how to be efficient and get the job done. These people are highly functional despite their addiction—until they burn out. Like many people who experience addiction, they can be masters at manipulating others and situations. They get angry easily; and if aggravated they may become malicious. They may have a mean streak and a history of violence in both the workplace and in the home.

Since these types are highly competitive, they can have a compulsive side and will obsess over small details. They are the micro-managers of the world. They are given to rage and jealousy and never forget a wrong that has been done to them. Unpredictable mood swings can produce a manic state. On the physical side we can see some of the reasons for the underlying emotional state.

This remedy has a physical presence in the gastro-intestinal tract. From constipation to diarrhea, nausea, and vomiting, these patients can live in an extremely uncomfortable physical state. Constant nausea and vomiting during and after eating and drinking creates a highly irritated person. Often because of an addiction to alcohol, the liver function becomes stressed and strained, and a toxic liver with signs of cirrhosis can occur frequently. Headaches are often caused by excessive drinking, and the resulting hangover is from a buildup of toxins throughout the body. Constriction in the chest, especially in the region of the heart, is made worse from the excessive use of coffee, tobacco, or alcohol. They love stimulants and use of such substances is often accompanied by great anxiety and overpowering panic attacks. These are people who have a difficult time unwinding and thus suffer from chronic insomnia. Their thoughts range from how their day had gone, to worrying about the day to come. Their on-edge paranoia results in them waking from the slightest noise and thinking that someone has come into their room. This alertness will keep them awake for hours on end.

*References* 1,2,4,9,10

## Case B

**Remedy:** Belladonna

**Addiction and/or related symptoms:** opiates or alcohol

**Personality:** Over-sensitive and delirious.

This person has lots of fears and anxieties. They have lots of delusions and hallucinations. The have visions of monsters, ghosts, and other scary things. They are scared of the dark.

All of their senses are heightened. Their moods are varied. They can be rage prone: they may hit, strike, bite, and/or spit on others.

They may engage in inappropriate behavior such as singing, dancing, or laughing at odd times. They are very quarrelsome, mistrustful, forgetful, and easily confused.

They are restless, always have to be moving (hands in constant movement), trying to catch things in the air, or picking at bedclothes, as if trying to find something. Often they sense they are dreaming when awake. They are hard to please. They rarely want to talk, and they fear they may die. Trying to console them makes it worse. They have suicidal tendencies; they are often tired of living and think they may be better off dead. They have lots of cramping in the stomach area, distention, pains come and go quickly. Feels better to bend backwards. They crave lemonade or lemons. They have pains and throbbing and cramping in the stomach. Their face can be red and hot to the touch. Glassy eyes and dilated pupils, and their conjunctiva red and dry.

Feeling a rush of blood to the head, head pains throbbing with hammering headache. Their head is sensitive to drafts, cold air and washing hair. They often get cramping feelings with swollen joints, jerks, and spasms or trembling. They don't sleep well due to fears and anxiety; they jerk and kick during sleep, kicks, and sometimes cry out. They have very vivid dreams.

*References* [1,2,4,9,10]

## Case C

**Remedy:** Syphilinum

**Addiction and/or related symptoms:** opiates or benzodiazepines

**Personality:** Self destructive/ suicidal, depression, muscle cramping penetrating the bones and restless legs.

This person has a destructive personality and sometimes suicidal tendencies. They are antisocial and peevish, and they do not want to be soothed or helped. They feel hopeless. They experience lots of sensations: they feel as if they are going insane, or their teeth are loose, or the top of their head is falling off; their tongue feels paralyzed, as if bitten by bugs. They have a fear of germs and are fastidious. They will wring their hands, and laugh or weep for seemingly no reason. They have extremely poor memory but remember everything before they were ill. They have severe insomnia. They are restless in bed at night; they may wake up after at midnight, for example, and can't fall asleep again. They have bad headaches and tend to hit their head against the wall repeatedly. The pains are stupefying: as if in the bones of the head. Can have hair loss. Their muscles contract and cramp and can feel like hard knots. They feel better from pouring cold water on sore parts of the body. They have excessive saliva, especially during sleep, and it can ooze out of the mouth while asleep. There is a copper-colored skin discoloration. They can have boils and blisters and warts. Dental caries and necrosis of bones may occur. Their bone pains feel deep, and there are tearing and burning sensations.

*References* 1,2,9,10

## Case D

**Remedy:** Fluoric acid

**Addiction and/or related symptoms:** sex, gambling, opiates, or benzodiazepines

**Personality**:
Their lives are maked by infrequent and broken relationships. They are often irresponsible, not wanting to do much, unless it's something like sex or gambling. They shun responsibility and are indifferent to business affairs. They are forgetful and generally absent minded. They have an aversion to their family and the ones they love the most. They think they have wrecked their relationship and that they have been betrayed and deeply hurt. They feel like they are the black sheep of the family and often run away as teens. They can form and break off relationships quickly, but the relationships they do form are superficial. They can be domineering and irritable. They will shun responsibilities and are indifferent to business affairs. They often have a surfeit of sexual energy and will have sex with anyone. They love to gamble and are always in a hurry. They are unhappy and unsatisfied people. They don't like heat, but their body temperature feels hot. They will get sweaty palms when anxious and apprehensive.

They will have a swollen abdomen from liver disorders and a feeling of emptiness in the stomach area, but they will often be hungry. They crave cold drinks and have an aversion to coffee but a love for spicy food. There is often swelling and edema of the limbs. They might have hepatic disorders from alcoholism, soreness in the liver area, possibly degeneration of the liver.

*References* 5,7,9,10

# Case E

**Remedy:** sulphur

**Addiction and/or related symptoms:** arrogance, entitlement, alcohol, or disorganized/scattered ADD symptoms

**Personality:** scatterbrained, selfish, and intelligent

Polycrest covers a lot of human traits, major ones includeselfishness and self-absorption, that come from ego. They like the idea of helping others as long as it is easy. They only like to do things that benefit themselves. This comes from a sense of entitlement. The feel they are always right and can do everything by themselves, so 12-step programs are not easy for this type of person to join: "Why do I need a sponsor I can stop drinking all by my self, I don't need anyone's help!" They love their material possessions and will collect things and can become hoarders. They don't like to share their possessions even if its something miniscule like a pencil sharpener; they will feel unsettled until it's returned. They are usually messy people and have papers all over their desks. They are intelligent but absent minded, and they can be quite forgetful. They will forget names, misspell words, and have brain fog (mental fatigue). They are lazy and can get bored easily. They don't like to do physical or mental work. But then sometimes they can be ambitious workaholics. They often repeat words said to them, as their powers of concentration can be weak.

They get irritated with advice, as they always seem to know better. They are quarrelsome and difficult to please. They can have very fixed ideas and be manic. They can have depression with thoughts of suicide by water or by leaping from a window. They have anxiety, especially at night; they have racing thoughts, which can prevent sleep. They like to drink a lot; yet when they realize that they have a problem, they try to overcome it but always experience relapses.

They often feel hot and can be hot to the touch, with hot palms and feet and can often have flashes of heat (male or female). They feel like they have a load on their chest, an oppressed feeling. May have a feeling of weakness in their chest, with difficult breathing, and they may want windows open. Loose rattling of mucus and heat in chest. Headaches with throbbing pains and a hot head to the touch. They have lots of skin issues, having unhealthy-looking, dry, scaly skin. Wounds take a long time to heal. Milk makes them worse and makes the person desire sweets. Acidity and sour eructations occur, and there is belching if pressure on the stomach area. Often these types have a sore liver need to urinate often and can wet the bed at night.

*References* 3,9

# Case F

**Remedy:** Arsenicum album

**Addiction and/or related symptoms:** high anxiety, OCD symptoms, alcohol, or stimulant use

**Personality:** Anxiety is the main disposition with this remedy, whether real or unreal, yesterday or tomorrow, molehill or mountain; for this patient it's a constant waterfall of worry. They have had worry/anxiety all of their lives. Being hypochondriacs, they will read up on every ailment they think they have, and then they think its something incurable. They can be very desperate, begging for help and complaining all the time. Not the easiest patient to deal with, these types will have 20 questions during a session and another 10 when their hand is on door to leave. They have OCD tendencies and lots of fears such as death, illness, cleanliness, virus's germs, ghosts, being left alone, and fear of being burglarized. Their obsession with cleanliness will lead them to wash the dishes as soon as they have finished eating, even if they have dinner guests. They think something bad will happen to them or a loved one. They can often turn to self-mutilation with picking and tearing at the skin and nail biting. They constantly move from place to place. They are melancholy and can have suicidal thoughts. It's hard for them to forgive, and they will hold grudges for years and become malicious. They are bossy, domineering, and demanding, having high standards; they are critical of themselves and others. A lot of their physical pains are burning sensations, like hot needles.

They have lots of GI issues often associated with anxiety, usually violent pains felt in the abdomen. Liver and spleen can be enlarged. Anxious dry cough, feeling tightness in chest worse with anxiety and restlessness. Photophobia, burning sensation in eyes with hot acrid lachrymation. Sunken or protruding eyes.

*References:* 3,9,10

# Case G

**Remedy:** Mercurius

**Addiction and/or related symptoms:** alcohol and stimulants

**Personality:** the "mercurial person" with mood swings

They are hurried, withdrawn people, and they feel the need to take care of their responsibilities. Their speech is hurried, with a nervous tremor and sometimes a stammer. The have violent tendencies; they may strike a person or cause them harm if offended. Often they have no appetite. Their acts can be foolish and some-times mischievous (and sometimes disgusting). They sometimes have deep anx-iety from thinking they are mentally ill; they are emotionally intense, suspicious, and paranoid people.

Often they have bad halitosis, with a metallic taste in mouth and excessive sa-liva that is worse at night in bed. The tongue is often imprinted with teeth marks. They have otitis media, otorrhea with thick yellow discharge. Sometimes they have tremors in the hands, which is worse when they write, type, or eat. They tend to have constipation with a sensation of incomplete bowel movements. They can have enlarged lymphatic glands. They can sometimes have an enlarged, sore liver and jaundice.

*References:* 8.9.10

# Case H

**Remedy:** Opium

**Addiction and/or related symptoms:** Opiate withdrawal/toxicity or Alcohol withdrawal/toxicity

**Personality:** These people are good at suppressing their emotions, and they are good at deception and can be master manipulators. Often they feel like victims. They lack will power, not wanting to do much. They can get into an apoplectic state when they are upset but can also be catatonic, dull, and sluggish. Their vivid imaginations can scare them, and they sometimes go into delirious rants. They have delusions that parts of their body are enlarged.

They can have delirium tremens and are susceptible to become comatose from a drug overdose. They have fainting spells often. They often jerking and twitch during sleep, or they might have epilepsy while sleeping or violent chills. They are very drowsy at night, but far-off noises will keep them awake.

Their abdomen is often hard and bloated, they have constipation with hard stool, and their bowels feel obstructed. Might have involuntary stool or urination after a fright. They can have staring, glassy eyes that are half closed. Pupils can be fixed, either dilated or contracted and non-reactive to light, and they may have cloudiness of vision. They feel that sometimes their eyeballs are too big for their sockets. There is twitching and coldness of limbs. It feels like their limbs belong to someone else, or they are severed. Hot perspiration is felt all over the body.

*References:* 9

# Case I

**Remedy:** Lachesis

**Addiction and/or related symptoms:** Alcohol, sex, or stimulants

**Personality:** vengeful, suspicious, mistrusting especially of doctors.

These types feel like they have two wills: an angel sitting on one shoulder and the devil on the other, both giving advice at the same time. They have a constant inner struggle going on. They have a highly disturbed mind; they are intense, and they can become hysterical and suffer from manic depression and anxiety.

They can be jealous and suspicious. They can even be schizophrenic. They have hasty speech with no editing process. They have rapid changes in thoughts, jumping from one topic to the next and often voice these thoughts in a loud, manic outburst.

They may have mental confusion and take on many tasks, but they can't finish them. They have a lot of anger and are often malicious and vindictive. Alcohol will bring on headaches and heart palpations at night, and they suffer from sleeplessness because of alcohol. They have a fear on going to sleep; they feel they will die in their sleep, and they wake often from bad dreams. They often suffer from flashes of heat and perspiration. They can't bear tight clothing, especially around their waist and neck. They feel sensitive around the liver area with inflammation and may have cirrhosis of the liver and hepatitis. Their hands will tremble from alcohol abuse. Their calves will cramp up. Most symptoms will appear on the left side. They are binge eaters who are addicted to sugar, and they never feel full.

*References:* 9,10

### Suggestions of Potency and Posology
An experienced homeopath will use their skills to determine the most efficacious manner to administer the remedy to the patient.

### Potency
The challenge in treating addiction is to calm the sympathetic nervous system, which has been over-stimulated by substance abuse itself. The homeopath must carefully choose a potency for the well-selected remedy.

For a highly over-stimulated system:

- Lower to medium potencies
- 12c–30c

To stimulate a depleted, low-functioning system:

- Medium to higher potencies
- 30c, 60c, 100c, 200c

### Administration of a Remedy
Ideally, the patient's mouth should be empty 15 minutes before and after taking the remedy, no matter what form the remedy is. In all forms of delivery, a homeopathic remedy works to stimulate the patient's vital force to start the healing process.

- Taken before bedtime allows the remedy to work right away while the body is at rest and repairing itself.
- Taken first thing in the morning helps keep the patient on track for the day.
- Remedies should not be handled or touched. Tap the remedy into the bottlecap, tip under the tongue, and let it dissolve.
- Dry dose: 4 pellets sublingually and let dissolve.
- Plussing method: 4 pellets in 4 ounces of water. Sip remedy solution for the next 24 hours, stirring the water before taking each sip.
- Split dose: remedy will be taken once every 12 hours for 36 hours.

### Frequency of a Remedy
Remedies can be given daily, every other day, weekly or monthly, depending on the strength of the patient's vital force.

- For a detoxifying patient, give the remedy more frequently: 1time daily for 7 days then 1 time every other day for 7 days then 3 times per week for 3 weeks.

Since homeopathic potency administration varies with each individual, knowing the method and amount to give may appear challenging. With careful observation a skilled practitioner will be able to judge the energy of the patient's vital force and understand which potency best matches the patient's state.

When a patient takes a homeopathic remedy, this helps to create a state of homeostasis in an otherwise over-reactive, agitated person.

### The First Follow-up
All follow-ups are used to evaluate the effectiveness of the chosen remedy and potency and the changes the patient has experienced and how they have managed those changes. There are numerous ways of evaluating the effect the remedy has had on the patient.

- Have the patient rate their improvement on a scale of 1 to 10, 10 being best.
- Ask what it was before the initial consultation. This enables the homeopath to gauge the patient's level of improvement.
- If the patient is doing well, keep them on the same remedy. Either keep the same potency or increase the dosage if you feel the patient is ready to take a higher dose.
- If the remedy is deemed correct, and there has been slight improvement, consider an increase in the dosage.
- If there is no change at all, then reevaluate the case and look for a different remedy.
- Follow up 3 to 4 weeks later to assess the action of the remedy.

### The Second Follow-up

Each follow-up is designed to evaluate the action of the remedy and how well the patient is progressing on the chosen remedy and potency. With each subsequent follow-up visit, the process is very much the same: to evaluate the action of the remedy and to observe the progress of the patient.

Once it has been determined that the remedy and potency are working, the patient will need less of the remedy over time. At this point, the patient is now on the road to recovery.

### Acute and Chronic Homeopathy

*Constitutional and symptom-based models.* It is imperative to clarify the difference between treating the whole person, as opposed to only one symptom the person may be experiencing. Addiction is only one part of the whole. One reason that homeopathy has been so successful in treating addictions is because of the nature of how a remedy opens up the patient to deep insights into their addictions.

Homeopathy looks to understand the nature of the whole, whereas allopathy, or Western-based medicine, looks to treat each individual symptom as something separate from rather than part of the whole. Evaluating the mental, emotional, and physical aspects of a person allows the homeopath to gain a deeper understanding of the reasons behind the addiction in the first place.

### Contraindications

Since homeopathy is an energy-based medicine it varies greatly from allopathic (often chemical-based) medicines.

Unless an extremely low potency is used (i.e., 1x-4x or 1c-4c), there are no contraindications for its usage with allopathic prescription or over-the-counter medicines. Herbs, vitamins, and supplements may interfere with allopathic medicines, but homeopathic remedies do not interact with these substances.

## Side Effects

In general, homeopathic remedies are safe for both children and adults. Recently, however, there have been many case reports showing the dangers of bella donna in infants and young children, and it should be avoided in these cases. In adults, under the supervision of a trained homeopath, bella donna can be used safely.

Homeopathic remedies can produce what is called a "healing aggravation." After a patient takes the remedy, it is possible that old symptoms may appear: this is considered a positive reaction. Old symptoms that have lain dormant or perhaps just under the surface are allowed to come forth and be removed for good, permitting the patient to experience a healing of old wounds (either physical and/or emotional). Depending on the severity, symptoms may be short lived and seldom return.

## Conclusion

One of the most important aspects of using homeopathic remedies for the treatment of addictions is that the remedies are non-addictive. There are no harmful side effects to contend with in most adults under the supervision of a trained homeopath. Remedies seek to be curative by addressing the totality of the person, not just the specific addiction and the parts of the body it immediately affects. This inclusiveness leads to improved patient care and wellness.

Perhaps some of these ideas may seem novelty-like alternative to allopathically trained physicians who may be accustomed to treating only the symptoms associated with a certain diagnosis. Homeopaths know that the outer symptoms of a malady are only superficial. With a thorough understanding of how a patient feels, physically and emotionally, homeopaths are able to help their patients recover. The insight a patient gains through the homeopathic consultation and homeopathic remedies enables each patient to travel a path to greater understanding and hence overcome their addiction. Through this healing process, a person is better able to become a productive, contributing member of society.

### REFERENCES

1. Boericke WM. *Pocket Manual of Homeopathic Materia Medica: Comprising Characteristic and Guiding Symptoms of All Remedies (Clinical and Pathogenic)*. Philadelphia: Boericke & Tafel; 1853:8–12.
2. Clark JH. *A Dictionary of Practical Materia Medica*. New Delhi, India: B.Jain; 1902:8–12.

3. Coulter CR. *Portraits of Homeopathic Medicines: Psychophysical Analyses of Selected Constitutional Types.* Berkeley, CA: North Atlantic; 1986:13–17.

4. Gallavardin JP. *Alcoholism: The Homeopathic Treatment of Alcoholism.* Philadelphia. Hahnemann; 1890:9, 11.

5. Kent JT. Lectures on Homeopathic Materia Medica. New Delhi, India. B. Jain; 1905:12–13.

6. Hahnemann SMD. Materia Medica Pura. New Delhi, India: B. Jain; 1811: 2

7. Sankaran R. Soul of Remedies Materia Medica. Bombay India: Homoeopathic Medical; 1997:12–13.

8. Morrison R. *Desktop Guide To Keynotes and Confirmatory Symptoms.* Albany, CA. Hahnemann Clinic; 1993:17–18.

9. Murphy R. Nature Materia Medica: *1,400 Homeopathic and Herbal Remedies.* 3rd ed. Pagosa Springs, CO: Lotus Star Academy; 2000:8 –20.

10. Phatak SR. Concise Materia Medica. Delhi, India. B. Jain; 1977:8–20.

# 15

## Ayurvedic Approach to Addiction

### SHAHLA J. MODIR

Ayurveda is one of the oldest systems of natural medicine in the world. Originating over 4,000 years ago, it is the root of several other branches of traditional medicine including the Chinese and Greek medical systems. As the traditional healing system of India, it is the medical aspect of the Vedic spiritual traditions of India and designed to keep aspirants in balance on their spiritual journey. The word "veda" means knowledge or science, and the term "ayus" means "life" or "life span" in Sanskrit. Thus, the term "ayurveda" means the knowledge or "science of life." Ayurveda follows the principle that living in harmony with the universal elements is important across the life span. In Ayurveda, there is a "scientific" aspect to creating and maintaining this balance. When a person is not living in tune with the season, time of day, and dietary considerations, then disease can occur.

On a spiritual level, Ayurveda views the body, mind, and soul (or "atman") of a person as connected to the universe. A disruption in the flow of life force or "prana" can create disease. Likewise, a state of health known in Sanskrit as "svastha" is not merely the absence of disease. A state of svastha is to be fully established in a spiritual higher self and to limit the attachment and fixation of the egoistic self. Ayurveda believes that individuals when connecting to their "higher" self-awareness will make choices that create balance and avoid disease.

## Cause of Disease

The original text of Ayurveda is known as the *Caraka Samhita*, which describes a threefold cause of disease. The "unwholesome conjunction of the senses with objects of their affections" is one of the main sources of imbalance. When a person loses a connection with their higher self-awareness, taking in objects of pleasure will become alluring. As one goes through life, the 5 senses are constantly presented with a variety of choices. Some of these options will bring the body and mind back into balance. Others will direct a person toward disease. Learning to manage the 5 senses to create balance and avoid disharmony is a way to prevent imbalance and bring health. Thus, the use of the 5 senses in an unmindful way addresses to the concept that eating and living in ways that only bring pleasure, at the expense of equanimity, can lead to disease.

According to the *Caraka Samhita*, the second major cause of disease is "prajnaparadha," or failure of the intellect. This concept explains that individuals inherently know what to do to bring their body and mind back into balance; however, they are often thrown off balance by the seductions of the senses. Ayurveda uses yoga and meditation to teach an individual how to listen to the advice of their higher self and how to train the mind to develop the discipline and concentration necessary to carry this into daily life choices.

"Parinama" is the third cause of disease in the *Caraka Samhita* and refers to an individual's experience of time. While life is experienced in the physical world through linear time and schedules, biological and mental time are subjective experiences and will affect aging and disease. The faster mental time is moving in Ayurveda, the quicker the degenerative processes in the body advance. When the mind is concentrated and calm, the decay of our human biology slows.

On a more physical level, these causes of disease manifest in the individual as a state of mind-body discord called "doshic imbalance." In Ayurveda, each person has a unique physical and mental makeup that is a microcosmic representation of the 5 elements. Each element or aggregated elements differs in quantity in each person. Thus, for each person, their psychological makeup, body structure, predisposition to disease, and treatment will be according to their individual makeup. In this model, prescribing the same treatment for a particular disease can be medicinal for one individual and have no effect (or negative effects) in another person: the exact opposite of standard treatment protocols followed by Western medical practitioners. Individualized dietary, lifestyle, and herbal prescriptions based on the mind-body constitutions (called "doshas") are essential to aligning the inner intelligence and natural healing ability of the individual.[1]

## Pancha Maha Bhuti: The 5-Element Theory

All matter in the universe is made of the 5 basic elements of air (vayu), fire (teja), water (jala), earth (prithivi), and ether or space (akasha). In Ayurveda, a fundamental concept is that the individual is a microcosmic manifestation of the elements of the universe. This relationship of the microcosmic human to the universe is reflected through the 5 basic elements. Each element has particular qualities inherent in its nature that are represented in the human body according to its properties. Air represents a cold, gaseous, mobile, unstable state. Fire represents heat, light, mobility, instability, and transformation. Water is cool, liquid, mobile; and earth is dense, thick, and stable. Ether is representative of space and is cold, light, unstable, and mobile.

As the elements manifest in the body, they represent the subtle aspect of the 5 senses: ether as hearing, air as touch, fire as vision, water as taste, and earth as smell. In addition, as an energetically dense expression, the 5 elements represent the 7 tissues of the body called "dhatus" and describe the nature of these tissues based on which element predominates. Ojas is the eighth dhatu layer. Ojas is the vital essence of all tissues; it is the central reserve energy of the body. When the ojas is of high quality and quantity, the internal strength of the body and its immunity is superior. Poor diet, stress, frequent changes in environment, chronic disease, physical trauma, over-indulgence in sex, drugs/alcohol/exercise, and exposure to toxins all deplete the ojas and reduce the body's natural healing reserve.[2]

## Tridosha Theory

In Ayurveda, the physiology of the human body is ruled by 3 forces known as the "doshas." The 3 doshas (vata, pitta, and kapha) are 3 specific combinations of the 5 basic elements that create the psycho-physiological characteristics of an individual based on their attributes. Vata is made up of air and ether. Pitta is created from fire and water, and kapha is the combination of the elements water and earth. They are the universe represented in the individual, and each person has a unique "fingerprint" combination of the 3 doshas, called the "prakruti" or "constitution." The prakruti (or individual balance of vata, pitta, and kapha) will describe the psycho-physiological characteristics of an individual and how the energy will move and function through their physical body and mind most harmoniously. The prakruti also predicts the types of diseases an individual will be predisposed to, as well as the treatments. One can have a prakruti with a relative dominance of any one dosha: vata, pitta, or kapha. It is also common to have a predominence of two doshas: vata-pitta, vata-kapha, or pitta-kapha. Rarely, there may also be an equal distribution of all the doshas. All of the doshas have strengths and weaknesses inherent in their qualities, and there is no best dosha. As individuals interface with the universe and the 5 elements in the outer world, they take in substances and sensory impressions that contain relative amounts of these elements that will interplay with their own doshic state and will lead to either harmony or disease. Increase and decrease of each dosha is also affected by diurnal, seasonal variations and stage of life. Table 15.1 reflects the relationship of these variations and which dosha predominates during a particular period.[3]

The vikruti of an individual represents the current state of the 3 doshas. If the vikruit is the same as the prakruti, then the person is balanced and healthy. When

Table 15.1  Balancing Tastes For Each Dosha

| Vata | Pitta | Kapha |
|------|-------|-------|
| Heavy/Sweet | Cold/Sweet | Light/Pungent |
| Oily/Sour | Heavy/Bitter | Dry/Bitter |
| Hot/Salt | Dry/Astringent | Hot/Astringent |

there is disease, the vikruti reflects a relative imbalance in the doshas that may illustrate how diet, lifestyle, emotions, age, and environment have impacted on the
prakruti. In Ayurveda, the physicians establish the difference between prakruti
and vikruti using the diagnostic procedures of taking a detailed history, analyzing
the face and tongue, and reading the pulse. The goal in Ayurveda is to maintain
one's prakruti, as it is the most balanced expression of the doshas in the individual.

Thus, as a subtle form of physiology, the doshas govern how the energy
will move through the body and affect the dhatus or "tissues." Although dosha
translates to "faulty" or "causing harm" in Sanskrit, the doshas only create disease
when they are functioning abnormally. Otherwise, they are important to maintain
good health.

Vata, pitta, and kapha each have their own attributes based on their elemental
makeup that dictate the psychology and physiology of the individual.

Vata dosha has dry, light, cold, rough, subtle, mobile, and clear attributes. In
Sanskrit, it means "that which moves things." Vata is the principle of air and mobility, and it regulates all activity in the body and mind such as circulation, respiration, digestion, elimination, and physical movement. Vata is the primary force in
the nervous system, governing sensory and motor function. It controls the expul-
sion of feces, urine, sweat, menstrual fluid, semen, and the fetus. The psychological
functions of creativity, imagination, spontaneity, and joy are also predicted from
vata's attributes. Individuals with vata predominance are easily excited and can be
impulsive or fickle decision makers. They are prone to emotions of fear, insecurity,
doubt, and worry when vata is in excess. Physical characteristics are also a product
of vata's attributes. Vata-predominant individuals are often light in weight with
thin tissues, dry skin, and thin hair. They may have small, dry eyes and irregular
appetite and thirst. Although vata is present throughout the body and mind, its
root is in the colon. Vata is increased in the body/mind by environmental factors
that have similar attributes such as old age, the fall season, and dry, light foods
such as salad. Conditions of vata imbalance are arthritis, tremors, anxiety, constipation, flatulence, and insomnia.[3]

The qualities of pitta are hot, sharp, light, liquid, mobile, and slightly oily.
The word "pitta" is derived from the Sanskrit root "tap," meaning to heat or be
austere, and it represents the principle of fire in the body. Pitta is responsible
for the digestion and assimilation of physical and mental phenomenon in the

body and mind through the metabolic activities of anabolism and catabolism. It is responsible for all the secretions of the gastrointestinal tract, the enzymes and hormones from the ductless glands, and for controlling body temperature. Individuals with pitta predominance have strong intellect, courage, confidence, articulation, organizing capacity, and natural leadership qualities. Emotions such as anger, jealousy, and hatred are signs of excess pitta in the mind, as is being judgmental and perfectionist. In the physical body, pitta types will have a sensitive and reactive body with a medium frame and average, stable weight. Since pitta is sour and associated with the colors red and yellow, pitta individuals may have yellowing of teeth, and their bodily fluids may have a pungent odor. Pitta dosha is primarily located in the small intestine. Pitta is increased in the body/mind during middle age and in the late spring and summer season—and by consuming spicy "hot" foods, such as chili peppers. Conditions of pitta excess reflect an inflammatory or feverish quality: heartburn, skin rashes, fevers, infections, and ulcers, for example.[3]

The attributes of kapha are heavy, slow, dull, cold, oily, smooth, dense, sticky, and cloudy. Kapha comes from two Sankrit roots "ka," meaning water, and "pha," which means "to flourish." The etymological meaning of kapha is that which is flourished by water. It is responsible for all of the activities pertaining to growth, stability, lubrication, and storage in the body. It is the principle of cohesion, structure, and lubrication. The physical structures of kapha are myelin sheath, connective tissues, and senses of taste and smell. It also protects the digestive and respiratory tracts, and it lubricates the joints. Kapha also regulates water and fat, builds tissues, and helps heal wounds. Individuals with kapha predominant have a strong long-term memory; they are tranquil, loyal, faithful, and have a natural capacity for forgiveness. Excess kapha in the mind leads to attachment, lethargy, depression, and greed. Kapha's primary location is in the lungs and upper stomach. Its maximum influence is during childhood and during winter and early spring. It can be increased during those vulnerable periods and with the intake of heavy, moist foods such as ice cream. Conditions caused by an imbalanced kapha dosha are obesity, lethargy, diabetes, swelling, and excessive mucus production.[3]

The activity of the body is governed by the doshas, and this is mediated onto the dhatus or tissues in part through an individual's agni. Agni, in Sanskrit, refers to "biofire," or the digestive power of the body/mind to metabolize inputs from emotional and sensory impressions to food. There are 40 different subtypes of agni in the body, and it is essential to have strong, balanced agni to maintain healthy metabolism and transformation on the subtle and dense tissue levels. If agni is too high, then tissues will be weak; if it is too low, tissues will build up and become hypertrophic. The balance of agni is an interplay between the individuals' doshas and what substances they are taking in through the 5 senses.

As tissues interact with the doshas thru the biofire of agni, metabolic waste is generated. This waste is called "mala," and each tissue level has a specific waste product associated with it. For example, sweat is a waste product from the metabolism of the medas (adipose) dhatu. Malas also are produced during the digestion of food. The buildup of waste materials and toxins in the body is called "ama." Ama is energetic, toxic "sludge" that can obstruct the flow through the communicating dosha channels or "srotas" and cause disease.[4]

Srotas are the channels of the body that are both energetically subtle and dense, which allows for the proper transfer of nutrients and waste products and maintains communication between different tissues and organs. Srota comes from the Sanskrit root "sru," meaning "to flow." In Western allopathic medicine, the dense expression of the srotas may be represented in the circulatory system as the arteries, veins, and the lymphatic system. They may also be the pathways of the nervous system, pulmonary system, digestive system, and systems of elimination. There are 7 major channels in Ayurveda, 1 for each tissue or dhatu level and a separate channel for the mind. In women, there are additional srotas for lactation and menstruation. However, the subtle aspect of the srotas, called the "nadis," is more like the meridian system of Chinese medicine. There are 14 chief nadis that connect with the 6 major energy centers in the body called the "chakras" and thousands of secondary nadis that form a vast energetic matrix in the body. Ama buildup in the srotas and nadis will cause disease through slowing or obstructing the movement of the doshas to the tissues or dhatus. In Ayurveda a balanced state of health is when the doshas, dhatus, and mala are in harmony.[4]

## Triguna

According to Ayurveda, there are 3 fundamental qualities of in the mind called the gunas. The 3 gunas are sattva, rajas, and tamas, meaning clarity, disturbance, and ignorance. Sattva, when present in the mind, is the clear, pure, alert state of awareness. Individuals with a sattvic predominant consciousness are peaceful, calm, and content. Rajas is the quality of turbulence and activity that leads to a mental state of distraction and desire. Rajasic characters are melodramatic and sensation seeking, with no end to their craving. Tamas is the quality of darkness and ignorance. Associated with the mental state is dullness and lethargy. Though this type of person may appear to be happy on the surface, they are often repressing their deeper feelings. In Ayurveda, these states of mind are shifting as the doshas shift and as the consciousness of the individual expands. The doshas provide a form that the energy of the gunas moves through. The interaction of an individual's dominant guna and their prakruti will determine their psychological nature. Assessing the dominant guna of a person's mind is important to the treatment process.[5]

# Diagnosis

Diagnosis in Ayurveda includes a detailed history and an 8-part physical exam or ashtavidha pariksha. It is important to first determine the individual constitution or prakruti before looking for the vikruti, or state of current imbalance. This requires an assessment of the long-term patterns of appetite, digestion, urination, sweat, menstruation, sexual function, and general energy level. Examining the nadi (pulse), jihva (tongue), shabda (speech), sparsha (touch), drig (eyes), and akruti (general form) is also completed. Often this may include an examination of the individual's mutra (urine) and mala (feces), for signs of ama and doshic imbalance. In addition, the fingernails should be examined, as they are significant indicators of prakruti and vikruti. It is essential to inquire as to whether these physical and historical traits are a long- or short-term tendencies, in order to tease out the prakruti from the vikruti. The mental and emotional nature with respect to memory, mood, and sleep will be examined, and the quality of the gunas will be assessed. There are currently forms widely available that help to assess and guide the practitioner through this initial process. The pulse is an essential component to the Ayurvedic assessment. Taking the pulse in Ayurveda is an art and takes many years to master. Currently, there are several systems of pulse diagnosis in Ayurveda. There are 7 levels of pulse that can be palpated. The topmost, superficial level expresses the individual's present imbalanced condition, or vikruti.[6]

The tongue is another important site for a practitioner to read the condition of the organs in body and digestive system. The presence and type of ama can be assessed from the tongue. Vata, pitta, and kapha will have differing qualities in their tongue according to each respective dosha that can also be useful for both prakruti and vikruti. A vata tongue is thin, small, brownish, and may be a little dry, with a fine tremor or twitching. A pitta tongue is broad at the base and tapered at the apex with a red tip and margins that are distinct and sharp. It may have a yellowish or reddish discoloration. A kapha tongue is large, round, glossy, thick, and relatively pale. It occupies the whole oral cavity, and it is moist.[6]

# Treatment

After assessing the prakruti and the current state of doshic imbalance, a unique treatment plan is designed to return the individual back to their natural state of balance (prakruti). Ayurvedic treatments have the effect of bringing the 5 elements into the body in a way that will counterbalance the doshic state of excess. For example, if vata dosha is increased in the digestive tract, leading to gas and constipation (due to its light, dry quality) then substances that have the inherent qualities of being warm and moist will be prescribed.

The treatment in Ayurveda consists of 2 main types. One form is called *shamana chikitsa* or "palliation," used to subdue the vitiated or excess doshas. Shamana uses a multilevel approach including a dosha-specific diet, medicinal herb-mineral preparations, bodywork, and physical exercise. Mind-body exercises such as the breathing technique called "pranayama," meditation, and yoga, along with daily/seasonal routines, are also emphasized. If the doshas are vitiated beyond a particular level, however, they give rise to various toxins (ama), which have a tendency to accumulate in the channels. These are beyond the level of pacification and need to be eliminated from the body. In this case, the second type of treatment, *shodhana chikitsa* (or "cleansing therapy") is indicated. Since shodana consists of 5 types of therapies, it is known as *panchakarma chikitsa*. The process of panchakarma will pull the excess doshas and ama out of the channels by means of the sweat glands, urinary tract, and intestines and into their sites of origin for elimination. Each shodana prescription is unique to the state of imbalance in the mental, physical, and spiritual body and usually only certain elements of the 5 therapies are needed. The five cleansing therapies are preceded by a preparation period called *purvakarma* and followed up by a rejuvenation treatment called *samajarna krama*. The five cleansing therapies include:

(1) *Vamana*: therapeutic vomiting or emesis; (2) *Virechana*: purgation through laxatives; (3) *Basti*: enemas (detoxifying and nutritive); (4) *Nasya*: elimination of toxins through the nose; (5) *Rakta moksha*: detoxification of the blood thorugh blood letting.[7]

Diet is an important preventative and treatment strategy in Ayurveda. Food is evaluated by its taste called the "rasa," in Sanskrit. There are 6 distinct tastes that are composed of the 5 elements. Understanding the elemental composition of each taste is the key to determining how the rasa of a food will affect the individual's doshas. Thus, according to the intake of the 6 tastes, the doshas, agni, and dhatus will be increased or decreased. The 6 tastes are: sweet, sour, pungent, bitter, salty, and astringent. The dietary prescriptions in Ayurveda use this concept to help alleviate imbalanced doshas and return the individual to an improved state of health (and to maintain it). Optimum health is obtained through counterbalancing the excess or deficiency with tastes that have an opposite or similar quality. During dosha aggravation, a certain taste may be emphasized to help pacify it. However, it is recommended that balanced meals contain all 6 tastes in moderation. There are several books on Ayurveda containing lists of foods for particular doshas emphasizing the optimal quantities of different types of foods. Thus, if any dosha is increased in the body, it can be reduced by taking in substances with the opposite qualities. If any of the dosha attributes are deficient, they can be supplemented by ingesting substances with similar properties. The use of herbs follows a similar philosophy, although special qualities of the herbs for a particular disorder called the *prabhva* are also considered.[8]

# Psychospiritual Treatment

In Ayurveda, the body and mind are interconnected through a subtle energetic highway. Treating the imbalanced doshas incorporates practices that use this energetic matrix to help an individual return to harmony. An individual prescription of meditation, yoga, and pranayama ensures that these exercises will help to alleviate disharmony rather than contribute to it.

Pranayama is translated as "prana" or breath control. It is used in Ayurveda to help balance the subtle nadi channels and the doshas. In the Yoga Sutras, the practices of pranayama and yoga postures called "asanas" are considered to be the highest form of purification and self-discipline for the mind and the body. There are several forms of pranayama, yoga, and meditation that are used for different doshas to activate or dissipate the energy, and an Ayurvedic specialist can assist in creating this prescription and teaching the techniques. In Ayurveda, the prescription of yoga is unique to the prakruti and vikruti of the individual.[9]

## ADDICTION

The root cause of addictions, as described by Dr. Vasant Lad in a personal interview, begins with the manas, or mind. The manas comprises the sensory mind, including thinking, perception, and emotion and the buddhi or intellect. The buddhi is made up of dhi (cognition), dhruti (retention), and smurti (memory). Prana facilitates the movement in the mind. As the object of perception is taken in through the retina it will be processed through all aspects of the manas and the buddhi and determined to be pleasurable or painful as an interaction between the object and past experiences with the object (smurti) occurs. This creates a karmic connection between the person and their perceptual experience of the object. If the experience is one of pleasure, it creates a seed of desire (vsana) for further interaction with that object. It may also be that a person has a karmic connection with a particular object of desire from a past life that causes vsana for the substance in their current lifetime.

For each of the major drug categories each drug will have elemental qualities that will interface with an individual's prakruti/vikruti. The stimulants will possess vata and pitta qualities. Cannabis will have a vata and kapha effect. Alcohol is pitta, and sedative hypnotics will enhance kapha. In the individual, this may have varied effects. With alcohol for example, there can be a variety of alcoholic types as a result of this interplay. The *Caraka Samhita* describes the vata, pitta, and kapha types of alcoholism and their respective treatments. The vata type of alcoholism arises in a person who is beset by grief, fear, overwork, and strenuous activity—and who eats a dry, scant diet and "takes in highly fermented wine in excess during the evening hours, losing his sleep." The symptoms range from hiccups and anxiety, to tremors of the head and insomnia.[10]

Pitta alcoholism develops in a person who consumes strong acid wines and a diet that is spicy and hot. The person may also be of irritable temperament and expose themselves to sun and fire. The symptoms will manifest as thirst, fainting, diarrhea, giddiness, and an icteric coloring to the body. A person who drinks fresh, sweet wine excessively, has a heavy, unctuous, and sweet diet, and who does not exercise (and naps during the day) will develop the kapha type of alcoholism. The symptoms will include vomiting, rigidity, heaviness, and feeling cold.[10]

The final section of the *Caraka Samhita* discusses the treatment of the three doshic types of alcoholism.

For the alleviation of vata alcoholism, the patient is prescribed a diet that should be unctuous (oily), sour, hot, and salty. They also recommend heavy foods prepared with black pepper and ginger. Thirst after meals will be quenched with pomegrante juice or a decoction of water boiled with coriander and dry ginger. It is also recommended that the patient eat appetizers and confections that make him or her relish food; the patient should also receive dry massage, take hot baths, cover themselves with eaglewood paste, and fumigate with the dense smoke of eaglewood. Additional treatment is to receive warm oil massage to subdue vata alcoholism.[10] Additional, grounded poses of hatha yoga or bikram yoga and particular forms of meditation meant to silence the mind will be prescribed along with aromatherapy and daily routines meant to decrease the vata.

For treatment of alcoholism of the pitta type, juice with added sugar or diluted with water and mixed with juices of dates, grapes, pomegranate should be given at the "proper time." Sweet and sour foods should be included in the diet. Demulcent drinks may be made out of grapes and dates. If there is thirst due to provocation of vata and pitta, grape juices will cool and regulate the humors. As the patient improves, he or she should receive a diet of cooling foods with sweet-and-sour foods. The juice of jujube, pomegranate, kokam butter, and yellow wood sorrel may be used as a mouth paste to quench thirst immediately. It is also advised to eat cool food and drinks, sleep on a cool bed, and experience cool breezes and water. Moreover, lotuses, water lilies, and pearls sprinkled with sandalwood water will help to relieve pitta. Massage with sandalwood paste is recommended for alcoholism of the pitta type. If the patient is suffering from "burning," the Caraka recommends devices that can shower water and blow breezes onto the patient. In addition, they advocate for painting the body with perfumed cherry, marshmallow, cinnamon leaves, and nutgrass mixed with sandalwood. A lathering of jujube sprouts, neem, and soapnut are also beneficial in burning.[10] There will also be cooling or lunar poses in yoga prescribed with cooling breath work and devotional forms of meditation aimed at reducing the fire in the body and mind.[10]

For treatment of alcoholism of the kapha type, the *Caraka Samhita* recommends fasting. If the patient is thirsty, they should be given water boiled with marshmallow or with yellow-berried nightshade mixed together with dry ginger; then the concoction should be cooled. The diet should be made up of barley and wheat with non-unctuous soups of dried radish. It should be thin and given in small quantities and mixed with pungent, acidic spices with a small amount of ghee. All meats must be prepared until completely dry, without heavy oils, and should be mixed with sour and pungent spices. For cleansing the body channels in kapha alcoholism, salt, cumin seeds, cinnamon, cardamom, and black pepper, a half part each, should be mixed with one part sugar. This can be added to meals or diluted and added to juices to help promote digestive heat. A chutney made from the same herbs can be created by adding grapes and mixing with vinegar. In general, the patient should eat hot, non-heavy, non-unctuous food, get proper exercise, and fast. They also should have systematic wakenings in the evenings and partake in dry baths and friction massagesHere also, a vigorous yoga such as ashtanga will be prescribed to generate heat and motion, and pranayama (meant to elevate vata) will be prescribed to counter the excess of water and earth along with the need to change routine.[10]

The environment where alcoholism is treated is mentioned in the *Caraka Samhita*. They state that "lovely woodlands, lakes, ponds full of lotuses" are important in the treatment. Furthermore, cheering companions, garlands, perfumes, music, humor, and stories act as curatives for alcoholism. This is believed to be due to the idea that alcohol agitates the mind and the body and so a mentally uplifting treatment should be given.

It is interesting how the Vedas approach the setting for the treatment of addiction in a similar way to modern rehabilitation centers and reflects the wisdom of this ancient science.

## REFERENCES

1. Halpren, M. *Principles of Ayurvedic Medicine. Teaching Syllabus California College of Ayurveda;* 2002; 5th Edition; Section 1; Introduction:1–15.
2. Halpren, M. *Principles of Ayurvedic Medicine. Teaching Syllabus California College of Ayurveda;* 2002; 5th Edition; Section 1; Ayurvedic anatomy and physiology:38–41.
3. Halpren, M. *Principles of Ayurvedic Medicine. Teaching Syllabus California College of Ayurveda;*2002;5th Edition;Section 1; Ayurvedic anatomy and physiology: 41–48.
4. Halpren, M. *Principles of Ayurvedic Medicine. Teaching Syllabus California College of Ayurveda;*2002;5th Edition;Section 3;Digestion and Srotas:1–37.
5. Halpren, M. *Principles of Ayurvedic Medicine. Teaching Syllabus California College of Ayurveda;*2002;5th Edition;Section 5;Pyscho-Spiritual Evaluation:83–86.
6. Halpren, M. *Principles of Ayurvedic Medicine. Teaching Syllabus California College of Ayurveda;*2002;5th Edition;Section 4;Diagnostics:28–42.

7. *Halpren, M. Principles of Ayurvedic Medicine. Teaching Syllabus California College of Ayurveda;2002;5th Edition;Section 8;Therapeutic Approaches and Pancha Karma: 1–50.*

8. *Halpren, M. Principles of Ayurvedic Medicine. Teaching Syllabus California College of Ayurveda;2002;5th Edition;Section 6;Ayurvedic Nutrition:32–40.*

9. *Halpren, M. Principles of Ayurvedic Medicine. Teaching Syllabus California College of Ayurveda;2002;5th Edition;Section 9;Daily routines and asana:22–30.*

10. *Sharma. P.V. (2000). Caraka-samhita Volume IV translated into English: Varanasi:Chaukhambha Orientalia.*

# 16

## Traditional Chinese Medicine (TCM) and Acupuncture Approach to Addiction

### SHAHLA J. MODIR AND JOEL MORRIS

While in China with the pre-Nixon table tennis team in 1971, *New York Times* columnist James Reston suffered an acute appendicitis. After his operation using only local anesthetics to remove his appendix, Reston suffered terrible pain post-surgery that was treated using acupuncture. Reston reported on his experience describing the house acupuncturist coming to his hospital bed to deliver pain relief using this method in an article detailing his acupuncture experience. This article appeared on the front page of the *New York Times*, generating a great deal of interest in acupuncture and TCM. In 1972, Nixon's physician confirmed Reston's reported analgesic effects of acupuncture. Today, there are 54 schools in the United States that belong to the Council of Colleges of Acupuncture and Oriental Medicine, which doesn't include the unaccredited schools that are functioning. Some insurance policies have included acupuncture as a legitimate modality for a variety of conditions. Within this 44-year period, the growth, interest, and public engagement in acupuncture has grown at an impressive if not explosive rate.

"Chinese Medicine is based on principles, theories, and applications of Chinese metaphysics."[57] The fundamental theories of Chinese Medicine can be traced back to the Zhou Dynasty (1045–2212 BC), the second historic period of China; the Zhou followed the Mandate of Heaven. Heaven is the guiding power; the rulers had a reciprocal responsibility with the divine to be given the right to rule, and needed to act accordingly. The major medical models then were: The Early Heaven Ba Gua, later Heaven Ba Gua, He Tu, and Luo Shu. Ancestors were placed as causative agents for disease by demons, which could be dispersed by acupuncture and herbal remedies. After the influence of demons, the causes of disease were due to exterior and interior causes. The major philosophies were yin-yang and the 5 elements, philosophies that have remained relevant into the 21st century. Though these systems contradicted each other in certain ways.[60] Unshuld points out that "the unique feature of the Chinese situation is the continuous tendency towards a syncretism of all ideas that exist (within accepted limits). Somehow a way was always found in China to reconcile opposing views and to build bridges-fragile as they may appear to the outside observer-permitting thinkers and practitioners to employ liberally all concepts available, as long as they were not regarded as destructive to society." Though there were multiple philosophical schools, acupuncture developed in China mostly under Confucian and Daoist philosophical influences. Two classics, *The Yellow Emperor's Inner Classic*, and *The Classic of Difficulties (Nan Jing)* remain available to the modern reader on the Internet.[58] Important features of these East Asian thought processes were to see the body and mind as necessarily interconnected and inseparable, and to see the connections and interactions of everything as equally if not more important than the individual elements of an illness or pathological process. During the Qing Dynasty (1644–1840) acupuncture was relegated to the "pavement physicians" with poor training, while the educated and respectable physicians practiced herbal and massage therapies.[59] There was a resurgence of interest in acupuncture in the 1930s. While surviving in rural China, Mao and the Communists relied on the available treatment modalities, thus having firsthand knowledge. Once in power, the Communists introduced the "Bare Foot" doctors, who were trained in a 3- to 6-month course and sent off with material interspersed with party rhetoric. Since the 1970s and 1980s, the Chinese study of acupuncture has become more evidence based, with "retrospective cohort studies and prospective, randomized comparison trials" that have been completed and published in Chinese journals.[59]

In the present forms that TCM has arrived, Birch and Lewith further point out some fundamental differences of thinking between TCM and Western science (Table 16.1).[62]

One of the implications of the above is that "the traditional model of practice is being assessed as more holistic. . . . then the RCT (research studies) must be designed around this assumption. It will then only be able to assess the "whole system," rather than evaluate the effects of various components within the system". This may mean that we require more pragmatic studies.

## Yin-Yang Theory

In Chinese medicine the theories of the yin-yang and the 5 elements underpin the theoretical framework of TCM. "Yin" and "yang" are the general terms for the opposing aspects of objects or phenomena of nature. An image of the yin-yang dynamic is the Tai Chi (see Table 16.1). The yang is the white area, which contains the seed of yin; the yin is the black area that contains the seed of the yang; and the

Table 16.1 Differences between Western Scientific Medicine and TCM

| Western Scientific Medicine | TCM |
| --- | --- |
| 1. General adoption of either-or assumptive approach | General adoption of a "both-and" assumptive approach |
| 2. Widespread effort at generating objective descriptions | Little to no effort at generating objective descriptions |
| 3. Widespread adoption of mind-body dualistic thinking | Widespread adoption of mind-body integrative thinking |
| 4. Widespread use of reductionistic-type thinking processes | General emphasis on holistic thinking processes |

"center curing line is called the Yuan line or force; it is the glue of force that contain Yin-Yang as one inseparable whole."[57]

Yin-Yang theory states that within all situations these concepts are interdependent; yin does not exist without yang. In opposing each other they create unity. The most influential schools of thought were the yin-yang school and the naturalistic school; they hoped to interpret laws of nature in terms of harmony and to relate this to the human body. (For a Western metaphysical view read chapter 10 of the *Kybalion*.)

## All Phenomenon are Either Yin or Yang

Any objects that have properties similar to fire (i.e., warmth, brightness, excitation, lightness, activity) are typically described as yang. All objects that are similar to water (i.e., cold, dim, inhibitory, heavy, and quiescent) are classified as yin.

## Yin and Yang are Relative Concepts

Though gray may be thought of as a yin color, relative to black it is yang. The amino acid tyrosine turns into dopamine, which in turn becomes norepinephrine and then epinephrine. Though each one of these important neurotransmitters tied in with addiction and may be considered yang, one can say that dopamine is yin to norepinephrine, which in turn is yin to epinephrine (or epinephrine is more yang than norepinephrine).

Regarding a different set of neurotransmitters, one can say that tryptophan turns into 5-HTP—and then serotonin and then melatonin. Each one is becoming progressively more yin. Serotonin would be yang to melatonin. However, relative to norepinephrine, serotonin would be considered yin.

## Yin and Yang are Interdependent

Without the concept of cold, we cannot speak of hot and so forth.

## The Relationship Between Yin and Yang is Constantly Changing

The waxing and waning of seasons is a typical example of this.

As one is losing weight, one becomes less yin as a person "burns" off adiposity to become thinner, and thus more yang.

## Under Certain Conditions, Yin May Transform into Yang and Yang into Yin

If someone is on opioids, one can say that person may be in a quiescent state: with slowed breathing, constricted pupils, constipation, less pain, and lethargy. Once that person goes into a state of withdrawal, the yin transforms into a state of yang: high excitability, enlarged pupils, diarrhea and cramping, increased respiration, anxiety, and agitation.

In the body, TCM refers to *substances* as corresponding to yin and the *functions* as yang. So, body organs (zang), body fluids, and blood are considered yin; while functional organs/fu (bladders, intestines), and qi are yang.

Exterior is yang, while interior is yin
The back is yang, while the abdomen is yin
The head is yang, while the foot is yin.

TCM recognizes 4 types of imbalance:

a. Yang impaired by preponderance of yin (e.g., heroin intoxication)
b. Yin consumed by a preponderance of yang (e.g., crystal meth intoxication)
c. An overabundance of yin, resulting from a deficiency of yang (e.g., Cushing's disease)
d. An overabundance of yang, caused by a deficiency of yin (e.g., menopause)

Additionally, there are 4 strategies to manage these imbalances:

- tonify yin
- tonify yang
- decrease excess yang
- decrease excess yin

# 5 Elements

The second model, the 5 elements or phases, underscores the relationship of each of the organs to each other, as also reflected in nature. Wood is characterized by bending and straightening and extends to phenomena that have properties of growing, stretching, or unfolding. Fire is characterized by upward flaring and heat and has properties of warmth and hotness, upward movement, and brightness. Earth, characterized by sowing and reaping, is extended to: producing, receiving, and harmonizing.

Metal is characterized as adaptable and extended to harshness, descending, purification, and condensing. Water is characterized by moistening and descending, and extended to moistening, going downward, coolness, and storage.[61]

The 5 phases of Chinese thought do not describe energy in an electrical circuit of the energy of a biochemical reaction; they describe the nature of the information exchanged.[62] The 5-phase theory can be thought of as describing the interaction between phases on more than one plane. Traditionally the 5 phases were described as interacting along 4 different pathways. The sheng or "engendering" cycle, and the ko, or "restraining cycle" are the most important. The counter-cycle pathways, and the counter-engendering and counter-restraining cycles are of secondary significance. However, taken as a whole, these four paths yield a model of interactions where each phase is always in relation to all other phase (Figures 16.1–16.3).

The engendering cycle shows a healthy human being. "In a well functioning body, any deficiency or excess in any one phase or element will be corrected by the balancing actions of other elements that come into play throughout the cycle."[61] The phase that is engendering is called the "mother," and the one being engendered is the child. The vital qualities of the mother are passed to her child.

There can be an over control of one phase onto another, i.e., Wood overacts on Earth or counteracts/insults. There are patterns of point selection to tonify or sedate, depending upon a deficiency or excess pattern. Herbs are used, depending upon their actions, colors, and flavors.

There are entire schools devoted to 5-element theory, and this theory is far more complex than this brief synopsis can show.

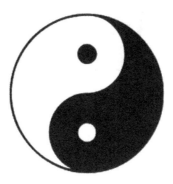

**FIGURE 16.1** Tai Chi, Showing the Yin-Yang Dynamic.

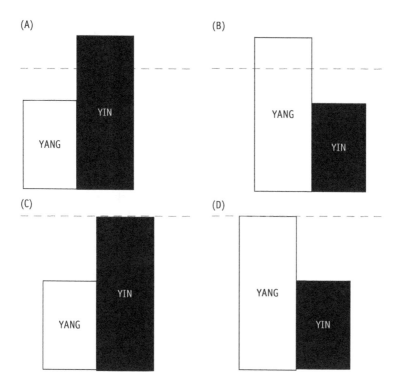

**FIGURE 16.2** The 4 types of imbalance between yin and yang. A) yang impaired by a preponderance of yin, B) Yin consumed by a preponderance of yang, C) An overabundance of yin, resulting from a deficiency of yang, D) An overabundance of yang, caused by a deficiency of yin.

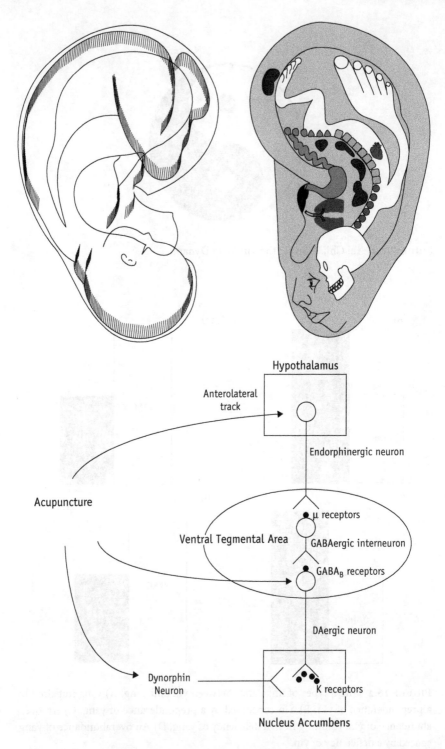

**FIGURE 16.3** A hypothetical model of possible bidirectional effects of acupuncture on dopamine release in the nucleus accumbens.

*Source:* Yang CH, Lee BH, Sohn SH. A possible mechanism underlying the effectiveness of acupuncture in the treatment of drug addiction. *Evidence-Based Complementary And Alternative Medicine: Ecam.* 2008;5:257–266.

# Zang Fu

There are certain important concepts in TCM, which are reflected in what is called the Zang-fu system, which is commonly taught in most Western and Eastern acupuncture schools. As Birch explains, each qi has its own source of production and origin, and these sources are centered in the traditional Chinese notions of Zang and Fu.[62] The Zang, the body's storage facilities, are variously called the "depots," "viscera," "solid organs," or "yin organs," and have the primary role of producing and storing vital substances, fluids, or qi. They are the organs of primary significance and to which attention is most commonly directed in diagnosis and treatment, because they perform the greatest number of functions.

The Fu, the body's grain collection centers, are variously called the "palaces," "bowels," "hollow organs," or "yang organs." Their primary role is transportation in the decomposition of food and the conveyance of waste.

Each yin organ is thought to be coupled to a yang organ:

lung-large intestine
spleen-stomach
heart-small intestine
kidney-bladder
pericardium-triple burner
liver-gallbladder

These pairings constitute the 12 primary channels. In addition to the channels, there are 3 primary substances, the "3 treasures," which are often difficult for Westerners to understand but fundamental to TCM. TCM considers *qi*/life force, *jing*/essence, and *shen*/mind/spirit as the 3 treasures. The interaction and interconnectedness of these processes/aspects are helpful to understand the interaction of the body/mind/spirit.

In the West, qi has become a common word in crosswords and Scrabble; it is often thought of simply as "energy." However, qi has multiple meanings and various forms. As Birch and Felt explain: "On the whole, qi was and is, too broad a concept to be covered by the idea of energy in either lay or scientific terms. The work "energy" is a convenient shorthand that allows us to talk about the responses we observe."[62] However, as Nathan Sivin states, "Qi is sometimes that which animates change in the material world." One way to describe qi in TCM is to see qi as sitting in the middle between more dense material and more rarefied material. It has 2 aspects: first, it indicates a refined essence produced by the internal organs; secondly, indicates the functional aspects of the organs. Qi is generally thought to be yang but has both a yin and yang aspect. Qi transforms, transports, holds, raises, protects, and warms. As Birch and Felt pointed out: "The ancient Chinese medical model posited the existence of 'Qi,' which is both the source of all material objects and all psychic and spiritual phenomena (which is in contrast to the West's tenuous distinctions between energy and matter, and between mind and body)."[62] Jing has multiple aspects, including pre-heavenly, post-heavenly, and kidney. The pre-heavenly can be thought of as genetic contributions from the parents and thus constitutional. This essence can be damaged by addictions and highly imbalanced behaviors. The post-heavenly essence is derived from the digestive processes post-birth. The kidney (where jing is stored) essence forms the basis for development; for males this flows in 8 year cycles and for females, 7 year cycles. The kidney yin assists with producing kidney-qi. Jing needs to be strong to enhance the shen/mind to be willful and confident.

The "shen," known as "spirit" or "mind" is "housed in the heart." Consequently the state of the heart and blood can impact mental activity, consciousness, memory, thinking, and sleep. One may see the state of the shen through the sparkle of the eyes.

The interplay of these 3 treasures, particularly when disrupted by severe addictions, has severe consequences for body, mind, and spirit.

## Recognition of Zang-Fu Patterns

Each of the organs has their own patterns. There are multiple ways to synthesize and conceptualize the patterns according to different schools of thought. Each method has their own strengths, and one typically learns how to use them all. Identification of patterns according to the 8 principles is based on interior/exterior, hot/cold, full/empty, and yin/yang. Then applying these principles to the internal organs is one of the more important systems for diagnosis and treatment.

## Principles of Treatment

Treatment is determined by the identified pattern and diagnosis. There may be both acute and chronic conditions that need to be addressed. The root, "ben," and manifestation, "biao," should be more closely studied. The practitioner must consider what to tonify and reduce. Understanding of the person's constitution and situation is are taken into consideration.

For example, John is a 29-year-old white male who has an 8-year history of crystal meth abuse, and he presents in a depressed state with low energy, poor concentration, irritability, anxiety, emaciation. He also has poor teeth, skin issues, and yellow phlegm production. He presents with both yin and yang deficiencies, manifested with a disturbance in his shen. He has phlegm-heat in the lungs, spleen-qi deficiency, liver-qi deficiency, kidney-qi, and jing deficiency. He would require tonification for his spleen, liver, and kidney, while dispersing the phlegm-heat manifesting in his lungs and restoring his shen.

Nutrition and herbs may typically be used when combining acupuncture points, distal and local points, balancing yin and yang points, and sometimes using front/mu points with back/shu points. There are other common treatments that employ points called "connecting points"/luo, which branch out into 2 directions with its source/yuan point. Thus the spleen connecting point would be used with the stomach source point (see coupled organ list). And there are points used to reduce, which are typically located between the fingers/toes and elbows/knees.

## Recognition of Patterns

Each of the organs has their own patterns, which constitute part of the study of TCM. There are multiple ways to synthesize and conceptualize the patterns according to different schools of thought. Each method has their own strengths, and one typically learns how to use them all. Identification of patterns according to the 8 principles is based on interior/exterior, hot/cold, full/empty, and yin/yang. Then applying these principles to the internal organs is one of the most important systems for diagnosis and treatment.

## Channel Systems

For TCM, the channel systems constitute half of the anatomy of the system.[63] If one thinks of the body constituting 3 concentric circles, the inner circle denotes the internal organs, the middle is the channel system, while the third is the surface layer of the body that is permeated by branches of the channel system. The channels do not consistently follow veins, arteries, lymph, or nerve. The channel systems are a map for the flow of qi/life force and blood and for the functionality of the body. The channel system has 3 primary functions:

1. **Communication** (the body's smartphone system) of parts to the whole
2. **Coordinator** (the body's symphony conductor) or manager of the body's activities, and
3. **Distribution** (the body's equivalent of a CEO) and infrastructure for the flow of qi and blood.

Both health and disease follow the channel systems.

There are 12 principal channels, 8 extraordinary channels, divergent channels, and connecting channels. For the purpose of this brief explanation, we will discuss the principal or primary channels and 2 commonly used extraordinary ones, the du and the ren.

The primary channels run lengthwise through the body. They follow yin-yang theory and have their own 24-hour rhythm. Each of the channels is associated with a yin/major organ or a yang/minor organ. The channels communicate with their respective organ. The yin channels are associated with the interior of the body, while the yang channels are associated with the exterior of the body.

There are 6 channels that are foot channels and 6 that are hand channels. The channels flow in a fixed manner. The 3 yin hand channels (lung, pericardium, and heart) begin and run from the chest to hands. The 3 yang hand ones (large intestine, triple burner, small intestine) start from the hand and flow to the head, where they meet the yang feet channels. The 3 yang feet channels (stomach, gallbladder, and urinary bladder) begin in the head and continue to the feet. In the feet the 3 yang feet channels connect with the 3 yin channels (spleen, liver, kidney). The latter flow to the torso, where they connect with the 3 hand yin channels.

The 2 extraordinary channels commonly used with the primary ones, the ren and the du, bifurcate the body. The ren flows from the perineum to the mouth, where is crosses over to the du channel. The du channel moves from above the anus up the spine and head and into the mouth. The ren is considered yin, while the du is yang. Each channel meets another channel and thus guarantees a flow of qi.

There is much evidence suggesting that acupuncture points have an electrical resistance lower than its surrounding area. As Birch and Felt suggest that the channels act "more like a signaling network that carries information throughout the body—like a computer network where messages that start, stop, and modify biological events are sent, routed, and received."[62] A review article in 2012 on the properties of acupuncture meridians concluded that "recent studies confirm that meridians and acupoints have many biophysical properties, which are different from those of nonacupuncture points.[63] The characteristics include electric, thermal, acoustic, optical, magnetic, isotopic, and myoelectric characteristics."

Western studies of acupuncture for addiction, unlike in China, for the most part have used auricular acupuncture. Ear acupuncture is a microsystem, with points that correspond to an image of a fetus. The ear has been thought to be important for acupuncture dating back to the Nei Jing in approximately 500 BC. In modern times, French physician Paul Nogier invented the auricular map in 1957. Both the Chinese and Nogier maps are similar with some exceptions.

TCM originates from within a complex history and survives through multiple streams of thought. The present-day practice remains with numerous cultural and theoretical underpinnings. It is less monolithic than multifaceted. As Birch and Felt have pointed out: "Again, because many people believe that the long history of continuous practice of acupuncture is proof of validity, they suppose it to be sufficient proof of the theories applied. The fact that good clinical results can be obtained is not precisely or absolutely linked to the veracity of the theory used."[62]

The scientific method is being applied worldwide. The Western mind not only needs to understand that acupuncture is effective but also needs to conceptualize how it works within a biomedical model. The challenges are great, but these are being addressed. The West has primarily focused on ear acupuncture for addiction. Though more complicated, the entire arena of somatic acupuncture remains a resource and creative model to better understand the complex and difficult-to-treat condition called addiction.

## MODERN SYSTEM: ACUPUNCTURE FOR TREATMENT OF ADDICTION

Serendipity or "fortunate luck" plays a role in medical advances. Examples of drugs whose effects were serendipitously discovered include lithium for mania, penicillin for bacterial infections, and sildenafil for erectile dysfunction. These drugs were all discovered based either on a false hypothesis or because the initial predictions about actions were incorrect.[1] The association of Lewy bodies and some forms of dementia was a serendipitous discovery by Kenji Kosaka.[2] Many other examples of serendipitous discoveries exist.[3-5]

# Serendipitous Discovery of Acupuncture in the Treatment of Addiction

The discovery of acupuncture as a treatment modality for addiction was a serendipitous discovery. In 1972, Dr. H. L. Wen, a neurosurgeon, serendipitously discovered that electro-acupuncture (EA) at 4 body points and 2 auricular points relieved symptoms of withdrawal in opiate-addicted surgical patients.[6] In a later study Wen used EA in combination with naloxone and found that 41 participants experienced symptom relief while 9 participants were counted as "failures."[7] In the same study Wen hypothesized that EA "increases endorphin and relieves abstinence syndrome, but also inhibits the autonomic nervous system, mainly the parasympathetic nervous system. The technique does not stop the craving."[7] In a somewhat larger study Wen et al measured ACTH, cAMP and cortisol levels in heroin addicts and normal controls. Participants with heroin addiction (N = 40) were given decreasing doses of methadone for 4 days. After the fourth day, no further methadone was given. Instead, both addicts and controls (N = 31) were given EA 3 times a day for 7 additional days. Urine levels of aldosterone, catecholamines, VMA, cortisol, and cAMP were also determined. Results indicated that ACTH and cortisol levels were significantly reduced in addicts after EA treatments, with no significant changes in the normal controls, suggesting a neuroendocrinological basis for the mechanism of EA action. cAMP levels were unchanged in both groups.[8] Further work suggested that β-endorphin was not involved in the alleviation of withdrawal symptoms.[9]

## Mechanisms of Acupuncture on Opiate Addiction

Ongoing research since the 1980s has indicated that both manual acupuncture and EA have multiple effects, particularly on endogenous opiates and their receptors.[10,11] For EA, these effects appear to be frequency dependent. Low frequency EA (2 Hz) accelerates the release of β-endorphins and enkephalins in the CNS. High frequency EA (100 Hz) induces the release of dynorphin. Early reports indicated that naloxone could reverse acupuncture-induced analgesia in manual acupuncture and low frequency EA.[12,13] Animal studies support the involvement of a number of different neurotransmitters in the basic mechanisms of acupuncture.[14]

Current understanding of the mechanism underlying the effects of EA involves the dopamine system of the nucleus accumbens and prefrontal cortex. Drugs of abuse induce changes in dopamine levels associated with feelings of euphoria, pleasure, and well-being and appear to provide positive reinforcement for the user.[15-17] Recent studies have indicated that high-frequency EA normalizes the activity of dopaminergic neurons specifically in the ventral tegmental area (VTA) and the nucleus accumbens.[17-20]

Additionally, evidence exists that EA may exert its effect via GABAergic and serotonergic neurons. EA has been shown to inhibit the sympathetic nervous system by affecting GABA activity in the rostral ventrolateral medulla, an effect that was reversible with GABA antagonists.[21] Serotonergic receptors in the nucleus accumbens have also been implicated. One working hypothesis is that the activation of hypothalamic serotonin receptors induces metenkephalin release, inhibiting GABAergic neurons with subsequent release of dopamine in the nucleus accumbens (Figure 16.4) (Since acupuncture has been shown to activate the descending serotonergic pathways via the anterolateral tract, acupuncture may possibly rebalance or normalize dopamine release.[16,22,23]

As mentioned, high- and low-frequency EA appear to function differently within the addiction continuum. Low frequency EA appears to be critical in reducing the risk of relapse, whereas high frequency EA may be most critical in ameliorating the withdrawal symptoms.[14-16,19-23]

## The NADA Protocol

NADA is the National Acupuncture Detoxification Association. NADA was founded in 1985 by Dr. Michael Smith and others to promote the integration of an addiction treatment. This protocol uses auricular acupuncture, which Dr. Smith and others have been developing since the 1970s.

The original protocol involved a single point: the lung point on the ear. But more points were added as it was determined that the anti-addictive effect could be prolonged and amplified by adding more points. The second point added was shen men, to help induce a sense of relaxation. Eventually, the NADA protocol became the "5 points": sympathetic, shen men, kidney, liver, and lung.[24-27]

In auricular acupuncture the external surface of the ear is believed to reflect a "map" of the body. The auricular acupuncturist visualizes an inverted fetus, while the points on the ear represent anatomic, physiologic, and emotional systems, organs, and responses. Auricular acupuncture, while originating in the background of TCM, was more fully developed in France and Germany.

The NADA protocol generally utilizes group sessions based on the concept that a group session builds rapport, trust, and comfort. These sessions break down various factors including denial, feelings of isolation, and anxiety. Acupuncture is applied bilaterally for 40 minutes. Patients are allowed to remove their own needles at the end of the treatment period. The NADA protocol is used throughout the world, with international organizations located in over 40 nations in Europe, the Middle East, Asia, Africa, and Asia. The protocol is utilized in locations as diverse as the Yale School of Medicine and the Nepali prison system. Currently, there are more than 1,000 programs in the United States and Canada with over 25,000 trained clinicians.

Despite the difficulties in acupuncture research (see below), NADA has produced an extensive literature supporting the use of auricular acupuncture for the treatment of addictions, particularly in community settings. The protocol has been used to treat heroin, cocaine, nicotine, and alcohol dependency. Importantly, the NADA protocol is designed to reduce the cravings and dysphoria associated with drug withdrawal as well as the generalized anxiety that accompanies withdrawal. The protocol is not designed to address a specific addictive substance. The NADA protocol in combination with standard care has been shown to be significantly more effective than standard care alone. Adverse effects reported include fainting, dizziness, and fatigue.[28]

The NADA protocol is composed of a number of components including: the integration of the protocol with other interventions (counseling, medical care, 12-step groups, peer mentoring); an emphasis on "barrier free" and regular treatments; a communal setting; cross-trained health-care providers; an emphasis on monitoring toxicologies to determine progress; and a collaboration with courts and court-related agencies.[29]

## Acupuncture and Research Design

Complementary and alternative medicine (CAM) systems often do not lend themselves well to the standard methodologies utilized in Western scientific research.

Acupuncture is viewed as a holistic, highly dynamic, and fluid practice that does not fit well with a standard static and reductionistic model of research. Some of the most critical issues cited in discussing clinical research in acupuncture include the selection of suitable controls, applying single- or double-blinded research designs, sham needling, and determining appropriate outcome measures. In addition acupuncture techniques vary, and there are significant physiological and emotional differences in patients' response to acupuncture. A significant number of clinical trials in acupuncture have been poorly designed, according to Western biomedical study standards, and have used "sham" needling as a placebo equivalent. Sham needling is particularly problematic in auricular acupuncture where the points are physically located extremely close to one another. The large number of variables such as treatment duration and frequency, number of points stimulated, blinding methods used (and including those variables already mentioned), make it extremely difficult to analyze the data generated.[30] It has often been argued that the Western models of biomedical research cannot be appropriately applied to CAM systems because these methods create an error in model fit validity; alternative methodologies must be used in order to properly assess the effectiveness of acupuncture within a clinical setting.[31-38] For example, at least four different types of sham methods have been utilized in clinical acupuncture studies. In the NADA protocol, practitioners are trained to use the same techniques, thus minimizing this variable. Work is ongoing in creating a set of recommendations and standards to report acupuncture research and improve clinical trial design: the STRICTA (Standards for Reporting Interventions in Controlled Trials of Acupuncture) recommendations. The STRICTA recommendations form 6 categories with 20 sub-categories covering choosing points, learning techniques of needling and stimulation, setting the frequency and number of treatments, designing controls, and setting up blinding.

## Opiate Detoxification Using Acupuncture

Pomeranz and Chiu showed that EA produced analgesia to heat stimuli in awake mice, an effect that was blocked by naloxone.[13] Also, the data suggested that endorphins are released at a basal rate in normal mice, and that rate is directly increased by EA. Other work by Ng et al showed that EA was able to mitigate naloxone-induced morphine withdrawal adult male Sprague-Dawley rats in whom subcutaneous morphine pellets had been implanted versus sham-implanted ones.[39,40]

In a single-blinded clinical trial of EA in heroin detoxification, Washburn et al randomly assigned heroin addicts to auricular acupuncture (N = 55) or sham acupuncture (N = 45) groups. The sham treatment consisted of points anatomically near standard points. The authors found that the addicts assigned to the treatment groups were more consistent in coming in for treatments. In addition, they found that treatment adherence was better in those for whom addiction was less long term and involved "lighter habits."[41] However, only 7% of the treatment group and 4% of the sham-treatment group appeared to be opiate-free at 2 weeks.

## Alcohol Detoxification Using Acupuncture

In a large randomized, single-blinded placebo controlled clinical study (N = 503), Bullock et al concluded that acupuncture was not significantly better than conventional treatment alone for the reduction of alcohol use.[42] In a more recent longitudinal study examining the effects or auricular acupuncture as a treatment for cocaine, heroin, and alcohol addiction, Verthein and colleagues studied 159 patients in a German outpatient clinic over 8 months, focusing on 30 patients who had been given at least 4 follow-up assessments. The results indicated a significant decrease in withdrawal symptoms, improvement in physical and mental states, and a decrease in alcohol and cocaine consumption.[43] Courbasson and colleagues evaluated the benefits of auricular acupuncture in a 21-day outpatient treatment center. Participants (all female) who received acupuncture (N = 185) reported a decrease in cravings, a decrease in depression and anxiety, and an increased level of problem-solving ability as compared to program participants not receiving acupuncture (N = 101).[44]

## Cocaine Detoxification Using Acupuncture

A single-blinded placebo study was done on cocaine detoxification in an outpatient setting.[45] Lipton et al randomly assigned individuals seeking treatment to either an acupuncture or a sham-acupuncture group. The sham-acupuncture group received acupuncture at anatomically discreet sites that were not related to detoxification. Treatments were provided for 30 days, and after each treatment session, urine samples were obtained for toxicologies. In pretreatment stage, cocaine and crack cocaine use averaged 20 days per month. Post-treatment (3-month) use averaged 5 days per month in both groups. The urinalysis profiles indicated that the experimental group had significantly lower cocaine metabolites. However, both groups reported a similar decrease in cocaine usage.

Margolin et al discussed the interpretation of clinical trials in acupuncture by comparing two trials conducted at the same site. In both trials individuals were randomly assigned to either the auricular acupuncture group, a "needle insertion" control group, or a no-needle relaxation group. Treatments were available 5 times a week for 2 months. In one study participants were paid for attendance, and the treatment did not include counseling sessions. In the other trial a total of 620 patients, 412 users and 208 methadone maintained users were studied. Cocaine use was assessed by weekly urine screens. An intent-to-treat analysis indicated that in only one trial

Table 16.2 Levels of Evidence for Therapeutic Studies

| Level | Type of Evidence |
| --- | --- |
| 1A | Systematic review (with homogeneity) of RCTs |
| 1B | Individual RCT (with narrow confidence intervals) |
| 1C | All or none study |
| 2A | Systematic review (with homogeneity) of cohort studies |
| 2B | Individual Cohort study (including low quality RCT, e.g., <80% follow-up) |
| 2C | "Outcomes" research; ecological studies |
| 3A | Systematic review (with homogeneity) of case-control studies |
| 3B | Individual Case-control study |
| 4 | Case series (and poor quality cohort and case-control study) |
| 5 | Expert opinion without explicit critical appraisal or based on physiology bench research or "first principles" |

Burna P, Rohrich R, Chung K. The levels of evidence and their role in evidence-based medicine. *Plast Reconstr Surg.* 2011;128:305–10.

positive effects were associated with the acupuncture group (p = 0.01; OR 3.41; 95% CI 1.33–8.72). The authors were unable to account for the differences in response but suggested that the lack of counseling and the payments were at least partly responsible for the discrepancy in the results.[46] Another larger study from the same group was undertaken using a similar design: acupuncture (N = 222), needle-insertion control (N= 203) and relaxation control (N = 195) concluded that the data did not support the use of acupuncture as a standalone treatment. As with the earlier study, treatments were available 5 times a week for 2 months. Counseling was also offered to all patients. Cocaine use was followed by urinalysis toxicology screens. An intent-to-treat analysis did show an overall reduction in cocaine use (p = 0.002; OR, 1.40; 95% CI, 1.11–1.74) but there was no significant difference between the groups (p = 0.90).[47] The authors concluded that the use of acupuncture as a standalone treatment for cocaine addiction is not effective. Level of Evidence 1B (Table 16.2).

# Methamphetamine Detoxification Using Acupuncture

There are few published studies of acupuncture to treat methamphetamine addiction. Liang and colleagues recently published a study of 90 male methamphetamine addicts. The men were randomly assigned to one of 3 groups equally: an electroacupuncture group, an auricular acupuncture, and a control group. Electroacupuncture was given at body points: neiguan (PC 6), shen men (HT 7), zusanli (ST 36), sanyinjiao (SP 6), jiaji (EX-B 2) at waigan (T5), and tai chong (L3)(bilaterally). Auricular acupuncture was at jiaogan (AH[6a]), shen men (TF4), fei (CO14), and gan (CO12) (unilaterally). Treatment was given 3 times a week for 1 month. The methamphetamine withdrawal syndrome score, Hamilton anxiety scale score, and Hamilton depression scale scores were taken before and after each week of treatment. All scores were decreased in the electroacupuncture and the auricular acupuncture groups (P<0.05). During the treatment period, the scores showed a gradual decline in both test groups. By weeks 3 and 4, the electroacupuncture group showed significantly lower anxiety and depression scores (All p<0.05) than the auricular acupuncture group.[48]

## Nicotine Detoxification Using Acupuncture

There have been few clinical trials using acupuncture for the treatment of nicotine addiction and nicotine withdrawal. A review of useful treatments in smoking cessation noted that "acupuncture and related techniques (including acupressure, laser acupuncture, and electrostimulation of acupuncture points ore acupuncture needles) are not helpful for stopping smoking compared to sham acupuncture treatment (in which needles do not penetrate the skin). Acupuncture seems to work better initially than no treatment at all."[49] Other studies have, however, shown positive responses to acupuncture especially when positive motivation exists combined with behavioral and/or pharmacologic therapy.[50–54]

## Summary of Literature

Acupuncture techniques appear to be beneficial for the detoxification from opiates and alcohol, reducing the craving for both of these addictive substances. There is less evidence that acupuncture can benefit cocaine addiction. Acupuncture is a somatic treatment that does not work as a substitute but rather as an adjunct treatment along with behavioral therapy, 12-step programs, and pharmacological treatments. The majority of the studies have shown that using acupuncture alone does not reduce relapse rates. Adding acupuncture to a complete psychosocial program keeps people enrolled for longer periods of time and reduces their discomfort during withdrawal, thereby improving overall outcomes.

### REFERENCES

1. Ban TA. The role of serendipity in drug discovery. *Dialogues in Clinical Neuroscience.* 2006;8:335–344.
2. Nunomura A. Serendipity and success: Asahi Prize awarded for discovery of dementia with Lewy bodies. *Psychiatry and Clinical Neurosciences.* 2014;68:390.

3. Szeto HH, Birk AV. Serendipity and the discovery of novel compounds that restore mitochondrial plasticity. *Clinical Pharmacology and Therapeutics.* 2014;96:672–683.

4. McMurray JJV. Neprilysin inhibition to treat heart failure: a tale of science, serendipity, and second chances. *European Journal of Heart Failure.* 2015;17:242–247.

5. Allegaert K. Paracetamol to close the patent ductus arteriosus: from serendipity toward evidence based medicine. *Journal of Postgraduate Medicine.* 2013;59:251–252.

6. Wen HL, Teo SW. Experience in the treatment of drug addiction by electro-acupuncture. *Xianggang Hu Li Za Zhi: The Hong Kong Nursing Journal.* 1975;19:33–35.

7. Wen HL. Fast detoxification of heroin addicts by acupuncture and electrical stimulation (AES) in combination with naloxone. *Comparative Medicine East & West.* 1977;5:257–263.

8. Wen HL, Ho WK, Wong HK, Mehal ZD, Ng YH, Ma L. Reduction of adrenocorticotropic hormone (ACTH) and cortisol in drug addicts treated by acupuncture and electrical stimulation (AES). *Comparative Medicine East and West.* 1978;6:61–66.

9. Wen HL, Ho WK, Ling N, Mehal ZD, Ng YH. Immunoassayable beta-endorphin level in the plasma and CSF of heroin addicted and normal subjects before and after electroacupuncture. *American Journal of Chinese Medicine.* 1980;8:154–159.

10. Hans JH. Acupuncture: neuropeptide release produced by electrical stimulation of different frequencies. *Trends in Neurosciences* 2003;26:17–22.

11. Hans JH. Acupuncture and endorphins. *Neuroscience Letters* 2004;361:258–61.

12. Mayer DJ, Price DD, Rafii A. Antagonism of acupuncture analgesia in man by the narcotic antagonist naloxone. *Brain Research.* 1977;121:368–372.

13. Pomeranz B, Chiu D. Naloxone blockade of acupuncture analgesia: Endorphin implicated. *Life Sciences.* 1976;19:1757–1762.

14. Kim KS, Lyu YS, Kim SH, et al. Effect of acupuncture on behavioral hyperactivity and dopamine release in the nucleus accumbens in rats sensitized to morphine. *Neuroscience Letters.* 2005;387:17–21.

15. Peoples UA, Guyette FX, West MO. Tonic inhibition of single nucleus accumbens neurons in the rat: a predominant but not exclusive firing pattern induced by cocaine self-administration sessions. *Neuroscience.* 1998;86:13–22.

16. Yang CH, Lee BH, Sohn SH. A possible mechanism underlying the effectiveness of acupuncture in the treatment of drug addiction. *Evidence-Based Complementary and Alternative Medicine: Ecam.* 2008;5:257–266.

17. Hu L, Chu N-N, Sun L-L, Zhang R, Han J-S, Cui C-L. Electroacupuncture treatment reverses morphine-induced physiological changes in dopaminergic neurons within the ventral tegmental area. *Addiction Biology.* 2009;14:431–437.

18. Hu L, Jing XH, Cui CL, Xing GG, Zhu B. NMDA receptors in the midbrain play a critical role in dopamine-mediated hippocampal synaptic potentiation caused by morphine. *Addiction Biology.* 2014;19:380–391.

19. Yoon SS, Yang EJ, Lee BH, et al. Effects of acupuncture on stress-induced relapse to cocaine-seeking in rats. *Psychopharmacology.* 2012;222:303–311.

20. Kim MR, Kim SJ, Lyu YS, et al. Effect of acupuncture on behavioral hyperactivity and dopamine release in the nucleus accumbens in rats sensitized to morphine. *Neuroscience Letters.* 2005;387:17–21.

21. Ku CY. Beta-Endorphin- and GABA-mediated depressor effect of specific electroacupuncture surpasses pressor response of emotional circuit. *Peptides* 2001;22:1465–1470.

22. Scott SW. A biochemical hypothesis for the effectiveness of acupuncture in the treatment of substance abuse: acupuncture and the reward cascade. *American Journal of Acupuncture.* 1997;25:33–40.

23. Ma S. Neurobiology of acupuncture: toward CAM. *Evidence-Based Complementary and Alternative Medicine.* 2004;1:41–47.

24. Kim Y-HJ, Schiff E, Waalen J, Hovell M. Efficacy of acupuncture for treating cocaine addiction: a review paper. *Journal of Addictive Diseases.* 2005;24:115–132.

25. D'Alberto A. Auricular acupuncture in the treatment of cocaine/crack abuse: a review of the efficacy, the use of the National Acupuncture Detoxification Association protocol, and the selection of sham points. *Journal of Alternative and Complementary Medicine.* 2004;10:985–1000.

26. Cui C-L, Wu L-Z, Li Y-J. Acupuncture for the treatment of drug addiction. *International Review of Neurobiology.* 2013;111:235–256.

27. NADA's Mission. *Guidepoints: News from NADA* 2004:10.

28. Carter KO, Olshan-Perlmutter M, Norton HJ, Smith MO. NADA acupuncture prospective trial in patients with substance use disorders and seven common health symptoms. *Medical Acupuncture.* 2011;23:131–135.

29. Ackerman R. Auricular Acupuncture Treatment for Chemical Dependency: A Review of the Literature. Laramie, WY: NADA Literature Clearinghouse; 1995.

30. Zhang CS, Yang AW, Zhang AL, May BH, Xue CC. Sham control methods used in ear-acupuncture/ear-acupressure randomized controlled trials: A systematic review. *Journal of Alternative & Complementary Medicine.* 2014;20:147–161.

31. Smith CA, Zaslawski CJ, Zheng Z, et al. Development of an instrument to assess the quality of acupuncture: results from a Delphi process. *Journal of Alternative and Complementary Medicine.* 2011;17:441–452.

32. Price S, Long AF, Godfrey M, Thomas KJ. Getting inside acupuncture trials—exploring intervention theory and rationale. *BMC Complementary and Alternative Medicine.* 2011;11:22.

33. Margolin A, Avants SK, Kleber HD. Rationale and design of the Cocaine Alternative Treatments Study (CATS): a randomized, controlled trial of acupuncture. *Journal of Alternative and Complementary Medicine.* 1998;4:405–418.

34. Lao L, Huang Y, Feng C, Berman BM, Tan MT. Evaluating traditional Chinese medicine using modern clinical trial design and statistical methodology: application to a randomized controlled acupuncture trial. *Statistics in Medicine.* 2012;31:619–627.

35. Kaptchuk TJ. Methodological issues in trials of acupuncture. *Journal of the American Medical Association.* 2001;285:1015.

36. Dorsher PT. The 2001 STRICTA recommendations for reporting acupuncture research: a review with implications for improving controlled clinical trial design. *Journal of Alternative and Complementary Medicine.* 2009;15:147–151.

37. Moroz A. Issues in acupuncture research: the failure of quantitative methodologies and the possibilities for viable, alternative solutions. *American Journal of Acupuncture.* 1999;27:95.

38. Cassidy CM. How acupuncture is actually practised, and why this matters to clinical research design. *European Journal of Oriental Medicine.* 2010;6:20.

39. Ng LK, Thoa NB, Douthitt TC, Albert CA. Experimental 'auricular electroacupuncture' in morphine-dependent rats: Behavioral and biochemical observations. *American Journal of Chinese Medicine.* 1975;3:335–341.

40. Ng LK, Douthitt TC, Thoa NB, Albert CA. Modification of morphine-withdrawal syndrome in rats following transauricular electrostimulation: an experimental paradigm for auricular electroacupuncture. *Biological Psychiatry.* 1975;10:575–580.

41. Washburn AM, Fullilove RE, Fullilove MT, et al. Acupuncture heroin detoxification: A single-blind clinical trial. *Journal of Substance Abuse Treatment.* 1993;10:345–351.

42. Bullock ML, Kiresuk TJ, Sherman RE, et al. A large randomized placebo controlled study of auricular acupuncture for alcohol dependence. *Journal of Substance Abuse Treatment.* 2002;22:71–77.

43. Verthein U, Haasen C, Krausz M. Auricular acupuncture as a treatment of cocaine, heroin, and alcohol addiction: a pilot study. *Addictive Disorders and Their Treatment.* 2002;1:11–66.

44. Courbasson CMA, de Sorkin AA, Dullerud B, Van Wyk L. Acupuncture treatment for women with concurrent substance use and anxiety/depression: an effective alternative therapy? *Family and Community Health.* 2007;30:112–120.

45. Lipton DS, Brewington V, Smith M. Acupuncture for crack-cocaine detoxification: experimental evaluation of efficacy. *Journal of Substance Abuse Treatment.* 1994;11:205–215.

46. Margolin A, Avants SK, Holford TR. Interpreting conflicting findings from clinical trials of auricular acupuncture for cocaine addiction: does treatment context influence outcome? *Journal of Alternative and Complementary Medicine-New York.* 2002;8:111.

47. Margolin A, Kleber HD, Avants SK, et al. Acupuncture for the treatment of cocaine addiction: a randomized controlled trial. *Journal of the American Medical Association.* 2002;287:55–63.

48. Liang Y, Xu B, Zhang X-C, Zong L, Chen Y-L. Comparative study on effects between electroacupuncture and auricular acupuncture for methamphetamine withdrawal syndrome. *Chinese Acupuncture and Moxibustion.* 2014;34:219–224.

49. Jain A. Treating nicotine addiction. *BMJ (Clinical Research Ed),* 2003;327:1394–1395.

50. White A, Resch K-L. Randomized trial of acupuncture for nicotine withdrawal symptoms. *Archives of Internal Medicine;*158:2251.

51. Stuyt E, Meeker J. Benefits of auricular acupuncture in tobacco-free inpatient dual-diagnosis treatment. *Journal of Dual Diagnosis*. 2006;2:41–52.
52. Roth JW. Curing nicotine addiction with acupuncture: A report on clinical experience. *Chinesische Medzine*. 2011;26:37.
53. Fuller JA. Smoking withdrawal and acupuncture. *Medical Journal of Australia*. 1982;1:28–29.
54. Cabioglu M, NeyhanTan Ü. Smoking cessation after acupuncture treatment. *International Journal of Neuroscience*. 2007;117:571–578.
55. Burna P, Rohrich R, Chung K. The levels of evidence and their role in evidence-based medicine. *Plastic and Reconstructive Surgery*. 2011;128:305–310.
56. Twicken D. *I Ching Acupuncture: The Balance Method*. London and Philadelphia: Singing Dragon; 2012.
57. Unschuld P. *Chinese Medicine*. Boston: Paradigm; 1998.
58. Flaws B. The Development of Modern Chinese Acupuncture and Why it Matters to Us in the West, Golden Needle Practitioner Library, Posted in Honora Wolfe's Blog.
59. Unschuld P. *Medicine in China, A History of Ideas*. Berkeley: University of California Press; 2010.
60. Sun G-R, Eisenstark D, Zhang Q-R. *Fundamentals of Chinese Medicine*. People's Medical; 2014.
61. Birch S, Felt R. *Understanding Acupuncture*. Edinburgh: Churchill Livingstone; 1999.
62. Maciocia G. *The Foundations of Chinese Medicine*. Edinburgh:Churchill Livingstone; 1989.
63. Juan Li, Qing Wang, Huiling Liang, et al. Biophysical Characteristics of Meridians and Acupoints: A Systematic Review. *Evidence-Based Complementary and Alternative Medicine*. 2012, Article ID 793841, 6 pages, 2012. doi:10.1155/2012/793841

# 17

## Nutritional Support and Addiction

### ROBERT KROCHMAL

## Introduction: Nutrition and the Addiction Disease Model

Nutrition plays a pivotal role (literally) in addiction treatment because it stands at the intersection between relapse and recovery. In asking the question, "What role does nutrition and a healthy diet play in the treatment of addictive disorders?" one must also ask the opposite question: "Can unbalanced nutritional intake actually play a role in *causing* addiction in the first place?" The answer to that question is *yes*, and evidence is mounting as to the biological mechanisms behind this. In chapter 4, this concept was explored, placing food squarely in the light of a potential addiction in and of itself. The focus of this chapter will be to sharpen the distinction between the particular characteristics of foods that amplify addictive behaviors and those that can provide a remedy. Thus we will be able to better answer what appears to be a simple question but that has befuddled modern practitioners and the lay public for years: "What to eat?"

For of course, not only must we eat, but we must enjoy it. Evolutionary mechanisms involved in our drive to eat food can be corrupted, but if we isolate the specific sources of that corruption, we can present a model by which food can be enjoyed without risk of addiction. In that sense, nutrition intersects with all aspects of the integrative philosophy: psychosocial, environmental, spiritual, *and* nutritional. In 2011, ASAM made a groundbreaking and much publicized impact on approaches to addiction when it redefined addiction as a neurobiological susceptibility involving many brain functions, particularly reward circuitry. The new definition, which was the result of a 4-year process involving more than 80 leading experts in the field, dealt a blow to a host of common conceptions about addiction: most specifically the question of whether addiction is a choice.

Understanding the role of nutrition across all spectrums of the addiction disease model is therefore critical, and this understanding must be expanded to include the role of the emerging fields of genetics and epigenetics. Environmental influences on our genes—of which nutrition is certainly foremost—are a leverage point to alter neurobiological susceptibilities. Other environmental factors, specifically socioeconomic factors, are known to affect access to healthy, nutrient-dense foods and increase the risk of obesity and its associated comorbidities, including addiction. Emerging new fields of research, such as the human microbiome and the gut-brain connection, provide further opportunities to understand and correct the imbalances that lead to increased neurobiological susceptibility. Additionally, more than a century after the discovery of vitamins, advances are being made in the understanding of phytonutrients, antioxidants, and other factors involved in the optimal functioning of our cellular machinery and the innumerable chemical reactions happening per second in our body.

## Whole Food Versus Isolated Nutrients/Biological Systems Model

### VITAMIN AND PHYTONUTRIENT DEFICIENCIES, INFLAMMATION, AND ILLNESS

In the late 1800s, it was discovered that when the principal components of food (carbohydrate, protein, fats) are separated from their "accessory factors," as was put by Sir Frederick Gowland Hopkins some 31 years before he was awarded the Nobel Prize in medicine for his discovery of vitamins, the result is disease. One example of this principle is the disease beriberi, now known to be caused by thiamine deficiency, and characterized by neurological and cardiovascular pathologies. Knowledge of the history and characteristics of this illness is a right of passage for all contemporary medical students. Interestingly, it is taught not in the context of clinical practice but medical history—no medical student is subsequently expected to diagnose this disease later in their clinical career. Though it is touted as a disease of the past, beriberi was still a modern disease. It was in the late 19th century that beriberi arguably reached its peak: many sailors were falling ill to its effects. In 1897 a Dutch physician by the name of Christiaan Eijkman found that feeding unpolished "brown" rice to chickens (as opposed to polished "white" rice) prevented beriberi. Thiamine (vitamin B1) was later found to be an inherent constituent in brown rice that was inadvertently discarded with the "whole grain" components removed in the polishing process.

Today, overt thiamine deficiency is almost unheard of in Western society except as occurs in Wernicke-Korsakoff syndrome in the case of alcohol abuse and its corresponding depletion of thiamine (although other related nutrients, such as magnesium and zinc, are gaining more recognition in alcoholic depletion, particularly in the integrative treatment approach). Given this discovery of thiamine and other B vitamins a century ago, processed foods are now universally enriched with these factors, so even with the dramatic increases in the proportion of processed food consumption through the latter 20th century, such overt deficiencies are greatly diminished.

However, we are now facing a new set of rising epidemics including diabetes, obesity, heart disease, cancer, Alzheimer's, mental health disorders, and substance addiction. While these problems have until this point not been generally recognized as nutrient related, medical schools are certainly scrambling to understand and institute training in integrative and nutritional approaches to disease. We must ask why 21st-century medicine has been dumbfounded by illnesses that are taking so many lives. What is beginning to emerge is that a common root cause of all these diseases is "inflammation." We are also beginning to understand some of the root causes of inflammation itself. These root causes can be seen as relating to the functional integrity of processes that occur on a cellular level. Among other factors, many of which will be discussed in this chapter, a basic one centers around the importance of "antioxidants" and "phytonutrients." Discoveries in this field provide a new frontier for the understanding of cellular function and take us deeper beyond our old friends from a century ago: the vitamins and minerals. More than 4,000 phytonutrients have now been identified and characterized, from carotenoids to alkaloids, flavonoids, tannins, terpenes, organosulfur compounds, anthocyanidins, glucosinolates, phenols, and others.

## METHYLATION, VITAMINS, AND PHYTONUTRIENTS

Looking back at another historical breakthrough in nutritional biochemistry, Sir Hans Adolf Krebs was awarded the Nobel Prize in Physiology in 1953 for the discovery of the tricarboxylic acid- or Krebs cycle as it is commonly known. The Krebs cycle involves reactions in living organisms by which substances formed by the breakdown of sugar, fats, and protein are converted to energy (ATP) in the presence of oxygen, leaving behind water and carbon dioxide. Another rite of passage for medical students, learning the Krebs cycle often involves many late nights. In recent years, a new cycle, methylation, has become popular. Particularly with the advent of inexpensive genetic tests available to the lay public, and an explosion of information about how genetic variations in methylation SNPs can affect health, the biochemistry of this process has come to the spotlight. Given its clinical relevance, the methylation cycle has thus become the new Krebs cycle.

Both cycles illustrate the need for factors (i.e., vitamins and minerals) that catalyze cellular reactions essential for anything from energy generation, to neurotransmitter production, to detoxification. Even with optimal vitamin and mineral status, by their very nature, these cellular functions produce metabolic and oxidative byproducts, such as free radicals. Here is where phytonutrients and antioxidants are especially relevant. Although phytonutrients are not classified as "essential nutrients" like the vitamins, we can look at these molecules as a deep layer of "accessory factors" important for buttressing cellular function, in particular, the potentially toxic byproducts of these chemical reactions.

Phytochemical extracts have been found to have strong antioxidant and antiproliferative activities, and combinations of phytochemicals have additive and synergistic effects.[1] This suggests that such compounds are best acquired through whole-food consumption, with an emphasis on diversity of food. However, at least two aspects of the modern food system create challenges to this goal. One is that phytonutrients often taste bitter, acrid, or astringent, and the food industry routinely removes these tastes either through selective breeding or other debittering processes.[2] Another reason has to do with the loss of ecological diversity itself. Research reveals that hunter-gatherers consumed upwards of 800 different types of plant foods and in significant quantities. However, Americans eat only 3 servings of plant food per day on average, and these servings tend to come from just a handful of different plant sources.[3]

There is also a more glaring reason that our modern food system is guilty of resulting in severe deficiencies of phytonutrients. As described above, even when supposedly phytonutrient-rich foods are consumed, quantity and variety of these substances appears to be minimal compared to historical levels. Compounding this problem is the increase in processed food consumption during the past half-century. Though processed foods are routinely "enriched" with a handful of vitamins, and here and there even a phytonutrient is thrown in, they are inevitably nutrient deficient foods.

It is also possible that consumption of processed carbohydrate and sugar actually *accelerates* the depletion of preexisting cellular nutrients. Take the example of thiamine deficiency in alcohol abuse. A prevailing theory of the past has been that alcohol is substituted for food as a percentage of the diet, progressively leading to deficiency. However, a recent study has shown that even in healthy, non-alcoholic, non-alcohol consuming volunteers, an intervention of 24 grams of red wine consumption for a mere 2 weeks (less than 2 drinks per day), caused statistically significant decreases in B12 and folate levels, and increases in homocysteine levels.[4]

A further illustration is provided by the example of native Inuit populations in Alaska. In what has been called the "Inuit Paradox," even a diet of exclusive consumption of meats and fats (with no food coming from plant sources) does *not* produce the vitamin C nutrient deficiency scurvy.[5] However, as is known during the 1700s to early 1800s, scurvy did become a prevalent issue for the British Mercantile Marine among sailors undergoing voyages where processed carbohydrates were the primary food source on board, suggesting a role for carbohydrates in accelerating the process of nutrient depletion in the body (particularly when they are in their processed form). Understanding of methylation and particularly the MTHFR SNP polymorphisms could help explain this observation. Specifically, increased metabolic and oxidative stress from increasing amounts of sugar and processed carbohydrates deplete and strain the vitamins and phytonutrients that catalyze and buffer our metabolic machinery. This can lead to the burn out of core energy systems like the Krebs or methylation cycle. In those suffering from polymorphisms that predispose to impaired methylation or other preexisting metabolic deficiencies, the modern food system can therefore have disproportionate and amplifying effects.

Given that we are only beginning to understand the complex interplay between not just vitamins and minerals but also phytonutrients and antioxidants we must assume that cellular function evolved to function best with optimal levels of all such factors. Such levels not only would depend on consumption of sufficient quantities of plant-based foods but also on some amount of animal-based foods that are rich in such nutrient sources, too. Grass-fed beef, as opposed to grain-fed beef, has been shown to have a higher prevalence not only of CLA and n-3 fatty acids, but also of vitamin precursors to vitamins A and E, as well as antioxidants glutathione (GT), superoxide dismutase (SOD), and catalase (CAT).[6]

## ISOLATED FOOD COMPONENTS AND ADDICTION

The increase in consumption of processed foods and sugar not only decreases phytonutrient levels but also creates another problem as well, one with even more direct relevance to addiction. Returning to the question of food addiction, what exactly is it about food that can produce addictive behaviors and imbalances in reward circuitry? In a word, sugar.

Sugar is certainly a component of food and could arguably be defined as a food itself. However, it has long been hypothesized that sugar—particularly refined sugar—triggers symptoms of addiction. William Duffy published the book, *Sugar Blues*, in 1975 and although it is just one example of many books that have collectively sold millions of copies, a common criticism has been lack of scientific support. Recently new evidence has emerged that supports the sugar-addiction hypothesis and has begun to elucidate its mechanisms. In fact, evidence is mounting that sugar might even be more addictive than some of the substances traditionally thought to be the most highly addictive. For example, in a much publicized recent study, researchers found that intense sweetness surpasses cocaine in drug-reward behavior.[7] An explanation for this finding may be evolutionary pressures that have created an innate hypersensitivity to sweet taste. Supranormal stimulation of sweet "receptors" that originally evolved in sugar-poor environments could override self-control mechanisms by overactivating reward centers. This is discussed further in the next section.

Despite warnings from the likes of individuals from William Duffy to Robert Atkins over the past half a century, there has been a dramatic escalation in sugar consumption, particularly in children and adolescents over the last few decades. Only recently has the scientific consensus belatedly shifted away from blaming obesity and its related comorbidities on fat consumption and toward sugar over-consumption. Even less recognized are the effects of sugar overconsumption on mental health. For example, major depression, bipolar disorder, schizophrenia, and obsessive compulsive disorder are significantly more prevalent among indus-trialized societies, and studies suggest the Western diet plays a significant role.[8,9]

## COMPULSIVE VERSUS HEALTHY EATING: SUGAR VERSUS FAT

We must ask why it has taken so long for evidence implicating sugar in addiction and other diseases to emerge. After all, as discussed above, an obvious potential explanation for these findings is that reward circuitry centered around our drive for food evolved ancestrally in sugar-poor environments and that overstimula-tion of these pathways as afforded by the modern diet could override evolutionary mechanisms for homeostasis.[10] In addition, not only was sugar (and carbohydrate) more scarce in ancestral diets than today, but where sugar was available, it was inseparable from phytonutrient molecules. In consuming berries for example, early humans would be rewarded by the taste of sugar, but methylation, neurolog-ical, antioxidant, and other pathways would be protected from overstimulation by the myriad phytonutrients carried along with the sugar. Furthermore, those very phytonutrients, which are often bitter, would have been present in higher quanti-ties in those foods than in berries selected for modern production and would act inherently as a counterbalance to sugar reward circuitry.

These suggestions are borne out by new studies showing overlapping neuronal circuits in compulsive versus healthy eating behavior.[11] In such a model, neuronal circuits, influenced by dopamine, interact with one another so that one circuit can be buffered by another. But resetting of thresholds, caused by repeated stimulation by drugs on the one hand or "palatable food" on the other, can overactivate the reward circuitry while inhibiting the cognitive control circuitry.

Furthermore, sugar not only appears to be an addiction in itself but also leads to increased risk of other drug dependencies. Sugar-addicted rats, for example, have been shown to be at increased risk of alcohol consumption.[12] Additional rat studies have shown that sugar bingeing followed by discontinuation produces a state of anxiety similar to opiate withdrawal.[13]

Such studies suggest an important distinction to be made in terms of defining what compulsive (or "unhealthy") eating behaviors actually are. In framing such unhealthy eating behavior, particularly as relates to obesity risk, most scholarly articles refer to the term "highly palatable, energy rich food" and go on to say that these are foods high in "sugar and fat."[14,15] Human and animal studies with palatable food equating to either sugar alone or sugar and fat combined, do result in addictive-like behaviors and symptoms.[16,17] However, when high fat palatable diets alone are studied, no such addictive symptoms are observed.[18]

## OFFICIAL DIETARY GUIDELINES AND IATROGENIC ILLNESS

These findings are only now emerging some 50 years after the cholesterol theory of disease became one of the cornerstones of the "success" of Western medicine treatments. In this model, it is fat that is theorized to lead to heart disease as well as the corresponding modern diseases including diabetes, all of which have only accelerated their rise to epidemic proportions during this time. Official medical guidelines as well as governmental policy have advocated a reduced consumption of fat, which has led to an increase in consumption of sugar and carbohydrates instead. In 2015, a systematic review looking at the same data that led to National Dietary Guidelines on Fat Intake in 1977 concluded there was no supporting evidence.[19] One must again ask why it took so long for these facts to come out. And now evidence continues to support this complete turnaround of conclusions. Even the American Heart Association is rushing to change their long-standing guidelines, while going through contortions to continue record numbers of statin prescriptions in the face of growing evidence of harm. Buried in their 85-page 2013 guideline on treatment of blood cholesterol, the ACC/AHA task force recommended increasing the acceptable blood limit of LDL-C to 190 from its nadir of 100, while producing 84 other pages of algorithms that have led to *increases* in statin use despite the mind- boggling LDL flip-flop.[20]

In addition, the American Diabetes Association (ADA) is also scrambling to revise their guidelines. However, in their summary of priority topics in 2013, the number 1 recommendation is "Portion Control" and their number 2 priority recommendation, in order to reduce the risk of hypoglycemia, is to eat frequent meals containing moderate amounts of carbohydrates, to "always carry a source of carbohydrates" with them, and to eat sugar (in the form of a glucose tablet) immediately if hypoglycemia occurs.[21]

Consider those statements in the context of addiction. Would we ever say that in order to prevent withdrawal symptoms from cocaine you must control your portions and always carry a source of cocaine and consume it immediately if symptoms occur? Again, it is with this background in mind that we must approach nutrition as relates to addiction, and why an integrative approach to addiction is paramount. In other words, could an integrative approach to nutrition not only be an adjunct to addiction treatment but also its cornerstone, given nutrition's role as both potential cause and cure? As an upstream regulator, or root causative factor, the answer might be yes.

## ADOLESCENT SUSCEPTIBILITY

Adolescents demonstrate a particular vulnerability to the neurobiological changes caused by sugar that lead to mental health and addictive risk. A 2010 study has shown that sugar overconsumption during adolescence induces alterations in reward processing centers that may contribute to an increased risk of addictive disorders in adulthood.[22] Much of the brain development that occurs during adolescence involves brain processes intimately tied to perception and decision making related to risk and reward. Sugar and other drug intake during this critical time of synaptic pruning could create significant alterations in the decision making, abstract reasoning, and response inhibition.[23] In essence, drug taking during adolescence is the riskiest period and predisposes to drug abuse during adulthood.[24,25]

## GENETICS AND EPIGENETICS

We have discussed overlapping pathways for food and drug addiction. Research is now beginning to expose addictive genes as a risk factor in relation to these findings. Polymorphisms in the dopamine receptor DRD2 gene, Leptin receptor Lep-R gene, and Mu-Opiod OPRM-1 gene, all suggest an overlapping risk between food addiction, obesity, and drug addiction.[26] Furthermore, and not surprisingly, there is evidence of an interaction between such receptors.[27] D2 receptor knock-out mice demonstrate leptin sensitivity, whereas wild type D2 mice are heavier and leptin resistant. Therefore, genetic variations contribute to neurotransmitter receptor differences as relates to reward circuitry but also potentially to differences in obesity-related systemic endocrine factors, such as leptin.

In addition to genetic variations in neurotransmitter-related reward pathways and hormone-related metabolic factors, there is evidence that genetic differences in methylation capacity also can contribute to addiction. For example, certain methylation polymorphisms can increase the risk of alcohol dependence.[28] It is probable that methylation deficits do interact with reward circuitry in terms of their direct effects on neurotransmitter levels, but this effect is a downstream result of decreased energy available for neurotransmitter production and regulation, rather than a direct effect. Decreased cellular energy has other downstream results as well, including increasing the risk for depression and other psychiatric disorders that are comorbid with addiction.[29]

To add to the complexity, epigenetic factors may be of even more importance than the underlying genes themselves. This is the case in terms of reward circuitry/neuronal plasticity[30] and related to alterations in gene expression through regulation of transcriptional machinery.[31] These mechanisms are multifaceted, influenced heavily and epigenetically by nutrition, and as is the case with the underlying genetics itself, involve more than just reward circuitry in the brain alone. In this regard, we turn to another emerging field of research intimately tied to nutrition, with implications across many disease spectrums including addiction: the importance of gut health.

# Nutrition, Digestion, and the Gut-Brain Connection

## STRUCTURE AND PHYSIOLOGY OF THE ENTERIC NERVOUS SYSTEM

The enteric nervous system is composed of some 100 million neurons, more than either the spinal cord or the peripheral nervous system, and it is second only to the brain itself with close to 100 billion neurons. Amazingly, 90% of the fibers in the vagus nerve carry messages *from* the gut *to* the brain—not the other way around. And unlike other organs, the intrinsic nervous system of the gut can display neuronal activity even when isolated from the central nervous system.[32] The brain and gut also share neurotransmitter systems. Serotonin is a particularly important gastrointestinal signaling molecule, and in fact 95% of the body's serotonin is not in the brain as might be expected, but in the gut.[33] It is therefore becoming increasingly apparent that gut health influences brain health in ways more profound than ever before imagined.

## GUT ROLE IN DETOXIFICATION

The liver is known as the principal organ of detoxification. Drugs and alcohol are just one example of compounds processed by the liver. From an evolutionary perspective, given that ancestral diets involved consumption of high quantities of phytonutrients (including potentially toxic phytonutrients), detoxification pathways evolved for the purpose of decreasing natural toxic burden. Today, we can add to the list contaminants/pollutants, food additives, pesticides and herbicides, and other chemicals. Phase I detoxification involves oxidation reduction and hydrolysis, catalyzed by the cytochrome P450 enzymes. Phase II detoxification—or conjugation—involves the addition of a molecular subunit to a molecule targeted for elimination, typically making it more water soluble so that it can be excreted via the bile or urine.

The small bowel and colon themselves also play direct and indirect roles in detoxification. Gut dysfunction, from simple constipation to inflammation, leaky gut, and other disturbances, can lead to increased toxic burden. Nutrition plays a critical role in a healthy gut and is therefore a starting point not only in suscepti- bility to addiction and relapse but certainly in optimizing acute substance detoxi- fication in the first place.

## IMPORTANCE OF THE GUT MICROBIOME
## AND CAUSES OF DYSFUNCTION

We have established that there are 100 million neurons in the gut and close to 100 billion neurons in the brain. The human body itself was originally estimated to contain 10 trillion total cells, but newer studies put the number at closer to 37.2 trillion.[34] And yet, these numbers are further dwarfed by the number of *non- human* cells occupying our human environs—namely the gut microbiome. We are host to over *100 trillion* organisms,[35] microbial cells that outnumber our own cells by a ratio of at least 3 to 1, and that boast an ecological diversity of 10,000 or more different species.

Although gut-brain interactions have been studied for decades, leading to discoveries about connections between the gut-associated immune system, en- teric nervous system, and gut-based endocrine system,[36] the clinical implications of such findings are only recently being recognized and integrated into psy- chiatric, neurological, or internal medicine practice (Figure 17.1). The Human Microbiome Project Consortium,[37] with its discovery and characterization of the human microbiome, has added a long overlooked component to such inquiry and triggered tremendous interest by professional and lay media. As of the time of this publication, findings on health and disease related to the gut microbiome are being released almost too quickly for clinical practice to keep up with their ramifications. The makeup of the microbiome has been shown to dramatically affect functional status and disease states, such as autism, mood, and other psy- chiatric disorders, as well as gut-related infections such as clostridium difficile,[38,39] and salmonella,[40] the immune system in general[41], and even obesity.

For example, gut microbes from an obese human twin transplanted into mice have been shown to cause them to gain fat, whereas microbes from the lean twin did not.[42] Studies are even beginning to show that the microbiome can play a role in altering the function of critical components of our metabolic machinery,[43] such as altering enzymes that regulate fatty acid release from circulating triglycerols. Another example would be that probiotics can diminish obesity by reducing gut permeability and inflammation however larger randomized prospective clinical trials are needed for definitive clinical intervention guidelines. In the opposite di- rection, on the other hand, evidence suggests that the introduction of high fruc- tose corn syrup into the US diet has led to an increase in the obesity-associated Firmicutes species in the microbiome.[44]

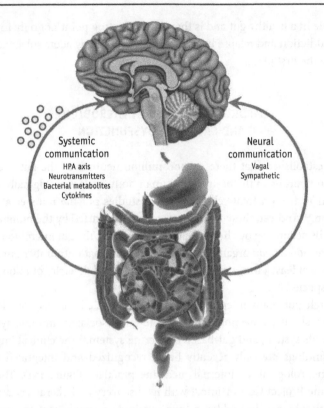

FIGURE 17.1 Bidirectional Communication Channels Between the Gut Microbiome, Gut, and Brain. Signals generated by the gut microbiota and specialized cells within the gut can affect the brain. In turn, the brain can influence microbial composition and function via endocrine and neural mechanisms.

## EVIDENCE FOR GUT-BRAIN-SYSTEMIC DYSFUNCTION

All of this information has also led to the intriguing theory that gut flora have developed ways to "hack" into our reward system, making us crave foods that are most beneficial to *them*.[45] Further evidence of the gut-brain connection is provided by emerging data in the field of autism. Researchers have found that mice with experimentally induced autism spectrum disorder (ASD) show marked improvement when fed the probiotic *Bacteroides fragilis*, and that this intervention is associated with repair of leaky gut.[46] One possible explanation for this is that increased gut permeability not only can be caused by a shift in bacterial populations in the direction of less beneficial organisms but that the permeability itself then causes bacterial metabolites to enter into the blood.[47] Many other psychiatric disorders have been linked to the gut as well, including anxiety and depression[48] and schizophrenia.[49] Thus, the emerging evidence leads to implications regarding the significance of gut health in cause and as well as treatment of addiction. In order to put some of these discoveries in the context of clinical decisions about treatment approaches, it is worth looking at some of the underlying root causes that may be contributing to the drastic changes in the gut microbiome we are seeing.

## CAUSES OF GUT MICROBIOME DYSFUNCTION

Inflammation is both a cause and effect of gut microbiome dysfunction. But inflammation itself has many root causes, even if we limit the discussion of inflammation just to the gut mucosa itself. One of these is food allergies. Given the fact that the lining of the gut consists of epithelial cells that are exposed to the outside world, the gut-associated immune system is faced with the task of recognizing and responding to pathological attacks while remaining passive to beneficial microflora and antigens in food. This ability appears to be deteriorating in the developed world with chronic inflammatory diseases of the gut on the rise even in the apparent absence of overt infection.[50]

In children with atopic eczema and intestinal inflammation due to food allergies, it appears there are more severe systemic immunological disturbances than previously thought, as evidenced by increased levels of tumor necrosis factor-α and eosinophil cationic protein in serum, as well as α-1 antitrypsin in feces of children challenged with oral cow's milk.[51] Interestingly, probiotics given to these children reduced concentrations of fecal α1-antitrypsin and tumor necrosis factor-α (though not eosinophil cationic protein) and also decreased atopic scores.[52] This suggests that the probiotic bacteria may be promoting endogenous barrier mechanisms and by alleviating intestinal inflammation may actually reduce the severity of the food allergy itself. Therefore, this is another example of inflammation both as cause and effect of illness.

While overt infection does not fully account for the rise in chronic inflammatory gut disease, there are certainly signs that infectious causes are on the rise as gut inflammation and microbiome collapse becomes more progressive. Decreasing diversity of the microbiome causes a loss of protective effect of the ecosystem against opportunistic pathogens. Cases of *C. difficile*, for example, increased between 2001 to 2010.[53] But it is not just overt infection with single identifiable species that is relevant. small intestinal bacterial overgrowth (SIBO) is also on the rise. SIBO is defined as a bacterial population in the small intestine exceeding $10^5$–$10^6$ organisms/mL whereas normally there are less than $10^3$ organisms/mL.[54] More significantly, this is caused by a transfer of organisms normally inhabiting the lower intestinal ecosystem upward in the digestive apparatus where the gut immune system reacts differently toward them. Estimates of SIBO prevalence have suggested rates as high as 20% in patients diagnosed with irritable bowel syndrome.[55]

USDA and Medical Association Guidelines recommending a low fat diet over the past 40 to 50 years are also a culprit in microbiome dysfunction. According to the USDA itself,[56] since 1970 (around the time when the low fat dietary guidelines were published) the consumption of added sugar and sweeteners increased by 19% through 2005. Since 1950, while the use of cane and beet sugar decreased by about 30%, the use of corn sweeteners increased by about 800%.[57] In contrast to the USDA data, however, the Sugar Association maintains that sugar consumption is on the decline, and that "continually eating too much food, and sedentary lifestyles are the major contributing factors to increasing rates of obesity—not sugar intake."[58] We have already discussed the particular increase in sugar consumption in adolescents, as well as their increased vulnerability to corruption of the reward system that interacts with drug addiction. Yet food industry advocates, including the sugar association, continue to push "individual responsibility" while aggressively marketing to children.

In addition to sugar itself, again according to the same USDA report cited above, total grain (carbohydrate) availability in the food supply grew by 41%, and more than 90% of grain consumption by 2005 was from refined grains. To be fair, meat consumption has also increased, but since 1970 meat production has been geared to the production of leaner animals and post-production is geared toward the trimming of extra fat before going to market. So in addition to guidelines officially recommending increased carbohydrate consumption and lower fat consumption, an inadvertent consequence has been the corruption of metabolic and reward centers (discussed earlier) to a physiological drive for more sugar and carbs.

## GMO FOODS

An underreported factor in microbiome demise is genetically modified foods, first approved in the United States and introduced to grocery markets in 1994 as the "Flavr Savr" tomato.[59] This step was arguably made possible by a 1980 5–4 Supreme Court ruling allowing the first patent on a living organism.[60] While the hallmark of the Flavr Savr tomato was its delayed ripening, what has particularly characterized the history of genetically modified foods are herbicide resistance genes. In true form to the classic evolutionary "Red Queen Hypothesis," which proposes that organisms must constantly adapt and evolve in order to survive in an ever-changing environment, there was evidence as early as 1996 of weeds resistant to the herbicide glyphosate.[61] By 1999, over a 100 million acres worldwide had been planted with GMO crops.[62] Since then, with increasing weed resistance to herbicides as well as pest resistance to pesticides (along with exponential increases in acreage dominated by GMOs) the amounts of these chemicals applied in food production have mounted.

Arguments for the safety of GMO foods take many forms, but a principal one is that human cells are not affected by the mechanisms of actions of herbicides and pesticides. On its face, this is arguably true. Glyphosate interferes with the shikimate pathway in creation of amino acids, and human cells do not have this pathway. Our gut bacteria, however, do.[63] Therefore, consuming foods with increasing quantities of the supposedly harmless glyphosate molecule would certainly be expected to affect the 100-trillion-cell ecosystem in our gut. Evidence not only suggests this is true but also shows that glyphosate appears to preferentially interfere with beneficial organisms rather than pathological ones, predisposing to SIBO as well as more severe outbreaks such as botulism.[64]

Returning to food allergies and their potential relation to the gut microbiome, according to a study released by the CDC in 2013, food allergies among children increased by a whopping 50% between 1997 (around the time GMOs came to market) and 2011.[65] Many theories are concurrently put forth as to why this may be the case. Some of these are changes in food macronutrient composition, genetics, vitamin status, and even the "hygeine hypothesis" (proposing that our over-sanitized modern societies cause a shift in early-life exposure that push our immune systems toward increased inflammatory response). But there is virtually no mention of GMO foods as a possible cause, at least among official institutions. New knowledge of the gut microbiome and genetically modified foods promises to change that.

## RESTORING GUT HEALTH

In the next section, we will discuss a broad practical framework as a starting point to evaluate and treat addictive imbalances and their root causes. Given the above considerations, any such approach should begin with the gut, taking into account its central role in nutrient assimilation, detoxification, inflammatory burden, and gut-brain communication—all in the context of the collective disintegration of the human microbiome.

A starting point therefore would be to encourage the reduction of antibiotic use, especially in newborns and children. A recent astounding finding has linked the absence of bacteria in the gut to celiac disease,[66] a severe example and harbinger of what happens when the gut can no longer distinguish food from foe. What is astounding about this study is that the bacteria tested is actually *H. pylori*. This lays bare our currently profound lack of understanding of the complex interplay of a microbiome in harmony that has served us for millions of years. *H. pylori* is bad, right? Wrong. The full details are beyond the scope of this discussion, but the bottom line is that it may be that *H. pylori* actually play a protective role in many ways. Here the study shows that the rate of *H. pylori* in patients who had signs of celiac disease was only 4.4% compared with 8.8% in those without. Given that this US study was large and nationwide, the researchers asked whether the same relationship was true in subjects of the 37 individual states that were studied. In each and every one of those 37 states, the same relationship held true.

In 2015, researchers were able to collect fecal samples from people deep in the Amazon rainforest that had previously never been exposed to antibiotics, or Western society at all. What they found was a microbiome more diverse than ever imagined, with species heretofore not seen.[67] Could it be that these samples may be our last hope of restoring from the brink of extinction a healthy ecological diversity to the collective human microbiome that may protect us from the calamity of burgeoning illness we are facing? This is a question we must ask and calls us to be bold about how to address gut healing.

Thus, we must look at everything from how we prescribe antibiotics, starting with newborns who are just acquiring their precious microbiome, to what food we eat, and even more importantly how that food is grown. No potential treatment breakthrough can ignore the question of how we are feeding ourselves. Probiotics for example, may be helpful, and there is some minimal evidence that they can help reduce the risk of antibiotic-induced *C. diff* infection.[68] But are we missing the big picture? We must be open to all ideas, gut healing diets that eliminate sugar and processed carbohydrates as well as food allergies, and even extending to the personal choice of whether to consume raw milk, for example. Although a recent CDC study found that raw milk was more likely to result in serious illness that pasteurized milk, that risk was only 1 in approximately 100,000.[69] Given local variations in how this milk is farmed, processed, and delivered to consumers, as well as taking into consideration the living nature of raw milk and beneficial microorganisms it contains, are we missing the potential benefits in the face of these risks?

Furthermore, we need to look at gut healing in the context of communication systems that allow its proper functioning, particularly in terms of the ever-important and constantly elusive determination between what is a food and what might be a potential poison or pathologic microbial invader. In this regard, the recently discovered (relative to modern medicine) endocannabanoid system appears to play a role unimagined until now.[70] Medicine has focused on single cause and effect relationships rather than complex interplays, but we need to take a step back and look at finer details of what might be causing pathology, and more importantly, how to fix it.

## A Practical Guide to Nutritional Evaluation and Treatment of Addiction

It is worth reviewing some of the principles of integrative medicine overall in introducing a hands-on clinical model for effective treatment of addiction. Of these principles, optimal health, innate healing power, individuality, wholeness, and root cause stand out. The World Health Organization defines health itself as "a state of optimal well-being, not merely the absence of disease and infirmity." With integrative medicine, the practitioner is encouraged to make use not only of Western medicine principles in promoting this state of optimal well-being but of other approaches and modalities where appropriate to the patient and informed by evidence. The goal is to promote the highest level of functioning and balance in order to be fully alive in appreciating the human experience.

To achieve optimal health, priority is placed on innate healing power. Examples of this are not hard to describe. Your finger gets a cut, it heals. Western medicine is often criticized for employing tactics that may get in the way of the body's natural healing capacity, with its "anti" approach: anti-inflammatory, anti-depressant, etc. However, when used in concert with innate healing power, conventional "anti" approaches are not to be discounted. Cut your finger while cleaning out your septic system, and it will probably heal better if you put some Neosporin on the cut. All medical students rotating through their nephology training learn the old saying: "The dumbest kidney is smarter than the smartest nephrologist." So integrative medicine is not anti-Western medicine, but integrative physicians do prioritize finding every opportunity to evoke innate healing power.

Integrative medicine also places a priority on individuality. While it is important to establish what disease may be present, optimal treatment approaches to the same disease in different people will diverge. Factors related to this include environment, genetics, spirituality and beliefs, nutrient status, and others. By the same token, where illness exists, it is related to the whole person rather than an isolated physical disorder or random event or occurrence. The concept of wholeness—that everything is connected—allows for healing opportunities to arise in unexpected ways. For example, constipation may be relieved by an herbal laxative, but if it is caused in the first place by a hypothyroid state, or even more specifically an iodine deficiency causing the hypothyroid state, the best (and simplest) treatment might be simply iodine replacement.

On that point, a root cause/biological systems model is perhaps the most important principle of integrative medicine, especially when it comes to evaluation and treatment approaches. Particularly in complex cases where comorbidity coexists with addictive disorders, finding a common root cause can be the simplest and most effective path toward resolving the addiction and reducing the risk of relapse.

## EVALUATION AND RESTORATION OF UNDERLYING IMBALANCES

### Routine Blood Tests

In addition to a comprehensive metabolic panel and CBC, the following tests are important and readily available through routine testing laboratories: vitamin D

25 (OH, GGT), magnesium (RBC), zinc (RBC), insulin, hemoglobin A1C, iron studies, homocysteine, TSH, and vitamin B12/ (RBC)folate.

Some of these nutrients and their values are discussed in more detail in the nutraceutical/botanical section but deserve mention here. Vitamin D is an example of a poorly understood and underestimated factor. In fact, it is not a vitamin at all, but a prohormone involved not just in regulation of skeletal composition and function but also immune, cardiovascular, neurological, and other systems. It has long been known to be an important factor in the prevention of the auto-immune inflammatory disease multiple sclerosis but is now known to be connected to other auto-immune diseases as well. It is also relevant to cancer prevention, cognition and Alzheimer's prevention, diabetes, mood disorders, allergies, and pain. While it is possible to accumulate to levels that cause symptoms of toxicity, cases are few in the literature and usually connected to accidental dosing. Evidence shows it tends to be most beneficial when dosed to blood levels of 60 to 80 ng/ml, and doses required to achieve this can vary greatly from individual to individual, ranging from 2,000 IU to 20,000 IU per day.

Magnesium and zinc must be measured within the RBC to be considered as more accurate markers of total body deficiency, since serum levels are tightly regulated independent of whole body stores. Again, both nutrients are covered in more detail in the nutraceutical chapter briefly mentioned here. Magnesium is involved in more than 200 different metabolic functions. In addition, it plays a role in the relaxation of smooth muscle and reduction in anxiety. Intravenous use has been employed as a first-line treatment in migraine as well as asthma. Prevalence of magnesium deficiency in the general population alone is as high as 7%.[71] In post-operative, ICU patients, one study found the prevalence to be a whopping 60%.[72] Magnesium (as well as zinc) are of particular risk for deficiency in alcohol use. Supplementation with various forms of oral magnesium, such as magnesium glycinate, magnesium threonate, and magnesium taurate, are well tolerated and can not only contribute to overall health but specifically reduce neuromuscular symptoms of withdrawal and well as anxiety and sleep problems. Intravenous magnesium can be reserved for more serious deficiency and/or symptomatology but is also safe, well tolerated, and effective.

The interaction between sugar and addictive reward center pathways has already been discussed. In addition to glucose levels, hemoglobin A1C and fasting insulin levels should be measured. Increases in either of these values suggests impaired metabolic pathways and a potential underlying trigger for addictive relapse, therefore making the importance of a low glycemic diet all the more important. Homocysteine is another marker for impaired metabolic pathways, specifically methylation, and can be affected not only by drug, sugar, and carbohydrate intake but also by genetic factors that can now be readily evaluated.

GGT is known to be elevated specifically with heavy alcohol exposure but can also be elevated with other drug use, inadvertent exposure to toxins such as pesticides, and with general illness itself. All of this relates to GGT's role in glutathione regeneration, and increased levels are therefore a marker of depleted intracellular glutathione levels. Of course, the first step in normalizing GGT is removal of the toxic offenders. Supplying depleted glutathione as a nutrient can be tricky but useful. Since glutathione is broken down by intestinal degradation, except possibly in the case of liposomal glutathione, intravenous glutathione administration can be a more effective method of restoring levels. More simply, N-acetylcysteine (NAC) administered orally as a glutathione precursor is often effective as well.

Iron studies through routine laboratory testing are an effective way to look for iron deficiency and hint at its potential causes, including drug addiction and chronic disease itself. Vitamin B12 and folate, although potentially worth checking through routine labs, may be better measured through specialized functional testing (see the section "Nutrient Status"), given the fact that serum levels do not necessarily reflect either cellular levels nor functionally active (methylated) forms of the vitamins versus their non-active (unmethylated) forms. Also, particularly in the case of B12, diagnosis of deficiency may be most accurate through clinical challenge, administration of intramuscular methylcobalamin (methylated B12), and determining deficiency based on response. Given the low-risk profile of methylcobalamin, and high potential for therapeutic benefit, allowing for a therapeutic trial as both potential treatment and diagnostic tool makes sense.

Low growth hormone is often the result of lack of deep sleep, so natural measures to restore optimal sleep function can restore this important hormone and its importance for restoration and repair. For women and men with laboratory and symptomatic evidence of sex-hormone deficiency related either to normal aging and/or to deterioration of function due to addictive disorders, bioidentical hormone replacement can be an effective therapy. It can not only restore levels but also combat symptoms of anxiety, sleeplessness, fatigue, low self-esteem, among others, that co-exist with drug abuse and withdrawal.

## Food Allergy Testing

The significance of the rising prevalence of food allergies has been growing. Various methodologies have been developed in order to test for food allergies, and it is important to choose the most accurate tests. Skin testing has often been used but relies exclusively on IgE reactivity, which is problematic for two reasons. One is that skin testing does not necessarily correlate with gut sensitivity, but more importantly IgE does not detect delayed food sensitivity, which can be more insidious. Further, immediate IgE sensitivity is more easily noticed by the patients on their own, reducing the need for laboratory confirmation in comparison with delayed sensitivity, which is not so easily noticeable, even when paying close attention.

Some non-conventional food allergy testing services have a particular appeal in integrative practice but are not necessarily accurate. For example, some labs utilize what is called the Coulter technique, where a small quantity of blood is separated into multiple alliquots and incubated with different food allergens. Following exposures, a change in the number and size of cells (such as leukocytes) is used as determination of an intolerant response for each relevant exposure. There is reason to think that this might be a more holistic way of measuring immune response than measuring individual components of the allergic response but may also lend itself to inaccuracies. At the current time, a combination of IgG and IgE testing through specialized laboratory services may offer the best chance for relevant and useful results. As with other testing, however, careful clinical analysis is necessary to put the results in context before recommending potential dietary changes.

## Genetic Tests

The importance of methylation and detoxification in treating addiction has already been discussed. Genetic testing has become more readily available as well as inexpensive. Whereas some routine labs now offer blood testing for the MTHFR SNPs for a relatively inexpensive pricetag, tests available to the lay public can test for these and thousands of other SNPs combined at affordable prices. Understanding an individual's underlying genetic machinery of methylation and detoxification, along with other potential gene interactions, can inform treatment decisions and epigenetic manipulation in the direction away from addiction and disease and toward optimal health.

## Nutrient Status

As mentioned earlier, while some nutritional factors can be assessed relatively simply through routine blood measurements, others cannot. As long as magnesium and zinc are measured through RBC levels, results are fairly reliable. Other vitamins such as B12 and additional members of the B-vitamin family, amino acids, certain healthful as well as toxic elements, fatty acids, and measures of antioxidant status may be best measured through functional assays available only through specialized labs.

### NUTRITIONAL GUIDANCE

We have discussed evidence that a low glycemic, anti-inflammatory diet can provide benefits in regulating reward behavior through central signaling pathways and indirectly through benefits to the gut and gut-brain connection and other factors. In addition, studies on a ketogenic (or modified) Atkins Diet reveal that in children with seizures refractory to conventional medications, 33% have more than a 50% reduction in seizures, and up to 20% become seizure free.[73] This would suggest that a diet eliminating or sharply reducing carbohydrates and sugar significantly decreases brain stress. As such, a low glycemic diet would be expected to assist in addiction treatment through reward behavior regulation by HPA axis rebalancing and decreasing central overstimulation.[74] Thus a low glycemic diet could act in a fashion similar to α2 agonists such as clonidine, in decreasing susceptibility to drug and alcohol relapse. It may also work in a fashion similar to naltrexone, which appears to help "reset" hypothalamic responsiveness in alcohol-dependent patients.[75]

A low glycemic, anti-inflammatory diet does not just mean high fat and protein, as with the Atkins Diet. In holding fast to the integrative principle of individuality, there are a variety of possible low glycemic diets. The predominantly plant-based, low fat Dean Ornish diet has, like the Atkins Diet, been shown to reduce or even reverse factors associated with heart disease. How can two such seemingly disparate approaches both boast research to this effect? A commonality between the two is that both approaches call for a strict elimination of processed sugar and carbohydrates. So again, if we take the examples of heart disease or obesity as related to an overall predisposition to illness including addiction, there are many possible variations of low glycemic dietary guidance that may be employed.

## Specific Considerations

### FOOD SECURITY

The paradox between food insecurity and obesity has been well studied.[76] Obesity rates are 37% for women in food-insecure households, versus 26% on households defined as food secure. Given that calories from sugar and processed carbohydrates are not only more readily available in poor neighborhoods (compared to nutrient-dense foods) but are also more inexpensive than calories from nutrient-dense foods—and given that such calories are now known to be at the root of the obesity epidemic—the paradox is thus explained. Once again, if we take obesity as a stand-in for generalized epidemics in other illnesses including addiction, we can extend the problem of food security to addiction risk as well. At least with alcohol, there is evidence that this is the case.[77]

Food quality is also a factor and intersects with socioeconomic status, although not always with food security per se. We have discussed evidence of food quality with regard to grass-finished versus grain-fed beef. Further, we have discussed potential evidence for genetically modified foods as a cause of microbiome collapse.

Both of these issues relate to agricultural consolidation in the hands of large industry. Just as integrative medicine calls for recognizing individual differences and rejects a one-size-fits-all approach, there is a need for local, individualized control over the food system and resulting nutritional choices available to consumers.[78] There is increasing evidence that the food industry is using the same "playbook" as the tobacco industry, which after decades of strategies to influence public opinion and even alter the conduct of science itself, was found to have led to the deaths of millions of people.[79] We must hope that the history of the food industry is written differently.

In further recognition of the principles of integrative medicine, such factors relate not just to nutritional choices, but to the bio-pycho-social-spiritual elements of existence as well. This is significant not just for consumers and the psychospiritual importance of access to enjoyable and healthy food but also to farmers themselves, among whom suicide rates are on the rise.[80] Recognition of the importance of nutrition and access to healthy food are therefore important in approaching not only addiction but in overall health and global well-being.

## REFERENCES

1. Liu RH. Potential synergy of phytochemicals in cancer prevention: mechanism of action. *Journal of Nutrition*. 2004;134:3479S–3485S.
2. Drenowski A, Gomez-Carneros C. Bitter taste, phytonutrients, and the consumer: a review. *American Journal of Clinical Nutrition*. 2000;72:1424–1435.
3. Brand-Miller JC, Holt SH. Australian Aboriginal plant foods: a consideration of their nutritional composition and health implications. *Nutrition Research Reviews*. 1998;11:5–23
4. Alcohol increases homocysteine and reduces B vitamin concentration in healthy male volunteers—a randomized, crossover intervention study.
5. The Inuit Paradox|DiscoverMagazine.com http://discovermagazine.com/2004/oct/inuit-paradox
6. Daley CA, et al. A review of fatty acid profiles and antioxidant content in grass-fed and grain-fed beef. *Nutrition Journal*. 2010; 9:10.
7. Lenoir M, Serre F, Cantin L, Ahmed, SH. Intense sweetness surpasses cocaine reward. *PloS ONE*. 2007;2(8):e698. doi:10.1371/journal.pone.0000698.
8. Lakhan SE, Vieira KF. Nutritional therapies for mental disorders. *Nutrition Journal*. 2008;7:2
9. Young SN. Clinical nutrition: 3. The fuzzy boundary between nutrition and psychopharmacology. *Canadian Medical Association Journal*. 2002;166(2).
10. Lutter M, Nestler EJ. Homeostatic and hedonic signals interact in the regulation of food intake. *Journal of Nutrition*. 2009;139:629–632

11. Volkow ND, Wang G-J, Fowler, J. S., Telang, F. Overlapping neuronal circuits in addiction and obesity: Evidence of systems pathology. *Philosophical Transactions of the Royal Society B: Biological Sciences.* 2008;363 (1507):3191–3200

12. Avena NM, Carrillo CA, Needham L, Hoebel BG. Sugar-dependent rats show enhanced intake of unsweetened ethanol. *Alcohol* 34:203–209

13. Avena NM, Bocarsly ME, Rada P, Kim A, Hoebel BG. After daily bingeing on a sucrose solution, food deprivation induces anxiety and accumbens dopamine/acetylcholine imbalance. *Physiology & Behavior.* 2008;94:309–315

14. Zhang, Yi, et al. Obesity: pathophysiology and intervention. *Nutrients.* 2014; 6(11):5153–5183.

15. Muele, Adrian. Back by Popular Demand: A narrative review on the history of food addiction research. *Yale Journal of Biology and Medicine.* 2015;88(3): 295/.–302.

16. Spring B, Schneider K, Smith M, Kendzor D, Appelhans B, Hedeker D, Pagoto S. Abuse potential of carbohydrates for overweight carbohydrate cravers. *Psychopharmacology (Berl).* 2008;197:637–647.

17. Wang GJ, Volkow ND, Telang F, et al. Exposure to appetitive food stimuli markedly activates the human brain. *Neuroimage.* 2004;21:1790–1797.

18. Avena NM, Rada P, Hoebel BG. Sugar and fat bingeing have notable differences in addictive-like behavior. *Journal of Nutrition.* 2009;139:623–628.

19. Harcombe Z, Baker JS, Cooper SM, et al. Evidence from randomised controlled trials did not support the introduction of dietary fat guidelines in 1977and 1983: a systematic review and meta-analysis. *Open Heart.* 2015;2:e000196.

20. Stone NJ, et al. 2013 ACC/AHA Guideline on the treatment of blood cholesterol to reduce atherosclerotic cardiovascular risk in adults: a report of the American College of Cardiology/American Heart Association Task Force on practice guidelines. *Circulation.* 2013;00:000

21. Evert AB, et al. Position statement: nutrition therapy recommendations for the management of adults with diabetes. *Diabetes Care.* 2013.

22. Sugar overconsumption induces a developmental stage-specific chronic depression in reward processing that may contribute to an increase in the vulnerability to reward-related psychiatric disorders.

23. Dahl RE. Biological, developmental, and neurobehavioral factors relevant to adolescent driving risks. *American Journal of Preventive Medicine.* 2008;35(3 Suppl):S278–S284.

24. Andersen SL. Trajectories of brain development: point of vulnerability or window of opportunity? *Neuroscience and Biobehavioral Reviews.* 2003;27(1–2):3–18.

25. Crews F, He J, Hodge C. Adolescent cortical development: a critical period of vulnerability for addiction. *Pharmacology Biochemistry and Behavior.* 2007;86(2):189–199.

26. Heber D, Carpenter CL. Addictive genes and the relationship to obesity and inflammation. *Molecular Neurobiology.* 2011;44:160–165

27. Kim KS, Yoon YR, Lee HJJ, et al. Enhanced hypothalamic leptin signaling in mice lacking dopamine D2 receptors. *Journal of Biological Chemistry.* 2010;285:8905–8917

28. Benyamina A, et al. Brief Report: Association between MTHFR 677C-T polymorphism and alcohol dependence according to Lesch and Babor typology. *Addiction Biology.* 2009;14(4):503–505

29. Gilbody S, Lewis S, Lightfoot T. Methylenetetrahydrofolate reductase (MTHFR) genetic polymorphisms and psychiatric disorders: A HuGE review. *American Journal of Epidemiology.* 2007;165(1):1–13.

30. Maze I, Nestler EJ. The epigenetic landscape of addiction. *Annals of the New York Academy of Sciences.* 2011;1216:99–113

31. Robison AJ, Nestler EJ. Transcriptional and epigenetic mechanisms of addiction. *Nature Reviews Neuroscience.* 2011;12(11):623–637

32. Gershon MD. Review article: serotonin receptors and transporters—roles in normal and abnormal gastrointestinal motility. *Alimentary Pharmacology and Therapeutics.* 2004;20(Suppl. 7):3–14.

33. Camilleri M. Serotonin in the gastrointestinal tract. *Current Opinion in Endocrinology, Diabetes and Obesity.* 2009;16(1):53–59

34. Bianconni E et al. An estimation of the number of cells in the human body. *Annals of Human Biology.* 2013;40(6):463–471

35. Potera C. Researchers find surprises in human microbiome. *BioScience.* 2014.

36. Mayer EA. Gut feelings: the emerging biology of gut-brain communication. *Nature Reviews Neuroscience.* 2011;12:453–466.

37. Human Microbiome Project Consortium. Structure, function and diversity of the healthy human microbiome. *Nature.* 2012;486:207–214.

38. Hickson M. Probiotics in the prevention of antibiotic-associated diarrhoea and Clostridium difficile infection. *Therapeutic Advances in Gastroenterology.* 2011;4(3):185–197.

39. Van Nood E, et al. Duodenal infusion of donor feces for recurrent Clostridium difficile. *New England Journal of Medicine.* 2013;368:407–415

40. Asahara T et al. Increased resistance of mice to Salmonella enterica serovar Typhimurium infection by synbiotic administration of Bifidobacteria and transgalactosylated oligosaccharides. *Journal of Applied Microbiology.* 2001;91(6):985–996.

41. Kau AL et al. Human nutrition, the gut microbiome and the immune system. *Nature.* 2011;474:327–336.

42. Turnbaugh PJ. et al. An obesity-associated gut microbiome with increased capacity for energy harvest. *Nature.* 2006;444;1027–1031.

43. Cani PD, Delzenne NM: The gut microbiome as therapeutic target. *Pharmacology & Therapeutics.* 2001;130:202–212.

44. Tsai F, Coyle WJ: The microbiome and obesity: is obesity linked to our gut flora? *Current Gastroenterology Reports.* 2009;11:307–313.

45. Alcock J, Maley CC, Aktipis CA. Is eating behavior manipulated by the gastrointestinal microbiota? Evolutionary pressures and potential mechanisms. *Bioessays.* 2014;36:940–949.

46. Hsiao EY, et al. Microbiota modulate behavioral and physiological abnormalities associated with neurodevelopmental disorders. *Cell.* 2013;155:1451–1463.

47. Finegold SM et al. Gastrointestinal microflora studies in late-onset autism. *Clinical Infectious Diseases.* 2002;35(Suppl 1):S6–S16.
48. Foster JA, McVey Neufeld KA. Gut–brain axis: how the microbiome influences anxiety and depression. *Trends in Neurosciences.* 2013;36(5):305–312.
49. Nemani K et al. Schizophrenia and the gut–brain axis. 2015;56:155–160.
50. MacDonald TT, and Monteleone G. Immunity, inflammation, and allergy in the gut. *Science.* 2005;307:1920–1925.
51. Majamaa H et al. Intestinal inflammation in children with atopic eczema: faecal eosinophil cationic protein and tumour necrosis factor-α as non-invasive indicators of food allergy. *Clinical and Experimental Allergy.* 1996;26(2):181–187.
52. Majamaa H et al. Probiotics: a novel approach in the management of food allergy. *Journal of Allergy and Clinical Immunology.* 1997;99(2):179–185.
53. Reveles KR et al. The rise in Clostridium difficile infection incidence among hospitalized adults in the United States: 2001–2010. *American Journal of Infection Control.* 2014;42(10):1028–1032.
54. Corrazza GR, Menozzi MG, Strocchi A, et al. The diagnosis of small bowel bacterial overgrowth: reliability of jejunal culture and inadequacy of breath hydrogen testing. *Gastroenterology.* 1990;98:302–309.
55. Dukowicz AC, Lacy BE, Levine GM. Small intestinal bacterial overgrowth: a comprehensive review. *Gastroenterology & Hepatology (NY).* 2007;3:112–122.
56. Wells HF, Buzby JC. *Dietary Assessment of Major Trends in US Food Consumption, 1970–2005,* Economic Information Bulletin No. 33. Economic Research Service, US Dept. of Agriculture. March 2008.
57. Profiling Food Consumption in America. Web site. http://www.usda.gov/factbook/chapter2.pdf
58. http://www.sugar.org/sugar-your-diet/caloric-intake/
59. Bruening G, Lyons JM. The case of the FLAVR SAVR tomato. *California Agriculture.* 2000;54(4):6–7..
60. *Association for Molecular Pathology v. Myriad Genetics*—Supreme Court Case
61. International Survey of Herbicide Resistant Weeds. Web site. http://weedscience.org/details/case.aspx?ResistID=380
62. Transgenic Crops: An Introduction and Resource Guide. Web site. http://cls.casa.colostate.edu/transgeniccrops/current.html
63. Samsel A, Seneff S. Glyphosate's suppression of cytochrome P450 enzymes and amino acid biosynthesis by the gut microbiome: Pathways to modern diseases. *Entropy.* 2013;15(4):1416–1463.
64. Ackermann W, Coenen M, Schroedl W, Shehata A, Krueger M. The influence of glyphosate on the microbiota and production of botulinum neurotoxin during ruminal fermentation. *Current Microbiology.* 2014.
65. Jackson KD et al. *Trends in Allergic Conditions among Children: United States,* 1997–2011. NCHS Data Brief No. 121 May 2013.
66. Lebwohl, B et al. Decreased risk of celiac disease in patients with helicobacter pylori colonization. *American Journal of Epidemiology.* 2013;178(12):1721–1730.

67. Clemente JC et al. The microbiome of uncontacted Amerindians. *Science Advances.* 2015;1(3).

68. Hickson, M. Probiotics in the prevention of antibiotic-associated diarrhoea and *Clostridium difficile* infection. *Therapeutic Advances in Gastroenterology.* 2011;4(3):185–197.

69. Majority of dairy-related disease outbreaks linked to raw milk. Press Release. February 21, 2012. https://www.cdc.gov/media/releases/2012/p0221_raw_milk_out-break.html

70. Storr MA, Sharkey KA. The endocannabinoid system and gut–brain signaling. *Current Opinion in Pharmacology.* 7(6):575–582.

71. Altura BM, Brodsky MA, Elin RJ, et al. Magnesium: growing in clinical importance. *Patient Care.* 1994;10:130–150.

72. Ryzen E, Elbaum N, Singer FR, et al. Parenteral magnesium tolerance testing in the evaluation of magnesium deficiency. *Magnesium.* 1985;4:137–147.

73. Sharma S, Jain P. The modified Atkins Diet in refractory epilepsy. *Epilepsy Research and Treatment.* 2014

74. Sinha R. The role of stress in addiction relapse. *Current Psychiatry Reports.* 2007;9(5):388–395.

75. Adinoff B, et al. Disturbances of the stress response: The role of the HPA axis during alcohol withdrawal and abstinence. *Alcohol Health and Research World.* 1998;22(1)

76. Dinour LM, et al. The food insecurity–obesity paradox: a review of the literature and the role food stamps may play. *Journal of the American Dietetic Association.* 2007;107(11):1952–1961.

77. Casswell S, et al. Socioeconomic status and drinking patterns in young adults. *Addiction.* 2003;98(5):601–610.

78. Horrigan L, et al. How sustainable agriculture can address the environmental and human health harms of industrial agriculture. *Environmental Health Perspectives.* 2002;110(5).

79. Brownell KD, Warner KE. The perils of ignoring history: big tobacco played dirty and millions died. How similar is big food? *Milbank Quarterly.* 2009;87(1):259–294..

80. Stone G. Biotechnology and suicide in India. *Anthropology News.* 2002;43(5)

# 18

## Functional Medicine Approach to Addiction

### GEORGE E. MUÑOZ AND ISABELLA LEONI GARCIA

This chapter is meant to expand the nutritional and functional approach covered in chapter 17. The concept here is to view analyze and deconstruct some of the underlying physiologic underpinnings that become disturbed in active addiction. Metabolic, inflammatory hormonal, and central nervous pathway effects will be discussed. The connection of mindfulness alterations to these pathway disturbances will also be reviewed. Using chapter 17 as a springboard, we will delve deeper into relevant areas in addiction and recovery, discussing vitamin deficiencies and nutraceuticals relevant to aiding the inflammatory processes activated and enhanced by addiction. Despite drug-of-choice abstinence, metabolic perturbations remain active in varying degrees during recovery phases, and this needs to be addressed.

## Anti-Inflammatory and Anti-Addiction Molecular Functional

### PHYSIOLOGY AND INTERVENTIONS

In food addiction, there is a loss of control over food consumption, where the hedonic/reward pathway can override the homeostatic pathway, leading to an increased desire to consume highly palatable foods. One might seek the fat/sugar food combination, despite being in a positive energy balance (energy or caloric abundance) and may be motivated to seek more after the exposure.[1]

Drugs and foods (specially sugar) both show activation in brain regions associated with the reward system. There are behavioral and neuronal (same neurochemical pathways) overlaps between over-consuming highly palatable foods (e.g., sugar and fat) and drug addiction.[2] Eating appetizing foods causes the firing of dopaminergic neurons in the ventra tegmental area (VTA), leading to a release of dopamine in the nucleus accumbens (NAcc), activating the reward circuit (increasing motivation to seek and eat food).[3] This activation of the reward pathway diminishes with repeated exposure to palatable foods. In contrast, sugar acts more like a drug, increasing dopamine in the NAcc, even after repeated exposures to it. Additionally, neuroimaging studies show that there is an activation of the anterior cingulate cortex, medial orbitofrontal cortex, and the amygdala in anticipation of the of consumption of sugar. These same areas are associated with increased motivation to seek and consume drugs.[4]

Furthermore, evidence suggests that chronic over-consumption of sugar alters the dopamine (specifically D2 dopamine receptors) and opioid mRNA levels, as well as their gene expression in the NAcc, which is similar to that seen in drug abusers. Moreover, studies have shown that obese and substance- abusing individuals have lower dorsal striatal dopamine D2 receptor availability, reducing their sensitivity to those rewards and leading them to strive for more.[5] All this evidence has led us to believe that food addiction and drug addiction have many commonalities and therefore relevance in treating food addiction.

## GUT HEALTH

The body is host to 30 to 50 trillion microbes, with the vast majority of them inhabiting the colon. These bacteria produce beneficial metabolites such as short-chain fatty acids (SCFAs) through bacterial fermentation of dietary fibers and neurotransmitters (e.g., serotonin, GABA, acetylcholine). The bacteria can also synthesize toxins, such as lipopolysaccharides (LPS) and peptidoglycans, which activate inflammatory pathways.[6] The production of different metabolites, depends on the type of bacteria that inhabit the gut, the number of bacteria, and also the presence of different pathogens (diversity) such as yeast, fungi, and pathogenic bacteria and viruses.

So, how do the bacteria and microbes in the gut play a role in addiction and recovery? Alcohol and drugs both change the functioning of our digestive system by increasing inflammation, reducing the absorption of nutrients, increasing intestinal permeability, and contributing to the production of toxic molecules. These changes give rise to cognitive issues, nutritional deficiencies, changes in mood, increasing cravings, and as a result increase the likelihood of relapsing.[7]

Research has shown how alcohol abuse can lead to an imbalance in the microbes inhabiting your gut (microbial dysbiosis), as well as an increase in intestinal permeability, intestinal inflammation, and toxins, such as LPS and peptidoglycans. The metabolism of alcohol by bacteria in the gut and by epithelial cells can generate a high concentration of acetaldehyde in the intestines. This causes an increase in tyrosine phosphorylation in the tight junction proteins (zonulin), leading to intestinal permeability (IP). Another mechanism for increases in IP is through the synthesis of nitric oxide (NO) in the intestines as a result from ingestion of alcohol, which interacts with tubulin, causing damage to the microtubule cytoskeleton of the intestinal barrier. As the gut's walls become more permeable, more endotoxins get released into the blood and transferred to the liver and other organs, leading to liver injury and an overall inflammation of the body.[8]

Additionally, the presence of different bacteria in the intestines can play a role in the development of depression and anxiety in active drinkers, which has been known to serve as a negative reinforcer in addicts, increasing the tendency to drink. Specifically, it has been seen that an increase in *bifidobacterium infanti* ("beneficial or good bacteria") can have an antidepressant effect in rats, through changes in the tryptophan/kynurenine pathway (down-regulating the ratio, leads to an increase in serotonin production and reduces related anxiety and psychosis).[9]

Dysbiosis can also lead to alcohol cravings, which can be significant predictors of relapse in addicts going throughout the detoxification process. Alcohol also contributes to the growth of yeast, most prominently *Candida*, as these species feed on sugars and alcohol. The presence of yeast such as *Candida albicans* in the gut is positively correlated with higher levels of anxiety, depression, and fatigue. Both yeast and fungi release toxins, which can be toxic to the brain causing imbalances in neurotransmitters. Additionally, these pathogens enhance gut inflammation, affecting micronutrient absorption and further contributing to neurotransmitter imbalances centrally.[10]

Recent research has demonstrated how long-term morphine use, which is commonly prescribed for pain management, can cause detrimental damages to microbiome of our gut. Abuse of opioids was associated with an increase in gram-positive bacteria, lower bacteroidetes/firmicutes ratio (correlated with an increase in systemic inflammation), translocation of commensal bacteria across the gut barrier, and stimulation of toll-like receptors (TLRs), resulting in changes in tight junction proteins and dysfunction of the gut barrier. Additionally, the microbial dysbiosis resulting from chronic morphine use causes changes in the metabolism of bile acids in the intestines and liver. This in turn leads the disruption in bile acids metabolism that can also lead to its own inflammatory state and alterations in the function of the gut barrier. Banerjee, et al went even further to study whether microbial transplant (fecal) in mice could reverse the effects of morphine in their gut. The fecal transplant was effective in restoring gut barrier function, the gut's microbiome, and gut immune homeostasis.[11]

In 2014 Leclecrcq and colleagues carried out a study to see the effects of intestinal permeability, dysbiosis, and endotoxins in alcohol-dependent subjects. They looked at 60 alcohol-dependent (AD) subjects during their first week of alcohol withdrawal. Of the subjects, 43% had high levels of IP, while 57% had low levels of IP. Both groups had high rates of depression, anxiety, and alcohol cravings. After just 19 days of withdrawal, their IP had been reduced significantly and the low IP group had lower scores of anxiety and depression. Those in the high IP group still had high depression, anxiety, and craving scores. This leads us to believe that gut-barrier function may play a significant role in psychological outcomes during and after the detoxification phase. Leclercq's study did not stop there. They also looked at the quantity and quality of the microbial population, as well as levels of inflammatory markers. They found that those with high IP had a lower number of total bacteria (reduced diversity), compared to the low IP and control group. Specifically, *Faecalibacterium prausnitzii* and *Bifidobacterium spp.*, bacteria with anti-inflammatory properties, were significantly lower in the high IP group. Also, they found that both groups of AD subject had high inflammatory markers (TNG-a, IL-1b, IL-6, IL-8, and IL-10) and a high CRP confirming the proinflammatory state of early alcohol and substance abuse abstinence and recovery phases. However, the level of IL-8 was significantly higher in the high IP group, a differentiating biomarker, correlated with abnormal intestinal permeability and a cytokine immune signature that is measurable and worth monitoring in the clinical setting. This study confirms that in this case, alcohol addiction, gut dysbiosis, and immunoregulatory signaling is associated with cravings, mood, anxiety, and depression enhancing relapse potential. The gut-brain connection has been demonstrated in alcohol addiction and potentially in therapeutics. Furthermore, this leads us to believe that the intestinal flora might be a good marker to measure likelihood of relapse in a significant subgroup of patients and simultaneously serve as another target for treatment. This viewpoint of microbiome distant immune-neural-metabolic-genomic effects is spreading to other subspecialties in medicine including immunology, rheumatology, and oncology to name a few.

Additional studies have shown a decrease in *Bifidobacterium* and *Lactobacillus* (beneficial bacteria) in the stool cultures of AD subjects, compared to control subjects with no AD.[12] Moreover, the dysbiosis is still present after 1 month of abstinence in a high percentage of patients,[13] which may be more of an indictment on persistently bad dietary patterns that persist.

As mentioned previously, bacteria in the gut can synthesize toxic molecules such as LPS (or lipopolysaccharides) or lipid and polysaccharide combinations. These endotoxins can activate inflammation in the intestines and remotely within the body. Additionally, high concentrations of LPS can increase intestinal permeability, therefore allowing toxins, undigested food, and microbes (or their immuno-stimulatory antigens) to "leak" into the blood initiating inflammatory cascades. LPS can affect brain chemistry by diminishing the activity of serotonin and decreasing the function of the serotonin transporter,[14] another biologic example of the gut-brain connection.

Functional medicine seeks to address core system issues that may be at the root of dysfunction of basic metabolic pathways affecting immunity, hormones, neurobiology, and inflammation and their integration in the systems biology of a whole person. Metabolic dysfunctions as part of the "whole person" approach to addiction and recovery therefore is an important aspect of patient- driven care with burgeoning science. The microbiome data explosion referencing the issue of dysbiosis, leaky gut (related to intestinal permeability [IP]), and inflammation in patients with classic inflammatory states such as rheumatoid arthritis or metabolic syndrome, also pertains to patients going through the process of recovery. A thorough assessment of microbial population and gut-barrier function should be part of the treatment plan. Specifically, advanced nutritional testing targeting functioning of the GI tract, analyzing for loss of variation in the gut microbiome, and identification of potential pathogens are part of this analysis. Various commercial laboratories* specialize in this approach to measure the gut's microbiology (beneficial bacteria, presence of pathogens, additional bacteria), gut metabolic markers (SCFAs, n-butyrate, b-glucoronidase, pH, SCFA distribution, fecal lactoferrin, occult blood), digestion and absorption chymotrypsin, putrefactive SCFAs, meat and vegetable fibers, and fecal fats). These tests will indicate how well the patient is digesting their macronutrients, if there is any malabsorption, presence of inflammation in the gut, presence of pathogens (dysbioisis), distribution of "bad and good" bacteria, and production of beneficial metabolites. Another valuable evaluation is the lactulose/mannitol assay (IP test), which measures creatinine, lactulose, and total urine volume. Identifying abnormalities in this testing allows one to identify individuals with "leaky gut" where the integrity of the columnar epithelial barrier tight junctions and the contiguous mucopolysaccharide barrier layer are not whole or functioning optimally enough to segregate foreign antigens, bacteria, viruses, etc., from coming into contact with the vast immune barrier lining the entire GI tract. The test analyzes urinary clearance of lactulose and mannitol (2 sugar molecules that cannot be metabolized by the intestines). Elevate lactulose indicates that there is permeability of the gut, while a decrease in mannitol suggests that absorption is impaired (specifically atrophy of the villi). Utilizing additional specialized intestinal permeability nutritional testing offers an understanding of this hyper-permeability by detecting "leaking" antigens for: intestinal cells' cytoskeleton (actomyosin IgA), tight junction proteins (occludin/zonulin IgG, IgA, and IgM), and endotoxins (LPS IgG, IgA, and IgM) as a tool in identifying these patient subsets. Again, these intestinal permeability antigen tests are commercially available for clinical use.**

** Cyrex Labs https://www.cyrexlabs.com/CyrexTestsArrays

## NUTRITIONAL DEFICIENCIES

Functional medicine also addresses the micronutrient deficiencies that results from substance abuse. For example, alcohol can lead to deficiencies in vitamin A, C, D, E, Bs, and K, as well as mineral deficiencies. Stimulants can suppress the appetite and thus may lead to a decrease in the consumption of foods containing the essential macro and micronutrients. Drugs such as cocaine and marijuana can cause problems with vitamin B and zinc absorption.[7] Zinc deficiency is also prevalent in alcohol-dependent individuals and closely related to high levels of reactive oxygen species (ROS), acetylaldehyde, and lipid peroxidation products. Low levels of zinc in the small intestine (ileum) can cause a disruption of the intestinal barrier, reducing the tight junction proteins and therefore increasing intestinal permeability.[15] Additionally, zinc has cytoprotective activity, which helps balance the mast cell (involved in defense against parasites and microbial infections) in the intestines.[16] As mentioned before, low vitamin-D levels are linked to use of narcotics, alcohol, and drug abuse in general. In fact, it has been observed that patients with low vitamin-D levels need higher doses of narcotics to manage the pain, compared to those with normal vitamin-D levels. Vitamin D has further benefits in the gut. Deficiencies are associated with contributing to or worsening dysbiosis and increasing permeability, neither of which are desirable and associated with multiple neuroendocrine and inflammatory sequelae. Today, vitamin D is being researched as a treatment for drug abuse and addiction because of its effect on the dopaminergic pathways. Animal studies looking at a vitamin-D treatment "showed significant attenuated methamphetamine-induced reductions in dopamine and metabolites when compared to control, indicating that vitamin D provides protection for the dopaminergic system against the depleting effects of methamphetamine."[17] Tocopherols and tocotrienols are fat-soluble vitamins (forms of vitamin E), which act as antioxidants and play an essential role in protecting the gut's lining from ROS. Clinical trials have shown that supplementing meals with vitamin E reduces inflammation of the lining of the colon and reduces bacterial translocation from the lumen of the intestines.[18]

Given the impact that drugs and substance abuse has on micronutrient deficiency and gut health, functional medicine seeks to evaluate the levels of these distinct factors to aid with healing process of drug detoxification. Again, advanced nutritional testing evaluating plasma or urine levels of amino acids, antioxidants, B vitamins, essential fatty acids, and minerals exist commercially for both whole blood and WBC intracellular determinations.*** These WBC micronutrients tests can measure 35 markers in white blood cells: vitamins, metabolites (choline, inositol, carnitine), CHO metabolism (chromium, fructose sensitivity, glucose-insulin metabolism), antioxidants, minerals, fatty acids (oleic acid), and amino acids. Treating these deficiencies appropriately reduces metabolic dysfunction, improves energy, aids in basic physiology important to the recovery process and helps reestablish normalization of neuroendocrine and immune function. In essence, this is part of the physiologic and systems recovery process needed.

***Spectra Cell Lab https://www.spectracell.com/

## GUT-BRAIN AXIS

In recent years there has been a growing amount of evidence about the connection between the gut and the brain, their communication through the autonomic nervous system, the enteric nervous system, and the HPA (hypothalamic-pituitary adrenal) axis. Through both neurons and hormones the brain can exert an effect on the intestine's immune cells, enteric neurons, smooth muscle cells, and entero-chromaffin cells. This, in turn, influences (and is influenced by) the gut microbiome in bidirectional modes. On the other hand, it has also been suggested that the microbes in the gut play an important role in the gut-brain axis: they interact not only with cells in the intestine but also directly with the central nervous system through the production of neurotransmitters (GABA, serotonin, dopamine), protection of the intestinal barrier, and tight junction integrity, bacterial metabolites, mucosal immune regulation, and modulation of enteric sensory afferents.[19]

To further explain this relationship, studies on mice have shown that gut microbes are of utmost importance for the development of the central and enteral nervous system. Germ-free mice resulted in an altered expression and synthesis of neurotransmitters, which affected brain as well as gut function (e.g., delayed gastric emptying, reduced migrating motor complex).[19] Other studies have shown how germ-free mice have memory dysfunction due to an altered expression of BDNF (brain-derived-neurotrophic factor) in the hippocampus and an increased HPA stress response.[20] Conversely, studies looking at supplementation with probiotics have shown a change in the CNS's biochemistry by altering the levels of BDNF, GABA, serotonin, and dopamine, therefore altering mood and brain function. Trials studying the effect of probiotics on the HPA response and immune system have also been promising. Probiotics have shown to attenuate the HPA response by decreasing production of ACTH and corticosteroids in both urine and saliva. Regarding the effects of probiotics on the immune systems, human studies have shown a decrease in pro-inflammatory cytokines (TNF-a, IL-6, and IL-12) and an increase in regulatory cytokine (Il-10, and increased NK cell activity.[20] An ever-expanding literature of both basic science, translational, and clinical evidence connecting the gut microbiome to both regulatory T-cell immunity, cytokine production, nutritional dysfunction, bowel inflammation, and neuroendocrine dysfunction all prove the importance of these systems on health, inflammation, and now being elucidated in addiction states involving all substances. Their role and interventional correction in clinical study open trials would be the next phase of the comprehensive approach to addiction and recovery that may be done independently or concurrently with classic approaches and indicated usual and customary pharmacotherapies. In the meantime, for the individual patient these functional medicine approaches remain generally safe, science grounded, and increasing in use in prominent academic centers (Cleveland Clinic) and a solid adjunctive option to the conventional framework of therapeutic options in addiction and recovery and in other subspecialties of medicine.

## FOOD SENSITIVITIES

Food allergies refer to the immediate IgE mediated response to a food or foreign substance, which results in release of histamine, leading to symptoms such as skin rash, abdominal pain, angioedema, and bronchoconstriction. There are also delayed response food allergies, which refers to the IgG-mediated food allergies. These "delayed response" allergies can occur a few hours to a couple of days after the person has been exposed to the antigen. On the other hand, a food sensitivity is an immune-mediated response to a particular food, which does not involve immunoglobulins but rather other aspects of the immune system. The last classification is "food intolerance," which refers to a non-immune-mediated food reaction driven by poor nutritional status or impaired detoxification.[21]

Food allergies and sensitivities can contribute to and result from inflammation and immune dysfunction. These can stimulate cytokine release, NF-KB activation, and an increase in intestinal permeability. When allergenic foods are consumed (delayed onset and IgE), there is an increase in damage to the intestinal lining, which in turn activates NF-KB, a potent inflammatory signal, resulting in the synthesis of inflammatory cytokines, therefore leading to immune dysfunction and overactivity. NF-KB and cytokines increase intestinal permeability, which leads to a vicious circle of inflammation and immune activation in our body.[21]

Adverse food reactions (allergies, sensitivity, or intolerance) all can be a cause or aggravate many health problems. These include migraines, inflammatory diseases, depression, asthma, attention deficit disorders, hypertensions, IBD, and many others.[22] Therefore, it is important to address the issue of adverse food reactions and identify the cause and effect relationship between ingestion of the food culprit and the reaction even if not Ig E mediated. This process can be difficult to interpret. Functional medicine relies on several tests and protocols to identify these types of potentially adverse food reactions and utilizes food elimination as an intervention. Hence, the "elimination diet" utility as an inexpensive protocol, which requires the patient to fast or eliminate the most allergenic foods (e.g., dairy, wheat, gluten, eggs, peanuts, soy, corn, chocolate, caffeine) for a period of time. The patient is instructed to eliminate the foods for at least 14 days (ideally 3 weeks). In the reintroduction phase, the patient starts adding one food at a time over varying periods of time such as 3 days to 3 weeks. The food being reintroduced is eaten several times in one day and then the patient waits for 2 more days, to see if any reaction to the food or symptoms appear. If no symptoms appear, then the patient adds a second food for testing.[23] If the patient reacts to a certain type of food, then it is identified and as an allergenic food and removed from the diet.

Other testing methods include: serum IgG4 assay, serum IgE assay, double-blind placebo-controlled food challenges, and skin-prick testing. Of special interest is the serum IgG4 testing, since it identifies delayed-onset food allergies (24 to 48 hours after ingesting the food), which we might not be able to identify otherwise. This test uses sensitive enzyme-linked-immunosorbent assay (ELISA) to assess the relative IgG antibody level response to different foods. If there are multiple foods, which cause a high IgG4 reactions, it might point to the idea that there is an intestinal permeability issue in the patient as many antigens are potentially traversing the increased permeable gut lining and interacting with surveillance immune cells in the lamina propria of the gut, replete with surveillance and T cells capable of up or down regulating immune responses (Treg). Activation leads to the production of IgG4 antibodies by lymphocytes.[24] The ALCAT**** test evaluates platelet aggregation and white blood cell movements.

****ALCAT https://cellsciencesystems.com/providers/alcat-test/food-panels/

After mixing the blood sample with food extracts. However, this last method has been controversial due to the many false positives (28%) presented in the results when tested for validity. To heal the gut and reduce symptoms possibly resulting from allergies and sensitivities, it is advisable to implement a rotation diet or plan while repairing the gut and replacing missing enzyme support, micronutrients, vitamins and aiding in microbiome optimization. The patient is encouraged to eliminate the most immune-reactive foods (as per test results or historical food log) and eat the less immuno-reactive foods once every 4 days (dietary rotation). This way, the patient diminishes the IgG response and gives the body a time to heal from the constant inflammatory state. It is also important to provide nutritional support for the leaky gut to help it heal during this phase.[24] This will be further explored in the functional protocol section. So how does addiction relate to adverse food reactions and our gut? The "second brain" as Michael Gershon referred to the gut, is lined with neurons and nerves (enteric nervous system), which produces neurotransmitters and is in constant communication with the brain.[25] These neurotransmitters and immunologically active substances produced by the gut microbiota can be transported by the blood, cross the blood-brain barrier, and influence the CNS.[26] Therefore, a "leaky gut," dysbiosis, and consequent microbiome changes associated with secondary immune and neural hormonal axis disturbances may adversely influence depression, anxiety, mood disorders, and chemical imbalances. With alcohol dependence, the existence of leaky gut and the effect on recovering individuals has been established by Leclercq and colleagues as previously mentioned.[6] Alcohol-dependent subjects frequently develop emotional symptoms that contribute to the persistence of alcohol associated GI disturbances in this study of 60 patients. Of the cohort, 46% had altered intestinal permeability and altered gut-microbiota composition as measured by advanced PCR RNA technology methods. This group remained with high scores of depression, anxiety, and alcohol craving after a short-term 3-week detoxification program. These results are consistent with the existence of a gut-brain axis disturbance in alcohol dependence, in which the GI microbiota altered the gut-barrier function and influenced behavior in alcohol dependence. Therefore, according to these authors the findings open a previously unidentified field of research for the treatment and the management of alcohol dependence, targeting the gut microbiota. An extrapolation from alcohol dependence to other substances can now realistically be entertained as another potential intervention point utilizing the GI functional approach to addiction and a whole person treatment perspective. Further studies of this nature are needed to make more substantial recommendations. Be that as it may, it is now scientifically proven that the microbiome has both primary and secondary immune, endocrine, and neurobiologic effects that may affect mood, sleep, anxiety levels, and furthermore be a target for clinical intervention in many specialties including addiction medicine.

## Hormones

Addiction to substances and drugs leads to hormonal imbalances. One example of these imbalances is the dysregulation of the HPA axis: specifically higher levels of cortisol and reduced inhibitory feedback control.[27] Alcohol and nicotine have been found to increase cortisol, cause a dysregulation of the HPA axis, and may cause a decrease in reactivity to other stressors (which can be a factor in the known high risk for relapse in drug addiction).[28] The glucocorticoid hormones facilitate DA (dopamine) transmission in the NAc (nucleus accumbens) and with chronic exposure to stress, the repeated increases in glucocorticoid hormones, and DA lead to a sensitization of the reward system. This sensitization, which continues long after the exposure to stress, can make the person more responsive to the drug and more likely to fuel the drug addiction. This stress can contribute to a predisposition to use drugs and can also make the person more vulnerable to relapse.[29]

As explained before, the emotional stress (increase in glucocorticoids) and negative affect have been shown to increase drug craving in addicts. Acute cortisol administration and a high level of stress have been found to increase cocaine craving. This has been linked to the activation of the DA system and an increase in receptor sensitivity, which leads to an enhancement of the
mesolimbic DA response to drugs. Not only does a hyper-responsive HPA axis contribute to drug addiction, but there are studies that show that a hypo-responsive HPA axis can contribute to enhanced drug consumption as apart of a maladaptive stress response.[29]

High levels of cortisol and HPA dysregulation may not only lead to increased risk of relapse but also several health consequences. For example, chronic high levels of cortisol can cause weight gain, memory loss, insulin resistance, obesity around the waist, hypertension, glucose intolerance, and an increase in inflammation in general.[21]

Another system greatly affected by drug and substance abuse is the gonadal function. The gonadotropin releasing hormone (GnRH = stimulated secretion of luteinizing hormone and follicle stimulating hormone) is in part inhibited by the endogenous opioids. Exogenous opioid use can also cause an inhibition of the GnRH, which in turn causes a dysfunction of the HPG (hypothalamic-pituitary-gonadal) and reduced levels of testosterone (in males) and menstrual cycle disruption (in females). Low levels of estrogen and testosterone have also a direct impact on cravings by reducing CNS opioid expression, which may contribute to relapse.[30]

Apart from the effects that hypogonadism can have on risk of relapse and craving in substance-dependent individuals, there are several other risks that arise from this issue. For example, hypogonadism can lead to fatigue, weakness, depression, slow healing, and low libido.[21]

Both acute and chronic consumption of alcohol has been seen to reduce GH (growth hormone) and IGF-1 (insulin growth factor-1) levels in humans. Additionally, alcohol blunts the GH response by suppressing the pituitary gland. This is very important, especially in adolescents who depend on GH for the puberty phase, as well as for older individuals for whom a deficiency in GH can lead to a suppressed immune system and muscle weakness. Additionally, well-known effects of chronic alcohol consumption such as metabolic bone disturbances, lipid and glucose balance in the body, and subsequent cardiovascular abnormalities are all well established. Brittle blood sugar homeostasis with chronic alcohol consumption may raise blood sugar in the fed state and conversely lowers blood glucose in a fasted state (leading to hypoglycemia and is some cases can cause neurological consequences).[31]

## Hormone Testing

Another aspect of the functional approach to addiction evaluation and treatment paradigm is hormonal assessment. Comprehensive hormone testing from commercially available labs are readily available for complete male and female panels. Whether urinary testing of metabolites and pathway is globally needed remains debatable but is obtainable from certain labs. Given the influence that substances and drugs have on the HPA axis, it is important to test the impact on cortisol as well as estrogen, progesterone, testosterone(free/total), DHEA sulfate and thyroid function (Free T3, Free T4, TSH, reverse T3), and gonadotropins (FSH/LH) in both men and women. Cortisol can be measured in blood, urine, and saliva as a helpful stress biomarker aside from its inherent adrenal function. Specifically, for cortisol, the most accurate testing is done by taking 4 samples of the saliva during a 24-hour period and mapping the levels throughout the day (showing the cortisol curve throughout the day) and in conjunction with DHEA, another adrenal hormone. This type of testing is informative of the diurnal physiology variations in individual patients and helpful in monitoring therapy.

## Addiction and Recovery Functional Protocol and Approach

As we have seen in the previous sections, the consequences of substance addiction and foods go beyond chemical imbalances in the brain. This complex process involves several organ systems and complex metabolic pathways, therefore addressing brain neurochemistry and the constellation of multisystem interactions within a person (hormonal, immune, gut, cardiovascular, nutrition, and secondary micronutrient deficiencies) in addiction will be the most comprehensive and optimal approach. Failing to treat other aspects mentioned previously (the gut, the immune system, and hormonal imbalances) is associated with a higher risk of relapse. For that reason, functional medicine seeks to treat the whole person through the lens of systems approach to illness attempting to identify root causes or dysfunctions and not only as a compartmentalized set of symptoms or solely a brain disease when addressing addiction and recovery.

## Nutrition Principles

As nutrition and an anti-inflammatory lifestyle and nutritional patterns have been reviewed in this book, we will limit discussion in this section to what is pertinent to the functional approaches relevant to addiction treatment. Essentially, as with other pro-inflammatory conditions (diabetes mellitus, insulin resistance, obesity, etc.) the approach to addiction would be similar. While there is no singular nutritional pattern or diet for addiction, the general principles remain the same. An anti-inflammatory Mediterranean diet minus any identified food sensitivities makes sense; this can be adjusted for carbohydrate intake and total caloric needs based on the patient's body composition and desired optimal body composition goals for healthy living. Of the most common sensitivities in inflamed populations, elimination of wheat, gluten, and dairy are primary considerations early on for a few weeks to 90 days and in some cases beyond. Balancing priority of recovery and food dietary changes is as important as drug abstinence, processed sugar intake reduction, and simultaneous elimination of excessive dairy and gluten.

Individualized and rational decisions for executing these changes are needed so as not to create an excessive burden on individual patients. This approach is useful and effective in inflammatory patient populations of all types, including systemic inflammatory rheumatic populations of both autoimmune and primary immune dysfunction or patients with chronic pain. Large randomized controlled trials of the AFMD in substance addiction do not yet exist, but the rationale for its use given the myriad of metabolic, immunologic, and microbiome similarities in the inflammatory systemic patient and addiction populations makes this approach intriguing, rational, and pragmatic. Other low glycemic index eating patterns with an abundance of healthy fats, fiber, and moderate clean protein allow patients individual variety and options to enhance enjoyment of eating rather than focusing on deprivation.

## Eliminating: Dysbiosis, Pathogens, and SIBO

Dysbiosis is defined as an imbalance of normal commensal bacteria diversity and numbers coupled with increased populations of abnormal or pathogenic bacteria. This imbalance leads to chronic inflammation, leaky gut, disturbed metabolism with changes in blood-brain barrier, metabolic endotoxemia, increased mood disorders, and immune dysfunction. The resulting myriad of biochemical, endocrine, neurologic, and secondary proinflammatory immune responses create havoc increasing cumulative disease burden on the cardiovascular system and potentially amplifying the addiction state in a closed loop setting. Treating the gut is a crucial step toward recovery of addiction as these secondary microbiome conditions can slow down recovery processes and exacerbate addiction related dysfunctions.[26,27,29] Even though it is not part of the traditional detoxification program, addressing dysbiosis is critical for restoring balance in the body.

Elimination of dysbiosis, pathogens, and SIBO involves several steps and different therapeutic treatments. Utilizing the functional medicine paradigm entails dietary change to

reduce the SIBO effect, and reference is made to FODMAPs dietary plans as an excellent starting point for implementation. However, this may not be sufficient in most individuals with severe SIBO, which can be a chronic or semi-chronic condition to consistently address in some patients both via diet, antibiotics, and antibacterial plant-based natural products such as berberine, oregano oil, and others. Using the concepts of recovery, cutting out offending foods such as high fructose corn syrup (HFCS)—with its addictive qualities, partially hydrogenated fats, and trans fats with pro-inflammatory effects—makes an excellent start.

Eliminating high FODMaps foods in individuals with SIBO suspected clinically or proven by formal GI nutritional testing (SIBO Breat test) is a recommended next step. Use of broad spectrum antibiotics for 10 to 14 days (tetracycline or derivative, neomycin, rifmaxin) when indicated along with probiotics and followed by plant-based antibacterial active compounds such as plant tannins, berberine, and others would be a preliminary alternative. GI sensitivity analysis of the microbiome, testing for existing pathogens, and improving diversity of bacterial populations with probiotics and suppression of pathogens is a helpful guide to manage a patient's symptoms with respect to flatulence, bloating, gas pain, and quality and quantity of stool and bowel movements. One such nutritional paradigm as, described by Dr. Alex Vasquez, calls for eradication of dysbiosis calls (i.e., "starve, poison, crowd, purge, and support immunity"). Recolonizing with healthy bacteria with consistent intake of adequate colonies and types of beneficial bacteria is desirable. While there are a wide market of probiotics available, randomized controlled trials for "the best" type is sorely lacking. A functional approach is recommended based on testing and clinical symptoms. In general, bifidobacteria, lactobacilli, and other live species colonies are recommended, many of which require refrigeration. Prebiotic foods (banana, chicory) and fermented foods should be part of the diet (sauerkraut, pickles, pickled ginger, kimchi, yogurt, etc.) to aid the microbiome. The paradigm refers to the following steps:

1. **Starve**: Entails starving the "bad bacteria" and pathogens, thus removing foods that bacteria feed on will be the aim of the diet prescribed. The patient should avoid sugar (fruits and sweeteners), grains, soluble fibers, gums (thickeners or stabilizing agents), prebiotic foods (beans, vegetables, roots/herbs, agave), and dairy. These all contain carbohydrates fermented by pathogens and lead to overgrowth of other pathogens and "bad bacteria."

2. **Poison**: This step involves "poisoning" the detrimental microbes in the gut by either killing them or inhibiting their growth. The presence of severe infections will require antimicrobial drugs (antibiotics), while in less severe cases a natural antibiotic botanical will suffice. The period of treatment can last from 1 to 3 months, depending on the response of the patient and adherence to the other steps of the protocol.

   - Botanical antibiotics: oregano oil, berberine, artemisia annua, St. John's Wort, bismuth, peppermint oil, uva vursi, garlic, thyme, anise, caprylic acid, and others.
   - Antibiotics: Rifaximin and Neomycin are the two most commonly used for treating SIBO and pathogens in the intestines, given the fact that they are non-absorbable and therefore will stay in the intestines. Addition of digestive enzymes: Supplementing with proteolytics, lipolytic, and amylolytic enzymes has several advantages during the functional protocol. These enzymes will aid in the digestion of carbohydrates, proteins, and fats. Besides helping with digestion, proteolytic enzymes can help reduce immune complexes, stimulate immune function, stimulate anti-inflammatory pathways, and inhibit the formation of microbial films. Specifically, proteolytic enzymes are

important for breaking up microbial films and allowing the antimicrobial agents (drugs and oils) to penetrate the films, therefore effectively attacking the pathogens.

3. **Crowd**: This step involves crowding out the "bad bacteria" with the "good bacteria." The use of probiotic supplements has been shown to boost the immune system (modulating IgA and IgG immune cells, B cells, T-killer cells, and inflammatory response), improve digestive function, reduce endotoxemia, and reduce the harmful effect of dysbiosis. As mentioned before, different strains of probiotics can have anti-inflammatory effects in the gut, therefore supplementing with *bifidobacteria, lactobacillus,* and *saccharomyces* will be a crucial step for normalizing the function of the gastrointestinal tract.

4. **Purge**: This step involves getting rid of impurities. Eating a low-fermentation fiber-rich diet is of utmost importance in order to allow for regular bowel movements. This one is the main means for eliminating toxins, microbial debris, and metabolites. If the diet is not sufficient for promoting bowel movement, the use of a magnesium supplement or ascorbic acid (laxative dose) is recommended.

5. **Support Immunity**: A diet free of sugars and "junk food" is ideal, since these promote inflammation and suppress the immune system. The use of vitamin and mineral supplements should be advised (at least for the initial stages), given the malabsorption and maldigestion issues that result from the dysbiosis, leaky gut, and pathogenic bacteria. Additionally, supplementation with L-glutamine, zinc, and vitamin A will provide the means for normalizing the intestinal permeability and immune function (refer to later sections for detailed uses and benefits of supplements).

## Supplements

The use of supplements for restoration of the brain, gut, and immune function, can serve as an aid in the functional protocol for addiction recovery.

## L-Glutamine

The purpose of glutamine supplementation is to aid in repairing the gut lining and decreasing intestinal permeability caused by stress, consumption of addictive substances, and foods. As mentioned before, glutamine is the preferred energy source for enterocytes and stimulates the growth of the epithelial cells. It has been shown to protect the epithelial cells by decreasing pathogens around them, decreasing cell apoptosis (due to DNA fragmentation), enhancing gut immune function, and enhancing its role as a barrier between the intestines and the bloodstream.

Furthermore, studies have shown that deprivation of glutamine can cause the villi to be atrophied, ulceration of the mucosal membrane, and injury to the cells.[32]

## L-theanine

L-Theanine is anon dietary amino acid (glutamate derivative), which has been shown to induce the elevation of glutathione. This is important because high levels of consumption of alcohol, increases the production of free radical, decreases GSH levels, and increases the LPOs in the liver.

L-theanine is converted to glutamate in the liver, which promotes the synthesis of glutathione (a powerful detoxifier and antioxidant). Sadzuka et al's study,[33] L-theanine administration was combined with alcohol consumption. L-theanine could reduce the synthesis of free radicals caused by alcohol consumption and suppressed their levels for up to 5 hours. In this study, researchers observed that L-theanine counteracted the loss of glutathione caused by the consumption of alcohol.[33] Additionally, this amino acid can directly impact brain chemistry and have a calming effect in the body. L-theanine crosses the blood-brain barrier and increases the levels of serotonin and GABA, which can help decrease anxiety and stress (due to their role in the pathophysiology of anxiety in the brain).[34]

## Vitamin D

The role of vitamin D3, really a prohormone more than a vitamin, has had an explosive effect in basic science immunology, cancer, cardiovascular, neurology, bone metabolism, and allergy and asthma literature to name a few. Its worldwide popularity is a paradox, as endemic deficiency and insufficiency of vitamin D3 exists. Couple these facts with the lack of uniformity in agreement on ideal Vitamin D3 blood levels, further adds confusion for both consumer patients and treating physicians. Here we will limit the commentary of Vitamin D3 to its role in addiction and recovery realms.

Using a mouse model, researchers have shown that Vitamin D3 modulates dopamine in the brain and can affect obesity and drug consumption with corresponding neuropharmacology changes modulated by both high fat diet and vitamin D3 deficiency and administration. Their findings suggest that reduced dietary D3 may be a contributing environmental factor enhancing diet induced obesity (DIO) as well as drug intake while eating a high-fat diet. Moreover, these data demonstrate that dopamine circuits are modulated by D3 signaling and may serve as direct or indirect targets for exogenous calcitriol.[35]

## Vitamin A

Supplementation with vitamin A helps support the immune system and gastro-intestinal tract. It has been shown to play a role in the growth and differentiation of intestinal cells. Deficiency of vitamin A is associated with shorter villi in the small bowel and higher rates of intestinal permeability.[36] Additionally, vitamin A is an important micronutrient for the proper function of the innate and adaptive immune systems. A deficiency in Vitamin A may result in reduction of NK cells, function of both neutrophils and macrophages, alteration of cytokine signaling, and compromises the first line of defense of the body.[37]

## Zinc

As mentioned before, zinc deficiency is highly prevalent in individuals with alcohol, opioid, and substance abuse. Zinc deficiency alters the microbial population of the intestines. Animal studies have shown how chronic consumption of alcohol can decrease concentration of zinc in the ileum, increase ROS and intestinal permeability, and reduce tight junction proteins.[38] A study on patients with Crohn's disease (high intestinal permeability), who added a supplement of zinc sulfate for 8 weeks, saw a significant improvement in intestinal barrier function. The importance of zinc in recovery is due to its antioxidant capacity and its anti-inflammatory effects, which help stabilize the membrane of mast cells (which release inflammatory cytokine when stimulated by allergies or injuries). Additionally, zinc is involved in anti-oxidant activity, hormone release, nerve impulse transmission in the CNS. Plus it regulates gene expression by acting as a DNA transcription factor and plays an important role in the immune response.[39]

## Omega-3 Fish Oil

Omega-3s are essential fatty acids, which have a plethora of benefits and functions. These polyunsaturated fatty acids (PUFAs) are essential for cognitive function, normal growth and development of the brain, as well as for the structure of the membrane of healthy cells. These PUFAs have been shown to help decrease overall inflammation in the body and may help reduce the risk of cardiovascular diseases. Despite this, the standard American diet (Sad Diet, i.e., one high in omega 6, trans fats, excessive processed sugar and salt and partially hydrogenated pro-inflammatory fats) is low in omega-3s and very high in omega-6s, which can result in a ration of up to 1:25 (omega-3 to omega:6), leading to a constant state of inflammation.[40] There are several types of omega-3s: DHA (part of cell membranes), EPA, and ALA (found in plants, this is less potent, and conversion of EPA and DHA is low). The EPA and DHA are found in higher concentration in coldwater fatty fish such as salmon, trout, sardines, anchovies, and mackerel. Given the fact that EPA and DHA are found only in seafood, supplementing with fish oil would be ideal. Fish has been studied for effects related to hyperlipidemia, hypertension, heart disease, diabetes, rheumatoid arthritis, SLE, MS, ADHD, cognitive decline, and many others. Several studies have looked at the role omega-3s play in addiction and recovery. Tajuddin et al saw a 90% decrease in neuroinflammation and cell apoptosis in cultures of rat brain cells exposed to alcohol and fish oil, compared to the cells exposed to alcohol only.[41]

Additionally, high consumption of alcohol and nicotine is linked to a lower level of omega-3 in the body affecting the membrane fluidity, integrity and neurotransmission. A deficiency in omega-3s results in a malfunction of the mesocorticolimbic pathways (the reward and cognitive control of behavior pathways), which may increase cravings.[42] Moreover, DHA and EPA deficiency can lead to an overactive HPA axis, which can translate to excessive stress and depression.

Using the articles obtained by a PubMed research, this article reviews 3 aspects of NF-κB/inflammatory inhibition by fish oil.[1] Inhibition of the NF-κB pathway at several subsequent steps: extracellular, free omega-3 inhibits the activation of the toll-like receptor 4 by endotoxin and free saturated fatty acids. In addition, EPA/DHA blocks the signaling cascade between toll-like/cytokine receptors and the activator of NF-κB, IKK. Oxidized omega-3 also interferes with the initiation of transcription by NF-κB.[2] The altered profile of lipid mediators generated during inflammation, with production of the newly identified, DHA-derived inflammation-resolving mediator classes (in addition to the formation of less pro-inflammatory eicosanoids from EPA) called Resolvin D1 and Protectin D, act as potent, endogenous, lipid mediators that attenuate neutrophil migration and tissue injury in peritonitis and ischemia-reperfusion injury. Their production is increased in the later stages of an inflammatory response, at which time they enhance the removal of neutrophils.[3] Modulation of vagal tone with potential anti-inflammatory effects: vagal fibers innervating the viscera down-regulate inflammation by activating nicotinic receptors upon infiltrating and resident macrophages. Stimulation of the efferent vagus is therapeutic in experimental septic shock. Fish oil supplementation increases vagal tone following myocardial infarction and in experimental human endotoxinemia.[43]

## Stress Reduction

Stress can be viewed in many ways and can originate from many different sources (emotional, environment, nutritional, physical, etc). For example, chronic sleep deprivation can lead to immune dysfunction, and chemical disruption can be the foundation for an impairment in the endocrine system through environmental endocrine disruptors (e.g., BisA plastics) with long-term effects. Emotional stress can lead to a cascade of inflammatory events, including elevated cortisol, reduced thyroid hormones, increased intestinal permeability, sleep disruption, dysbiosis, decreased production of IgA, suppression of the immune system and NK cells, and an increase in nutritional needs (vitamins, minerals, and amino acids).[21]

Stress has been regarded as one of the major causes of relapse (even after a long time in abstinence), and it is the most common trigger for every type of addiction. Drug users are more sensitive to stress, making them more likely to seek drugs when under stress. For this reason, it is vital to include stress management in the recovery for addiction.[44]

Therefore, we seek natural stress reduction techniques that can help the patient cope with the emotional stress we deal with every day. These include using methods such as journaling, meditation, mind-body interventions, botanicals, aromatherapy (refer to Chapter 22 - Aromatherapy chapter), homeopathy (refer to Chapter 14 - Homeopathy chapter), and breath work.

Studies have looked at the effect of mindfulness practice on the brain, inflammation, and stress. A study by Bhasin, et al showed how an 8-week intervention in which they taught subjects how to implement the relaxation response techniques (mindfulness meditation, breathing, and body scan) reduced the expression of genes related to inflammatory response and stress-related pathways. The intervention also enhanced expression of genes linked to mitochondrial function, insulin signaling, energy metabolism, and telomere length.[44]

## Journaling

Expressive writing or journaling on a daily or recurring basis has been used as technique to help reduce stress. In journaling the patient is asked to write about a stressful experience, the current situation they are dealing with, or a traumatic event. Often, patients find that writing about their feelings and thoughts about the situation is a way to self-exploration, releasing emotions, and even a way to cope with the traumatic events themselves. There are several reasons why journaling is thought to help patients. For example, simply thinking about the experience and expressing everything the person is feeling helps the patient organize his/her thoughts about the event. Also, the act of taking the first step to rationalize their feelings privately often leads the person to be more open to talking about the event or situation with others.[45]

Expressive writing has been studied for its impact on different health conditions, including sleep apnea, rheumatoid arthritis, migraine headaches, depression, PTSD, and cancer. Dr. James W. Pennebajer (University of Texas at Austin, Chief of Division of Psychology) has done several studies with a 20-minute expressive writing intervention, which has shown promising results in reduction of stress, anxiety, depression, and decreasing number of sick days. Using this same 20-minute intervention, Meshberg-Cohen and her team studied 149 women who were being treated for substance-use disorder in a residential facility. The participants attended 4 writing sessions in 4 days and were followed up 2 weeks and 1 month later. After 2 weeks, the writing intervention reduced depression, anxiety, and trauma symptom severity compared to control. Yet there was no difference between the 2 groups after 1 month, which is probably because both groups were in a residential recovery facility. Regardless of this second outcome, the intervention proved successful when helping patients work through stressful events and deal with their emotions in a safe and private environment.[46]

## Meditation

One goal of yoga is meditation. Deepak Chopra has stated that "Meditation is not forcing your mind to be quiet; it's finding the quiet that is already there".[47] Through it we bring awareness to the silence and expand this awareness into our daily lives. Meditation entails directing one's attention on a single point, be it: a mantra (word or phrase repetition), breath, drishti (focus point), and bodily sensations. It involves turning one's attention from the worldly distractions, ruminating thoughts, and outward senses to the present moment and our internal world. As Baer describes, through meditation there is a cognitive change where the person realizes that the meanings associated with a thought may be inaccurate.

So, how does this translate to recovery from addiction? Meditation has been shown to decrease inflammation at the cellular level; increase immune function; decrease stress, anxiety, and depression; reduce activation of the amygdala; increase gyrification of the brain; reduce cortisol levels; and many other benefits.[48] Additionally, from changes seen at the physical levels, meditation also has a great impact at the emotional and spiritual level. It has been proven to help with anger management skills, emotion regulation, coping skills, motivation, stress management, and self-confidence; it can also alleviate tension and give greater psychological balance in general.[49] These components are negatively correlated with drug craving, relapse, and drug use.[50]

## Vagus Nerve Immunology and Addiction

The role of parasympathetic stimulation in health, wellness, immunology, and now in the field of addiction as an integrative modality, is worth mentioning here in concert and following the "Mind-Body" section on breathwork. Inhibition of inflammatory pathways has been discussed, and the state of active inflammation created by addiction is an important healing and treatment focus. Given this, the role of parasympathetic activity on the brain, behavior, and immunity is discussed by Pavlov in this citation from 2005 that demonstrated that the efferent vagus nerve inhibits pro-inflammatory cytokine release and protects against systemic inflammation; this vagal function was termed **"the cholinergic anti-inflammatory pathway."** The discovery that the innate immune response is regulated partially through this neural pathway provides a new understanding of the mechanisms that control inflammation.[51]

Furthermore, from a critical review of the evidence on the cholinergic anti-inflammatory pathway and its mode of action, the following conclusions were reached by D. Martelli in their 2014[52] review of this topic that included the following points dissecting the complex nature of this neural immune network as the following points are emphasized:

(1) Both local and systemic inflammation may be suppressed by electrical stimulation of the peripheral cut end of either vagus.

(2) The spleen mediates most of the systemic inflammatory response (measured by TNF-α production) to systemic endotoxin and is also the site where that response is suppressed by vagal stimulation.

(3) The anti-inflammatory effect of vagal stimulation depends on the presence of noradrenaline-containing nerve terminals in the spleen.

(4) There is no disynaptic connection from the vagus to the spleen via the splenic sympathetic nerve: vagal stimulation does not drive action potentials in the splenic nerve.

(5) Acetylcholine-synthesizing T lymphocytes provide an essential non-neural link in the anti-inflammatory pathway from vagus to spleen.

(6) Alpha-7 subunit-containing nicotinic receptors are essential for the vagal anti-inflammatory action: their critical location is uncertain but is suggested here to be on splenic sympathetic nerve terminals.

(7) The vagal anti-inflammatory pathway can be activated electrically or pharmacologically, but it is not the efferent arm of the inflammatory reflex response to endotoxemia.

Thus from a practical standpoint it makes sense to address and consider all practices and activities that stimulate the parasympathetic neural immune pathways. This should be an adjunct to the total approach to recovery in addiction from an immunology, neural, hormonal, and psychologic perspective replete with science- and evidence-based solutions. Yoga, breathwork, mediation, exercise, vagal stimulation, and parasympathetic stimulation all re-create these sets of desirable physiologic beneficial effects in translational biologic and functional neural perspectives.

## REFERENCES

1. Lutter M, Nestler EJ. Homeostatic and hedonic signals interact in the regulation of food intake. *Journal of Nutrition.* 2009;139(3):629–632.
2. Avena NM, Gold MS. Food and addiction—sugars, fats and hedonic overeating. *Addiction.* 2011;106;1214–1215.
3. Volkow ND, Wang G, Volkow ND, Wang G, Baler RD. Reward, dopamine and the control of food intake: Implications for obesity. *Trends in Cognitive Sciences.* 2010;15(1), 37–46.
4. Gearhardt A, Yokum S, Orr PL, Stice E, Corbin W, Brownell K. Neural correlates of food addiction. *Archives of General Psychiatry.* 2011;68(8). http://archpsyc.jamanetwork.com/article.aspx?articleid=1107239#ArticleInformation
5. Spangler R, Wittkowski KM, Goddard NL, Avena NM, Hoebel BG, Leibowitz SF. Opiate-like effects of sugar on gene expression in reward areas of the rat brain. *Molecular Brain Research.* 2004;124(2):134–142.
6. Leclercq S., Matamoros S, Cani PD, et al. Intestinal permeability, gut- bacterial dysbiosis, and behavioral markers of alcohol-dependence severity. *Proceedings of the National Academy of Sciences of the United States of America.* 2004;111(42):E4485.
7. Ross CC. Is alcohol or drug abuse taking a toll on your digestion? *Psychology Today,* April 10, 2016. https://www.psychologytoday.com/blog/real-healing/201604/is-alcohol-or-drug-abuse-taking-toll-your-digestion. Accessed September 15, 2016.
8. Purohit V, Bode JC, Bode C, et al. Alcohol, intestinal bacterial growth, intestinal permeability to endotoxin, and medical consequences: Summary of a symposium. *Alcohol.* 2008;42(5):349–361.
9. Oxenkrug G. Insulin resistance and dysregulation of tryptophan–kynurenine and Kynurenine–Nicotinamide adenine dinucleotide metabolic pathways. *Molecular Neurobiology.* 2010;48(2):294–301
10. Macedo D, Filho AJMC, Soares de Sousa, CN, et al. Antidepressants, antimicrobials or both? Gut microbiota dysbiosis in depression and possible implications of the antimicrobial effects of antidepressant drugs for antidepressant effectiveness, *Journal of Affective Disorders.* 2017;208: 22–32.
11. Banerjee S., Sindberg G., Wang F, et al. Opioid- induced gut microbial disruption and bile dysregulation leads to gut barrier compromise and sustained systemic inflammation. *Mucosal Immunology,* 2016 Nov;9(6):1418–1428.

12. Kirpich IA, Solovieva NV, Leikhter SN, et al. Probiotics restore bowel flora and improve liver enzymes in human alcohol-induced liver injury: a pilot study. *Alcohol.* 2008;42(8):675–682.

13. Mutlu EA, Gillevet PM, Rangwala H, et al. Colonic microbiome is altered in alcoholism. *American Journal of Physiology-Gastrointestinal and Liver Physiology.* 2012;302(9):G966–G978.

14. Mendoza C, Matheus N, Iceta R, Mesonero JE, Alcalde A I. Lipopolysaccharide induces alteration of serotonin transporter in human intestinal epithelial cells. *Innate Immunity.* 2009 Aug;15(4):243–50.

15. Zhong W, McClain C, Cave M, Kang Y, Zhou Z. The role of zinc deficiency in alcohol- induced intestinal barrier dysfunction. *American Journal of Physiology.* 2010;298(5): G625.

16. Penissi AB, Rudolph MI, Piezzi RS. Role of mast cells in gastrointestinal mucosal defense. *Biocell: Official Journal of the Sociedades Latinoamericanas De Microscopía Electronica.* 2003;27(2):163.

17. Eserian JK. Vitamin D as an effective treatment approach for drug abuse and addiction. *Journal of Medical Hypotheses and Ideas.* 2013;7(2):35–39.

18. Resnick C. Nutritional protocol for the treatment of intestinal permeability defects and related condition. *Natural Medicine Journal,* 2010;2(3):14–23.

19. Carabotti M, Scirocco A, Maselli MA, Severi C. The gut- brain axis: Interactions between enteric microbiota, central and enteric nervous systems. *Annals of Gastroenterology: Quarterly Publication of the Hellenic Society of Gastroenterology.* 2015;28(2):203–209.

20. Wang H, Lee I, Braun C, Enck P. Effect of probiotics on central nervous system functions in animals and humans—a systematic review. *Journal of Neurogastroenterology and Motility,* 2016 Oct 30;22(4):589–605.

21. Vazquez A. Food allergy and adverse food reactions: A few considerations and perspectives. Inflammation mastery: Introduction to functional inflammology and integrative pain management (pp. 376). Barcelona, Spain: International College of Human Nutrition and Functional Medicine; 2014. http://www.ichnfm.org/product-page/inflammation-mastery-4th-edition-2015

22. Alpay K, Ertaş M, Orhan EK, Üstay DK, Lieners C, Baykan, B. Diet restriction in migraine, based on IgG against foods: A clinical double-blind, randomised, crossover trial. *Cephalalgia.* 2010;30(7):829–837.

23. Rakel D. *Integrative Medicine.* 3rd ed. Philadelphia: Elsevier, 2015.

24. Grisanti R. *Insider's Guide—Interpretation of Food Allergy, Sensitivity, and Intolerance.* Functional Medicine University; 2008.

25. Gershon, Michael, The Second Brain: A New Groundbreaking Underastanding of Nervous disorders of the Stomach and Intestine, Harper collins, 1998.

26. Petra AI, Panagiotidou S, Hatziagelaki E, Stewart JM, Conti P, Theoharides TC. Gut- microbiota- brain axis and its effect on neuropsychiatric disorders with suspected immune dysregulation. *Clinical Therapeutics.* 2015;37(5): 984–995.

27. Thayer JF, Hall M, Sollers JJ 3rd, Fischer JE. Alcohol use, urinary cortisol, and heart rate variability in apparently healthy men: Evidence for impaired inhibitory control of the HPA axis in heavy drinkers. *International Journal of Psychophysiology.* 2006;59(3):244–250.

28. Lovallo WR. Cortisol secretion patterns in addiction and addiction risk. *International Journal of Psychophysiology.* 2006;59(3):195–202.

29. Goodman A. Neurobiology of addiction: an integrative review. *Biochemical Pharmacology.* 2008;75(1):266–322.

30. Brown TT, Wisniewski AB, Dobs, AS. Gonadal and adrenal abnormalities in drug users: Cause or consequence of drug use behavior and poor health outcomes. *American Journal of Infectious Diseases.* 2006;2(3):130.

31. Emanuele MA, Emanuele NV. Alcohol's effects on male reproduction. *Alcohol Health and Research World.* 1998;22(3):195–201

32. Larson SD, Li J, Chung DH, Evers BM. Molecular mechanisms contributing to glutamine-mediated intestinal cell survival. *American Journal of Physiology Gastrointestinal and Liver Physiology.* 2007;293(6):G1262.

33. Sadzuka Y, Inoue C, Hirooka S, Sugiyama T, Umegaki K, Sonobe T. Effects of theanine on alcohol metabolism and hepatic toxicity. *Biological and Pharmaceutical Bulletin.* 2005;28(9):1702–1706.

34. Nathan PJ, Lu K, Gray M, Oliver C. The neuropharmacology of L- theanine (N-ethyl- L- glutamine): a possible neuroprotective and cognitive enhancing agent. *Journal of Herbal Pharmacotherapy.* 2006;6(2):21.

35. Trinko JR, Land BB, Solecki WB, et al. Vitamin D3: A role in dopamine circuit regulation, diet-induced obesity, and drug consumption. *eNeuro.* 2016;3(3): ENEURO.0122-15.2016.

36. Bischoff S. "Gut health": a new objective in medicine? *BMC Medicine.* 2011;9:24.

37. Drake VJ, Angelo, G, Gombart AF, Immunity. 2016. Web site. http://lpi.oregonstate.edu/mic/health-disease/immunity#macronutrients.

38. Zhong W, McClain C, Cave M, Kang Y, Zhou Z. The role of zinc deficiency in alcohol- induced intestinal barrier dysfunction. *American Journal of Physiology.* 2010;298(5):G625.

39. Ciubotariu D, Ghiciuc CM, Lupusoru CE. Zinc involvement in opioid addiction and analgesia—should zinc supplementation be recommended for opioid- treated persons? Substance Abuse Treatment, Prevention, and Policy. 2015;10:29.

41. Ehrlich S. Omega-3 fatty acids. University of Maryland Medical Center. Web site. http://umm.edu/health/medical/altmed/supplement/omega3-fatty-acids. Accessed October 10, 2016.

41. Tajuddin N, Moon K, Marshall SA, et al. Neuroinflammation and neurodegeneration in adult rat brain from binge ethanol exposure: abrogation by docosahexaenoic acid.(research article). *Plos ONE.* 2014;9(7).

42. Rabinovitz S. Effects of omega-3 fatty acids on tobacco craving in cigarette smokers: a double- blind, randomized, placebo-controlled pilot study. *Journal of Psychopharmacology.* 2014;28(8):804–809.

43. Singer P, Shapiro H, Theilla M,et al. Anti-inflammatory properties of omega-3 fatty acids in critical illness: novel mechanisms and an integrative perspective. *Intensive Care Medicine.* 2008;34:1580.

44. Bhasin M, Dusek JA, Chang, B-H, et al. Relaxation response induces temporal transcriptome changes in energy metabolism, insulin secretion and inflammatory pathways. *PLoS ONE.* 2013;8(5):E62817.

45. Robb-Nicholson CMD. Writing about emotions may ease stress and trauma. Harvard Health Publishing. Harvard Medical School. http://www.health.harvard.edu/healthbeat/writing-about-emotions-may-ease-stress-and-trauma. Accessed October 17, 2016.

46. Meshberg-Cohen S, Svikis D, McMahon TJ. Expressive writing as a therapeutic process for drug-dependent women. *Substance Abuse.* 2014;35:80–88.

47. https://www.goodreads.com/quotes/345259-meditation-is-not-a-way-of-making-your-mind-quiet

48. Pace TWW, Negi LT, Adame DD, et al. Effect of compassion meditation on neuroendocrine, innate immune and behavioral responses to psychosocial stress. *Psychoneuroendocrinology.* 2009;34(1):87–98.

49. Tang Y-Y, Tang R, Posner MI. Mindfulness meditation improves emotion regulation and reduces drug abuse. *Drug and Alcohol Dependence.* 2016;163:S13–18.

50. Young SN. Biologic effects of mindfulness meditation: Growing insights into neurobiologic aspects of the prevention of depression. *Journal of Psychiatry and Neuroscience.* 2011;36(2):75–77.

51. Pavlov VA, Tracey KJ, The vagus nerve and the inflammatory reflex—linking immunity and metabolism. *Nature Reviews Endocrinology.* 2012;8(12):743–754.

52. Martelli D, McKinley MJ, McAllen RM, The cholinergic anti-inflammatory pathway: a critical review. *Autonomic Neuroscience.* 2014;182:65–69.

*Laboratory Commercial References*

Specialty And Advanced Nutritional Labs
*Genova Diagnostic Lab https://www.gdx.net/
**Cyrex Labs https://www.cyrexlabs.com/CyrexTestsArrays
***Spectra Cell Lab https://www.spectracell.com/
****ALCAT https://cellsciencesystems.com/providers/alcat-test/food-panels/
*****IMMUNOLAB http://www.immunolabs.com/patients/

Commercial Labs
a. Quest Diagnostic http://www.questdiagnostics.com/home.html
b. Lab Corp https://www.labcorp.com
c. MDP labs http://www.mdp-worldwide.com/index.html

# 19

## Exercise for Addiction and Recovery

### GEORGE E. MUÑOZ

## The Inevitable Question: Why Exercise?

The benefits of activity and structured exercise in particular are numerous and well documented in many bodies of literature.[1] For general health purposes it is a mainstay and consistent with the integrative medicine model. In alcohol addiction, the literature shows that exercise benefits long-term recovery.[2] In fact, active addiction and its consequent deleterious metabolic changes, while obviously present during the active addiction phase of the disease, continue in early recovery and abstinence phases. These changes have the potential to endure for long periods and even a lifetime if the proper lifestyle recovery measures are not adopted. The metabolic consequences have potential for catastrophic results including increased risks of cancer and cardiovascular disease. And all-cause mortality increases with secondary metabolic derangements, including insulin resistance and proinflammatory cytokine activation. These inflammatory and neuroendocrine changes not only enhance systemic inflammation but also affect brain function in a deleterious manner. Specifically, activated microglial cells now become the hunting macrophage type of cell in the CNS ready to release more pro-inflammatory cytokines to further the immune response cascade. That depression, mood changes, and the addicted brain neurochemistry is predisposed and primed by an inflammatory milieu is now being touted in the basic sciences as part and parcel of the addiction pathophysiology at the brain cellular level. That lack of exercise and unhealthy eating patterns may add fuel to this fire is now understood and needs to be addressed along with the usual interventions in an overall recovery program. However, the timing, type amount, and duration of exercise in relation to the phase of addiction and recovery matters as neurochemical differences do exist. For example, during drug-use initiation and withdrawal, its efficacy may be related to its ability to facilitate dopaminergic transmission; once addiction develops, its efficacy may be related to its ability to normalize glutamatergic and dopaminergic signaling and reverse drug-induced changes in chromatin via epigenetic interactions with brain-derived neurotrophic factor (BDNF) in the reward pathway.[5] This could explain the observations that exercise generally decreases the reinforcing effects of drugs of abuse, but its efficacy is variable. Specific cytokines that are activated in addiction including NFK-B, TNF, Il-6, and upregulation of proinflammatory pathways.[6] Moderate exercise will help counter this proinflammatory state along with an anti-inflammatory patterned diet and appropriate supplementation of omega-3 fatty acids. One can even make a case to monitor several surrogate systemic inflammatory markers in the newly recovering construct utilized in the mind, body, spirit, and whole person approach to health and disease prevention. Let's take a look at some other reasons and associated positive outcomes related to exercise including effects on inflammation, neurobiology, mood, depression, sleep, energy, and obvious cardiovascular and bone benefits.

## GENERAL HEALTH

From a general health perspective, exercise is as important as eating properly and at the summit of preventative and personal care priorities to reduce cancer and cardiovascular risk significantly. Its effect on all-cause mortality is well established and more effective than any single pill or drug that exists to date.[2] Exercise habits form a construct for a healthy lifestyle, creating a base for stress reduction, improved sleep, and maintenance of a sound physical and biomechanical body. Muscle mass development helps reduce inflammation and improve bone mass over time in spite of biologic aging.[3] An active stretching, core strengthening and balance program help reduce the chance of injury with falls as well as induce positive neurocognitive signals for brain vitality.[4] All in all, the benefits of exercise are numerous, varied, and applicable to all ages. In the recovering individual this is an essential part of the whole person recovery and positively impacts not only the physical aspects of health but also the secondary benefits.

## INFLAMMATION REDUCTION

Addiction is an inflammatory state. As such assessment of an individual's inflammatory burden makes sense clinically and could include basic inflammation markers such as CRP, fasting insulin, and cortisol as stress response markers. More sophisticated cytokine evaluations of TNF, IL6, VCAM-1, EGF (endothelial growth factors) various matrix metalloproteinases (MMP-1 and MMP-3), and hormones including Leptin and Resistin provide more in-depth profiling of the inflammatory cascades that may be activated in an individual. These markers may herald premature vascular inflammation of potential life-threatening degree but also are part and parcel of the brain inflammatory state of active addiction and its consequent deranged metabolomic states.

## EXERCISE AND NEUROBIOLOGY

The concept that exercise and physical activity can help shape, maintain, and even improve neurologic function is now well described and accepted within science. Stimulation of the neuroadaptive mechanisms by movement, balance exercises, and feedback proprioceptive both play important roles in reshaping for neuro-regenerative capacity. Whether this effect is through stem-cell activity within the sanctuary CNS or through cross-talk communication from the outside is irrelevant. The fact is that it works; therefore, exercise is a critical piece of the pre-scriptive whole person approach for recovering individuals in all phases of their recovery. As such, the health-care team involved in addiction and recovery must be well informed as to not only benefit but also some nuances: these include warning signs of potential red flags with respect to overuse, over-exercising, and obsessive behaviors including body image and eating disorders that may manifest or be unmasked with increased exercise. This obviously is most relevant once the chemicals are removed and the individual patient is in abstinence mode. Neurobiological systems affected by exercise include improved cytokine markers, rebalancing of dopaminergic pathways, and improved glial and dendritic function. Additionally, peripheral endocrine and metabolism function that improves with exercise also helps the CNS. Specifically, reduced insulin levels and improved glucose metabolism help brain metabolic pathways.

## MOOD EFFECTS—DEPRESSION, ANXIETY, HELPS SLEEP

The effect of consistent exercise on mood is another well-recognized benefit of this healthy lifestyle habit. There is significant data on its benefits in treating depression and anxiety.[5] Consistent exercise regimens of 3 to 5 days per week for 45–60 minutes with combinations of cardiovascular and resistive weight training seem to be best for overall benefits. These health effects are not only limited to mood but also reduced all-cause mortality, cardiovascular mortality, and cancer risks (7,8)as has been previously alluded. Furthermore, anxiety or GAD are extremely common in the recovering population. Exercise plays an important role in addressing this situation as well. The anxiolytic benefits once again are well documented in the scientific literature and the same types and amount of exercise as noted above apply for this purpose as well.

Finally, insomnia and sleep disturbances of various forms exist in active addiction, early recovery, abstinence phases, and in middle- and long-term recovering individuals. The causes of these disturbances are varied and can include anxiety, neurochemical withdrawal responses, medication effects, sleep-cycle reversals, brain-ophthalmic and hypothalamic dysfunctions, and deep-seated GAD or PTSD to name a few. Whatever the cause, balanced consistent forms of exercise reap benefits irrespective of the hour they are performed. So if one is dealing with a recovering patient (addict/recovering individual) who is dealing with insomnia as their baseline, exercise should be prescribed during their reversed phase of sleep in order to begin the shift of the metabolic and neurobiochemical processes back toward normalcy. It doesn't matter what time one exercises. Secondary sleep patterns will improve over time as anxiety, stress, metabolic pathways, and inflammation are all improved. The increase in vagal or parasympathetic activity further aids in reduction of an overactive "fight or flight" state common in active addiction, early recovery, or anxiety states including PTSD, GAD, etc.

## EXERCISE AND THE MIND-BODY SPIRITS PARADIGM

As part of the whole person or integrative approach to health, healing, and wellness, exercise easily is categorized in at least two if not all three of these categories: mind, body, and spirit. If one wishes to remain strict and reductionist, it clearly falls into the "body" aspect; and for purposes of this rendering, a few of these points will be touched on now. The other effects of exercise with respect to the effect of the mind and spirit are interspersed within this chapter. Having said this, the state of addiction is obviously the antithesis of the healthy balanced state. Lack of coordinated cardiovascular exercise, resistive programs for strength and adequate hydration, nutrition, sleep, and a flexibility program all lay the groundwork for creating the exact opposite of optimal health. Once again, the state of addiction has its roots not only in the substance or dual diagnosis references but in the "dis-ease" of the mind-body-spirit paradigm. Consequently, regaining the mere intention to take care of oneself, exercise, hydrate, and fuel the body adequately (and have enough rest to repeat these activities) in and of itself has high-value target results in the war on addiction. The metaphor is militaristic, which implies that a regimented commitment of this aspect of the whole person recovery state is needed in addition to psychotherapy, pharmacotherapy, and specific addiction protocols appropriate for the treatment setting. In other words, the benefit and effects of exercise are so important and profound that they should start as soon as possible and be considered an integral part of the treatment paradigm in addiction settings.

## What Kind of Exercise?

According to the National Institute of Health (NIH), the 4 main types of physical activity are aerobic, muscle strengthening, bone strengthening, and stretching.[9] Examples of aerobic activity include running, swimming, walking, bicycling, dancing. Aerobic activity is also called "endurance" activity. When aerobic exercise is performed beyond a certain amount and time, physiologic changes occur that are associated with endorphin release and a "natural high" or -"sense of well-being" attributable to endogenous endorphin release. The interplay of this endogenous opioid system and its blunted or accentuated effects on individuals is varied. Nevertheless, the cardiovascular and mental benefits are definite and a gradual aerobic program to build up to 30 to 60 minutes maximum 3 to 4 days per week of a cardiovascular program is recommended for reduction in all-cause mortality and as part of wellness and cancer-risk reduction.[10] Muscle strengthening, typically thought of as resistive weight training with free weights, machines, or resistive bands are the next main category of exercise. Again, a gradual build up over weeks or months is recommended depending on the degree of deconditioning. The point is to start and to build upon it either by time or number of exercises (sets) and repetitions (or "reps"). Decreasing the amount of rest time between sets and reps and maintaining a slow, medium, or fast pace are other variables to consider in resistive weight muscular training. Again, the suggestion to start slowly with adequate rest periods and hydration throughout a session are good training principles. By decreasing the interval rest periods, a combination of cardiovascular and resistive muscle strengthening can be performed simultaneously so as to reduce the total amount of training to 45 to 60 minutes to include both critical types of exercise: aerobic cardio and muscle strengthening. Doing this 3 to 5 days per week would be a goal, and consistency once again is key for optimal benefit and total health, stress reduction, mental, balance and aiding in stress reduction, and improved sleep. All of these points are obviously important for anyone but especially for recovering individuals.

Bone-strengthening activities are covered in all muscle and resistive weight training but may overlap into some cardio-type exercises such as running and especially sprinting or shorter higher intensity interval trainings (HIIT) where moderate-to-high levels of exertion for relatively brief 1 to 2 minutes are expended at near max capacity of effort in sets of 5 to 10 with 1-to-2-minute rest periods and adjustments made for optimal heart rate and recovery. This takes time to accomplish and should not be attempted in the beginning; the goal should be to perform this type of exercise gradually over a 90- to 180-day adaption period. Finally, the fourth category of exercise is flexibility. Stretching and flexibility activity and formal exercises that include yoga, pilates, and therapeutic band stretching are examples. They should be incorporated into the formal exercise program either on a daily or weekly basis or other time interval: whatever suits the overall goals and exercise schedule of a patient or individual. Brief stretching stints after the main cardiovascular and resistive weight-training sessions make sense; stretching helps relieve soreness and tightness and also reduces the chance of injury. Formal use of aids to manually reduce muscle spasm including foam rolling are being utilized more in both competitive and recreational venues to help in such endeavors.

## BALANCE EXERCISES

Balance exercises are effective in helping to retool neuromuscular patterns that are generally diminished with inactivity, deconditioning, or with neurologic or blunt physical trauma of any type. Firing patterns can be corrected and restored with repetitive, structured movements that elicit proprioceptive, balance, and neuro-muscular re-education by controlled, deliberate movements including balancing on one foot and leg. Squatting with or without assistance, and walking a line, much like a sobriety test, is also good. Doing some of these activities with eyes open and eyes closed further stimulates the neocortex, ocular, cerebellar, and midbrain pathways involved in these complex integrated systems. Yoga and tai qi once again encompass this health benefit.[11]

## BREATHWORK

How to breathe during exercise is of interest as is the art of breathwork as a disci-pline, which includes various mind-body interventions such as yoga, meditation, Tai Qigong, and other contemplative still or moving martial arts. What we are discussing here is more of a "how do I breathe with movement and running?" question. While there is no one way to answer this, we can give some useful suggestions for breathing while running.

Essentially the concept is that we in the West do not perform what is called tan-tien breathing and instead limit our capacity and airflow by moving on the chest. In the tan-tien model, we inhale from the belly, pushing out the belly button and exhale by bringing the belly back in and sucking the belly button in toward the spine. This creates enhanced airflow and lung expansion that is not usually obtained.[12] This can be performed while walking, jogging, and running. With running, a cadence will be developed so that an inhale could be 3 steps and an exhale at 2 steps; however, this may be adjusted to an individual's preference. Another style of breathing is to alternate the inhalation through the nose and the exhale portion through the mouth while keeping the belly breathing pattern active. Some individuals breathe through both the nose and mouth simultaneously while running. An individual should try various patterns and utilize what fits their particular physiology and preference. As long as there is a consciousness to the breathwork in both stillness and in motion, the health benefits are maximized.

## YING VERSUS YANG

Both hard and soft exercises are recommended to form a cross-training construct. This is both energetically preferred but also reduces muscle memory adaptation and injury by reducing overuse in single anatomic areas. An example of this would be to begin to lift heavier weights after a 3-month adaption phase of gradually lower-level exercise and weights. The concept here is not to lift the same weight every day but to vary the workload so as to increase the number of reps with lower weights, which is also safer for injury and tendon protection. The following day, changing the focus on what part of the body will be exercised while doing more flexibility and cardiovascular work makes sense. This way, body fatigue and boredom are minimized. Utilizing a trainer or workout buddy makes sense also for the group motivation benefit. Again, the idea is to change one's workout and balance harder with softer, yin and yang, as this is how we and the universe are wired. Combining mind-body exercises such as yoga, pilates, Tai Chi, and Qigong are also helpful in this regard in between the traditional exercise regimens involving straight resistive or interval cardio training. Examples of the "harder" (or yang) types of exercise activities could include kickboxing or crossfit training where the intensity is much higher and requires basic fitness. This is not how a novice or someone new to addiction and recovery should generally begin, however. Hard yoga with an emphasis on strength more than finesse, balance, and mindfulness is another example of hard exercise without excessive movement or contact.

## WEIGHTS VERSUS BODYWEIGHT EXERCISES

Finally, a word about resistive exercise from the point of view of utilizing weights or bodyweight exercise. Again, there is no right or wrong here. It comes down to preference and availability. One should have a functional body weight exercise regimen as an option if traveling or time constraints limit access to a gym. The concept here is a mindfulness and preplanning of this healthy lifestyle habit so it is transferable, mobile, and readily accessible. Examples of bodyweight exercises would be pushups, situps, pullups, dips, leg lifts, jumping jacks, jumping rope, or body weight squat transitioning to a jump (then down to the floor for a single pushup, or burpie). These done in sequence and in repetitive sets of 10 to 120 comprise an excellent, well-rounded regimen that is easily performed indoors or outdoors.

## The How to Exercise Section

### CV GUIDELINES

The American heart Association guidelines for individuals 18 to 65 years old is for moderate exercise 30 minutes, 5 days per week or high-intensity activities 3 days per week for 20 minutes in order to reduce cardiovascular mortality and maintain optimal health. In order to reduce cardiovascular risk in this highly inflamed population, it makes sense to mirror these recommendations for maximum protection.[13]

### CANCER PREVENTION

Similarly, the risk of cancer is also reduced with a regular exercise program that appears to be similar, if not identical, to the CV risk reduction paradigm.[14] Specifics regarding types of exercise and cancer risk reduction for various types of cancer are discussed and known throughout the literature and may be viewed at the NIH cancer site.[15]

### OSTEOPOROSIS

The exercise benefits on bone health are also well recognized and replete with literature examples. The National Osteoporosis Foundation is a reliable source for benefit of exercise in risk reduction and prevention of osteoporosis in all aged individuals.[16]

### EXERCISE AS PART OF ADDICTION

What distinguishes the everyday gym enthusiast from someone addicted to exercise? An excellent review on this topic with breakdown by incidence, diagnostic dilemma and presenting a 4-phase diagnostic criteria, in order to identify and stratify patients with exercise addiction into a more cogent grouping.[17] This is a pivotal question and raises the possibility of other co-existing eating disorders and the associated obsessive compulsive behaviors linked with them. Hausenblas and Downs[18,19] identify exercise addiction based on the following criteria that are modifications of the *DSM-4 TR*[20] criteria for substance dependence:

- *Tolerance*: increasing the amount of exercise in order to feel the desired effect, be it a "buzz" or sense of accomplishment;
- *Withdrawal*: in the absence of exercise the person experiences negative effects such as anxiety, irritability, restlessness, and sleep problems;
- *Lack of control*: unsuccessful at attempts to reduce exercise level or cease exercising for a certain period of time;
- *Intention effects*: unable to stick to one's intended routine as evidenced by exceeding the amount of time devoted to exercise or consistently going beyond the intended amount;
- *Time:* a great deal of time is spent preparing for, engaging in, and recovering from exercise;
- *Reduction in other activities*: as a direct result of exercise social, occupational, and/or recreational activities occur less often or are stopped;
- *Continuance*: continuing to exercise despite knowing that this activity is creating or exacerbating physical, psychological, and/or interpersonal problems.

These criteria are more consistent with a *DSM-5* classification for exercise addiction that includes the behavioral addictions of the prior *DSM-4*.[20,21] The general incidence in the general population appears to be about 3%, but this percentage is much higher in subgroups that represent at-risk populations by the mere definition of their involvement or engagement in more elite athletic forums, such as marathoners, or Division 1 athletes, and the like. Similarly, a failure to distinguish exercise addiction from exercise done with high frequency and intensity has been a source of confusion in the literature.[22] In defining exercise addiction, the question becomes how to distinguish healthy exercise from exercise addiction; and a model of how to approach this dilemma is set forth by Freimruth.[23] Clinical assessment of each phase of the exercise addiction continuum can be broken down utilizing this grid approach evaluating three components: motivation (referring to the person's motivation for exercising in that stage), consequences, and frequency/control. In this construct, three phases will be laid out below.

**Phase 1: Recreational Exercise**. This primarily occurs because it is a pleasurable and rewarding activity.

**Phase 2: At-Risk Exercise**. This can comprise a large group of individuals. So who exactly is at risk in this cohort? Again, motivation may play a key role in identifying the at-risk individual in addition to the usual genetics, family history, peer pressure, etc. Thornton and Scott have shown this effect for exercise. The likelihood of an addiction increases for those who exercise with the goal of escaping unpleasant feelings or transforming their appearance to improve self-esteem—compared to those who exercise with the goal of improving performance and fitness.[24]

**Phase 3: Problematic Exercise**. Here, recreational exercisers integrate their daily physical activity into their lives. Those for whom exercise is becoming problematic begin to organize their day around their exercise regimen, which is becoming increasingly rigid.[25] Once in the problematic phase, the behavior continues despite having met the stated goal similar to other addictive substance behaviors.

Maintaining control over the behavior becomes more difficult in the problematic phase. This is because when the behavior ceases, withdrawal symptoms set in with resultant stressors and secondary backlash. This withdrawal phenomenon from exercise has been demonstrated via biochemical changes associated with increased exercise: the body down regulates endorphin production in response to exercise. Consequently, the absence of exercise can be associated with withdrawal.[26]

**Phase 4: Exercise Addiction**. The frequency and intensity of exercise continues until this behavior becomes life's main organizing principle. As the life of the addicted person revolves around exercise, the pleasure of the behavior recedes as the primary motivation becomes avoiding withdrawal symptoms.

Direct and secondary negative consequences continue to mount, which leads to tertiary negative consequences in the form of impairments in daily functioning and inability to meet role obligations. Other metrics exist to assess exercise behavior as normal engagement versus addiction behavior including the 2 metric systems commonly cited in the literature: the Exercise Dependence Scale (EDS-R) based on modification of the criteria for substance dependence[21] and the Exercise Addiction Inventory (EAI)[27] represents another measurement tool based on Griffiths's modification of Brown's model of addiction. Both the EDS-R and EAI have good validity and reliability. Whether assessing or treating exercise addiction, it is important to be attuned to the common co-occurring disorders, especially if it is an eating disorder or food-related problem—and vice versa with primary eating disorders and a balanced exercise regimen. Although exercise addiction is not included in *DSM-5*, it is imperative that many kinds of health-care providers become familiar with its attributes. Distinguishing exercise addiction versus balanced lifestyle will challenge all types of health-care personnel and physicians of all specialties, not just psychologists, psychiatrists, or addiction specialists. The physician may see repetitive injuries and not recognize this as a sign that the compulsion to exercise prevents an injury from fully healing.[17]

## WRITING THE EXERCISE PRESCRIPTION IN RECOVERY

Exercise should be prescribed just like any other medication or therapeutic intervention. The reasons for doing so are various, including telling the patient that this exercise prescription is as important as their conventional therapeutic prescriptives and should be followed accordingly. Additionally, precision as to amount, type, and frequency of exercise is needed to avoid confusion and limit the addiction or other obsessive compulsive behaviors. It is generally recommended that this process be part of the overall treatment program along with pharmacotherapy, stress-reduction techniques, mind-body intervention, meditation, and nutraceutical directives for the recovering individual in any phase. The use of trainers or athletic wellness specialists, if available for compliance and establishment of a routine, would be wise options if available. Once again, the written exercise prescription aids in communicating with the health-care team, the patient, and their family.

## Understanding Risk Stratification in Exercise Prescription

In the general wellness setting, writing the exercise prescription requires situating a patient into 1 of 3 categories to determine if they may exercise alone or if they must be monitored by a paraprofessional. In the addiction setting, the same principles will apply to the general population, with their exercise-risk stratification being based on age and the presence of the following: hypertension, smoking, diabetes, obesity, sedentary lifestyle or family history, premature CV disease, and dyslipidemia. The presence of 2 or more of these requires a more comprehensive medical or cardiovascular evaluation before a general exercise prescription can be written. A negative risk factor or protective factor is HDL > 60 mg/ml and would negate any single positive risk factor. Moderate-risk individuals would be males >45 or women >55 years old or who have 2 or more positive risk

factors. These moderate-risk individuals need further medical clearance before vigorous exercise is prescribed; but clearance is not necessary for low or moderate vigorous activity. Any patient with cardiovascular, pulmonary (COPD, asthma) or metabolic diseases (Type 1 or 2 diabetes) and signs or symptoms including dyspnea and edema, would be classified as high risk. These individuals could only exercise with professional medical supervision for all levels of exercise intensity and would not be the patient target population for this book. Examples of moderate activity would be walking briskly, water aerobics, ballroom dancing, and general gardening. Vigorous activity examples include race walking, jogging, running, swimming laps, jumping rope, and hiking uphill or with a heavy jumping rope.[29,30]

### MANAGING PAIN BEFORE AND AFTER EXERCISE

The issue of managing pain in the recovering patient either before after initiating exercise should follow some obvious tenets. Since the use of narcotics is for the most part not a consideration unless no other option exists, the following strategies work well. Generally speaking nonsteroidal OTC are used commonly for mild skeletal discomfort, but the use of some localized creams (including Tiger Balm with menthol), analgesic-containing compounds with salicylate or other camphor-containing topicals (along with massage) often prove effective. Oral NSAID as prescriptives would be the next pharmaceutical option, but anti-inflammatory botanicals including turmeric, holy basil, and ginger root extracts are also quite effective generally around 500 mg for use as analgesia and anti-inflammatory agents. Flavococid compounds by prescription are another safe alternative that practitioners may prescribe; these have no GI ulcer, bleeding, or renal hypertensive or cardiovascular risk and are sold in the United States under the trade name Limbrel by medical prescription. Homeopathics including Arnica montana, Rhus toxicodendron, Ruta graveolens, and Kali bichromatum 9c or 30 c 5 tabs S/L tid-qid may be useful in treating the exercise-associated sports injury with muscular or tendinous injury as the source of pain. Finally, manual modalities and physical medicine work well with exercise-induced pain including classic massage, neuromuscular therapy, and of course acupuncture and TCM modalities. Maintenance therapies to prevent injury include adequate stretching and foam-rolling techniques after exercise to avoid common injuries and nagging discomfort.

## "Fueling" Before, During, and After Exercise

Adequate energy, proper calories, and carbohydrate (carbs) intake before exercise will assure adequate energy during the 45- to 60-minute period of movement and energy consumption required for an adequate workout session. Like many other activities in early and later recovery, pre-planning and some basic structure help maintain this good habit. Inadequate energy intake at least 1 hour prior to exertion could allow for a "weak" feeling: this could be hypoglycemia in some cases, or a simple case of running out of adequate body stores via glycogen in the liver and muscles. The goal in the beginning is simply to get to the exercise venue and develop good habits. Over time, this can progress to a more moderately intense session and both adequate hydration (1 to 1.5) gallons of preferably mineralized and electrolyte-containing water is recommended. Building the good habit of drinking water throughout the day as a main beverage sets the stage to avoid mildly dehydrated states during athletic activity. Consciousness of one's meals, timing, hunger, or pre-hunger sensations takes time but is important for everyone on a consistent exercise regimen. During activity, consistent water intake without filling up too suddenly is recommended, especially once cardiovascular activities have started. Insensible water losses, or water loss through the skin or respiration, will increase during these segments, and constant low-grade hydration following the pre-activity hydration is needed. If an individual has consumed enough useable calories before activity, consuming more energy during the activity is not needed. Exemptions would be lightheadedness, sensation of hunger or knowing that not enough nutrients have preceded the exercise session. In the latter case, a banana slowly consumed during weight training or a protein shake with a banana work well to maintain euglycemia and enough energy to complete a session. After exercise, it is equally important to fuel the body and brain. Obviously for a recovering individual, this may be even more essential as the "hungry" component of HALT (acronym for Hungry, Angry, Lonely, Tired) needs to be avoided however a good "TIRED" feeling could be expected post-workout and possessing many physiologic benefits. Eating high complex carbs (brown or basmati rice, sweet potato, quinoa), broccoli, and other cruciferous veggies) with "lean protein" (chicken, turkey, oily wild fish, eggs, or egg whites are some examples of food groupings that are recommended post-workout. If a meal can't be consumed, a protein shake with about 20 to 30 grams of protein and 80 to 120 grams of carbs will suffice, all within the first hour post-workout. This assures adequate fueling of muscles and body stores of glycogen so as to avoid any hypoglycemia later and secondary mood changes (including fatigue and poor eating choices, etc.). This all becomes a normal sequence of healthy habits versus obsessive compulsive ritualism and enhances the post-exercise sense of well being, which is one of the benefits of a balanced healthy lifestyle. Multiple resources exist for further detailed approaches on pre-, during- and post-exercise meal planning and hydration, but the aforementioned plans a good starting point.[32,33]

## Exercise Supplements in Recovery: What to Avoid

Numerous supplements exist to improve exercise performance, muscle function, fat burning, among others. Many of these products have fat burning as a primary intent and fall under the "weight loss" rubric. Unfortunately, some of these "supplement" or "exercise aids" have stimulants or other adulterants that are not clearly stated on labels, which makes it difficult for the consumer to identify. Additional to caffeine, stimulants (e.g., Mu Hung) containing ephedra have been associated with cardiovascular deaths due to arrhythmia and or malignant hyperthermia. Under the Dietary Supplement Health and Education Act (DSHEA), it is difficult for the FDA to put together strong enough evidence to take products off the market. To date, it has banned only one ingredient: ephedrine alkaloids. That effort dragged on for a decade, during which ephedra weight-loss products were implicated in thousands of adverse events, including deaths.[34] Additionally, epinephrine is another stimulant that is sometimes used for purposes that should be avoided, especially in the recovering individual; a "fight or flight" response is no longer conducive to recovery. These substances have not been banned by the FDA, and should be avoided. In fact, all stimulants should be avoided. Effects and perceived benefits of branched chain amino acids and L-glutamine can be achieved by following adequate hydration, meal and protein supplementation, as well as adjustment in the training regimens, intensity, frequency, and workloads. Consuming branched chain amino acids, L-glutamine, and arginine along with vitamins such as C, D, B12, and B6 are generally considered safe, however. Omega-3 fatty acids and Alpha linoleic acid are fine and not associated with any toxicity when used in conventional doses for health purposes. In general, patients should avoid products containing words such as "ripped," "boosters," "fat burners," etc. Most of these contain varying amounts of caffeine and use of either coffee or tea in moderation or normal usage before a workout: using a trusted caffeine source is safer than taking supplements where the exact amounts are difficult to assess or contain other poorly labeled substances.

## REFERENCES

1. Warburton DER, Nicol CW and Bredin SSD, Health benefits of physical activity: the evidence. *Canadian Medical Association Journal.* March 14, 2006;174(6):801–809.
2. Brown R, Abrantes AM, Read, JP, et al. Aerobic exercise for alcohol recovery: rationale, program description, and preliminary findings. *Behavior Modification.* 2009;33(2):220–249.
3. Lynch WJ, Peterson AB. Exercise as a novel treatment for drug addiction: a neurobiological and stage-dependent hypothesis. *Neuroscience and Biobehavioral Reviews.* 2013;37(8):1622–1644.
4. Nelson ME, Rejeski WJ, Blair SN, Duncan PW, Judge JO., King, A. C., . . . Castaneda-Sceppa, C. (2007). Physical activity and public health in older adults: Recommendation from the American College of Sports Medicine and the American Heart Association. *Circulation, 116*(9), 1094–110.
5. Salmon P. Effects of physical exercise on anxiety, depression, and sensitivity to stress: a unifying theory. *Clinical Psychology Review.* 2001.
6. Crews FT. Induction of innate immune genes in brain create the neurobiology of addiction. *Brain, Behavior, and Immunity.* 2011;25(Suppl 1):S4–S12.
7. Stamatakis E, Bennie I -Min Lee, Freeston J, American, Does Strength Promoting exercise Confer Unique Benefits? A pooled analysis of data on 11 population cohorts with All-Cause, Cancer, and Cardiovascular Mortality Endpoints. *Journal of Epidemiology,* October 2017, https://academic.oup.com/aje/advance-article/doi/10.1093/aje/kwx345/4582884
8. Leitzmann MF, Park Y, Blair A, et al., Physical Activity Recommendation and decreased Risk of Mortality, Arch *Internal Medicine.* 2007:167(22):2453–2460.
9. http://www.nhlbi.nih.gov/health/health-topics/topics/phys/types
10. http://www.nhlbi.nih.gov/health/health-topics/topics/phys/benefits

11. http://www.heart.org/HEARTORG/HealthyLiving/PhysicalActivity/FitnessBasics/Balance-Exercise_UCM_464001_Article.jsp#.V26mSbgrJeU

12. http://www.wikihow.com/Breathe-While-Running

13. Haskell WL, Lee Pate R, Powell K, et al. Physical activity and public health: Updated recommendation for adults from the American College of Sports Medicine and the American Heart Association. *Circulation*. 2007;116(9):1081–1093.

14. Friendenreich C, Orenstein M, Physical activity and cancer prevention: Etiologic evidence and biologic mechanisms. *Journal of Nutrition*. 2002;132:3456S-3464S.

15. http://www.cancer.gov/about-cancer/causes-prevention/risk/obesity/physical-activity-fact-sheet

16. https://www.nof.org

17. Freimuth M, Moniz S, Kim SR. Clarifying exercise addiction: differential diagnosis, co-occurring disorders, and phases of addiction. *International Journal of Environmental Research and Public Health*. 2011;8(10):4069–4081.

18. Hausenblas HA, Downs DS. How much is too much? The development and validation of the exercise addiction scale. *Psychology and Health*. 2002;17:387–404.

19. Downs DS, Hausenblas HA, Nigg CR. Factorial validity and psychometric examination of the Exercise Dependence Scale-Revised. *Measurement in Physical Education and Exercise Science*. 2004;8:183–201.

20. APA. *Diagnostic and Statistical Manual of Mental Disorders*. 4th ed. Washington, DC: American Psychiatric Association; 2000.

21. APA. *DSM 5 Development*. http://www.dsm5.org/Pages/Default.aspx. Accessed on September 30, 2011.

22. Allegre B, Therme P, Griffiths M. Individual factors and the context of physical activity in exercise dependence: a prospective study of "ultra-marathoners." *International Journal of Mental Health and Addiction*. 2007;5:233–243.

23. Freimuth M. *Addicted? Recognizing Destructive Behavior Before It's Too Late*. Lanham, MD: Rowman & Littlefield: 2008.

24. Thornton EW, Scott SE. Motivation in the committed runner: correlation between self-report scales and behavior. *Health Promotion International*. 1995;10:177–184.

25. Johnston O, Reilly J, Kremer J. Excessive exercise: from quantitative categorisation to a qualitative continuum approach. *European Eating Disorders Review*. 2011;19:237–248.

26. Adams J, Kirkby RJ. Excessive exercise as an addiction: a review. *Addiction Research & Theory*. 2002;10:415–437.

27. Terry A, Szabo A, Griffiths M. The exercise addiction inventory: A new brief screening tool. *Addiction Research & Theory*. 2004;12:489–499.

28. Brown RIF. A theoretical model of the behavioural addictions—applied to offending. In: Hodge JE, McMurran M, Hollins CM, eds. *Addicted to Crime?* Chichester, UK: Wiley; 1997.

29. http://www.health.gov/PAguidelines

30. Jonas S, Phillips EM. Exercise is Medicine™: A Clinician's Guide to Exercise Prescription. Philadelphia: Lippincott, Williams, and Wilkins; 2009

31. Pharmacology and Homeopathic Materia Medica, Denis D, Jaques J, Bernard P, Yves Saint-Jean, 2008, 3rd Edition, CEDH reference.

32. Wataru A, Naito Y, Yoshikawa T Exercise and unctional foods. *Nutrition Journal.* 2006;5–15.

33. http://www.cdc.gov/nccdphp/dnpao/

34. http://www.consumerreports.org/cro/2012/05/dangerous-supplements/index.htm

# 20

## Nutraceutical Treatments for Addiction Recovery

### JEFFREY BECKER

## Introduction

S tudies examining medication treatment outcomes in substance-use
disorders (SUDs) often report disappointing results, which is not surprising
given that addiction-related pathophysiology and molecular deficiencies are
rarely directly addressed by medications. Treatment focused upon damaging biochemical processes that undermine early and sustained recovery should include
rational incorporation of nutrients, vitamins, and herbal treatments supported by
research. Natural treatments can help support physical recovery in early sobriety.
Many natural treatments have been shown to support sustained recovery and risk
reduction.

However, a relative shortage of research on sobriety outcomes with complimentary molecular options can necessitate extrapolation of data across different drug
classes to craft natural treatment approaches for a variety of patients. Wherever
research into natural options is lacking, the clinician must turn to their understanding of addiction-related nutrient depletions, inflammation, neurotransmitter
depletions, and reward system down-regulation. While specific evidence may be
lacking in a given case, the addiction mechanisms and toxicity can be similar across
various drugs of abuse. So extrapolation of data can be a reasonable approach.

Each patient presents with both particular and universal principles regarding the pathophysiology of their addiction and recovery. An understanding
of the mechanisms of drug toxicity and addiction can inform natural treatment
recommendations that address post-acute recovery symptoms and/or chronic
underlying comorbid psychiatric symptoms. A complex interrelation of factors
is at work in addiction, and studies investigating the benefits of a single amino
acid or vitamin are likely to fail where more complex treatment might succeed.

This model does not easily bend to single-parameter DBPC research. Synergistic benefits through multiple, rational, natural treatments is a reasonable goal in the treatment of such a difficult set of disorders.

To this point, a wide range of valuable research into natural addiction treatments has focused upon repletion of essential nutrients without relation to sobriety measurements. efficacy, and safety in repletion of toxic deficiencies. Given the substance-abuse treatment community's growing appreciation for the value of harm-reduction treatment models, these studies can inform treatment planning to address a wider array of recovery parameters in patients. As such, treatments reasonably expected to reduce harm or support recovery at any level are presented in good faith for the mindful practitioner (Box 20.1).

Sustained abuse of psychoactive substances can derange neurological signaling and health through many mechanisms, but 3 categories of pathophysiology can inform and anchor treatment with natural options: inflammation and antioxidant system degradation, stress activation and reward deficiency, and vitamin and nutrient deficiency.

It is clear that despite the detrimental effect these pathologies have upon recovery they are generally unaddressed by medications. And while natural treatment options fulfill a deep need in this regard, it is likely that simultaneous address of all 3 categories is necessary to achieve comprehensive outcomes in recovery through natural treatments.

# Inflammation and Antioxodant System Degredation

## PATHOPHYSIOLOGIC BASIS

Drug-induced oxidative stress and inflammation may inhibit recovery by damaging molecular health and homeostasis and neurological function. The mechanisms underlying cellular damage and aging that occur with reactive oxygen species (ROS) and inflammation are well established in many diseases and conditions. However, removing the offending agent with sobriety is sometimes not enough to restore natural physiology. Elevations in TNF-α have been shown in alcoholics long after sustained recovery, implying that other mechanisms may be maintaining brain dysfunction.

Inflammation and degraded antioxidant systems are especially common in stimulant and alcohol dependence. Chronic alcohol use produces enzymatic deficits in RBC superoxide dismutase, catalase, and glutathione peroxidase[1] and increases ROS levels (e.g., superoxide, hydroxyl) through oxidation of NADH and CoQ10 degradation and decreased mitochondrial protein synthesis and oxidative

### Box 20.1 Pathophysiologic Basis for Natural Treatment Planning and Intervention in Alcohol and SUDs

ALCOHOL
Reward-system deficits
Nutritional deficiencies
Neurological inflammation
DNA damage[5]
Stress-system hyperactivation
Glutamate/NMDA receptor upregulation and hyperactivation[145]
GABA receptor downregulation
Altered carbohydrate metabolism
Altered methylation pathways[145,146,5]
Gastrointestinal damage and leaky gut

STIMULANTS
Reward-system deficits
Nutritional deficiencies
Neurological inflammation
Stress system hyperactivation: during use[147]
Stress system hypoactivation: post-withdrawal
Acute neurotransmitter depletion: dopamine, norepinephrine, serotonin
Chronic neurological damage: dopaminergic
Sex hormone deficiencies[148]

OPIATES
Reward-system deficits
Nutritional deficiencies
Rebound inflammation
Stress-system hyperactivation: post-withdrawal
Sex hormone deficiencies[148,149]

TOBACCO
Nicotinic receptor blunting
Reward-system deficits
MAO-inhibitor withdrawal

CANNABIS
Reward-system deficits
Nutritional deficiencies
Hormonal effects/deficiencies[150]
Stress system hyperactivation – post-withdrawal

phosphorylation.[2] Increased levels of TNF-α, IL-8, and malondialdehyde, a marker for lipid peroxidation and oxidative stress are reported.[3] Neuronal death in the context of chronic alcohol use may be due to an accumulation of DNA damage due increased ROS and weakened repair systems.[4,5] Neurological damage due to alcohol use may persist long after sobriety, inducing long-term decrement in cholinergic neurons,[6] and loss of gray and white matter.[4] Brain levels of TNF-α can remain elevated long after sobriety, revealing the broad, sustained neuroinflammatory effects of alcohol.

Some of the inflammatory effects of alcohol may stem from gastrointestinal toxicity, intestinal permeability, and increased growth of pathogenic bacteria. Alcohol promotes growth of gram-negative bacteria and gut-related acetaldehyde, both of which damage enterocytic tight-junctions through tyrosine phosphorylation. Subsequent increases in circulating endotoxin and peptidoglycans initiate a strong systemic inflammatory response that may substantially contribute to alcohol's addictive mechanism and toxicity.[7] Compared to controls, alcoholics with liver disease showed marked increases in oral lactulose absorption, a sign of increased intestinal permeability.[8] Thus, treatments oriented toward restoring gut integrity and ecology may be of particular use in recovering alcoholics.

Stimulants increase DA turnover and MAO-B related production of peroxide and hydroxyl after reuptake. These ROS damage DA neurons by overwhelming the antioxidant capacities of these already-fragile neurons. Neuronal aging and apoptosis may explain deficits related to cognitive, mood, and motivational domains that persist even after sustained recovery. Tobacco's free-radical and toxic effects are notorious.

## TREATMENT APPROACHES

### Prebiotics and Probiotics

Lactulose is a prescription prebiotic sugar derived from lactose that can substantially improve bowel flora composition.[9,10] In addition to its capacity to reduce serum ammonia levels, lactulose was reported to significantly reduce TNF-α, IL-6, IL-18, and serum endotoxin levels in cirrhotic patients with minimal encephalopathy.[11] No human trials with naturally derived prebiotic sugars (e.g., inulin, fructooligosaccharide) are available, but it is possible that benefits might be derived from these as well.

In alcoholism prebiotics may possess a distinct advantage over probiotics in that they support the individual's naturally existent probiotic bacterial strains rather than introducing exogenous bacteria. Despite reports that probiotic supplements lowered ALT and AST levels in hospitalized alcoholics with reduced probiotic genera,[12] comorbid disease burden is of critical importance in assessing research given that another study reported a two-fold increased risk of mortality in patients with pancreatitis.[13]

## Resveratrol

Resveratrol is a powerful antioxidant with anti-inflammatory qualities through nuclear factor kappa beta (NFKß) blockade, of particular importance in alcohol-related brain inflammation. NFKß is a protein complex found in B-cells that stimulates the innate immune system in rapid response to increases in oxidized glutathione,[14] TNF-α,[15] ROS, lipopolysaccharide (LPS),[16,17] and elevated glutaminergic neurotransmission.[18] Given that many of these are elevated in alcohol and stimulant abuse, resveratrol might be expected to provide anti-inflammatory relief in acute and sustained recovery.

But, the potential of this NFKß-antagonist may go even deeper. A Fos family protein, ΔFosB, has been implicated as a likely transcriptional factor involved in the development of addiction through stimulus-reward linkages in the nucleus acumbens (NA).[19] Increases in ΔFosB are seen in multiple brain regions with cocaine, morphine, ethanol, and cannabinoids. But while ΔFosB has many actions, upregulation of NFKß in the NA is believed to contribute to the development of addiction[20] specifically through increased drug-reward signaling.[21]

In short, resveratrol positively affects multiple pathophysiologic mechanisms involved in the inflammation and addiction associated with multiple drugs of frequent abuse. While there are no human studies to date, animal research is very promising. In alcohol-fed rats, resveratrol completely reversed elevations in AST, ALT, and GGT. It also inhibited lipid peroxidation and reversed alcohol-related deficiencies in superoxide dismutase, catalase, and glutathione peroxidase activity.[22] Resveratrol prevented alcohol-related cognitive deficits, improved SOD, GPx and catalase activity and restored normal acetylcholinesterase activity in alcohol-fed rats.[23] It reduced alcohol-induced TNF-α, IL-1, lipid peroxides and NFKß, even though blood alcohol levels were unchanged.[23] Low concentrations of trans-resveratrol applied to in-vitro cultures of rat astrocytes reduced the cytotoxic and genotoxic damage associated with alcohol,[24] and others have reported in vitro benefits in animal[25] and human cells.[26] There are no in vivo human clinical trials to date.

## Taurine

Taurine is a natural endogenous antioxidant, a sulfonic acid derivative of the amino acid cysteine. It is essential for cardiac function and within the central nervous system displays inhibitory effects on neurotransmission and protection against glutamate excitotoxicity.[27] It also has receptor effects that naturally overlap with the effects of alcohol, including potentiation of GABA and glycine receptors and inhibition of excitatory amino acid receptors and calcium channels.[28] The homotaurine derivative acamprosate is FDA-approved for use in alcohol treatment.

While there are a number of animal studies showing varying potential benefits in alcohol treatment,[28] there is only one human study to date. In chronic alcoholics with elevated liver enzymes, 2 grams of Taurine 3 times daily for 3 months significantly reduced liver enzyme levels, improved B-vitamin status, reduced TBARS (a marker for ROS), and increased the activities of alcohol dehydrogenase and aldehyde dehydrogenase compared to placebo.[29] Taurine supplementation reduced hepatic steatosis and abolished lipid peroxidation in Sprague-Dawley rats.[30]

## N-Acetyl Cysteine and Glutathione

N-Acetyl Cysteine (NAC) has established utility in multiple arenas of SUD treatment and psychiatry in general.[31] As a cysteine substrate with high bioavailability, NAC quickly and affordably provides a highly limited resource that increases glutathione, which protects tissues from ROS and positively modulates NMDA receptor directly and through improving the neurological re-dox environment. Through a variety of mechanisms, glutathione depletion occurs commonly in alcoholism and SUDs through a variety of interconnected mechanisms. Indeed, gamma-glutamyltransferase or GGT, used to monitor alcohol intake through lab values, specifically measures an enzyme that upregulates during shortages of cysteine: the rate-limiting substrate for glutathione production. As such, supplementation with NAC in active alcoholism and recovery is rational and likely warranted, though clinical studies are surprisingly lacking, and some research in rats even calls into question the breadth of the antioxidant value of NAC in alcoholism.[32]

Recent research with NAC in other categories of addiction has been promising. AMPA glutamate receptors have been implicated in the mechanism of cocaine craving,[33] and cocaine-addicted rats given NAC during extinction and abstinence experienced substantial anti-relapse protection during re-exposure that continued even after treatment was discontinued.[34] In an open-label trial, cocaine users taking from 1.2 to 3.6 grams of NAC per day reported substantial reductions in money spent on cocaine and total days using over 4 weeks,[35] and within 3 days, it was found that 1,200 mg/day of NAC reduced interest in and desire to use cocaine in a small hospital-based DBPC study.[36] Compared to controls, cocaine-dependent subjects taking NAC showed reductions in in anterior cingulate cortex glutamate levels within an hour.[37]

NAC supplementation at 2.4 grams per day also doubled the chances of a negative urine screen for cannabinoids in n 8-week, DBPC study with 116 subjects.[38] It is worth noting that a shorter-term pilot study reported positive but underwhelming results[39], thus longer periods of treatment with NAC may be necessary to achieve benefits (as has been established in other psychiatric conditions).

NAC also improved the extinction process produced an anti-relapse effect during reinstatement of heroin in addicted rats,[40] and in tobacco cessation research there have been reported benefits.[41] Finally, NAC is reported to have protective effects against methamphetamine neurotoxicity in animal studies,[42,43] and an 8-week DBPC crossover study found that 1,200 mg of NAC substantially reduced methamphetamine craving during recovery[44] (although other methamphetamine research results have been underwhelming).

## Mitochondrial Protection: CoQ10, Acetyl-L-Carnitine, and Lipoic Acid

Mitochondrial damage with drug abuse and alcoholism is likely to contribute to addiction-related mechanisms and generalized comorbidity,[45] and strategies to improve function in recovery may be helpful. CoQ10 supplementation successfully attenuated neurobehavioral changes, striatal dopamine depletion, and lipid peroxidation associated with methamphetamine and cocaine administration to rats.[46] Lipoic acid dose dependently reduced self-administration in alcohol addicted rats.[47] Two in-vitro studies report that acetyl-L-carnitine reverses the toxic effect of methamphetamine to blood-brain-barrier and microtubular function.[48,49]

## Turmeric/Curcumin

In mice fed excessive alcohol over 24 weeks, diets containing 0.016% curcumin reversed the elevation in MDA (marker for ROS) compared to controls, though it did not increase antioxidant enzyme activity.[50] A different group reported improvements in liver injury and endogenous antioxidants in alcohol-fed mice with high curcumin doses.[51] Curcumin also reduced ROS levels in alcohol-fed rats and improved endogenous antioxidant systems when zinc was chelated to the curcumin, an effect attributed to the added value of zinc.[52]

## Danshen/Salvia Miltiorrhiza

Danshen is widely used in traditional Chinese medicine in treatment of cardiovascular and cerebrovascular diseases, including coronary artery disease, angina pectoris, and stroke. While many chemical constituents have been isolated from this herb, preclinical research has isolated 3 that have shown promise in animal studies: tanshinone IIA, cryptotanshinone, and miltirone.[53] Pure miltirone

reduced acquisition and maintenance of alcohol use in sP rats, and effect correlated to miltirone levels.[54] No human research in this regard has been reported.

## Stress Activation and Reward Deficiency

### PATHOPHYSIOLOGIC BASIS

Drug abuse may also damage stress-system homeostasis and key executive and
reward neurotransmitter systems, affecting judgment, and sapping volition during
the "white-knuckle" stage of recovery. Even short-term use of stimulants may be
associated with depleted neurotransmitter levels and decreased post-synaptic
DA receptor densities in early recovery, which explains symptoms commonly
seen in the initial stages of recovery (e.g., lethargy, depression, cognitive deficits,
irritability).

Reward deficiency syndrome refers to deficits in key neurotransmitter signaling due to damage, receptor down-regulation, and neurotransmitter depletion,
with specific attention directed to the HPA axis, the DA system,[55,56] and dopamine
receptor genetics (Table 20.1).[57] This hypothesis provides a rational basis for neurotransmitter and stress-system treatment support in the form of adaptogenic herbs,
essential amino acids, vitamins and minerals, and neurotransmitter breakdown
inhibitors. It also supports a principle of treatment synergy as illustrated by a proprietary mixture containing Rhodiola rosea, essential amino acids (5HTP, DLPA,
Glutamine, L-tyrosine), and cholinergic support (DMAE, huperzine-A) that was
reported to produce benefits in alcohol treatment.[58] As this study was not blinded,
randomized, or placebo controlled, it should be interpreted with caution; however,
the benefits of rationally layered natural treatments will likely be revealed in future
research.

### TREATMENT APPROACHES

### Rhodiola rosea

Rhodiola rosea is an herbal adaptogen with energizing qualities useful in asthenia and fatigue, which are common characteristics in early recovery. Actions
likely stem from effects on catecholamine neurotransmitters and possibly
through endogenous opiate production and opiate-receptor effects.[59] While
rosavin is often the constituent cited in extract standardization, Rhodiola
contains a variety of antioxidants and flavonoids with monoamine oxidase
(MAO) inhibition. The Rosiridin component inhibits MAO-b by 83.8%, and

**Table 20.1  Natural Modulators of Reward Deficiency Syndrome and HPA-Axis Hyperactivation**

| Compound | Mechanism and Effects | Potential Clinical Targets |
|---|---|---|
| L-phenylalanine | DA and NE precursor. Increased BH4, DA, NE and mild MAO-B inhibition | Increased focus, initiative, drive, memory. Increased energy. Mood elevation. |
| D-phenylalanine | Enkephalinase inhibitor | Anti-nociceptive. Mood elevator |
| L-tyrosine | DA and NE precursor, Increased DA, NE | Increased focus, initiative, drive, memory. Increased energy. Antidepressant. |
| 5-Hydroxytyrptophan | serotonin precursor | Calming agent, anxiolytic, sleep |
| Lecithin, Choline and DMAE | Acetylcholine precursor | Increased focus, initiative, drive, memory. Increased energy. Mood elevation. |
| B-Vitamins/ activated B6 | Increased production of catacholamines and GABA | Increased focus, initiative, drive, memory. Increased energy. Antidepressant. Anxiolytic, sleep. |
| Huperzine-A | Acetylcholinesterase inhibition, increased acetylcholine | Increased focus, initiative, drive, memory. Increased energy. Mood elevation. |
| N-acetyl-L-tyrosine | DA and NE precursor with potentially enhanced BBB penetration | Increased DA, NE |
| Phosphatidylserine | HPA Axis downregulation | Calming agent, anxiolytic, sleep |
| *Rhodiola rosea* | Catecholamine reuptake inhibition and MAO inhibition | Increased focus, initiative, drive, memory. Increased energy. Mood elevation. |
| *Mucuna puriens* | L-Dopa source increases DA and NE production | Increased focus, initiative, drive, memory. Increased energy. Mood elevation. |
| *Bacopa monnieri* | Unclear | Nootropic and anti-nociceptive. Mood elevation |

Abbreviations: DA-dopamine, NE-norepinephrine, BBB-blood brain barrier, DMAE-Dimethylaminoethanol, HPA-hypothalamic-pituitary-adrenal, GABA-gamma-aminobutyric acid

MAO-A is inhibited by other extract isolates, although to a substantially lesser degree.[60] These findings are consistent with reported serotonin effects in a nicotine withdrawal study in rats.[61] Rhodiola also significantly reduced serum norepinephrine in food-deprived rats while substantially elevating dopamine levels in the frontal cortex but not the striatum,[62] effects that warrant further study in addiction treatment.

### *St. John's Wort (SJW)/Hypericum perforatum*

St. John's Wort was first described by Hippocrates in the fifth-century BCE and is now accepted as a natural treatment for depression, anxiety, and obsessive compulsive disorder. High doses of SJW $CO_2$ extract (31 or 125 mg/kg) were reported to reduce self-administered ethanol intake over 2 hours by approximately 30% and 60% (p<0.01) respectively in alcohol-preferring rats who had not undergone deprivation. A lower dose of SJW (7 mg/kg) in conjunction with 1 mg/kg naltrexone produced a synergistic effect, lowering intake by approximately 30%, while neither treatment alone produced significant effects.[63] SJW at 31 and 125 mg/kg also significantly reduced alcohol lever-presses (i.e., requests for alcohol) by 37% and 82% in rats withdrawn for 10 days before reintroduction.[64] In chronic treatment models, SJW at 31 and 125 mg/kg attenuated self-administered alcohol in dependent rats over 12 days by approximately 50% and 75% respectively. When researchers held treatment on day 8, they reported a rapid return to previous levels of alcohol intake, implying a clear continuing treatment effect.[65]

Clinical- and animal-based evidence support hyperforin, hypericin, and bioflavinoids for general clinical effects,[66–68] and other researchers have also reported attenuation of alcohol use in rats treated with SJW.[69,70] However, no human studies have been reported. While the lack of research on effects in humans is disappointing, the safety of SJW is reassuring. Mechanism of action likely involves interplay between serotonin and norepinephrine reuptake inhibition and properties that increase extracellular glutamic acid, GABA, and acetycholine levels.[53] Medications with potentially similar actions (antidepressants, anxiolytics) have been disappointing in AUD research,[71] and thus an alternative option may have distinct value.

SJW is typically standardized to contain a consistent level of 1 or both of 2 naturally occurring chemicals found in the plant—hypericin (0.3%) and hyperforin (3% to 5%).[72] Total daily dosing of standardized extract ranges from 600 to 1,200 mg, administered in thrice daily dosing due to a short T½. Because products vary widely, clinicians may wish to prescribe proprietary formulations with supporting research. Hyperforin can cause photosensitization in fair-skinned individuals.[72] It is also an inducer of CYP3A4 and may potentially change the levels and/or efficacy of other medications including:

- oral contraceptives
- statins
- quetiapine
- lurasidone
- buspirone
- midazolam
- Triazolam
- omeprazole
- astemizole
- pimozide
- quinidine
- tacrolimus
- sirolimus
- digoxin
- protease inhibitors
- reverse transcriptase inhibitors
- warfarin
- fentanyl
- dihydroergotamine

## Citicoline

Citicoline, also known as CDP-Choline, is an intermediate molecule in the production of phosphatidylcholine that reduces memory impairment in aging and may have specific effects upon the dopaminergic system. Citicoline increased dopamine membrane transporters in the rat-brain frontal lobe,[73] dopamine levels in rabbit retina,[74] and dopamine receptor densities in rat striatum.[75] It also protected cultured mesenchephalic cells from MPP(+)-induced death,[76] increased phosphocreatine and triphosphates/ATP energetics in human anterior cingulate cells by 7% and 32%,[77] and improved function in Parkinson's patients when added to levodopa.[78]

A review of 9 clinical studies reported promising results in cocaine abuse with citicoline supplementation from 500 to 2,000 mg/day, especially in subjects with comorbid bipolar disorder.[79] A large clinical trial following this review reported approximately 15% decrease in positive urine screens in bipolar cocaine users receiving 2,000 mg/day.[80] And, although self-reported methamphetamine use did not differ between active treatment versus placebo, increased treatment retention time, completion rates, and improvements in depression scales were reported when 2,000 mg/day of citicoline was given to users with unipolar or bipolar depression.[81]

## Amino Acids

Various neurotransmitter depletions and essential amino acid deficiencies contribute to many acute and chronic withdrawal symptoms associated with substance abuse. Multiple and various amino acids (AA) are commonly depleted in alcoholism[82] and other SUDs due to a combination of malnutrition, excessive neurotransmitter turnover/breakdown, and the directly toxic effects. Treatment of many wide-reaching psychiatric disorders with L-type amino acids have become relatively mainstream. And AA treatment benefits in alcoholism and SUDs are likely to be proven in coming years. Potential benefits of AA supplementation may go beyond neurotransmitter repletion with L-type amino acids; D-type amino acids also have a potential role to play. For example, though there is conflict in the literature, D-phenylalanine has anti-nociceptive properties that may be mediated through enkephalinase inhibition. And a combination of D-phenylalanine, L-glutamine and L-5-hydroxytryptophan reduced symptom checklist-90-R scores and improved immune system parameters in recovering alcoholics over a 40-day period.[83] Route of administration may matter, as intravenous AA therapy produced improved outcomes over oral administration in one report.[84]

## Bacopa monnieri

*Bacopa monnieri* is a renowned ayurvedic medicine with established nootropic, anti-nociceptive, and anti-inflammatory properties with reported benefits in opiate withdrawal and tobacco cessation. It may have a role to play in SUDs marked by cognitive dysfunction and/or mitochondrial fatigue due to ROS overload. In mice, bacopasides reduced morphine-withdrawal-related depression,[85] as well as the development of morphine tolerance.[86] It also reduced morphine-induced hyperactivity, striatal dopamine, and serotonin turnover.[87] Bacoside-A provided substantial protection against brain mitochondrial dysfunction[88] and reduced heat shock protein 70 kDa expression and apoptosis in rats exposed to tobacco smoke.[89]

# Vitamin and Nutrient Deficiency

### PATHOPHYSIOLOGIC BASIS

The severe nutrient depletions commonly reported in AUDs and SADs are likely to affect recovery and physical health post-recovery. Depletions present through multiple mechanisms including direct nutrient wasting effects, poor nutrition and anorexic effects, and altered absorption and homeostasis. When metabolic needs are not supported in the recovery period, disability may extend beyond that caused by the abused substance alone, potentially contributing to relapse or serious comorbidities. Alcoholism is notorious for inducing severe and interactive nutrient deficiencies that require sustained repletion efforts at high dosages.

Documented deficiencies in AUDs include: thiamine/B1,[90,91] niacin/B3,[92,93] folate/B9,[94] cobalamin/B12,[95–98] zinc [92,99–103], magnesium,[97,98,101,104,105] phosphate,[97,106] vitamin D,[97,98,101,103,104,106,107] vitamin A,[3,100,103,108] iron,[98] CoQ10,[2,109] carnitine,[110] vitamin C,[91,103,111,112] and vitamin E.[13,103] As such, prescriptions for vitamins, herbs, minerals, and nutrients are rational in the recovery period, are not likely to harm the patient, and may improve outcome measures at many levels. In particular, a number of nutrients discussed below warrant specific attention given how poorly they are understood and how severely they can affect SUD-related comorbidity.

## TREATMENT APPROACHES

### General Vitamins and Nutrients

Clinicians tailoring baseline nutrient recommendations in SUDs should feel comfortable with empiric decisions based on the substance(s) abused, the severity and length of addiction, associated comorbidities, and presenting clinical signs or symptoms. Generally, a broad and relatively aggressive nutrient support regimen can be offered with little fear of overloading patients within reasonable time frames. In assessing which nutrients might be depleted in chronic alcoholism, the right question is actually, "Which nutrients are not depleted?" The only nutrient consistently elevated in uncomplicated alcoholism is copper; this is likely due to the ubiquity of zinc deficiency, which inhibits copper excretion. Tobacco use severely depletes multiple B vitamins and vitamin C.

### Zinc

Severe zinc deficiency commonly occurs in alcoholism through multiple mechanisms, including sharply decreased intake, decreased intestinal absorption, decreased albumin-related carrying capacity,[108] and substantially increased urinary losses.[99,100] Serum zinc levels were much lower in patients with cirrhosis compared to controls and were even worse in patients with encephalopathy.[102] Liver biopsy revealed severe zinc depletion in alcoholics with (–55%) and without cirrhosis (–30%) compared to controls.[113] In addition, zinc deficiency affects the production of other essential nutrients, such as niacin implicated in alcoholic pellagra.[92]

Given that alcohol-induced zinc deficiency is implicated in many comorbid conditions including skin lesions, retinal dysfunction, hypogonadism, anorexia, congenital malformations, immune dysfunction, and cancer,[99] deficiencies clearly warrant attention at any stage of treatment.

It is important to note that both zinc and magnesium are primarily intracellular ions that buffer out to plasma during long-term depletion. As such, plasma levels can normalize despite severe intracellular depletion. One study reports severely depleted intracellular levels of zinc in the alveolar macrophages of healthy alcoholics despite normal serum levels.[114] Another study reports that while plasma zinc levels normalized in heroin addicts after 10 days of hospitalization, intracellular zinc levels (i.e., RBC levels) deteriorated to less than 80% of controls—and similar outcomes occurred with magnesium.[115] Because plasma testing is common, many clinicians fail to prescribe appropriate and adequate supplementation by inadvertently providing themselves false laboratory reassurance. This phenomena should be considered when assessing research that reports serum levels of any primarily intracellular nutrient.

It is also clear that an improved post-recovery diet is insufficient to replete whole-body zinc deficiency within a reasonable timeframe. Serum zinc and selenium levels did not improve without supplementation during a 21-day alcohol rehabilitation program,[116] and alcohol rehab patients still exhibited significantly lower zinc levels compared to controls after 30 days of sobriety.[117]

Regarding zinc repletion in chronic alcoholism, animal studies are encouraging. In alcoholic mice, zinc supplementation restored normal zinc and metallothionein levels in the liver, reduced histologically confirmed steatosis and inflammation, reduced elevations in alanine aminotransferase (ALT) and tumor necrosis factor-alpha, prevented glutathione depletion, and reduced lipid and protein oxidation products due to reactive oxygen species.[118] Supplementary zinc has been associated with inhibition of alcohol-related TNF-α, oxidative liver injury and apoptosis, and circulating endotoxin due to alcohol-related gastrointestinal permeability.[119] Human studies are highly positive, except where small doses or insufficient repletion time was provided. While 3 days of zinc at 40 mg/day did not affect acute withdrawal outcome parameters,[120] 1 month of repletion at 400 mg/day of zinc sulfate improved visual capacity in patients with visual neuropathy related to tobacco and alcohol use.[121] Significant improvements in delayed hypersensitivity was reported in patients with alcoholic cirrhosis with 200 mg of zinc sulfate for 2 months,[122] and 200 mg of zinc sulfate thrice daily in 30 patients with alcoholic cirrhosis restored taste function, raised prothrombin and alkaline phosphatase levels, and lowered levels of bilirubin and carotene over 6 weeks compared to controls.[123]

Finally, some forms of zinc are poorly absorbed or tolerated, and research into optimal forms for supplementation is needed. Zinc repletion can generally occur through oral supplementation, though repletion dosing in alcoholism should be higher than many clinicians are generally comfortable with. Chelated forms of zinc (e.g., orotate, picolinate, and glycinate) may be better tolerated and absorbed, although they can be more expensive per milligram.

## Thiamine

Thiamine deficiency occurs in 30% to 80% of alcoholics, due to reduced intake[124,125] and alcohol-induced malabsorption through transcriptional inhibition of the thiamine transporter.[126] Liver injury directly reduces natural stores of thiamine and thiamine phosphorylation, while direct damage to the blood-brain barrier may substantially slow brain uptake.[127] Genetic susceptibility may also play a role through variations in the SLC19A3 thiamine transporters,[128] a factor that has been associated in non-alcoholic Wernicke encephalopathy in children and adolescents.[129] This water soluble vitamin is already poorly absorbed and transported across membranes in the gut and the blood-brain barrier, a quality that can produce vast differences between blood and brain levels.[130] Thiamine deficiency leads to impaired lead detoxification[124] and massive oxidative stress, inflammation, and excitotoxicity that ultimately cause the characteristic histological lesions in the mammillary bodies and thalamus of Wernicke-Korsakoff syndrome, a severe, progressive dementia and encephalopathy associated with high morbidity and acute mortality of 20%.[131]

Many factors point toward substantially increased need for repletion in alcoholics beyond the initial recovery period, yet even basic guidelines regarding thiamine repletion in AUD are often ignored by clinicians. American hospitals often neglect to prescribe thiamine to patients with AUD or prescribe oral dosing at inadequate strength.[90] Many clinicians are not aware that IM dosing of thiamine at 100 mg/day is warranted for many weeks, in much the same way that B12 injections should occur more frequently during initial periods of repletion. Down-regulated thiamine-dependent enzymes in the brain and other tissues persist after detoxification requiring concentrations of thiamine that are difficult to achieve orally.[127]

Natural high-potency analogs (e.g., benfotiamine, sulbutiamine, fursultiamine) have a role to play in recovery given thiamine's poor absorption. Benfotiamine (S-benzoylthiamine-O-monophosphate) is the most studied and most potent of the allithiamines, found in trace amounts in allium-family vegetables such as garlic, onions, and leeks.[130] Indeed, a small study reports that women (but not men) prescribed 600 m daily oral benfotiamine reduced their total mean alcohol intake over 6 months by 611 drinks compared to 159 in controls.[125]

## Magnesium

Magnesium deficiency has been reported in 30% to 60% of alcoholics, increasing to 90% for those in withdrawal.[132,104] Magnesium is involved in over 2,000 metabolic reactions and is a natural intracellular NMDA receptor antagonist. Chronic alcohol intake induces NMDA receptor upregulation; hypomagnesemia during early sobriety may compound the alcohol craving and physical agitation believed to be related to rebound NMDA receptor hyperactivity.

Deficiency is associated with reduced intake and absorption, and sharply increased urinary loses seen within minutes of alcohol ingestion[133,104] by renal tubular reabsorption. Hypomagnesemia has been associated with the osteoporosis and cardiovascular disease of alcoholism,[104,134] and may contribute to the psychiatric profile of early sobriety. Similar to zinc, initial, and ongoing assessment of magnesium status through serum levels will frequently underestimate the prevalence and severity of magnesium deficiency. Intracellular levels (RBC levels) must be used.[104]

While short-term studies examining repletion benefits have been disappointing, longer clinical trails have shown substantial benefits. Recently sober alcoholics receiving 500 mg of magnesium (as magnesium carbonate, magnesium acetate, and magnesium hydroxide) had greater reduction in serum AST levels, a factor associated with all cause mortality in alcoholism.[135] In addition, hypomagnesemia is generally associated with depression, and replacement can have rapid antidepressant effects[136] and may be useful in recovery.

Magnesium is frequently used as an osmotic laxative due to its resistance to gastrointestinal absorption. Thus, whole body repletion often requires long-term, high-dose oral repletion with chelated forms of magnesium that are more easily absorbed (e.g., magnesium glycinate, magnesium taurinate). Highly effective IV magnesium treatments are sometimes offered in inpatient rehab settings. Magnesium citrate can be the right choice if co-occurring constipation requires treatment.

## Other Herbal Interventions

### KUDZU/*PUERARIA LOBATE*

Kudzu should only be recommended with caution in the treatment of alcoholism. Despite use in traditional Chinese medicine for issues pertaining to alcohol use, evidence for kudzu only supports an anti-alcohol effect based on pro-intoxication pharmacodynamics and increased acetaldehyde levels. This combination of effects may reduce the rate of drinking by increasing toxicity, while having little effect upon total 24-hour consumption. While the flower component of kudzu (Pueraria flos) indeed enhances acetaldehyde removal, the root component (Pueraria lobata) is being used in many herbal preparations instead. Because concentrated root extract may inhibit ALDH2 by 70%, concurrent use with alcohol (as is recommended by the manufacturer) may increase risk of aldehyde-related complications and neoplasm.[137] This is especially pertinent given that aldehyde can produce a reinforcing euphoria in some individuals.[138]

Human studies with kudzu are underpowered, misleading, and potentially compromised by commercial interests. One group does not compare to placebo,[139] while another reports substantial anti-alcohol effects of a proprietary kudzu extract when total reductions in drinking were insignificant compared to placebo.[140] Other studies are either underwhelming[141] or blatantly misleading, with one group concluding that concurrent use of alcohol and kudzu extract had no adverse consequences despite reporting 70% increases in blood-alcohol level BAL, as well as dizziness, accelerated heart rate, and a 3.1°C increase in skin temperature,[142] all likely signs of high blood acetaldehyde levels.[138,143]

## IBOGAINE/*TABERNANTHE IBOGA*

Ibogaine, a principal alkaloid found in the African shrub *Tabernanthe iboga*, has been associated in some preliminary research with anti-addiction effects in multiple forms of drug abuse, including alcohol, opiates, and cocaine. However, ibogaine's potential to induce seizures limits its usefulness as a treatment option. Research into analogs with reduced toxicity are occurring.[144]

## REFERENCES

1. Zhou JF, Chen P. Studies on the oxidative stress in alcohol abusers in China. *Biomedical and Environmental Sciences.* 2001;14(3):180–188.
2. Cunningham CC, Bailey SM. Ethanol consumption and liver mitochondria function. *Biological Signals and Receptors.* 2001;10(3–4):271–282.
3. González-Reimers E, Fernández-Rodríguez CM, Candelaria Martín-González M, et al. Antioxidant vitamins and brain dysfunction in alcoholics. *Alcohol and Alcoholism.* 2014;49(1):45–50. doi:10.1093/alcalc/agt150.
4. Brooks PJ. Brain atrophy and neuronal loss in alcoholism: a role for DNA damage? *Neurochemistry International.* 2000;37(5–6):403–412.
5. Kruman II, Henderson GI, Bergeson SE. DNA damage and neurotoxicity of chronic alcohol abuse. *Experimental biology and medicine (Maywood NJ).* 2012;237(7):740–747. doi:10.1258/ebm.2012.011421.
6. Arendt T. Impairment in memory function and neurodegenerative changes in the cholinergic basal forebrain system induced by chronic intake of ethanol. *Journal of Neural Transmission. Supplementa.* 1994;44:173–187.
7. Purohit V, Bode JC, Bode C, et al. Alcohol, intestinal bacterial growth, intestinal permeability to endotoxin, and medical consequences: summary of a symposium. *Alcohol.* 2008;42(5):349–361. doi:10.1016/j.alcohol.2008.03.131.
8. Keshavarzian A, Holmes EW, Patel M, Iber F, Fields JZ, Pethkar S. Leaky gut in alcoholic cirrhosis: a possible mechanism for alcohol-induced liver damage. *The American Journal of Gastroenterology.* 1999;94(1):200–207. doi:10.1111/j.1572-0241.1999.00797.x.

9. Bouhnik Y, Neut C, Raskine L, et al. Prospective, randomized, parallel-group trial to evaluate the effects of lactulose and polyethylene glycol-4000 on colonic flora in chronic idiopathic constipation. *Alimentary Pharmacology & Therapeutics.* 2004;19(8):889–899. doi:10.1111/j.1365-2036.2004.01918.x.

10. Riggio O, Varriale M, Testore GP, et al. Effect of lactitol and lactulose administration on the fecal flora in cirrhotic patients. *Journal of Clinical Gastroenterology.* 1990;12(4):433–436.

11. Jain L, Sharma BC, Srivastava S, Puri SK, Sharma P, Sarin S. Serum endotoxin, inflammatory mediators, and magnetic resonance spectroscopy before and after treatment in patients with minimal hepatic encephalopathy. *Journal of Gastroenterology and Hepatology.* 2013;28(7):1187–1193. doi:10.1111/jgh.12160.

12. Kirpich IA, Solovieva NV, Leikhter SN, et al. Probiotics restore bowel flora and improve liver enzymes in human alcohol-induced liver injury: A pilot study. *Alcohol.* 2008;42(8):675–682. doi:10.1016/j.alcohol.2008.08.006.

13. Besselink MGH, van Santvoort HC, Buskens E, et al. [Probiotic prophylaxis in patients with predicted severe acute pancreatitis: a randomised, double-blind, placebo-controlled trial]. *Nederlands Tijdschrift Voor Geneeskunde.* 2008;152(12):685–696.

14. Renard P, Zachary MD, Bougelet C, et al. Effects of antioxidant enzyme modulations on interleukin-1-induced nuclear factor kappa B activation. *Biochemical Pharmacology.* 1997;53(2):149–160.

15. Fitzgerald DC, Meade KG, McEvoy AN, et al. Tumour necrosis factor-alpha (TNF-alpha) increases nuclear factor kappaB (NFkappaB) activity in and interleukin-8 (IL-8) release from bovine mammary epithelial cells. *Veterinary Immunology and Immunopathology.* 2007;116(1–2):59–68. doi:10.1016/j.vetimm.2006.12.008.

16. Chandel NS, Trzyna WC, McClintock DS, Schumacker PT. Role of oxidants in NF-kappa B activation and TNF-alpha gene transcription induced by hypoxia and endotoxin. *Journal of immunology.* 2000;165(2):1013–1021.

17. Qin H, Wilson CA, Lee SJ, Zhao X, Benveniste EN. LPS induces CD40 gene expression through the activation of NF-kappaB and STAT-1alpha in macrophages and microglia. *Blood.* 2005;106(9):3114–3122. doi:10.1182/blood-2005-02-0759.

18. Meffert MK, Chang JM, Wiltgen BJ, Fanselow MS, Baltimore D. NF-kappa B functions in synaptic signaling and behavior. *Nature Neuroscience.* 2003;6(10):1072–1078. doi:10.1038/nn1110.

19. Ruffle JK. Molecular neurobiology of addiction: what's all the (Δ)FosB about? *American Journal of Drug and Alcohol Abuse.* 2014;40(6):428–437. doi:10.3109/00952990.2014.933840.

20. Nestler EJ. Review. Transcriptional mechanisms of addiction: role of DeltaFosB. *Philosophical transactions of the Royal Society of London.* 2008;363(1507):3245–3255. doi:10.1098/rstb.2008.0067.

21. Russo SJ, Wilkinson M, Mazei-Robison M, et al. NFκB signaling regulates neuronal morphology and cocaine reward. *Journal of neuroscience: the official journal of the Society for Neuroscience.* 2009;29(11):3529–3537. doi:10.1523/JNEUROSCI.6173-08.2009.

22. Kasdallah-Grissa A, Mornagui B, Aouani E, et al. Resveratrol, a red wine poly-phenol, attenuates ethanol-induced oxidative stress in rat liver. *Life Sciences.* 2007;80(11):1033–1039. doi:10.1016/j.lfs.2006.11.044.

23. Tiwari V, Chopra K. Resveratrol prevents alcohol-induced cognitive deficits and brain damage by blocking inflammatory signaling and cell death cascade in neonatal rat brain. *Journal of Neurochemistry.* 2011;117(4):678–690. doi:10.1111/j.1471-4159.2011.07236.x.

24. Gonthier B, Allibe N, Cottet-Rousselle C, Lamarche F, Nuiry L, Barret L. Specific conditions for resveratrol neuroprotection against ethanol-induced toxicity. *Journal of Toxicology.* 2012;2012:973134. doi:10.1155/2012/973134.

25. Yuan H, Zhang W, Li H, Chen C, Liu H, Li Z. Neuroprotective effects of resveratrol on embryonic dorsal root ganglion neurons with neurotoxicity induced by ethanol. *Food and Chemical Toxicology.* 2013;55:192–201. doi:10.1016/j.fct.2012.12.052.

26. Chan W-H, Chang Y-J. Dosage effects of resveratrol on ethanol-induced cell death in the human K562 cell line. *Toxicology Letters.* 2006;161(1):1–9. doi:10.1016/j.toxlet.2005.07.010.

27. Leon R, Wu H, Jin Y, et al. Protective function of taurine in glutamate-induced apoptosis in cultured neurons. *Journal of Neuroscience Research.* 2009;87(5):1185–1194. doi:10.1002/jnr.21926.

28. Olive MF. Interactions between taurine and ethanol in the central nervous system. *Amino Acids.* 2002;23(4):345–357. doi:10.1007/s00726-002-0203-1.

29. Hsieh Y-L, Yeh Y-H, Lee Y-T, Huang C-Y. Effect of taurine in chronic alcoholic patients. *Food Function.* 2014;5(7):1529–1535. doi:10.1039/c3fo60597c.

30. Kerai MDJ, Waterfield DCJ, Kenyon SH, Asker DS, Timbrell JA. Taurine: Protective properties against ethanol-induced hepatic steatosis and lipid peroxidation during chronic ethanol consumption in rats. *Amino Acids.* 1998;15(1–2):53–76. doi:10.1007/BF01345280.

31. Deepmala null, Slattery J, Kumar N, et al. Clinical trials of N-acetylcysteine in psychiatry and neurology: A systematic review. *Neuroscience and Biobehavioral Reviews.* 2015;55:294–321. doi:10.1016/j.neubiorev.2015.04.015.

32. Caro AA, Bell M, Ejiofor S, Zurcher G, Petersen DR, Ronis MJJ. N-acetylcysteine inhibits the up-regulation of mitochondrial biogenesis genes in livers from rats fed ethanol chronically. *Alcoholism: Clinical and Experimental Research.* 2014;38(12):2896–2906. doi:10.1111/acer.12576.

33. Loweth JA, Tseng KY, Wolf ME. Adaptations in AMPA receptor transmission in the nucleus accumbens contributing to incubation of cocaine craving. *Neuropharmacology.* 2014;76:287–300. doi:10.1016/j.neuropharm.2013.04.061.

34. Reichel CM, Moussawi K, Do PH, Kalivas PW, See RE. Chronic N-acetylcysteine during abstinence or extinction after cocaine self-administration produces enduring reductions in drug seeking. *Journal of Pharmacology and Experimental Therapeutics.* 2011;337(2):487–493. doi:10.1124/jpet.111.179317.

35. Mardikian PN, LaRowe SD, Hedden S, Kalivas PW, Malcolm RJ. An open-label trial of N-acetylcysteine for the treatment of cocaine dependence: a pilot study.

*Progress in Neuro-Psychopharmacology & Biological Psychiatry.* 2007;31(2):389–394. doi:10.1016/j.pnpbp.2006.10.001.

36. LaRowe SD, Myrick H, Hedden S, et al. Is cocaine desire reduced by N-acetylcysteine? *American Journal of Psychiatry.* 2007;164(7):1115–1117. doi:10.1176/ajp.2007.164.7.1115.

37. Schmaal L, Veltman DJ, Nederveen A, van den Brink W, Goudriaan AE. N-acetylcysteine normalizes glutamate levels in cocaine-dependent patients: a randomized crossover magnetic resonance spectroscopy study. *Neuropsychopharmacol Off Publ Am Coll Neuropsychopharmacol.* 2012;37(9):2143–2152. doi:10.1038/npp.2012.66.

38. Gray KM, Carpenter MJ, Baker NL, et al. A double-blind randomized controlled trial of N-acetylcysteine in cannabis-dependent adolescents. *American Journal of Psychiatry.* 2012;169(8):805–812. doi:10.1176/appi.ajp.2012.12010055.

39. Gray KM, Watson NL, Carpenter MJ, Larowe SD. N-acetylcysteine (NAC) in young marijuana users: an open-label pilot study. *American Journal on Addictions.* 2010;19(2):187–189. doi:10.1111/j.1521-0391.2009.00027.x.

40. Zhou W, Kalivas PW. N-acetylcysteine reduces extinction responding and induces enduring reductions in cue- and heroin-induced drug-seeking. *Biological Psychiatry.* 2008;63(3):338–340. doi:10.1016/j.biopsych.2007.06.008.

41. Prado E, Maes M, Piccoli LG, et al. N-acetylcysteine for therapy-resistant tobacco use disorder: a pilot study. *Redox Report: Communications in Free Radical Research.* 2015;20(5):215–222. doi:10.1179/1351000215Y.0000000004.

42. Hashimoto K, Tsukada H, Nishiyama S, et al. Protective effects of N-acetyl-L-cysteine on the reduction of dopamine transporters in the striatum of monkeys treated with methamphetamine. *Neuropsychopharmacology.* 2004;29(11):2018–2023. doi:10.1038/sj.npp.1300512.

43. Fukami G, Hashimoto K, Koike K, Okamura N, Shimizu E, Iyo M. Effect of antioxidant N-acetyl-L-cysteine on behavioral changes and neurotoxicity in rats after administration of methamphetamine. *Brain Research.* 2004;1016(1):90–95. doi:10.1016/j.brainres.2004.04.072.

44. Mousavi SG, Sharbafchi MR, Salehi M, Peykanpour M, Karimian Sichani N, Maracy M. The efficacy of N-acetylcysteine in the treatment of methamphetamine dependence: a double-blind controlled, crossover study. *Archives of Iranian Medicine.* 2015;18(1):28–33. doi:0151801/AIM.008.

45. Haorah J, Rump TJ, Xiong H. Reduction of brain mitochondrial β-oxidation impairs complex I and V in chronic alcohol intake: the underlying mechanism for neurodegeneration. *PloS ONE.* 2013;8(8):e70833. doi:10.1371/journal.pone.0070833.

46. Klongpanichapak S, Govitrapong P, Sharma SK, Ebadi M. Attenuation of cocaine and methamphetamine neurotoxicity by coenzyme Q10. *Neurochemical Research.* 2006;31(3):303–311. doi:10.1007/s11064-005-9025-3.

47. Peana AT, Muggironi G, Fois G, Diana M. Alpha-lipoic acid reduces ethanol self-administration in rats. *Alcoholism, Clinical and Experimental Research.* 2013;37(11):1816–1822. doi:10.1111/acer.12169.

48. Fernandes S, Salta S, Bravo J, Silva AP, Summavielle T. Acetyl-L-Carnitine prevents methamphetamine-induced structural damage on endothelial cells via ILK-related MMP-9 activity. *Molecular Neurobiology.* 53(1), 408–422.2014. doi:10.1007/s12035-014-8973-5.

49. Fernandes S, Salta S, Summavielle T. Methamphetamine promotes α-tubulin deacetylation in endothelial cells: the protective role of acetyl-l-carnitine. *Toxicology Letters.* 2015;234(2):131–138. doi:10.1016/j.toxlet.2015.02.011.

50. Pyun C-W, Kim J-H, Han K-H, Hong G-E, Lee C-H. In vivo protective effects of dietary curcumin and capsaicin against alcohol-induced oxidative stress. *BioFactors.* 2014;40(5):494–500. doi:10.1002/biof.1172.

51. Zeng Y, Liu J, Huang Z, Pan X, Zhang L. Effect of curcumin on antioxidant function in the mice with acute alcoholic liver injury. *Wei Sheng Yan Jiu.* 2014;43(2):282–285.

52. Yu C, Mei X-T, Zheng Y-P, Xu D-H. Zn(II)-curcumin protects against hemorheological alterations, oxidative stress and liver injury in a rat model of acute alcoholism. *Environmental Toxicology and Pharmacology.* 2014;37(2):729–737. doi:10.1016/j.etap.2014.02.011.

53. Abenavoli L, Capasso F, Addolorato G. Phytotherapeutic approach to alcohol dependence: New old way? *Phytomedicine.* 2009;16(6–7):638–644. doi:10.1016/j.phymed.2008.12.013.

54. Colombo G, Serra S, Vacca G, et al. Identification of miltirone as active ingredient of Salvia miltiorrhiza responsible for the reducing effect of root extracts on alcohol intake in rats. *Alcoholism, Clinical and Experimental Research.* 2006;30(5):754–762. doi:10.1111/j.1530-0277.2006.00088.x.

55. Comings DE, Blum K. Reward deficiency syndrome: genetic aspects of behavioral disorders. In: *Research B-P in B, ed. Vol 126. Cognition, Emotion and Autonomic Responses: The Integrative Role of the Prefrontal Cortex and Limbic Structures.* Netherlands Institute for Brain Research, Amsterdam, The Netherlands: Elsevier; 2000:325–341.http://www.sciencedirect.com/science/article/pii/S0079612300260226. Accessed October 18, 2015.

56. Blum K, Braverman ER, Holder JM, et al. Reward deficiency syndrome: a biogenetic model for the diagnosis and treatment of impulsive, addictive, and compulsive behaviors. *Journal of Psychoactive Drugs.* 2000;32(Suppl:i–iv): 1–112.

57. Blum K, Sheridan PJ, Wood RC, et al. The D2 dopamine receptor gene as a determinant of reward deficiency syndrome. *Journal of the Royal Society of Medicine.* 1996;89(7):396–400.

58. Chen TJH, Blum K, Waite RL, et al. Gene\Narcotic Attenuation Program attenuates substance use disorder, a clinical subtype of reward deficiency syndrome. *Advances in Therapy.* 2007;24(2):402–414.

59. Rhodiola rosea. Monograph. Alternative Medicine Review : A Journal of Clinical Therapeutic. 2002;7(5):421–423.

60. van Diermen D, Marston A, Bravo J, Reist M, Carrupt P-A, Hostettmann K. Monoamine oxidase inhibition by Rhodiola rosea L. roots. *Journal of Ethnopharmacology.* 2009;122(2):397–401. doi:10.1016/j.jep.2009.01.007.

61. Mannucci C, Navarra M, Calzavara E, Caputi AP, Calapai G. Serotonin involvement in Rhodiola rosea attenuation of nicotine withdrawal signs in rats. *Phytomedicine: International Journal of Phytotherapy and Phytopharmacology.* 2012;19(12):1117–1124. doi:10.1016/jphymed.2012.07.001.

62. Verpeut JL, Walters AL, Bello NT. Citrus aurantium and Rhodiola rosea in combination reduce visceral white adipose tissue and increase hypothalamic norepinephrine in a rat model of diet-induced obesity. *Nutrition Research.* 2013;33(6):503–512. doi:10.1016/j.nutres.2013.04.001.

63. Perfumi M, Santoni M, Cippitelli A, Ciccocioppo R, Froldi R, Massi M. Hypericum perforatum $CO_2$ extract and opioid receptor antagonists act synergistically to reduce ethanol intake in alcohol-preferring rats. *Alcoholism, Clinical and Experimental Research.* 2003;27(10):1554–1562. doi:10.1097/01.ALC.0000092062.60924.56.

64. Perfumi M, Mattioli L, Forti L, Massi M, Ciccocioppo R. Effect of Hypericum perforatum $CO_2$ extract on the motivational properties of ethanol in alcohol-preferring rats. *Alcohol Alcohol.* 2005;40(4):291–296. doi:10.1093/alcalc/agh133.

65. Perfumi M, Mattioli L, Cucculelli M, Massi M. Reduction of ethanol intake by chronic treatment with Hypericum perforatum, alone or combined with naltrexone in rats. *Journal of Psychopharmacology.* 2005;19(5):448–454. doi:10.1177/0269881105056519.

66. Franklin M, Cowen PJ. Researching the antidepressant actions of Hypericum perforatum (St. John's wort) in animals and man. *Pharmacopsychiatry.* 2001;34(Suppl 1):S29–S37.

67. Butterweck V, Schmidt M. St. John's wort: role of active compounds for its mechanism of action and efficacy. *Wiener Medizinische Wochenschrift.* 2007;157(13–14):356–361. doi:10.1007/s10354-007-0440-8.

68. Butterweck V, Christoffel V, Nahrstedt A, Petereit F, Spengler B, Winterhoff H. Step by step removal of hyperforin and hypericin: activity profile of different Hypericum preparations in behavioral models. *Life Sciences.* 2003;73(5):627–639.

69. Rezvani AH, Overstreet DH, Yang Y, Clark E. Attenuation of alcohol intake by extract of Hypericum perforatum (St. John's Wort) in two different strains of alcohol-preferring rats. *Alcohol Alcohol.* 1999;34(5):699–705.

70. De Vry J, Maurel S, Schreiber R, de Beun R, Jentzsch KR. Comparison of hypericum extracts with imipramine and fluoxetine in animal models of depression and alcoholism. *European Neuropsychopharmacology.* 1999;9(6):461–468.

71. Aubin H-J, Daeppen J-B. Emerging pharmacotherapies for alcohol dependence: a systematic review focusing on reduction in consumption. *Drug and Alcohol Dependence.* 2013;133(1):15–29. doi:10.1016/j.drugalcdep.2013.04.025.

72. Blumenthal M. *The ABC Clinical Guide to Herbs.* 1st edition. American Botanical Council; 2003.

73. Tayebati SK, Tomassoni D, Nwankwo IE, et al. Modulation of monoaminergic transporters by choline-containing phospholipids in rat brain. *CNS & Neurological Disorders Drug Targets.* 2013;12(1):94–103.

74. Rejdak R, Toczołowski J, Solski J, Duma D, Grieb P. Citicoline treatment increases retinal dopamine content in rabbits. *Ophthalmic Research.* 2002;34(3):146–149. doi:63658.

75. Giménez R, Raïch J, Aguilar J. Changes in brain striatum dopamine and acetylcho-line receptors induced by chronic CDP-choline treatment of aging mice. *British Journal of Pharmacology*. 1991;104(3):575–578.

76. Radad K, Gille G, Xiaojing J, Durany N, Rausch W-D. CDP-choline reduces dopa-minergic cell loss induced by MPP(+) and glutamate in primary mesencephalic cell culture. *International Journal of Neuroscience*. 2007;117(7):985–998. doi:10.1080/10623320600934341.

77. Silveri MM, Dikan J, Ross AJ, et al. Citicoline enhances frontal lobe bioenergetics as measured by phosphorus magnetic resonance spectroscopy. *NMR Biomed.* 2008;21(10):1066–1075. doi:10.1002/nbm.1281.

78. Cubells JM, Hernando C. Clinical trial on the use of cytidine diphosphate choline in Parkinson's disease. *Clinical Therapeutics*. 1988;10(6):664–671.

79. Wignall ND, Brown ES. Citicoline in addictive disorders: a review of the litera-ture. *American Journal of Drug and Alcohol Abuse*. 2014;40(4):262–268. doi:10.3109/00952990.2014.925467.

80. Brown ES, Todd JP, Hu LT, et al. A randomized, double-blind, placebo-controlled trial of citicoline for cocaine dependence in bipolar I disorder. *American Journal of Psychiatry*. 2015;172(10):1014–1021. doi:10.1176/appi.ajp.2015.14070857.

81. Brown ES, Gabrielson B. A randomized, double-blind, placebo-controlled trial of citicoline for bipolar and unipolar depression and methamphetamine de-pendence. *Journal of Affective Disorders*. 2012;143(1–3):257–260. doi:10.1016/j.jad.2012.05.006.

82. Vannucchi H, Moreno FS, Amarante AR, de Oliveira JE, Marchini JS. Plasma amino acid patterns in alcoholic pellagra patients. *Alcohol Alcohol.* 1991;26(4):431–436.

83. Jukić T, Rojc B, Boben-Bardutzky D, Hafner M, Ihan A. The use of a food sup-plementation with D-phenylalanine, L-glutamine and L-5-hydroxytriptophan in the alleviation of alcohol withdrawal symptoms. *Collegium Antropologicum*. 2011;35(4):1225–1230.

84. Miller M, Chen ALC, Stokes SD, et al. Early intervention of intravenous KB220IV--neuroadaptagen amino-acid therapy (NAAT) improves behavioral outcomes in a residential addiction treatment program: a pilot study. *Journal of Psychoactive Drugs*. 2012;44(5):398–409. doi:10.1080/02791072.2012.737727.

85. Rauf K, Subhan F, Abbas M, et al. Inhibitory effect of bacopasides on spontaneous morphine withdrawal induced depression in mice. *Phytotherapy Research : PTR.* 2014;28(6):937–939. doi:10.1002/ptr.5081.

86. Rauf K, Subhan F, Abbas M, Badshah A, Ullah I, Ullah S. Effect of bacopasides on acquisition and expression of morphine tolerance. *Phytomedicine: International Journal of Phytotherapy and Phytopharmacology*. 2011;18(10):836–842. doi:10.1016/j.phymed.2011.01.023.

87. Rauf K, Subhan F, Sewell RDE. A Bacoside containing Bacopa monnieri extract reduces both morphine hyperactivity plus the elevated striatal dopamine and ser-otonin turnover. *Phytotherapy Research : PTR.* 2012;26(5):758–763. doi:10.1002/ptr.3631.

88. Anbarasi K, Vani G, Devi CSS. Protective effect of bacoside A on cigarette smoking-induced brain mitochondrial dysfunction in rats. *Journal of Environmental Pathology, Toxicology and Oncology.* 2005;24(3):225–234.

89. Anbarasi K, Kathirvel G, Vani G, Jayaraman G, Shyamala Devi CS. Cigarette smoking induces heat shock protein 70 kDa expression and apoptosis in rat brain: modulation by bacoside A. *Neuroscience.* 2006;138(4):1127–1135. doi:10.1016/j.neuroscience.2005.11.029.

90. Isenberg-Grzeda E, Chabon B, Nicolson SE. Prescribing thiamine to inpatients with alcohol use disorders: how well are we doing? *Journal of Addiction Medicine.* 2014;8(1):1–5. doi:10.1097/01.ADM.0000435320.72857.c8.

91. Baines M. Detection and incidence of B and C vitamin deficiency in alcohol-related illness. *Annals of Clinical Biochemistry.* 1978;15(6):307–312.

92. Vannucchi H, Moreno FS. Interaction of niacin and zinc metabolism in patients with alcoholic pellagra. *American Journal of Clinical Nutrition.* 1989;50(2):364–369.

93. Badawy AA-B. Pellagra and alcoholism: a biochemical perspective. *Alcohol Alcohol.* 2014;49(3):238–250. doi:10.1093/alcalc/agu010.

94. Blasco C, Caballería J, Deulofeu R, et al. Prevalence and mechanisms of hyperhomocysteinemia in chronic alcoholics. *Alcoholism, Clinical and Experimental Research.* 2005;29(6):1044–1048.

95. Fragasso A, Mannarella C, Ciancio A, Sacco A. Functional vitamin B12 deficiency in alcoholics: an intriguing finding in a retrospective study of megaloblastic anemic patients. *European Journal of Internal Medicine.* 2010;21(2):97–100. doi:10.1016/j.ejim.2009.11.012.

96. Cylwik B, Czygier M, Daniluk M, Chrostek L, Szmitkowski M. Vitamin B12 concentration in the blood of alcoholics. *Polski Merkuriusz Lekarski: Organ Polskiego Towarzystwa Lekarskiego.* 2010;28(164):122–125.

97. Wijnia JW, Wielders JPM, Lips P, van de Wiel A, Mulder CL, Nieuwenhuis KGA. Is vitamin D deficiency a confounder in alcoholic skeletal muscle myopathy? *Alcoholism, Clinical and Experimental Research.* 2013;37(Suppl 1):E209–E215. doi:10.1111/j.1530-0277.2012.01902.x.

98. Sobral-Oliveira MB, Faintuch J, Guarita DR, Oliveira CP, Carrilho FJ. Nutritional profile of asymptomatic alcoholic patients. *Arquivos de Gastroenterologia.* 2011;48(2):112–118.

99. McClain CJ, Su LC. Zinc deficiency in the alcoholic: a review. *Alcoholism, Clinical and Experimental Research.* 1983;7(1):5–10.

100. Russell RM. Vitamin A and zinc metabolism in alcoholism. *American Journal of Clinical Nutrition.* 1980;33(12):2741–2749.

101. Wilkens Knudsen A, Jensen J-EB, Nordgaard-Lassen I, Almdal T, Kondrup J, Becker U. Nutritional intake and status in persons with alcohol dependency: data from an outpatient treatment programme. *European Journal of Nutrition.* 2014;53(7):1483–1492. doi:10.1007/s00394-014-0651-x.

102. Rahelić D, Kujundzić M, Romić Z, Brkić K, Petrovecki M. Serum concentration of zinc, copper, manganese and magnesium in patients with liver cirrhosis. *Collegium Antropologicum.* 2006;30(3):523–528.

103. Maillot F, Farad S, Lamisse F. [Alcohol and nutrition]. *Pathologie-Biologie.* 2001;49(9):683–688.

104. Abbott L, Nadler J, Rude RK. Magnesium deficiency in alcoholism: possible contribution to osteoporosis and cardiovascular disease in alcoholics. *Alcoholism, Clinical and Experimental Research.* 1994;18(5):1076–1082.

105. Turecky L, Kupcova V, Szantova M, Uhlikova E, Viktorinova A, Czirfusz A. Serum magnesium levels in patients with alcoholic and non-alcoholic fatty liver. *Bratisl Lekárske Listy.* 2006;107(3):58–61.

106. Vandemergel X, Simon F. Evolution of metabolic abnormalities in alcoholic patients during withdrawal. *Journal on Addictions.* 2015;2015:541536. doi:10.1155/2015/541536.

107. Neupane SP, Lien L, Hilberg T, Bramness JG. Vitamin D deficiency in alcohol-use disorders and its relationship to comorbid major depression: a cross-sectional study of inpatients in Nepal. *Drug and Alcohol Dependence.* 2013;133(2):480–485. doi:10.1016/j.drugalcdep.2013.07.006.

108. McClain CJ, Van Thiel DH, Parker S, Badzin LK, Gilbert H. Alterations in zinc, vitamin A, and retinol-binding protein in chronic alcoholics: a possible mechanism for night blindness and hypogonadism. *Alcoholism, Clinical and Experimental Research.* 1979;3(2):135–141.

109. Bianchi GP, Fiorella PL, Bargossi AM, Grossi G, Marchesini G. Reduced ubiquinone plasma levels in patients with liver cirrhosis and in chronic alcoholics. *Liver.* 1994;14(3):138–140.

110. Kępka A, Waszkiewicz N, Zalewska-Szajda B, et al. Plasma carnitine concentrations after chronic alcohol intoxication. *Postępy Higieny I Medycyny Doświadczalnej.* 2013;67:548–552.

111. Ong J, Randhawa R. Scurvy in an alcoholic patient treated with intravenous vitamins. *BMJ Case Reports.* 2014;2014. doi:10.1136/bcr-2013-009479.

112. Shugaleĭ IS. Features of vitamin C metabolism and the functional status of the liver in alcoholism and alcoholic delirium in the stage of detoxification therapy. *Zhurnal Nevropatol Psikhiatrii Im SS Korsakova Mosc Russ 1952.* 1987;87(2):240–243.

113. Rodriguez-Moreno F, González-Reimers E, Santolaria-Fernandez F, et al. Zinc, copper, manganese, and iron in chronic alcoholic liver disease. *Alcohol.* 1997;14(1):39–44. doi:10.1016/S0741-8329(96)00103-6.

114. Mehta AJ, Yeligar SM, Elon L, Brown LA, Guidot DM. Alcoholism causes alveolar macrophage zinc deficiency and immune dysfunction. *American Journal of Respiratory and Critical Care Medicine.* 2013;188(6):716–723. doi:10.1164/rccm.201301-0061OC.

115. Ruiz Martínez M, Gil Extremera B, Maldonado Martín A, Cantero-Hinojosa J, Moreno-Abadía V. Trace elements in drug addicts. *Klin Wochenschr.* 1990;68(10):507–511.

116. Gueguen S, Pirollet P, Leroy P, et al. Changes in serum retinol, alpha-tocopherol, vitamin C, carotenoids, xinc and selenium after micronutrient supplementation during alcohol rehabilitation. *Journal of the American College of Nutrition.* 2003;22(4):303–310.

117. De Vos N, Song C, Lin A, et al. Lower serum zinc in relation to serum albumin and proinflammatory cytokines in detoxified alcohol-dependent patients without apparent liver disease. *Neuropsychobiology*. 1999;39(3):144–150. doi:26574.

118. Zhou Z, Wang L, Song Z, Saari JT, McClain CJ, Kang YJ. Zinc supplementation prevents alcoholic liver injury in mice through attenuation of oxidative stress. *American Journal of Pathology*. 2005;166(6):1681–1690. doi:10.1016/S0002-9440(10)62478-9.

119. Kang YJ, Zhou Z. Zinc prevention and treatment of alcoholic liver disease. *Molecular Aspects of Medicine*. 2005;26(4–5):391–404. doi:10.1016/j.mam.2005.07.002.

120. Iber FL. Evaluation of an oral solution to accelerate alcoholism detoxification. *Alcoholism, Clinical and Experimental Research*. 1987;11(3):305–308.

121. Béchetoille A, Ebran JM, Allain P, Mauras Y. Therapeutic affect of zinc sulfate on central scotoma due to optic neuropathy of alcohol and tobacco abuse. *Journal Français D'Ophtalmologie*. 1983;6(3):237–242.

122. Labadie H, Verneau A, Trinchet JC, Beaugrand M. Does oral zinc improve the cellular immunity of patients with alcoholic cirrhosis?. *Gastroentérologie Clinique et Biologique*. 1986;10(12):799–803.

123. Weismann K, Christensen E, Dreyer V. Zinc supplementation in alcoholic cirrhosis. A double-blind clinical trial. *Acta Medica Scandinavica*. 1979;205(5):361–366.

124. Mancinelli R, Barlocci E, Ciprotti M, et al. Blood thiamine, zinc, selenium, lead and oxidative stress in a population of male and female alcoholics: clinical evidence and gender differences. *Annali dell'Istituto Superiore di Sanità*. 2013;49(1):65–72. doi:DOI: 10.4415/ANN_13_01_11.

125. Manzardo AM, He J, Poje A, Penick EC, Campbell J, Butler MG. Double-blind, randomized placebo-controlled clinical trial of benfotiamine for severe alcohol dependence. *Drug and Alcohol Dependence*. 2013;133(2):562–570. doi:10.1016/j.drugalcdep.2013.07.035.

126. Subramanian VS, Subramanya SB, Tsukamoto H, Said HM. Effect of chronic alcohol feeding on physiological and molecular parameters of renal thiamin transport. *American Journal of Physiology-Renal Physiology*. 2010;299(1):F28–F34. doi:10.1152/ajprenal.00140.2010.

127. Thomson AD, Guerrini I, Marshall EJ. The evolution and treatment of Korsakoff's syndrome. *Neuropsychology Review*. 2012;22(2):81–92. doi:10.1007/s11065-012-9196-z.

128. Guerrini I, Thomson AD, Gurling HM. Molecular genetics of alcohol-related brain damage. *Alcohol Alcohol*. 2009;44(2):166–170. doi:10.1093/alcalc/agn101.

129. Lallas M, Desai J. Wernicke encephalopathy in children and adolescents. *World Journal of Pediatrics*. 2014;10(4):293–298. doi:10.1007/s12519-014-0506-9.

130. Gibson GE, Hirsch JA, Cirio RT, Jordan BD, Fonzetti P, Elder J. Abnormal thiamine-dependent processes in Alzheimer's disease: lessons from diabetes. *Molecular and Cellular Neuroscience*. 2013;55:17–25. doi:10.1016/j.mcn.2012.09.001.

131. Hazell AS, Faim S, Wertheimer G, Silva VR, Marques CS. The impact of oxidative stress in thiamine deficiency: a multifactorial targeting issue. *Neurochemistry International*. 2013;62(5):796–802. doi:10.1016/j.neuint.2013.01.009.

132. Elisaf M, Merkouropoulos M, Tsianos EV, Siamopoulos KC. Pathogenetic mechanisms of hypomagnesemia in alcoholic patients. *Journal of Trace Elements in Medicine and Biology: Organ of the Society for Minerals and Trace Elements (GMS)*. 1995;9(4):210–214. doi:10.1016/S0946-672X(11)80026-X.

133. Laitinen K, Lamberg-Allardt C, Tunninen R, et al. Transient hypoparathyroidism during acute alcohol intoxication. *New England Journal of Medicine*. 1991;324(11):721–727. doi:10.1056/NEJM199103143241103.

134. Brown RA, Crawford M, Natavio M, Petrovski P, Ren J. Dietary magnesium supplementation attenuates ethanol-induced myocardial dysfunction. *Alcoholism, Clinical and Experimental Research*. 1998;22(9):2062–2072.

135. Poikolainen K, Alho H. Magnesium treatment in alcoholics: a randomized clinical trial. *Substance Abuse Treatment, Prevention, and Policy*. 2008;3:1. doi:10.1186/1747-597X-3-1.

136. Eby GA, Eby KL. Rapid recovery from major depression using magnesium treatment. *Medical Hypotheses*. 2006;67(2):362–370. doi:10.1016/j.mehy.2006.01.047.

137. McGregor NR. Pueraria lobata (kudzu root) hangover remedies and acetaldehyde-associated neoplasm risk. *Alcohol*. 2007;41(7):469–478. doi:10.1016/j.alcohol.2007.07.009.

138. Eriksson CJ. The role of acetaldehyde in the actions of alcohol (update 2000). *Alcoholism, Clinical and Experimental Research*. 2001;25(5 Suppl ISBRA):15S–32S.

139. Kushner S, Han D, Oscar-Berman M, et al. Declinol, a complex containing kudzu, bitter herbs (gentian, tangerine peel) and bupleurum, significantly reduced alcohol use disorders identification test (AUDIT) scores in moderate to heavy drinkers: A pilot study. *Journal of Addiction Research and Therapy*. 2013;4(3). doi:10.4172/2155-6105.1000153.

140. Lukas SE, Penetar D, Su Z, et al. A standardized kudzu extract (NPI-031) reduces alcohol consumption in nontreatment-seeking male heavy drinkers. *Psychopharmacology (Berl)*. 2013;226(1):65–73. doi:10.1007/s00213-012-2884-9.

141. Penetar DM, Toto LH, Farmer SL, et al. The isoflavone puerarin reduces alcohol intake in heavy drinkers: a pilot study. *Drug and Alcohol Dependence*. 2012;126(1–2):251–256. doi:10.1016/j.drugalcdep.2012.04.012.

142. Penetar DM, MacLean RR, McNeil JF, Lukas SE. Kudzu extract treatment does not increase the intoxicating effects of acute alcohol in human volunteers. *Alcoholism, Clinical and Experimental Research*. 2011;35(4):726–734. doi:10.1111/j.1530-0277.2010.01390.x.

143. Bae K-Y, Kim S-W, Shin H-Y, et al. The acute effects of ethanol and acetaldehyde on physiological responses after ethanol ingestion in young healthy men with different ALDH2 genotypes. *Clinical Toxicology*. 2012;50(4):242–249. doi:10.3109/15563650.2012.672743.

144. Rezvani AH, Overstreet DH, Perfumi M, Massi M. Plant derivatives in the treatment of alcohol dependency. *Pharmacology Biochemistry and Behavior*. 2003;75(3):593–606. doi:10.1016/S0091-3057(03)00124-2.

145. Bleich S, Degner D, Sperling W, Bönsch D, Thürauf N, Kornhuber J. Homocysteine as a neurotoxin in chronic alcoholism. *Progress in Neuro-Psychopharmacology and Biological Psychiatry.* 2004;28(3):453–464. doi:10.1016/j.pnpbp.2003.11.019.

146. Bleich S, Spilker K, Kurth C, et al. Oxidative stress and an altered methionine metabolism in alcoholism. *Neuroscience Letters.* 2000;293(3):171–174.

147. Manetti L, Cavagnini F, Martino E, Ambrogio A. Effects of cocaine on the hypothalamic-pituitary-adrenal axis. *Journal of Endocrinological Investigation.* 2014;37(8):701–708. doi:10.1007/s40618-014-0091-8.

148. Wisniewski AB, Brown TT, John M, et al. Hypothalamic-pituitary-gonadal function in men and women using heroin and cocaine, stratified by HIV status. *Gender Medicine.* 2007;4(1):35–44.

149. Elliott JA, Horton E, Fibuch EE. The endocrine effects of long-term oral opioid therapy: a case report and review of the literature. *Journal of Opioid Management.* 2011;7(2):145–154.

150. Brown TT, Dobs AS. Endocrine effects of marijuana. *Journal of Clinical Pharmacology.* 2002;42(Suppl. 11):90S–96S.

# 21

## Interaction of Spirituality and Religion with Health, Mental Health, and Substance Abuse

### BRUCE Y. LEE, ANDREW B. NEWBERG, AND SHAHLA J. MODIR

## Introduction

Throughout history, religion and health care have oscillated between co-operation and antagonism. In ancient times, many of the world's most advanced civilizations (such as the Assyrians, Chinese, Egyptians, Mesopotamians, and Persians) equated physical illnesses with evil spirits and demonic possessions and devised treatments to exorcize these spirits. Since then, religious groups have labeled physicians and other health-care providers as everything from evil sorcerers to charlatans to conduits of God's healing powers. Similarly, views on religion of physicians, scientists, and health-care providers have ranged from interest to disinterest to disdain.

In the 21st century, the medical and scientific communities have grown increasingly interested in the effects of religion on health.[1] Coverage of the interplay of religion and health has become much more frequent in popular magazines, such as *Time* and *Newsweek*, and on television shows.[2-5] There has been a surge in the popularity of spiritual activities, such as yoga, that aim to improve or maintain health.[6,7] Moreover, many patients consider religion to be important and have indicated that they would like their physicians to discuss religious issues with them. We will review what is currently known about clinical effects of religious and spiritual practices, as well as the challenges that researchers and health-care practitioners may face in designing appropriate studies and translating results to clinical practice. We also will discuss future directions in the roles of religion and spirituality in health care.

# The Importance of Religion and Spirituality to Patients and Physicians

Religion and spirituality play significant roles in many people's lives. Over 90% of Americans believe in God or a higher power, 90% pray, 67%–75% pray on a daily basis, 69% are members of a church or synagogue, 40% attend a church or synagogue regularly, 60% consider religion to be important in their lives, and 82% acknowledge a personal need for spiritual growth.[8–12] Additionally, many patients seem interested in integrating religion with their health care. Over 75% of surveyed patients want physicians to include spiritual issues in their medical care, approximately 40% want physicians to discuss their religious faith with them, and nearly 50% would like physicians to pray with them.[13–16] Although many physicians seem to agree that spiritual well-being is an important component of health that should be addressed with patients, only a minority (less than 20%) do so with any regularity.[17,18] According to surveyed physicians, lack of time, inadequate training, discomfort in addressing the topics, and difficulty in identifying patients who want to discuss spiritual issues are responsible for this discrepancy.[19–21]

Educators have responded by offering courses, conferences, and curricula in medical schools, postgraduate training, and continuing medical education.[22] However, some question the relevance and appropriateness of discussing religion and spirituality in the health-care setting, fearing that health-care workers may impose personal religious beliefs on others and replace necessary medical interventions with religious interventions. Sloan and colleagues cautioned that patients may be forced to believe that their illnesses are due solely to poor faith.[23,24] Moreover, there is considerable debate over how religion should be integrated with health care and who should be responsible, especially when health-care providers are agnostic or atheist.[25]

# The Role of Religion in Health Care

Despite this controversy, the role of religion in health care seems to be growing. For instance, the *DMS-4* recognizes religion and spirituality as relevant sources of either emotional distress or support.[26–28] Also, the guidelines of the Joint Commission on Accreditation of Health Care Organizations (JCAHO) require hospitals to meet the spiritual needs of patients.[29] The medical literature reflects this trend as well. The frequency of studies on religion and spirituality and health has increased over the past decade.[30] Stefanek and colleagues tallied a 600%

increase in spirituality and health publications and a 27% increase in religion and health publications from 1993 to 2002.[31]

Some have recommended that physicians and other health-care providers routinely take religious and spiritual histories of their patients to better understand the patients' religious background, determine how he or she may be using religion to cope with illness, open the door for future discussions about any spiritual or religious issues, and help detect potentially deleterious side effects from religious and spiritual activities.[32-35] It may also be a way of detecting spiritual distress:[36] There has also been greater emphasis in integrating various religious resources and professionals into patient care, especially when the patient is near the end-of-life stage.[33] Some effort has been made to train health- care providers to listen to patients' religious concerns, perform clergylike duties when religious professionals are not available, and better understand spiritual practices.[37,38]

## Methodological Issues with Clinical Studies

Like most nascent research areas, the study of religion and health has had to contend with lack of adequate funding, institutional support, and training for investigators. These challenges have helped limit the number of well-designed studies in the medical literature. Rather than true scientific studies, many "studies" actually have been anecdotes and editorials, which can galvanize discussions, germinate ideas, and fuel future studies but cannot establish causality or scientifically justify the use of specific interventions. In fact, many of the "scientific" studies have only been correlational, and while they have demonstrated interesting associations, they have not always adjusted for all possible confounding variables, such as socioeconomic status, ethnicity, and different lifestyles or diets. As a result, they have not clearly established causality. In some cases, religious variables were included in a larger study that did not focus on the effects of religion. Since these studies were not necessarily designed and powered primarily to study the religious variables, results must be considered cautiously. There have been a limited number of randomized controlled trials (RCTs). For example, in a systematic review of studies from 1966 to 1999, Townsend and colleagues counted 9 RCTs. But as the study of religion and health progresses, the number and sophistication of scientific studies should continue to grow.

In addition to external challenges, the clinical study of religion has some inherent challenges as well. Understanding these inherent challenges is crucial when either designing or interpreting studies. Otherwise, you may conduct significantly flawed studies, draw inappropriate conclusions, administer unnecessary or even dangerous interventions, pursue the wrong research questions, or neglect to pursue further necessary research.

# The Positive Effects of Religion on Health

## GENERAL BEHAVIOR AND LIFESTYLES

Studies have looked at whether people with high religiosity live generally healthier and less risky lifestyles than those with lower religiosity, which may account for some of the observed health benefits of religion. One hypothesis is that religion may provide structure, teaching, role models, and support to individuals, so that they do not have the desire or time to engage in risky behavior. Some studies have supported this hypothesis. The study of Texas adults by Hill and colleagues showed that regular religious activity attendance correlated with use of preventive care, vitamins, and seatbelts, and decreased smoking and drinking; and, there was more walking, strenuous exercise, and sound sleep quality.[39, 41] Oleckno and Blacconiere's study of college students revealed an inverse correlation between religiosity and behaviors that adversely affect health.[40] Compared to the general population, Mormons and Seventh-day Adventists have been found to have lower incidence of (and mortality rates from) cancers that have been linked to tobacco and alcohol.[42,43] However, other studies have shown no relationship, or even an inverse relationship, between religiosity and certain risky behaviors.[44,45]

## DIET AND NUTRITION

Could dietary differences explain some of the observed health benefits of religion? A 2005 study found that African American women with high religiosity consumed more fruits and vegetables than those with low religiosity.[46] Studies in Israel showed that compared to religious residents, secular residents had diets higher in total fat and saturated fatty acids,[47] and higher plasma levels of cholesterol, triglyceride, and low-density lipoprotein.[48] Some religions enforce certain specific diets, such as periodic fasting or vegetarianism.[49,50] For example, a large, prospective epidemiologic study of Seventh-day Adventists revealed that a diet rich in nuts, as advocated by Adventists, was associated with a lower risk of cardiovascular disease.[51] However, the benefits and harms of specific religious diets have not been clearly established.

## ALCOHOL, TOBACCO, AND DRUG ABUSE

Religion can affect alcohol and substance use at several stages. It may affect whether a person initiates use, how significant the use becomes, how the use affects the person's life, and whether the person is able to quit and recover.[52] The attitudes of religions toward alcohol and substance use vary considerably. Some religious sects strictly prohibit alcohol and substance use.[53] Others are less stringent but discourage excessive use. Some allow the use of alcohol and have incorporated drinking wine into their rituals, and others use psychoactive substances, such as peyote, khat, and hashish to achieve spiritual goals.[54]

Indeed, some evidence suggests that individuals involved in religion are less likely to use alcohol and other substances.[55-57] Even among alcohol and drug users, religious individuals are more likely to use them moderately.[52,58] Leigh and colleagues' study of college students revealed that students with higher spirituality scores smoked and binge drank less frequently.[59] In a nationally representative sample of adolescents, Miller and colleagues determined that personal devotion—which they defined as a personal relationship with the Divine—and affiliation with more fundamentalist denominations were inversely associated with alcohol and illicit drug use.[60] This effect was seen outside the United States as well, in Latin America.[61] There are a number of possible reasons for these findings. Fear of violating religious principles and doctrines can have a powerful effect. Religions can play a role in educating people about the dangers of alcohol and drugs.[62] Religious involvement and the accompanying positive externalities may keep people occupied and prevent idleness and boredom that can lead to substance abuse. There may be peer pressure from other members of the church to remain abstinent, and there may be less peer pressure to try alcohol and other substances. Moreover, religious involvement could be the effect rather than the cause. Substance abuse may prevent religious involvement. Larson and Wilson noted that alcoholics compared to nonalcoholic subjects had less involvement in religious practices, less exposure to religious teachings, and fewer religious experiences.[63]

Many, including patients, believe that incorporating religion and spirituality into alcohol, tobacco, and drug cessation programs may enhance their efficacy.[64,65] Indeed, spirituality already permeates many established programs, such as AA.[66-69] Studies have suggested that religious and spiritual practices may aid recovery.[70-72]

Research on spirituality and alcohol use has been focused on participant engagement in 12-step programs such as AA. This is because one of the major tenets of AA is founded on participants having a spiritual transformation through awakening to one's higher power. Accordingly, researchers have used spiritual growth and transformation to explore the connection of AA and alcoholic recovery. In a recent study by Tonigan et al in 2013, spiritual growth was found to positively mediate the effects of AA on increased abstinence and decreased drinking on a group of new AA members. Spiritual growth, in this study, was shown to correlate with increased abstinence rates.[73] Kelly et al studied the effect of AA attendance on abstinence and drinking intensity and found these were both partially mediated by participants increase in spirituality.[74] Additionally, having increased participation in AA through obtaining a sponsor and attending regular meetings has also been shown to predict improved drinking outcomes and increase the likelihood of a spiritual experience versus AA attendance alone.[75]

Additionally, in a study by Matzger in 2005 in data that examined 659 adults with problem drinking split into treatment seeking groups and the general public it was determined that a "spiritual awakening" was essential to predict reduced drinking rates and sustained remission from alcohol. This is an intriguing finding that having a spiritual awakening was needed to modify problem drinking in both the treatment seeking and the general public.[76]

Not all studies have used spirituality in AA as a means to evaluate the effect of this on recovery. In a 2011 study by Robinson, researchers examined religious and spiritual participation in AUD patients who were either part of AA or those who did not use AA as part of their recovery. Findings suggested that a 6-month increase in personal and spiritual practices that included self-forgiveness were the highest predictors of drinking outcomes independent of any participation in AA.[77] These findings suggest that spirituality can exert a positive influence on drinking outcomes independent of AA participation. A broad understanding regarding which spiritual practices and principles exert the most robust effect on AUD outcomes can be a helpful future direction of inquiry.

Data suggests that patients often experience spiritual awakenings or religious conversion during recovery.[78] A significant number of recovering intravenous drug abusers use religious healing, relaxation techniques, and meditation.[79] Recent research on meditation and substance abuse supports the use of mindfulness meditation for treating SUD.[80,81] MBRP is a new type of cognitive behavioral therapy designed to target cravings and negative emotions by using mindfulness meditation exercises along with cognitive behavioral prevention and coping skills. MBRP teaches addicted individuals how to become more aware of their external triggers, their internal thought processes, and how to better tolerate physical and emotional experiences. One systematic review of the effectiveness of MBRP showed that individuals who used MBRP reported reduced substance use, reduction in cravings, and reduced reactivity to environmental cues.[82] The MBRP group also reported a significantly higher level of awareness and self-acceptance, as well as significant decreases in cravings over a 4-month follow-up period.[82] A large randomized clinical trial showed that compared to treatment as usual, MBRP led to lower risk of relapse to substance use and heavy drinking. Among participants who continued to use substances, there were significantly fewer days of substance use and drinking at the 6-month follow-up. At the 12-month follow-up, the MBRP group reported statistically significant fewer days of substance use and significantly decreased heavy drinking compared to the treatment-as-usual group.[83]

However, not all studies showed that religiously involved patients have better outcomes. The first randomized controlled trials failed to demonstrate sufficient clinical benefit from meditation[84] or intercessory prayer.[85] In a study by Tonigan and colleagues, while subjects self-labeled as religious were more likely than agnostics and atheists to initiate and continue attending AA meetings, their outcomes were not clearly better.[86]

## SEXUAL BEHAVIOR

Some religions may play a role in preventing risky sexual behavior. In a study of African American adolescent females, religiosity correlated with more frank discussions about the risks of sex and avoidance of unsafe sexual situations.[87] Miller and Gur's study of over 3,000 adolescent girls found positive associations between personal devotion and fewer sexual partners outside a romantic relationship, religious event attendance and proper birth control use, and religious event attendance and a better understanding of human immunodeficiency virus or pregnancy risks from unprotected intercourse.[88] But these findings are not universal. Some have found no relationship between religiosity and sexual practices.[89,90] Based on data from the 1995 National Survey of Family Growth, Jones and colleagues concluded that young women with more frequent religious service attendance tended to have delayed first intercourse but did not exhibit significantly different sexual behavior from others once they began having sex.[91] In fact, religious traditions or environments may actually suppress open discussion of sex and contraception. Lefkowitz and colleagues found that adolescents who discussed safe sex with their mothers tended to be less religious.[92]

## EXERCISE

Some religious or spiritual practices promote or even involve exercise. Religious activities can motivate people to leave their homes, walk to different locations, and participate in physical activities. Some church-related activities, such as softball leagues or dances, involve even more strenuous exercise. Among Utah residents, Merill and Thygerson found that people who attended church weekly were more likely to exercise regularly. However, differences in smoking and general health status seemed to account for this effect.[93] A study by McLane and colleagues suggested incorporating faith-based practices in exercise programs may be attractive to certain people and improve participation in physical activity.[94] To date, church-based initiatives to promote exercise have yielded mixed results.[95,96]

## GENERAL MENTAL HEALTH

The impact of religion on mental health has been studied more extensively than the impact of religion on physical health. Studies have demonstrated religiosity to be positively associated with feelings of well-being in white American, Mexican American,[97] and African American populations,[98] as well as in different age groups.[99] Krause observed that older African American individuals were more likely than similarly aged white Americans to derive life satisfaction from religion.[100] Religious service attendance was predictive of higher life satisfaction among elderly Chinese Hong Kong residents[101] and elderly Mexican American women.[102] Members of religious kibutzes in Israel reported a higher sense of coherence and less hostility and were more likely to engage in volunteer work than nonmembers.[103] Similar findings occurred in a population of nursing home residents.[104] Hope and optimism seemed to run higher among religious individuals than nonreligious individuals in some study populations.[105-107] Using religious attendance as one of the markers of social engagement, Bassuk and colleagues determined that social disengagement was linked with cognitive decline in the noninstitutionalized elderly.[108]

A few studies compared different religions. For example, one study showed that among elderly women in Hong Kong, Catholics and Buddhists enjoyed better mental health status than Protestants.[109] However, not enough data exist to generate meaningful conclusions.

## DEPRESSION

A number of investigators have looked at the effects of religion on depression. Prospective cohort studies have shown religious activity to be associated with remission of depression in Protestant and Catholic Netherlanders[110] and in ill older adults.[111] Prospective studies have also found religious activity to be strongly protective against depression in Protestant and Catholic offspring who share the same religion as their mother[112] and weakly protective in female twins.[113] Cross-sectional studies have yielded significant[114] and[115-117] associations among different indicators of religiosity and a lower prevalence of depression in various populations. Chen and colleagues found that in patients already diagnosed with depression, religious participation may lead to better outcomes.[118]

Studies also have suggested an inverse correlation between religiosity and suicide. This was found to be the case in Nisbet's analysis of 1993 National Mortality Followback Survey data[119] and Neeleman and colleagues' analysis of cross-sectional data of Judaeo-Christian older adults from 26 countries.[120] Suicide may be less acceptable to people with high religious devotion and orthodox religious beliefs.[121,122] But again, it is unclear whether suicidal individuals are less likely to hold strong religious beliefs or individuals with strong religious beliefs are less likely to be suicidal.

Several RCTs have been performed. One RCT demonstrated that directed and nondirected intercessory prayer correlated favorably with multiple measures of self-esteem, anxiety, and depression but did not clearly state the randomization technique and did not account for multiple confounders.[123] Another RCT suggested that using religion-based cognitive therapy had a favorable impact on Christian patients with clinical depression but may have contained too many comparison groups for strong cause-and-effect relationships to be established.[124] Three RCTs suggested that religious (Islamic-based) psychotherapy appeared to speed recovery from anxiety and depression in Muslim Malays but did not control for the use of antidepressants and benzodiazepines.[125–127]

## The Negative Effects of Religion on Health

Although most studies have shown positive effects, religion and spirituality also may negatively impact health. For example, religious groups may directly oppose certain health-care interventions, such as transfusions or contraception, and convince patients that their ailments are due to noncompliance with religious doctrines rather than to organic disease.[128] Asser and colleagues demonstrated that a large number of child fatalities could have been prevented had medical care not been withheld for religious reasons.[129] After interviewing 682 North Carolina women, Mitchell and colleagues concluded that belief in religious intervention may delay African American women from seeing their physicians for breast lumps.[130] In addition, religions can stigmatize those with certain diseases to the point that they do not seek proper medical care.[131,132]

Moreover, as history has shown, religion can be the source of military conflicts, prejudice, violent behaviors, and other social problems. Religions may ignore, sterotype, ostracize, or abuse those who do not belong to their church. Those not belonging to a dominant religion may face obstacles to obtaining resources hardships and stress that deleteriously affect their health.[133,134] Religious leaders may abuse their own members physically, emotionally, or sexually.[135,136] Religious laws or dictums may be invoked to justify harmful, oppressive, and injurious behavior.[137]

Additionally, perceived religious transgressions can cause emotional and psychological anguish, manifesting as physical discomfort. This "religious" and "spiritual pain" can be difficult to distinguish from pure physical pain.[138] In extreme cases, spiritual abuse—convincing people that they are going to suffer eternal purgatory—and spiritual terrorism (an extreme form of spiritual abuse) can occur either overtly or insidiously (i.e., it can be implied, though not actually stated, that a patient will be doomed).[139,140] When a mix of religious, spiritual, and organic sources is causing physical illness, treatment can become complicated. Health-care workers must properly balance treating each source.

## Conclusions and Future Directions

Existing evidence suggests that religious and spiritual practices may have beneficial effects on health. But the reasons behind these findings are not clearly understood. We know that religious and spiritual practices can bring social and emotional support, motivation, healthy lifestyles, and health-care resources to their practitioners. However, are there other mechanisms involved? The medical world is just starting to answer this question.

In general, performing clinical studies that can establish cause-and-effect relationships is difficult. This is especially true in the study of religion and health. Confounding factors abound. Religious and spiritual doctrines and practices vary significantly among and within different sects and denominations. It is challenging not only to measure religious and spiritual activity but also to monitor and ensure compliance among study subjects. Moreover there has been a paucity of available resources, properly trained investigators, and institutional support for clinical studies. As a result, the current body of medical literature is short on well-designed clinical studies.

Future studies should address a number of different issues. What are the roles of different potential confounding factors? What physiologic mechanisms may be involved? What are the clinical implications of existing physiologic studies? How much does a person's health affect his or her ability to engage in religious and spiritual activities? Do findings hold across different practices, sects, and denominations? Existing studies have only looked at a limited population of religious groups and sects. What are the effects of varying demographic parameters, such as age, gender, and location? How do different practices affect different diseases? Many practices and diseases have not been studied. How should religious and spiritual issues be incorporated into the health-care system?

The findings to date already have clinical implications. Religion is clearly important to many patients. Health-care providers may need to better address patients' religious concerns and be aware of how religious involvement can affect patients' symptoms, quality of life, and willingness to receive treatment. Moreover, religious and spiritual activities may serve as adjunct therapy in various disease and addiction treatment programs. The future may see the development of more specific spiritual interventions for particular medical problems.

In the coming years, the study of religion and health, as well as the integration of religion into health care, should continue to grow. New research methods, designs, techniques, and instruments may emerge. As long as the worlds of religion, science, and health care cooperate, many exciting new findings could appear in coming decades, hopefully for the betterment of all.

# REFERENCES

1. Levin JS. How religion influences morbidity and health: reflections on natural history, salutogenesis and host resistance. *Social Science & Medicine*. 1996;43:849–864.
2. Begley S. Religion and the brain. *Newsweek*. 2001;137:50–57.
3. Begley S. Searching for the God within. *Newsweek*. 2001;137:59.
4. Greenwald J. Alternative medicine. A new breed of healers. *Time*. 2001;157:62–5, 8–9.
5. Woodward KL. Faith is more than a feeling. *Newsweek*. 2001;137:58.
6. Corliss R. The power of yoga. *Time*. 2001;157:54–63.
7. van Montfrans GA, Karemaker JM, Wieling W, Dunning AJ. Yoga and massage: If it's physical, it's therapy. *Newsweek*. 1990b;140:74–75.
8. Bezilla R., ed. *Religion in America*. Princeton, NJ: Princeton Religious Center (Gallup Organization); 1992–1993.
9. Miller, WR, Thoresen CE. Spirituality, religion, and health. An emerging research field. *American Psychologist*. 2003;58:24–35.
10. Poloma M, Pendleton B. The effects of prayer and prayer experience on measures of general well being. *Journal of Psychology and Theology*. 2001;10:71–83.
11. Shuler PA, Gelberg L, Brown M. The effects of spiritual/religious practices on psychological well-being among inner city homeless women. *Nurse Practitioner Forum*. 1994;5:106–113.
12. *The Gallup Report: Religion in America: 1993–1994*. Princeton, NJ: Gallup Poll; 1994.
13. Daaleman TP, Nease DE, Jr. Patient attitudes regarding physician inquiry into spiritual and religious issues. *Journal of Family Practice*. 1994;39:564–568.
14. King DE, Bushwick B. Beliefs and attitudes of hospital inpatients about faith healing and prayer. *Journal of Family Practice*. 1994;39:349–352.
15. King DE, Hueston W, Rudy M. Religious affiliation and obstetric outcome. *Southern Medical Journal*. 1994;87:1125–1128.
16. Matthews DA, Clark C. *The Faith Factor: Proof of the Healing Power of Prayer*. New York: Viking; 1998.
17. MacLean CD, Susi B, Phifer N, et al. Patient preference for physician discussion and practice of spirituality. *Journal of General Internal Medicine*. 2003;18:38–43.
18. Monroe MH, Bynum D, Susi B, et al. Primary care physician preferences regarding spiritual behavior in medical practice. *Archives of Internal Medicine*. 2003;163:2751–2756.
19. Armbruster CA, Chibnall JT, Legett S. Pediatrician beliefs about spirituality and religion in medicine: associations with clinical practice. *Pediatrics*. 2003;111:e227–e235.
20. Chibnall JT, Brooks, CA. Religion in the clinic: the role of physician beliefs. *Southern Medical Journal*. 2001;94:374–379.
21. Ellis MR, Vinson DC, Ewigman B. Addressing spiritual concerns of patients: family physicians' attitudes and practices. *Journal of Family Practice*. 1999;48:105–109.
22. Pettus MC. Implementing a medicine-spirituality curriculum in a community-based internal medicine residency program. *Academic Medicine*. 2002;77:745.

23. Sloan RP, Bagiella E. Claims about religious involvement and health outcomes. *Annals of Behavioral Medicine.* 2002;24:14–21.

24. Sloan RP, Bagiella E, Powell T. Religion, spirituality, and medicine. *Lancet.* 1999;353:664–667.

25. Levin JS, Larson DB, Puchalski CM. Religion and spirituality in medicine: research and education. *Journal of the American Medical Association.* 1997;278:792–793.

26. Kutz I. Samson, the Bible, and the *DSM. Archives of General Psychiatry.* 2002;59:565.

27. Lukoff D, Lu F, Turner R. Toward a more culturally sensitive *DSM-IV.* Psychoreligious and psychospiritual problems. *Journal of Nervous and Mental Disease.* 1992;180:673–682.

28. Turner RP, Lukoff D, Barnhouse RT, Lu FG. Religious or spiritual problem: a culturally sensitive diagnostic category in the *DSM-IV. Journal of Nervous and Mental Disease.* 1995; 183:435–444.

29. La Pierre LL. JCAHO safeguards spiritual care. *Holistic Nursing Practice.* 2003;17:219.

30. Levin JS, Larson DB, Puchalski CM. Religion and spirituality in medicine: research and education. *Journal of the American Medical Association.* 1997;278:792–793.

31. Stefanek M, McDonald PG, Hess SA. Religion, spirituality and cancer: Current status and methodological challenges. *Psycho-oncology.* 2004;14:450–463.

32. Kuhn CC. A spiritual inventory of the medically ill patient. *Psychiatric Medicine.* 1988; 6:87–100.

33. Lo B, Ruston D, Kates LW, et al. Discussing religious and spiritual issues at the end of life: a practical guide for physicians. *Journal of American Medical Association.* 2002;287:749–754.

34. Lo B, Quill T, Tulsky J. Discussing palliative care with patients. ACP-ASIM End-of-Life Care Consensus Panel. American College of Physicians-American Society of Internal Medicine. *Annals of Internal Medicine.* 1999;130:744–749.

35. Matthews DA, Clark, C. *The Faith Factor: Proof of the Healing Power of Prayer.* New York: Viking;1990.

36. Abrahm J. Pain management for dying patients. How to assess needs and provide pharmacologic relief. *Postgraduate Medicine.* 2001;110: 99–100, 8–9, 13–14.

37. Morse JM, Proctor A. Maintaining patient endurance. The comfort work of trauma nurses. *Clinical Nursing Research.* 1998;7:250–274.

38. Proctor A, Morse JM, Khonsari, ES. Sounds of comfort in the trauma center: how nurses talk to patients in pain. *Social Science & Medicine.* 1996;42:1669–1680.

39. Hill TD, Burdette AM, Ellison CG, Musick MA. Religious attendance and the health behaviors of Texas adults. *Preventive Medicine.* 2006;42:309–312.

40. Oleckno WA, Blacconiere MJ. Relationship of religiosity to wellness and other health-related behaviors and outcomes. *Psychological Reports.* 1991;68:819–826.

41. Comstock GW, Partridge KB. Church attendance and health. *Journal of Chronic Diseases.* 1972;25:665–672.

42. Grundmann E. Cancer morbidity and mortality in USA Mormons and Seventh-day Adventists. *Archives d'Anatomie Et De Cytologie Pathologiques.* 1992;40:73–78.

43. Fraser GE. Associations between diet and cancer, ischemic heart disease, and all-cause mortality in non-Hispanic white California Seventh-day Adventists. *American Journal of Clinical Nutrition.* 1999;70: 532S–538S.

44. Hasnain M, Sinacore JM, Mensah EK, Levy, JA. Influence of religiosity on HIV risk behaviors in active injection drug users. *AIDS Care.* 2005;17:892–901.

45. Poulson RL, Eppler MA, Satterwhite TN, Wuensch KL, Bass LA. Alcohol consumption, strength of religious beliefs, and risky sexual behavior in college students. *Journal of American College Health.* 1998;46:227–232.

46. Holt CL, Haire-Joshu DL, Lukwago SN, Lewellyn LA, Kreuter MW. The role of religiosity in dietary beliefs and behaviors among urban African American women. *Cancer Control.* 2005;12(Suppl. 2):84–90.

47. Friedlander Y, Kark JD, Kaufmann NA, Stein Y. Coronary heart disease risk factors among religious groupings in a Jewish population sample in Jerusalem. *American Journal of Clinical Nutrition.* 1985;42:511–521.

48. Friedlander Y, Kark JD, Stein Y. Religious observance and plasma lipids and lipoproteins among 17-year-old Jewish residents of Jerusalem. *Preventive Medicine.* 1987;16:70–79.

49. Roky R, Houti I, Moussamih S, Qotbi S, Aadil N. Physiological and chronobiological changes during Ramadan intermittent fasting. *Annals of Nutrition & Metabolism.* 2004;48:296–303.

50. Sarri K, Linardakis M, Codrington C, Kafatos A. Does the periodic vegetarianism of Greek Orthodox Christians benefit blood pressure? *Preventive Medicine.* 2007;44:341–348.

51. Sabate J. Nut consumption, vegetarian diets, ischemic heart disease risk, and all-cause mortality: evidence from epidemiologic studies. *American Journal of Clinical Nutrition.* 1999;70(3 Suppl.):500S–503S.

52. Miller WR. Researching the spiritual dimensions of alcohol and other drug problems. *Addiction.* 1998;93: 979–990.

53. Enstrom JE, Breslow L. Lifestyle and reduced mortality among active California Mormons, 1980–2004. *Preventive Medicine.* 2007;(2):133–136.

54. Lyttle T. Drug based religions and contemporary drug taking. *Journal of Drug Issues.* 1988;18:271–284.

55. Heath AC, Madden PA, Grant JD, McLaughlin TL, Todorov AA, Bucholz KK. Resiliency factors protecting against teenage alcohol use and smoking: influences of religion, religious involvement and values, and ethnicity in the Missouri Adolescent Female Twin Study. *Twin Research.* 1999;2:145–155.

56. Luczak SE, Shea SH, Carr LG, Li TK, Wall TL. Binge drinking in Jewish and non-Jewish white college students. *Alcoholism, Clinical and Experimental Research.* 2012; 26:1773–1778.

57. Stewart C. The influence of spirituality on substance use of college students. *Journal of Drug Education.* 2001;31:343–351.

58. Gorsuch RL, Butler MC. Initial drug abuse: a review of predisposing social psychological factors. *Psychological Bulletin.* 1976;83:120–137.

59. Leigh J, Bowen S, Marlatt GA. Spirituality, mindfulness and substance abuse. *Addictive Behaviors*. 2005;30:1335–1341.

60. Miller L, Davies M, Greenwald S. Religiosity and substance use and abuse among adolescents in the National Comorbidity Survey. *Journal of the American Academy of Child and Adolescent Psychiatry*. 2000;39:1190–1197.

61. Chen CY, Dormitzer CM, Bejarano J, Anthony JC. Religiosity and the earliest stages of adolescent drug involvement in seven countries of Latin America. *American Journal of Epidemiology*. 2004;159:1180–1188.

62. Stylianou S. The role of religiosity in the opposition to drug use. *International Journal of Offender Therapy and Comparative Criminology*. 2004;48:429–448.

63. Larson DB, Wilson WP. Religious life of alcoholics. *Southern Medical Journal*. 1980;73:723–727.

64. Arnold R, Avants SK, Margolin A, Marcotte D. Patient attitudes concerning the inclusion of spirituality into addiction treatment. *Journal of Substance Abuse Treatment*. 2002;23:319–326.

65. Dermatis H, Guschwan MT, Galanter M, Bunt G. Orientation toward spirituality and self-help approaches in the therapeutic community. *Journal of Addictive Diseases*. 2004;23:39–54.

66. Brush BL, McGee EM. Evaluating the spiritual perspectives of homeless men in recovery. *Applied Nursing Research*. 2000;13:181–186.

67. Forcehimes AA. De profundis: spiritual transformations in Alcoholics Anonymous. *Journal of Clinical Psychology*. 2004;60:503–517.

68. Li EC, Feifer C, Strohm M. A pilot study: locus of control and spiritual beliefs in alcoholics anonymous and smart recovery members. *Addictive Behaviors*. 2000;25:633–640.

69. Moriarity J. The spiritual roots of AA. *Minnesota Medicine*. 2001;84:10.

70. Aron A, Aron EN. The transcendental meditation program's effect on addictive behavior. *Addictive Behaviors*. 1980;5:3–12.

71. Avants SK, Warburton LA, Margolin A. Spiritual and religious support in recovery from addiction among HIV-positive injection drug users. *Journal of Psychoactive Drugs*. 2001;33:39–45.

72. Carter TM. The effects of spiritual practices on recovery from substance abuse. *Journal of Psychiatric and Mental Health Nursing*. 1998;5:409–413.

73. Tonigan JS, Rynes KN, McCrady BS. Spirituality as a change mechanism in 12-step programs: A replication, extension, and refinement. *Substance Use & Misuse*. 2013;48(12):1161–1173.

74. Kelly JF, Stout RL, Magill M, et al. Spirituality in recovery: A lagged mediational analysis of Alcoholics Anonymous' principal theoretical mechanism of behavior change. *Alcoholism: Clinical and Experimental Research*. 2011;35(3): 454–463.

75. Krentzman AR, Cranford JA, Robinson EA. Multiple dimensions of spirituality in recovery: A lagged mediational analysis of Alcoholics Anonymous' principal theoretical mechanism of behavior change. *Substance Abuse*. 2013;34(1):20–32.

76. Matzger H, Kaskutas LA, Weisner C. Reasons for drinking less and their relationship to sustained remission from problem drinking. *Addiction.* 2005;100(11):1637–1646.

77. Robinson EA, Krentzman AR, Webb JR, Brower KJ. Six-month changes in spirituality and religiousness in alcoholics predict drinking outcomes at nine months. *Journal of Studies on Alcohol and Drugs.* 2011;72(4):660–668.

78. Green LL, Fullilove MT, Fullilove RE. Stories of spiritual awakening. The nature of spirituality in recovery. *Journal of Substance Abuse Treatment.* 1998;15:325–331.

79. Manheimer E, Anderson BJ, Stein MD. Use and assessment of complementary and alternative therapies by intravenous drug users. *American Journal of Drug Alcohol Abuse.* 2003; 29:401–413.

80. Witkiewitz K, Warner K, Sully B, et al. Randomized trial comparing mindfulness-based relapse prevention with relapse prevention for women offenders at a residential addiction treatment center. *Substance Use & Misuse.* 2014;49(5):536–546.

81. Zgierska A, Rabago D, Chawla N, et al. Mindfulness meditation for substance use disorders: A systematic review. *Substance Abuse.* 2009;30(4):266–294.

82. Witkiewitz K, Lustyk K, Bowen S. Re-training the addicted brain: A review of hypothesized neurobiological mechanisms of mindfulness-based relapse. *Psychological Addictive Behaviors.* 2013; 27(2):351–365.

83. Bowen S, Witkiewitz K, Clifasefi S, et al. Relative efficacy of mindfulness-bassed relapse prevention, standard relapse prevention, and treatment as usual for substance use disorders: a randomized clinical trial. *JAMA Psychiatry.* 2014:71(5):547–556.

84. Murphy TJ, Pagano RR, Marlatt GA. Lifestyle modification with heavy alcohol drinkers: effects of aerobic exercise and meditation. *Addictive Behaviors.* 1986;11:175–186.

85. Walker SR, Tonigan JS, Miller WR, Corner S, Kahlich L. Intercessory prayer in the treatment of alcohol abuse and dependence: a pilot investigation. *Alternative Therapies in Health and Medicine.* 1997;3:79–86.

86. Tonigan JS, Miller WR, Schermer C. Atheists, agnostics and Alcoholics Anonymous. *Journal of Studies on Alcohol.* 2002;63:534–541.

87. McCree DH, Wingood GM, DiClemente R, Davies S, Harrington KF. Religiosity and risky sexual behavior in African-American adolescent females. *Journal of Adolescent Health.* 2003;33:2–8.

88. Miller L, Gur M. Religiousness and sexual responsibility in adolescent girls. *Journal of Adolescent Health.* 2002;31:401–406.

89. Dunne MP, Edwards R, Lucke J, Donald M, Raphael B. Religiosity, sexual intercourse and condom use among university students. *Australian Journal of Public Health.* 1994;18:339–341.

90. McCormick N, Izzo A, Folcik J. Adolescents' values, sexuality, and contraception in a rural New York county. *Adolescence.* 1985;20:385–395.

91. Jones RK, Darroch JE, Singh S. Religious differentials in the sexual and reproductive behaviors of young women in the United States. *Journal of Adolescent Health.* 2005;36:279–288.

92. Lefkowitz ES, Boone TL, Au TK, Sigman M. No sex or safe sex? Mothers' and adolescents' discussions about sexuality and AIDS/HIV. *Health Education and Research.* 2003;18:341–351.

93. Merrill RM, & Thygerson AL. Religious preference, church activity, and physical exercise. *Preventive Medicine.* 2001;33:38–45.

94. McLane S, Lox CL, Butki B, Stern L. An investigation of the relation between religion and exercise motivation. *Perceptual and Motor Skills.* 2003;97:1043–1048.

95. Wilcox S, Laken M, Bopp M, et al. Increasing physical activity among church members: community-based participatory research. *American Journal of Preventive Medicine.* 2007;32:131–138.

96. Young DR, Stewart KJ. A church-based physical activity intervention for African American women. *Family Community Health.* 2006;29:103–117.

97. Markides KS, Levin JS, Ray LA. Religion, aging, and life satisfaction: an eight-year, three-wave longitudinal study. *Gerontologist.* 1987; 27: 660–665.

98. Coke MM. Correlates of life satisfaction among elderly African Americans. *Journal of Gerontology.* 1992;47:P316–P320.

99. Yoon DP, Lee EK. The impact of religiousness, spirituality, and social support on psychological well-being among older adults in rural areas. *Journal of Gerontology and Social Work.* 2007;48:281–298.

100. Krause N. Religious meaning and subjective well-being in late life. *Journals of Gerontology. Series B Psychological Sciences and Social Sciences.* 2003;58:S160–S170.

101. Ho SC, Woo J, Lau J, et al. Life satisfaction and associated factors in older Hong Kong Chinese. *Journal of the American Geriatrics Society.* 1995;43:252–255.

102. Levin J, Markides K. Religious attendance and psychological well-being in middle-aged and older Mexican Americans. *Sociological Analysis.* 2008;49:66–72.

103. Kark JD, Carmel S, Sinnreich R, Goldberger N, Friedlander, Y. Psychosocial factors among members of religious and secular kibbutzim. *Israel Journal of Medical Sciences.* 1996;32:185–194.

104. House JS, Robbins C, Metzner HL. The association of social relationships and activities with mortality: prospective evidence from the Tecumseh Community Health Study. *American Journal of Epidemiology.* 1982;116:123–140.

105. Idler E, Kasl SV. Religion among disabled and nondisabled persons II: attendance at religious services as a predictor of the course of disability. *Journals of Gerontology. Series B Psychological Sciences and Social Sciences.* 1997;52:S306–S316.

106. Idler EL, Kasl SV. Religion among disabled and nondisabled persons I: cross-sectional patterns in health practices, social activities, and well-being. *Journals of Gerontology. Series B Psychological Sciences and Social Sciences.* 1997;52:S294–S305.

107. Raleigh ED. Sources of hope in chronic illness. *Oncology Nursing Forum.* 1992;19:443–448.

108. Bassuk SS, Glass TA, Berkman LF. Social disengagement and incident cognitive decline in community-dwelling elderly persons. *Annals of Internal Medicine.* 1999;131:165–173.

109. Boey KW. Religiosity and psychological well-being of older women in Hong Kong. *International Journal of Psychiatric Nursing Research.* 2003;8: 921–935.

110. Braam AW, Beekman AT, Deeg DJ, Smit JH, van Tilburg W. Religiosity as a protective or prognostic factor of depression in later life; results from a community survey in The Netherlands. *Acta Psychiatrica Scandinavica.* 1997; 96:199–205.

111. Koenig HG, George LK, Peterson BL. Religiosity and remission of depression in medically ill older patients. *American Journal of Psychiatry.* 1998;155:536–542.

112. Miller L, Warner V, Wickramaratne P, Weissman M. Religiosity and depression: ten-year follow-up of depressed mothers and offspring. *Journal of the American Academy of Child and Adolescent Psychiatry.* 1997;36:1416–1425.

113. Kennedy GJ, Kelman HR, Thomas C, Chen J. The relation of religious preference and practice to depressive symptoms among 1,855 older adults. *Journals of Gerontology. Series B Psychological Sciences and Social Sciences.* 1996;51:P301–P308.

114. Koenig HG, Hays JC, George LK, Blazer DG, Larson DB, Landerman LR. Modeling the cross-sectional relationships between religion, physical health, social support, and depressive symptoms. *American Journal of Geriatric Psychiatry.* 1997;5:131–144.

115. Bienenfeld D, Koenig HG, Larson DB, Sherrill KA. Psychosocial predictors of mental health in a population of elderly women. Test of an explanatory model. *American Journal of Geriatric Psychiatry.* 1997;5:43–53.

116. Koenig HG. Religious attitudes and practices of hospitalized medically ill older adults. *International Journal of Geriatric Psychiatry.* 1998;13:213–224.

117. Musick MA, Koenig HG, Hays JC, Cohen HJ. Religious activity and depression among community-dwelling elderly persons with cancer: the moderating effect of race. *Journals of Gerontology. Series B Psychological Sciences and Social Sciences.* 1998;53:S218–S227.

118. Chen H, Cheal K, McDonel Herr EC, Zubritsky C, Levkoff SE. Religious participation as a predictor of mental health status and treatment outcomes in older persons. *International Journal of Geriatric Psychiatry.* 2007;22:144–153.

119. Nisbet PA, Duberstein PR, Conwell Y, Seidlitz L. The effect of participation in religious activities on suicide versus natural death in adults 50 and older. *Journal of Nervous and Mental Disease.* 2000;188:543–546.

120. Neeleman J, Lewis G. Suicide, religion, and socioeconomic conditions. An ecological study in 26 countries, 1990. *Journal of Epidemiology and Community Health.* 1999;53:204–210.

121. Neeleman J, Halpern D, Leon D, Lewis G. Tolerance of suicide, religion and suicide rates: an ecological and individual study in 19 Western countries. *Psychological Medicine.* 1997;27:1165–1171.

122. Neeleman J, Wessely S, Lewis G. Suicide acceptability in African- and white Americans: the role of religion. *Journal of Nervous and Mental Disease.* 1998;186:12–16.

123. O'Laoire S. An experimental study of the effects of distant, intercessory prayer on self-esteem, anxiety, and depression. *Alternative Therapies in Health and Medicine.* 1997;3:38–53.

124. Propst LR, Ostrom R, Watkins P, Dean T, Mashburn D. Comparative efficacy of religious and nonreligious cognitive-behavioral therapy for the treatment of clinical depression in religious individuals. *Journal of Consulting and Clinical Psychology*. 1992;60:94–103.

125. Azhar MZ, Varma SL. Religious psychotherapy in depressive patients. *Psychotherapy and Psychosomatics*. 1995;63:165–168.

126. Azhar MZ, Varma SL, Dharap AS. Religious psychotherapy in anxiety disorder patients. *Acta Psychiatrica Scandinavica*. 1994;90:1–3.

127. Razali SM, Hasanah CI, Aminah K, Subramaniam M. Religious-sociocultural psychotherapy in patients with anxiety and depression. *Australian and New Zealand Journal of Psychiatry*. 1998;32:867–872.

128. Donahue MJ. Intrinsic and extrinsic religiousness: review and meta-analysis. *Journal of Personality and Social Psychology*. 1985;48:400–419.

129. Asser SM, Swan R. Child fatalities from religion-motivated medical neglect. *Pediatrics*. 1998;101:625–629.

130. Mitchell J, Lannin DR, Mathews HF, Swanson MS. Religious beliefs and breast cancer screening. *Journal of Womens Health (Larchmt)*. 2011;11:907–915.

131. Lichtenstein B. Stigma as a barrier to treatment of sexually transmitted infection in the American deep south: issues of race, gender and poverty. *Social Science & Medicine*. 2003;57:2435–2445.

132. Madru N. Stigma and HIV: does the social response affect the natural course of the epidemic? *Journal of the Association of Nurses in AIDS Care*. 2003;14:39–48.

133. Bywaters P, Ali Z, Fazil Q, Wallace LM, Singh G. Attitudes towards disability amongst Pakistani and Bangladeshi parents of disabled children in the UK: considerations for service providers and the disability movement. *Journal of Health Care for the Poor and Underserved*. 2003;11:502–509.

134. Walls P, Williams R. Accounting for Irish Catholic ill health in Scotland: a qualitative exploration of some links between "religion," class and health. *Sociology of Health & Illness*. 2004;26:527–556.

135. Rossetti SJ. The impact of child sexual abuse on attitudes toward God and the Catholic Church. *Child Abuse & Neglect*.1995;19:1469–1481.

136. Tieman J. Priest scandal hits hospitals. As pedophilia reports grow, church officials suspend at least six hospital chaplains in an effort to address alleged sexual abuse. *Modern Healthcare*. 2002;32:6–7, 14, 1.

137. Kernberg OF. Sanctioned social violence: a psychoanalytic view. Part II. *International Journal of Psycho-analysis*. 2003; 84:953–968.

138. Satterly L. Guilt, shame, and religious and spiritual pain. *Holistic Nursing Practice*. 2001;15:30–39.

139. Purcell BC. Spiritual abuse. *American Journal of Hospice & Palliative Care*. 1998;15:227–231.

140. Purcell BC. Spiritual terrorism. *American Journal of Hospice & Palliative Care*. 1998;15:167–173.

# 22

## Three Dynamic Healing Modalities for the Treatment of Substance Use and Co-Occurring Disorders: Aromatherapy, Equine Therapy, and Creative Arts Therapies

### E. HITCHCOCK SCOTT

## Introduction

This chapter introduces 3 dynamic and widely divergent treatments: aromatherapy, equine therapy, and the creative arts therapies. All of these healing modalities are found to be useful by culturally disparate—age, gender, and race—clinical populations. The usefulness of these interventions is known and supported via reports by patient participants and via observations by professional staff members.

Anecdotal and empirical observations by patients and staff members, while not at all equivalent to experimental research, has merit especially when supported by valid research studies. Each subchapter's theoretical discipline is supported by a variety of research studies. Additionally, there is great promise that once more well-designed, large-scale, and randomized controlled trials are held that all 3 will be validated.

The problem with determining the efficacy of a treatment process with only anecdotal and empirical patient reports is a complex one. There are times when patients may deny that they have benefited from one particular intervention, even when patient peers and staff can see dramatic results. The converse is also true: patients may declare dramatic healing, and staff may view the claims as a detour from important clinical issues.

This author of this chapter acts as a consultant to various treatment programs. In one session, a patient expressed virulent contempt for art therapy. At first, she was not able to articulate why this was. She was asked, "What are you calling art therapy?" The client explained that every week, the patients were given mandala coloring books by staff members. This activity, with mandala coloring books, was billed to patients and insurance companies as if an art therapy group. Her disclosure was met with, "That is not art therapy, and if your example was a true representation of art therapy, I would hate it, too."

Caution is suggested and warranted with regard to the hiring practices by treatment program administrators. For example, allowing a massage therapist to administer aromatherapy is not sufficient, nor is hiring a skilled equestrian to facilitate equine therapy. A talented artist inadequately trained in issues of addiction, mental health, and trauma may not be able to manage an art therapy group.

This is why it is strongly recommended that only skilled, trained, and certified practitioners motivated to uphold clinical standards of ethics, practice, and care be chosen.

There are two more anecdotal stories we need to include here to further illuminate the possible positive impact of equine therapy and aromatherapy.

The first story involves a past patient who had admitted herself to a program for SUD and trauma. This female client was middle-aged, poised, perfectly coiffed (hair, nails, designer outfits), and an accomplished athlete. It was difficult to determine why she was in treatment. She was able to dismiss the need for treatment until she had equine therapy: the horse she was assigned to chased her around the corral. Apparently, as she was running in high heels, she looked back over her shoulder and asked the staff, "What is this about?" The equine therapy staff gently suggested that the horse chased her because she was not congruent. By this statement they meant that her inside experience or world did not match her external presentation. At that moment the patient gained a new understanding of the meaning and purpose of psychotherapy in an experiential and holistic way. This experience opened up her ability to be more fully proactive, willing, and engaged in the therapeutic process, which allowed her to meet her treatment goals.

The last story is a brief anecdotal vignette. My deceased husband was a lunar and planetary scientist for NASA. He was well educated, brilliant, and had a negative opinion of alternative or complimentary medicines. Therefore it was a surprise to me when in 1998 he suggested that I try aromatherapy to calm my nerves for my doctoral dissertation defense. Apparently, it had been recommended to him for his defense and he had found it to be helpful. Since before that time, I have encouraged those with substance-abuse problems, especially those at risk to abuse prescriptions, to consult with an aromatherapists. The goal of a referral to an aromatherapist is help patients address issues of anxiety, grief, and even self-esteem while they are focused on establishing long-term sobriety. Jerrold Berstein, author of *Handbook of Drug Therapy in Psychiatry*, *suggests aromatherapy in the last chapter of his book for those who may be overly sensitive to traditional medications.

Today, clinicians rarely see uncomplicated cases arrive for the intake process, whether or not the intake is for an admission to residential or outpatient care. Therefore a multimodal or multimodal type of treatment program design is ideal. Offering multiple processes and services within each program will be essential, in order to be able—as a profession—to raise our success rates for long-term sobriety. With a variety of interventions embedded into a treatment program, there is a better chance to find at least one that will reach a patient, regardless of cultural differences or how high the patients' resistance to the need for therapeutic help.

This chapter is an introduction to 3 interventions that are able to bring insight, awareness, clarity, greater accountability, creativity, strength, connection, soothing, and even joy to the recovery process for the patients, and sometimes even the health care practitioners.

## REFERENCE

*Bernstein JG. *Handbook of Drug Therapy in Psychiatry*. New York: Mosby; 1995.

# 22.1

## Creative Arts Therapies: An Integrative Modality for Addiction and Trauma Treatment

### E. HITCHCOCK SCOTT

A rt therapy is provided in many residential addiction programs. The quality of that service varies widely from clinically sound and professional to something more akin to arts and crafts activities that are primarily used to entertain clients. The differential may be due to a lack of understanding by agency administrators and therapists of the discipline of the arts in psychotherapy and addiction treatment (and therefore ignorance of the greater potential for art therapy to enhance treatment success). Although visual art therapy is not considered to be evidence based due to the lack of large quantitative studies, there are plenty of small, statistically valid studies that support the efficacy of art therapy for psychological, emotional, and physical healing. In a comprehensive review of published research studies from several countries and disciplines from January 1999 to December 2007, Slayton et al (2010) remarked:

> The results of these 35 studies provide varying degrees of support that art therapy does work. Compared to 10 years ago when Reynolds et al. (2000) found only 17 studies that met the criteria in their review, the fact that there are 35 studies in our review provides clear evidence of improvement. Although most of the studies do not meet the highest standard in efficacy research, they do serve to add support to the few that do. (p. 115)

When addiction programs hire staff members without specialized credentials in art therapy, the definition, meaning, and efficacy of art therapy and the profession become questionable. Yet, the number of certified art therapists and/or expressive art therapists is growing significantly. In addition, the quality and number of academic journals are also growing: for example, *The Arts in Psychotherapy*,

*Art Therapy: Journal of the American Art Therapy Association, Arteterapie (Czech Republic), Canadian Journal of Art Therapy,* and *International Journal of Art Therapy.*

Although the power of art therapy is not benign, in skilled hands that power can intervene upon the denial of addiction and trauma, motivate and inspire clients to be proactive in their treatment and complete treatment goals prior to discharge, provide cathartic relief and resolution of trauma (a common driving force behind addiction), and transform lives (Scott, 1999; Scott & Ross, 2006; Springham, 2008; Wilson, 2003; Malchiodi, 2003)

Malchiodi's (2003) definition of art therapy embodies a spectrum of theory and thought:

> Some therapists see it as a modality that helps individuals to verbalize their thoughts and feelings, beliefs, problems and world views. By this definition, art therapy is an adjunct to psychotherapy, facilitating the process through both image making and verbal exchange with the therapist. Others see art itself as the therapy; that is, the creative process involved in art making, whether it be drawing, painting, sculpting or some other art form, that is life enhancing and ultimately therapeutic.
>
> In actuality, both aspects contribute to art therapy's effectiveness as a form of treatment and most art therapists subscribe to both definitions in their work. (p. 2)

For the purpose of this article, the term "expressive arts therapies" might be best, since a fluid and overlapping multimodal and multimedia approach was used.

*Case Study:* This case study is of an adult married man, separated, who was 40 years old at the time of admission to a hospital 15 years ago. At the time of admission he was a late-stage alcoholic and drug addict with a history of multiple overdoses, a suicide attempt, previous self-mutilation, extreme piercings, accidents, a cut artery via a knife attack by a stranger, and near-death experiences. His tolerance for illicit drugs had become so elevated that people have overdosed and died at much lower levels of inebriation than he sustained on a regular basis for years. Prior to this admission, he had engaged in one short-term failed treatment program and left "against medical advice" (AMA) followed by 4 months of treatment at a residential addiction treatment center, which was immediately followed by a door-to-door transfer to a residential sober living environment where he lived for 6 months. During this time, he maintained sobriety in spite of extreme psychological discomfort. He voluntarily chose to return to intensive treatment due to a realistic concern that he was at risk for relapse. He returned sober to treatment as a form of relapse prevention. He stated that he was at risk for relapse because, "the latent shame disappears when I am high."

## Processes Used in Treatment

During his treatment trajectory, the client completed various creative arts assignments in a psychodynamic group and on his own personal time. Throughout his treatment, he completed several written first-step guides for chemical addiction and related issues, wrote in his journal on a consistent basis, drew a comprehensive lifespan timeline (7 feet long), painted a "life-sized silhouette mandala" (a body map tracing), created a sand tray with miniature figurines, painted blind contour self-portraits, wrote Haikus, and participated in several psychodramas. At the end of his stay he used the artwork as mnemonic to help him tell a 2-hour integrated personal life story to his group peers and therapist. As a client addresses the fragmentation and compartmentalization of memory and life experience, the psyche follows and also becomes more integrated.

Of the activities listed above, this paper will explore the processes and client perceptions of journal writing in treatment and a painting made prior to recovery; this will be followed by the life-sized silhouette mandala and a Haiku poem.

The first painting (Figure 22.1) is a self-portrait completed while still using substantial amounts of drugs and alcohol, prior to any attempt to achieve sobriety.

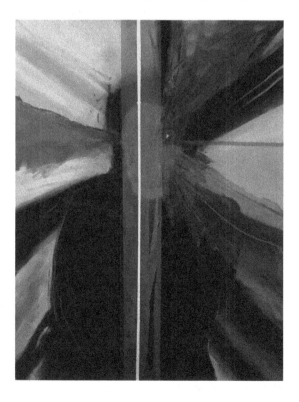

FIGURE 22.1   Self-Portrait Prior to Sobriety and Treatment JPEG.

Per the client's report, the straight white line down the middle of the canvas is a reference to the use of cocaine and the split of both a strong desire to use and to quit, as well as a split down the middle of his own psyche. When asked about the predominantly red color of the portrait, the client referenced his experience of a knife attack, which severed an artery, and the volume of blood lost. In this sense, red is a reference to death, the possibility of death, not only from the knife attack but also chemical addiction.

Soon after the client's admission to treatment, the client was asked to remove some or all of his piercings that, by anyone's standards, were extreme. This request was not mandated; the choice to remove the piercings was left up to him. It was presented to the client that the piercings may serve as a "fixed or temporary remedy" for intrapsychic pain. He was offered a chance to go deeper into his emotional process while safe in a residential setting. Readers will see parallels between the journal entry below and sentiments often associated with giving up alcohol and drugs, both the piercings and the chemicals can be framed as idealized objects.

> I don't want the holes to close, I feel naked without my piercings. I am really pissed about my nipple piercings being removed. I am seething. THIS IS MINE and somebody took it away. I want my pain, I want my blood. My heart is racing and I can't breathe. I like my piercings. I don't care if any one else likes them. Each one means something to me and I can remember how each one felt . . . I can feel the holes closing and sticking to together, reconnecting, connecting with myself. The holes seem empty like there is some thing missing. But I have the scars to remind me of what was there. My body feels smooth and free of the pain from the jewelry, nothing to catch fingers on, nothing to pull, no bumps on my body. It's a fond farewell, but frightful resignation, I am reclaiming my body and becoming whole again.

It is normative and understandable that the client returned to treatment to address the obvious and socially acceptable trauma—the shame- and guilt-free—knife attack. Yet, after experiencing a chemical addiction history that often flirted with death, along with observing the extreme nature of the piercings and his reaction to their removal, the client was asked if he had ever been sexually abused in childhood. It turns out that this was a secret he had planned to take to his grave, a grave that would have arrived sooner than later, if he had kept the secret.

The life-sized silhouette mandala (body map tracing) (Scott, 1999) (Figure 22.2), is a common assignment in many rehabilitation centers, especially for those with eating disorders. This assignment has been used as an integrative approach to help clients gain an understanding of how addiction, trauma, and mental health issues overlap and affect the body, mind, and spirit (Scott 1999, 2006). At first the client thought this assignment was trivial and was unable to start. Once he started to paint, what emerged was a surge of intense suppressed emotions that he did not

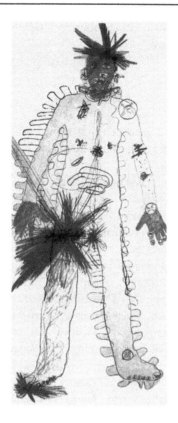

FIGURE 22.2   Life-Sized Silhouette Mandala (Body Tracing) Exercise: A Visual First
Step in Powerlessness and Unmanageability.
(Image reference: to article in *Renew*) TIFF

expect. For those with a profound addiction history and whose lives have been
extremely intense for years, and for counseling to be successful for them, that intensity needs to be safely replicated as cathartic process during treatment; if not,
clients will not be able to relate or maintain interest. Art therapy is a perfect tool
for providing intense cathartic process, as well as bilateral neurological processing,
which soothes and calms the autonomic nervous system's trauma activation. Even
though this client had painted self-portraits prior to treatment, regarding the silhouette he states, "The body map was the most pivotal and effective exercise because I could see myself It . . . was almost overwhelming but for the first time,
I saw the real me. I realized, I have been through so much, but I am still here." This
statement was followed by a renewed will to live.

This brief overview of art therapy for addiction and trauma is more like an hors
d'oeuvre than a proper dinner. It is hoped that the reader will be tempted by this
first taste to seek out more information regarding art therapy. The client's Haiku

foreshadows his long-term success in sobriety: "Gentle sun kisses/softly stir my sleeping soul/awake and alive."

## REFERENCES

Anderson SL, Teicher MH. Desperately driven and no brakes: Developmental stress exposure and subsequent risk for substance abuse. *Neuroscience and Biobehavioral Reviews*. 2008;33:516–524.

Glover NM. Play therapy and art therapy for substance abuse clients who have a history of incest victimization. *Journal of Substance Abuse Treatment*. 1999;16(4):281–287.

Holt E, Kaiser DH. The first step series: art therapy for early substance abuse treatment. *The Arts in Psychotherapy*. 2009;36:245–250.

Korlin D, Nyback H, Goldberg FS. Creative arts groups in psychiatric care: development and evaluation of a therapeutic alternative. *Nord J. Psychiatry*. 2000;54:333–340.

Malchiodi CA., ed. Handbook of Art Therapy. New York: Guilford; 2003.

Morrison R. Poetry as Therapy. New York: Human Sciences; 1987:24.

Scott EH. Healing Through Art. *Renew Magazine*. Deerfield Beach, FL: HCI; 2015:74–79.

Scott EH, Ross, CJ. Integrating the creative arts into trauma and addiction treatment: eight essential processes. In: *Psychological Trauma and Addiction Recovery*. New York: Haworth; 2006a.

Scott EH, Ross CJ. Integrating the creative arts into trauma and addiction treatment: Eight essential processes. *Journal of Chemical Dependency Treatment*. 2006b;8(2):207–226. doi.org/10.1300/J034v08n02_11.

Scott EH. The body as a testament: A phenomenological case study of an adult woman who self-mutilates. *The Arts in Psychotherapy*. 1999;26(3):149–164.

Slayton SC, D'Archer J, Kaplan F. Outcome studies on the efficacy of art therapy: A review of findings. *Art Therapy: Journal of the American Art Therapy Association*. 2010;27(3):108–118.

Springham N. Through the eyes of the law: what is it about art that can harm people? *International Journal of Art Therapy: Formerly Inscape*. 2008;13(2):65–73. doi: 10.1080/17454830802489141.

Wilson M. Art therapy in addictions treatment: creativity and shame reduction. In: Malchiodi, C., ed. *Handbook of Art Therapy*. New York: Guilford: 2000:281–293

# 22.2

## The Role of Aromatherapy in the Treatment of Substance Use and Co-Occurring Disorders

CATHY SKIPPER AND FLORIAN BIRKMAYER

## Essential Oils and the Central Nervous System

Perfumed oils and aromatic plants have been used for thousands of years to alter states of mind. All over the world, complicated and often secret aromatic formulas were used regularly in religious ceremonies. The Bible has over 200 references to perfumed oils, incense, and aromatic substances that were used for healing the mind, body, and soul. Since the 1970s the use of essential oils both by laypeople and professionals has grown dramatically. In Germany for example, aromatherapy is now commonly used in medical settings to support clients through cancer treatments, to reduce pre-procedural anxiety as well as in mental health and palliative care.[1] The basis for the use and choice of essential oils today still relies on traditional and experiential knowledge. Even though scientific studies on the effect of essential oils on the nervous system are becoming more common, there are still relatively few studies about their mechanism of action on states such as anxiety, restlessness, insomnia, and depression.

The effects of an essential oil are influenced both by the constituents as well as the route of administration. Essential oils are thought to have 3 different modes of action. First, there is a pharmacological action (i.e., a direct biochemical interaction between essential oil molecules and different tissues). Second, there is a physiological action, via the endocrine and nervous systems. Third is psychological action, which happens either indirectly through the first 2, or directly via the olfactory system. Although these 3 modes are distinct from each other, they often occur simultaneously. It is thought that the therapeutic effect of essential oils on the mind and nervous system occur by both the pharmacological and physiological modes of the inhaled or absorbed aromatic molecules and the psychological effects from the actual odor of the essential oils via the limbic system.[2]

The different aromatic molecules an essential oil contains, called constituents, each have unique actions based on their structure. Many essential oils contain tens and sometimes hundreds of constituents that have synergistic effects. Although there are a few studies on the synergistic effects of certain essential oil constituents in simple situations (e.g., antibacterial efficacy),[3] it is difficult to elucidate all the potential synergies in an essential oil that contains dozens of different constituents. Blending different essential oils adds even more complexity.[4] While these limited studies suggest positive synergies (i.e., increased activity and decreased side effects), it is possible that there are negative synergies (i.e., worsened or novel side effects).

## Mechanisms of Action of Essential Oils

The pathway for the psychological effects of essential oils is generally thought to be olfaction, even at low concentrations below the threshold of conscious scent detection. Olfaction is the most archaic sense. And unlike all other senses, olfactory pathways do not pass through the thalamus and reach the limbic system without thalamic modulation. The amygdala and olfactory tubercle are implicated in emotional reactions to odors.[5] Over 900 genes code for olfactory receptors, which are G-protein coupled receptors and account for more than 50% of the G-protein coupled receptor genes in the human genome, hinting at the importance of olfaction.[6] Olfactory receptors are found in any organs of the human body.[7] In the CNS, olfactory receptors are found in the olfactory bulb, limbic system, hippocampus, hypothalamus, and in dopaminergic neurons in the ventral tegmental area,[8] which plays a central role in addiction. The other receptor family for which certain essential oil constituents are ligands are the Transient Receptor Potential (TRP) channels, which play a role in anxiety, conditioned fear and hippocampal long-term potentiation,[9] and which appear to be modified by drug treatment, addiction, anxiety, and depression.[10] For example, incensole acetate, a constituent of Frankincense (*Boswellia carterii*) essential oil, has been shown in animal models to have anxiolytic and antidepressant effects that are mediated by TRP-V3 channels found in the CNS.[11] With the recent discoveries about the role of gut flora on anxiety, depression and other conditions, and since essential oils have profound effects on bacteria, including influencing virulence, it is tempting to speculate whether the gut flora represent another, indirect mechanism of action of essential oils on the CNS.

## Aromatherapy for Addiction Symptoms

Essential oils can be used "psychiatrically" (i.e., to alleviate specific symptoms) as well as "psychologically" (i.e., as cues or grounding strategies in CBT & EMDR) to set intentions, facilitate meditation, and increase self-awareness. They can even be used spiritually to transform consciousness, reconnect clients with their spirit and the spirits of the plants in their environment, their self-healing powers, and for shamanic soul-retrieval work. In South America, shamans who use scents for ceremony are called *perfumeros*.

Essential oils have shown promise in a number of addiction-related symptoms, including withdrawal, irritability, anxiety, difficulties with concentration, lack of energy, as well as common co-occurring symptoms such as anxiety and depression.

Essential oils of black pepper (*Piper nigrum*) and angelica (*Angelica archangelica*) have been show to decrease nicotine cravings[12] and withdrawals.[13] In an animal model, dihydromyricitin, a constituent of Himalayan cedar (*Cedrus deodara*) essential oil, has been shown to counteract acute alcohol intoxication and withdrawal signs, including tolerance, increased anxiety, and seizure susceptibility.[14] Aniseed (*Pimpinella anisum*) essential oil relieves muscle tension and GI distress, as commonly seen in withdrawal from opiates and other substances and has GABAergic activity.[15]

A number of essential oils, including Neroli (*Citrus aurantium var. amara*),[6,17] Lemon balm (*Melissa officinalis*),[18] Sandalwood (*Santalum album*),[19] fennel (*Foeniculum vulgare*)[20] as well as others[21] (xx10) have shown to have anxiolytic properties.

Lavender (*Lavandula angustifolia*) essential oil, traditionally used for regulating the nervous system and its calming sedative and anti-depressive qualities, is the most common essential oil used for anxiety. Studies have shown that even when taken internally in capsule form, to avoid olfactory cues it decreases both blood pressure and pulse rate and possibly modulates the parasympathetic system to alleviate anxiety. This may in part be due to *Linalyl acetate*, one of the principal constituents of lavender essential oil. Studies on linalool, another major component of lavender oil, have also been shown to have sedative qualities as well.[22] Other studies on lavender show that it can significantly lower cortisol levels and provoke shifts in EEG readings signifying a state of relaxation.[23]

Essential oils can be both calming or stimulating or both simultaneously on the nervous system. Rosemary (*Rosmarinus officinalis*) essential oil, for example, has been shown to significantly increase blood pressure and rate of breathing, indicating a stimulating effect, while subjects also showed higher levels of alertness, concentration and joy.[24] Another study of inhaled rosemary (*Rosmarinus officinalis*) and lavender (*Lavandula angustifolia*) essential oils showed that lavender oil calms and relaxes while rosemary is stimulating and improves performance on memory tasks.[25] A number of essential oils that increase relaxation or decrease anxiety in studies have also been shown to simultaneously increase alertness and mental performance.[5] Ylang-ylang (*Canaga odorata*) essential oil reduces blood pressures and pulse rate indicating a more relaxed state, while subjects felt more alert and attentive in an inverse correlation.[26] Incensole acetate, a constituent of Frankincense (*Boswellia carterii*) essential oil, has anxiolytic and antidepressant effects and increases hippocampal Brain-derived neurotrophic factor (BDNF) expression while decreasing Corticotropin-releasing factor (CRF) expression in animal models.[11,27] Spikenard (*Nardostachys jatamansi*) has been shown to have sedative effects and can provide relief of insomnia.[28,29] PTSD is the most common co-occurring disorder and has a profound negative impact on outcomes in substance-abuse treatment. Sylla Sheppard-Hanger has described her successes in relieving PTSD symptoms in a variety of populations, including 9/11 responders and people impacted by Hurricanes Katrina and Rita.[30]

## Routes of Administration for Essential Oils

Essential oil constituents are small, lipophilic molecules that are easily and rapidly absorbed through the skin and mucous membranes, both in liquid and vapor form. Understanding the different routes and the influence of each oil's unique composition on absorption and action is important for their safe and effective use.

To limit absorption to the *olfactory pathway* only, which is considered the most rapid and most focused on the CNS and mental effects, there are several options. An ultrasonic diffuser can fill an entire room with healing scents rapidly and the duration of the scent can be prolonged if needed. Usually operating a diffuser for 15 minutes every 2 hours provides a continuous scent. Diffusers should not be left on overnight or in a room with an infant or young child. Heat-based diffusers should be avoided as this can degrade essential oils. Another route for brief and personal, as-needed use is to take whiffs from a small bottle of essential oil or a drop put on a handkerchief or tissue.

The *cutaneous pathway* combines absorption through the skin and olfactory pathways. Before using an essential oil on the skin for the first time, a patch test is strongly recommended (e.g., putting a drop of the oil blend on the skin of the forearm and observing the area for 48 hours to see if there are any adverse reactions). In general, essential oils must be diluted to be safely applied to the skin, although a few essential oils, such as lavender (*Lavandula angustifolia*), helichrysum (*Helichrysum italicum*) and tea tree (*Melaleuca alternifolia*) are considered safe to be applied to skin undiluted. There are several methods for transdermal application of essential oils. *Massage* is very popular, especially in medical settings, and the relaxing effects of massage synergize with the properties of the oils. Essential oils should be diluted to 2% to 5% concentration by volume. A client's allergies need to be assessed in the choice of carrier oil, of which there are several choices (e.g., sesame, almond kernel, coconut). A massage can be overall or focused on certain parts of the body such as back, feet, or hands, which may be more convenient in certain settings.

*Aromatic baths* combine the cutaneous and olfactory routes. A bath can be of the whole body or just hands or feet, which have a lot of nerve endings. The water should be between 30 to 42C (86 to 103F) depending on individual preference for a relaxing bath. Thirty drops of essential oil in a full bathtub are necessary for a therapeutic effect. Before being put in the bathwater, an essential oil needs to be mixed with a dispersant, such as table salt, liquid soap or milk.

Although there is growing interest in taking essential oils internally, this should only be done under the close supervision of a well-trained aromatherapist since there can be significant side effects. Also, based on clinical experience, when taken orally, essential oils seem to work more on viral and bacterial infections and seem to be less effective for mental and emotional symptoms. When ingesting essential oils they should always be in a medium such as honey or oil or put in special capsules and never ingested undiluted, since severe irritation of the mucous membranes can occur. Essential oils should never be taken internally for prolonged periods of time, only for a few days at most. No one should ever ingest more than 6 to 12 drops in a 24-hour period. Oral administration should never be done with children under age 7.

## Safety/Precautions

Essential oil use is extremely effective and safe as long as it's administered by someone with the proper training, which means at least one year of training from a certified aromatherapy therapy training program.

The safety profiles and potential side effects of essential oils have been described in encyclopedic detail by Robert Tisserand in *Essential Oil Safety* (2014), which covers over 400 essential oils.[31]

## Conclusion

Essential oils are an important element in a bio-psycho-social-environmental-Spiritual approach to healing addictions. They can be allies in deep personal transformation by reawakening the senses and reconnecting humans to the consciousness of the ecosystem they are merely a part of. If we allow ourselves to see our entire ecosystem as one system in which all the different participants (i.e., plants, animals and humans) are in constant, mostly unconscious communication, the volatile aromatic molecules found in essential oils can be viewed as analogous to neurotransmitters or neurohormones in this network that is larger than any individual or species While addictions cut us off from ourselves, our loved ones and our environment and spirit, essential oils reawaken the senses and awareness. They truly are the "molecules of connectedness."

## REFERENCES

1. Dunwoody L, Smyth A, Davidson R. Cancer patients' experiences and evaluations of aromatherapy massage in palliative care. *International Journal of Palliative Nursery*. 2002;8(10):497–504. doi:10.12968/ijpn.2002.8.10.10696

2. Herz RS. Aromatherapy facts and fictions: A scientific analysis of olfactory effects on mood, physiology and behavior. *International Journal of Neuroscience*. 2009;119(2):263–290. doi: 10.1080/00207450802333953

3. Onawunmi, GO, Yisak WA, Ogunlana EO. Antibacterial constituents in the essential oil of cymbopogon citratus. *Journal of Ethnopharmacology*. 1984;12(3):279–286.

4. Fu, YJ, Zu Y, Chen L, Shi X, et al. Antimicrobial activity of clove and rosemary essential oils alone and in combination. *Phytotherapy Research*. 2007;21(10):989–994.

5. Royet JP, Plailly J, Delon-Martin C, Kareken DA, Segebarth C. fMRI of emotional responses to odors: influence of hedonic valence and judgment, handedness, and gender. *Neuroimage*. 2003:20(2):713–728.

6. Georgina GJ, Hindmarch CC, Pope GR, et al. G protein-coupled receptors in the hypothalamic paraventricular and supraoptic nuclei—serpentine gateways to neuroendocrine homeostasis *Front Neuroendocrinology*. 2012;33(1):45–66.

7. Pluznick JL Zou DJ, Zhang X, Yan Q, et al. Functional expression of the olfactory signaling system in the kidney. *PNAS*. 2009;106(6):2059–2064.

8. Grison A, Zucchelli S, Urzì A, Zamparo I, et al. Mesencephalic dopaminergic neurons express a repertoire of olfactory receptors and respond to odorant-like molecules. *BMC Genomics*. 2014;15(1): 729.

9. Marsch R, Foeller E, Rammes G, Bunck M, et al. Reduced anxiety, conditioned fear, and hippocampal long-term potentiation in transient receptor potential vanilloid type 1 receptor-deficient mice. *Journal of Neuroscience*. 2007;27(4):832–839.

10. Ho KW, Ward NJ, Calkins DJ. TRPV1: a stress response protein in the central nervous system. *American Journal of Neurodegener Disorder*. 2012;1(1):1–14.

11. Moussaieff A, Rimmerman N, Bregman T, et al. Incensole acetate, an incense component, elicits psychoactivity by activating TRPV3 channels in the brain. *FASEB J*. 2008;22(8):3024–3034.

12. Cordell B, Buckle J. The effects of aromatherapy on nicotine craving on a U.S. campus: a small comparison study. *Journal of Alternative Complement Medicine*. 2013;19(8):709–713.

13. Rose JE, Behm FM. Inhalation of vapor from black pepper extract reduces smoking withdrawal symptoms. *Drug Alcohol Depend*. 1994;34(3):225–229.

14. Shen Y, Lindemeyer AK, Gonzalez C, Shao XM, Spigelman I, et al. Dihydromyricetin As a novel anti-alcohol intoxication medication. *Journal of Neuroscience.* 2012;32(1):390–401. doi: 10.1523/JNEUROSCI.4639-11.2012.

15. Shojaii A, Fard MA. Review of pharmacological properties and chemical constituents of *Pimpinella anisum. ISRN Pharmacotherapy.* 2012; 2012: 510795. doi: 10.5402/2012/510795

16. Ying-Ju C et al. Inhalation of neroli essential oil and its anxiolytic effects in animals. In: Spi Spink A, Ballintjin M, Bogers N, eds. *Proceedings of Measuring Behavior 2008, 6th International Conference on Methods and Techniques in Behavioral Research (Maastricht, The Netherlands, August 26–29, 2008).* Wageningen, The Netherlands; 2008:256–257.

17. Namazi M, Ali Akbari SA, Mojab F, et al. Aromatherapy with citrus aurantium oil and anxiety during the first stage of labor. *Iranian Red Crescent Medical Journal.* 2014;16(6):e18371. doi: 10.5812/ircmj.18371

18. Ulbricht C, Brendler T, Gruenwald J, Kligler B, et al. Lemon balm (Melissa officinalis L.): an evidence-based systematic review by the Natural Standard Research Collaboration. *Journal of Herbal Pharmacotherapy.* 2005;5(4):71–114.

19. Satou T, Miyagawa M, Seimiya H, et al. Prolonged anxiolytic-like activity of sandalwood (Santalum album L.) oil in stress-loaded mice. *Flavour Frag J.* 2014;29(1):35–38. doi:10.1002/ffj.3176

20. Mesfin M, Asres K, Shibeshi W. Evaluation of anxiolytic activity of the essential oil of the aerial part of Foeniculum vulgare Miller in mice. *BMC Complement Alternative Medicine.* 2014;14:310. doi: 10.1186/1472-6882-14-310

21. Cooke B, Ernst E. Aromatherapy: a systematic review. *British Journal of General Practice.* 2000;50:493–496.

22. Bradley BF, Brown SL, Lea RW. Effects of orally administered lavender essential oil on responses to anxiety-provoking film clips. *Human Psychopharmacology.* 2009;24(4):319–330. doi: 10.1002/hup.1016

23. Field T, Cullen C, Largie S, et al. Lavender bath oil reduces stress and crying and enhances sleep in very young infants. *Early Human Development.* 2008;84(6):399–401.

24. Hongratanaworakit T. Simultaneous aromatherapy massage with rosemary oil on humans. *Science Pharmaceutical.* 2009;77:375–387. doi:10.3797/scipharm.0903-12

25. Moss M, Cook J, Wesnes K, Ducket P. Aromas of rosemary and lavender essential oils differentially affect cognition and mood in healthy adults. *International Journal of Neuroscience.* 2003;113(1):15–38. doi: 10.1080/00207450390161903

26. Hongratanaworakit T, Buchbauer G. Evaluation of the harmonizing effect of ylang-ylang oil on humans after inhalation. *Planta Medica.* 2004;70(7):632–636.

27. A. Moussaieff, Gross M, Nesher E, et al. Incensole acetate reduces depressive-like behavior and modulates hippocampal BDNF and CRF expression of submissive animals. *Journal of Psychopharmacology.* 2012;26(12):1584–1593. doi:10.1177/0269881112458729

28. Takemoto H, Ito M, Shiraki T, Yagura T, Honda G. Sedative effects of vapor inhalation of agarwood oil and spikenard extract and identification of their active components. *Journal of Natural Medicines.* 2008;62(1):41–46. doi: 10.1007/s11418-007-0177-0

29. Takemoto H, Yagura T, Ito M. Evaluation of volatile components from spikenard: valerena-4,7(11)-diene is a highly active sedative compound. *Journal of Natural Medicines.* 2009;63(4): 380–385.

30. United Aromatherapy Effort Helping Our Heros. http://unitedmatherapy.org/ 2001-2016. Accessed March 29, 2016.

31. Tisserand R, Young R. *Essential Oil Safety.* 2nd ed. Edinburgh: Churchill Livingstone Elsevier; 2014.

# 22.3

## Equine-Assisted Psychotherapy for Substance Use and Co-Occurring Disorders

### FLORIAN BIRKMAYER

## Background

The horse (*Equus ferus caballus*) evolved over approximately 50 million years, and humans began domesticating horses around 4000 BC, which led to evolutionary leaps in hunting, agriculture, transportation, and warfare—all of which profoundly shaped human history. In several European languages the word for knight or nobleman is the word for rider (e.g., *ritter* [German], *chevalier* [French], *caballero* [Spanish]), indicating the cultural importance of a deep relationship with horses. Although the horse species native to North America became extinct 10,000 years ago, it became important to Native Americans once it was reintroduced by the Spanish colonizers. Among hundreds of large mammalian species, the horse is one of only a handful that are domesticatable, allowing humans to exploit it. This willingness to interact with humans also makes horses uniquely suited to be a powerful therapeutic partner.

## Horse Characteristics Suitable for Psychotherapy

The horse, being the largest prey animal in North America, has evolved a highly acute ability to assess the intentions of beings (specifically predators) around it. The evolutionary advantage of this is that instead of reacting in flight-or-fight mode to every disturbance in its surroundings—which expends a lot of energy and would constantly interrupt other vital activities—a horse can preserve its energy and return to homeostasis faster; this appears to impact longevity and survival. This also appears to allow horses to develop lasting bonds and relationships with humans. It is speculated that horses are able to do this by utilizing their exquisite olfaction[1] as well as their vision. Horses have been shown to recognize human emotional facial expressions as well as dogs can.[2]

Horses are herd animals. A herd has a different dynamic from a pack, such as wolves or dogs. In a herd, the well-being of the individual depends on the well-being of the group, and horses are constantly aware of the state of each herd member: they frequently "check in" with one another, and there is a continuous drive to homeostasis. When horses react to external threats or when 2 herd members are working out a conflict, they rapidly release the build-up of stress through movement, breath, and vocalizations and return to calm homeostasis.

What distinguishes equine therapy from other forms of animal-assisted therapy is that the horse is a prey animal and not a predator or "cute parasite," a herd animal and not a pack animal, and much larger than a human, all of which changes the dynamics of the interaction. Establishing a connection with a horse requires that the client is fully present, authentic, and calmly assertive. This gives clients the opportunity to become aware of (and let go of) dissociative and "numbing out" patterns; dissonance between their thoughts, attitudes, and behaviors; and self-defeating, threatening, and self-victimizing. Many clients describe that their inability to tolerate severely negative feelings, common in trauma-spectrum disorders as well as anxiety and other severe mental illnesses, is what led to escalating and problematic substance use to "self-medicate." The view among professionals has evolved to match this.[3]

## Models and Standards of Practice

There is a wide range of approaches to EAP from hippotherapy, which focuses on children with developmental delays, to therapeutic riding, to EAP for adolescents and adults for a variety of conditions including SUDs and PTSD. Several EAP training organizations have adopted standards of practice and codes of ethics. For example, Eponaquest Worldwide Best Practice Guidelines[4] emphasize collaboration between humans and horses; authenticity; thriving instead of surviving; and integrating body, mind, spirit, and emotion to advance human development and teach assertiveness, empowerment, and relationship and emotional/social fitness skills. EAGALA, the Equine Assisted Growth and Learning Association[5], emphasizes a client-centered and solution-oriented approach, a team approach, and ground- based work (i.e., no riding). In both of these examples, the focus is holistic and client-centered instead of symptom or pathology focused. Importantly, EAP is not simply learning horsemanship. EAP can be done with individuals, families, and groups. A survey of over 200 EAP programs found that the primary orientation was experiential theory and that horses were considered essential because specific characteristics of the species facilitate key therapeutic processes.[6] Because the emphasis is on interacting with the horse in the present and less on talking about the past, EAP seems uniquely suited to clients struggling with talking about their feelings such as adolescents, people with trauma, and other groups that are frustrated by and frequently fail talk-based, office-based group and individual psychotherapies.

## Evidence

A 2011 review of the literature on the efficacy of EAP[7] states that most of the literature has been practice based rather than research and theory oriented, and there is a lack of randomized controlled studies. Schultz et al[8] showed that in a pilot study of 63 children aged 4 to 16, children with a history of intra-family violence and familial substance abuse showed greater improvement in Global Assessment of Functioning (GAF) score, and there was a statistically significant correlation between improvement in GAF score and number of treatments, although the study suffered from a number of methodological issues. While there has been concern about the cost of and time required for equine therapy, an unpublished study by Mann and Williams[7] suggests that there is faster progress in some adolescents with conduct, mood, and psychiatric disorders (82% of a cohort showed significant clinical improvement over 5 sessions) that failed conventional therapies. Another review[9] states that there is strong clinical evidence that equine-facilitated psychotherapy reduces impulsivity, improves self-concept, and increases both the subjects' sense of responsibility and their ability to engage in emotional relationships. In a 2011 interview Cody and Szymandera[10] discuss their clinical experience with EAP for clients with SUD. Although controlled studies are still lacking, there are many promising reports[11] about the benefits of EAP for clients with PTSD, which is the most common co-occurring disorder, and it is frequently undiagnosed and adversely impacts outcomes in substance-abuse treatment.

An informal survey by the author found that over the past 5 years multiple residential substance-abuse treatments have added equine therapy, although this may be more common outside of large urban settings. In discussions with staff at several programs, it appears that the majority of clients are eager to participate in EAP, report benefit, and appear to gain more out of the residential programs overall.

In a cohort of women (n = 48) in a community corrections (jail diversion) program for DUI/DWI (mean age 45, median number of DUI arrests 4) that participated in equine-assisted group psychotherapy (1.5 hours weekly for 4 weeks) in Albuquerque New Mexico, the re-arrest rate for violations of the community corrections program, i.e. relapse, decreased by 70% compared to baseline, i.e. the cohort members themselves before starting equine assisted group therapy had been in the community corrections longer than initially ordered due to repeated relapses. (Birkmayer F, Simon W unpublished data[12]. For more information http://www.eagala.org/node/7748)

# Conclusion

While much research still needs to be done, equine-assisted therapy appears to offer rapid, deep transformation and improved outcomes for clients with substance use and co-occuring disorders.

## REFERENCES

1. Briggs K Equine Sense of Smell http://www.thehorse.com/articles/10055/equine-sense-of-smell Published Dec 11, 2013. Accessed March 29, 2016.
2. Smith AV, Proops L, Grounds K, Wathan J, McComb K. *Functionally relevant responses to human facial expressions of emotion in the domestic horse (Equus caballus). Biology Letters.* 2016;12(2). Published 10 February 2016. doi:10.1098/rsbl.2015.0907
3. Khantzian E. *The Self-Medication Hypothesis of Substance Use Disorders: A Reconsideration and Recent Applications. Harvard Review of Psychiatry.* 1997;4(5):231–244. doi:10.3109/10673229709030550
4. Eponaquest Worldwide Best Practice Guidelines http://eponaquest.com/ethics-standards-of-practice/ Published 2015. Accessed March 29, 2016.
5. EAGALA Model http://www.eagala.org/about/model Accessed March 29, 2016.
6. McConnell PJ. *National Survey on equine assisted therapy: An exploratory study of current practitioners and programs* Walden University 2010 UMI Number: 3412302
7. Cantin A, Marshall-Lucette S. *Examining the Literature on the Efficacy of Equine Assisted Therapy for People with Mental Health and Behavioural Disorders. Mental Health and Learning Disabilities Research and Practice.* 2011;8(1):51–61.
8. Schultz PN, Remick-Barlow GA, Robbins L. Equine-assisted psychotherapy: a mental health promotion/intervention modality for children who have experienced intra-family violence. *Health & Social Care in the Community.* 2007;15(3):265–271. doi:10.1111/j.1365-2524.2006.00684.x
9. Bates A. *Of Patients & Horses: Equine-Facilitated Psychotherapy. Journal of Psychosocial Nursing and Mental Health Services.* 2002;40(5):16–19.
10. Cody P, Steiker LH, Szymandera ML. Equine Therapy: Substance Abusers' "Healing Through Horses". *Journal of Social Work Practice in the Addictions.* 2011;11(2):198–204.
11. Selected Articles on Equine Therapy with Military EAGALA http://www.eagala.org/military_articles Accessed March 29, 2016.
12. WT Equestrian/SW Horsepower http://www.eagala.org/node/7748 Accessed March 29, 2016.

# 23

## Shamanism: Addiction and Soul Sickness

DEAN TARABORELLI, ALBERTO VILLOLDO, AND GEORGE E. MUÑOZ

## Medical Anthropology Perspective in Addiction and Recovery

The fusion of pure science and the healing arts poses the greatest challenge to the conventional thinker, science, and conventional medicine. The aim of this chapter is to present the paradox of a cutting-edge yet timeless approach noteworthy in the context of healing applicable to the field of addiction. Dr. Munoz would like to express deep gratitude to Dr. Alberto Villoldo and his colleague Dean Taraborelli, both of whom have been ideal collaborators here, accepting the calling to tell the story of the shamanic healer approach. Theirs is an oral tradition passed on through the millennia by some of the greatest planetary healers and shamans that Dr. Villoldo has had the opportunity to study for close to 30 years at first as a medical anthropologist but then as a friend and protector of these great indigenous peoples, the Quero. They are direct Inca descendants, Quechua speaking, and are the prime focus of his anthropologic studies. Dean Taraborelli is an accomplished healer and shaman and highly experienced in the field of addiction treatment utilizing the Quero's techniques. Through the processes of initiation, discovery, and self-healing Dean exemplifies the "hero's journey," which Joseph Campbell speaks about in his timeless works on spirituality and the quest for wholeness implicit throughout time and synonymous with disparate cultures. The complexities of the biologic disturbances at both the molecular, receptor, and neuroendocrine levels of addiction are as undeniable as their scientific constructs. However, in the jungle of the Amazon or in the highlands of the Andes, where the air is thin and the Sumi energy of the planet dominates, the spirit of Mother Earth or Pacha Mama resides as the purest primal energy on the planet to the Quero. Their healing traditions transcend our Western thinking—our classic conception of science and its constructs of reality and probability.

## The Dawn of the Shamans

One of the earliest bits of evidence of shamanic practice comes from the Middle Paleolithic period some 35,000 years ago, from a deliberate burial ritual performed in a cave in Shanidar, Iraq. Here, archeologists discovered flowers and medicinal plants carefully laid around the body of the deceased, together with stone tools to accompany them in their journey to the afterlife.

We can see earlier traces of shamanic art in the cave paintings at Lascaux and Altamira. In these magnificent frescoes we observe how humans are just one of many different creatures that populate the earth, and we do not hold a privileged place in creation. The hunter-gatherers that practiced this form of animism believed that the plants and animals, as well as the spirits of the invisible world, are equal in stature to humans. The interests of the plants and the animals had to be taken into consideration, the balance of the invisible world had to be maintained, and the natural order of the cosmos had to be kept in equilibrium.

The dawn of agriculture at the end of the Paleolithic brought with it a new set of beliefs that were championed by religion. With farming, man became the owner of the plants and the animals, which no longer had equal footing in the grand scheme of creation. The corn in the granary and the sheep and horses in the stable became *property*. They were there to serve and delight man.

Today we are testing the limits of the belief that man reigns supreme above all creatures. Planetary over-population, global climate change, environmental toxins, and the illnesses of civilization (including cancer, Alzheimer's, and heart disease) are making us reconsider our position in the cosmos. Many of us have been called to more sustainable and ecological relationships with ourselves and with nature. We are returning to the ways of the shaman.

While most religions are theistic, or centered around the idea of a god that created the heavens and the earth, shamans insists that your sacred relationship is not with your god but with nature. Shamanism recognizes laws or underlying principles that inform all of creation. When you have the right relationship with these natural laws, you have health. Disease results when you break these natural laws or cease to respect them.

Just like modern scientists who identify the laws of physics and biology, shamans identified certain laws of nature. For example, it is obvious to any modern person that Einstein's equation $E = MC^2$ explains how that energy (E) and mass (M) are intimately related to each other. Likewise it was obvious to the shaman that the world of energy and the material world are interwoven and mirror each other. In fact, the shaman learns to dance on top of the equal sign in Einstein's famous equation. She is the midwife to those things that need transferrence from the world of energy into the world of matter, and the shaman helps those things (and persons) that needed to return to the invisible world of energy.

In our materialistic society we have come up with extraordinary physical tools for changing the world. We can move mountains with our bulldozers, and perform brain surgery. Similarly, shamans devised subtle tools for working in the invisible realms. These tools allowed them to change the matrix or blueprint of the energetic realm and to bring about healing in their patients. They learned to fix things in the world of energy before they became broken in the physical.

Today our Western paradigms about health, disease, aging, and recovery from trauma and addiction are being reexamined. As we test the limits of allopathic medicine, we are faced with the need for new paradigms founded on maintaining health rather than treating disease so that our healthspan can equal our lifespan and of stewardship of the body and nature. Many of us have been called to rediscover the ancient shamanic beliefs.

In my own case, I went from being a medical anthropologist who spent many years in the Amazon and Andes researching the shamans to becoming a practicing shaman-healer. In fact, all of the authors of this article have become practicing shamans, mediating between the visible world of matter and the invisible world of energy. We have learned to heal things at the source and at the matrix level of creation. We have stopped treating symptoms and have begun treating causes. We discovered that the body is an energy system and that we are sunlight that is tightly bound into matter.

We practice shamanic energy medicine. We apply the tools of the shaman to treat conditions that do not respond to conventional medical interventions. At the heart of shamanic energy medicine is the notion that when you create the conditions for health, disease disappears. When we create the physical (nutritional and biochemical), emotional, and spiritual conditions for health disease goes away. We tend to the spirit and know that it will repair the mind that in turn will help us create psychosomatic health. And we help our patients, many who have given up hope by the time they reach us, dream their world and their health into being each day.

## Addiction and Soul Sickness

### THE NEED FOR A DEEPER UNDERSTANDING OF ILLNESS, HEALTH, AND HEALING

The United States currently spends more on health care than any other country on earth, yet ranks 34th in the general health of its people.[1] Despite our science and our technology, there are still over 400 different mental diagnoses used to describe the various ways people are not well.[2] Countless other diagnoses identify non-psychiatric illnesses.

While the United States has some of the best emergency medicine in the world, we are not a nation that demonstrates good overall health and mental well-being. Clearly, our system has room to broaden its view beyond the typical symptom management approach to a holistic approach in which symptoms are clues of distress bubbling up from deeper problems. We have to focus on interrelated systems within an individual and in their relationship to the world around them.

It seems that people in need are already seeking such methods. As our medical system falls short, many use alternatives to mainstream health care. For example, we find that the words "shaman" and "shamanism" have even eased into the awareness of our culture at large as people look for more effective methods of healing.[3]

### THE SHAMAN—A TECHNICIAN OF THE SOUL

Shamanism's history is ancient and worldwide. It has been practiced on every continent on earth for 10,000 to 20,000 years. Some think it is even an older path. Shamanic cave glyphs have been discovered, for example, that are estimated to be 40,000 years old.

Shamanism goes beyond a body of knowledge used for healing; it is a way of being, thinking, feeling, and looking at the world. The Shaman knows that all life on earth is related, and the health and well-being of each life depends on the cooperation and balance of the whole. In addition to the need for a vital body and mind, the Shaman knows that every person yearns for love, meaning, belonging, expression, creativity, truth, and beauty. This is the domain of the soul. When we become disconnected from it, we eventually become ill. For the Shaman, every disease, including addiction, has its roots in soul sickness and energetic imbalance.

Shamanism is not a religion or a belief system. It is not based on a doctrine but rather a body of wisdom informed by the direct experience of the natural world. Viewing everything as part of the natural world, there is no concept of the natural versus the supernatural. There is only the visible and the invisible.

A Shaman is trained through experiential rituals, ceremonies, trials, and initiations. These lead to a mastery of awareness in both the physical and energetic realms of the natural world—the seen and the unseen. She is learned in both the natural/material world (plants, animals, humans, minerals, elements) and the "hidden"/immaterial world (the subconscious, unconscious, and energetic realms). This knowledge has many applications in helping and healing.

As an observer of universal patterns and lessons found in the natural world, the Shaman understands there is a vast world of information beyond the five senses in the invisible realm we call energy. Consequently, Shamanism understands that people are more than body and mind; they are unified fields of energy that live and interact in a much larger energetic field.[4,5] This is an ancient paradigm, but also the science of quantum physics that is a modern world discovery.

## THE NEWTONIAN WORLD AND A SPLINTERED VISION

Until about 100 years ago, modern science, including medicine, was informed primarily by Newtonian physics—the most credible scientific view of the time. This was a mechanistic model in which the universe was believed to consist of matter ruled by cause and effect. In this paradigm, all reality could be seen and measured. Objects in space could be observed, and their movements could be predicted. Objects on earth could similarly be observed and explained. Any issue of invisible forces at work was dismissed in favor of a more "modern" and machine-like construct.[5]

Eventually medicine adopted this view in its understanding of health and disease. However, the Newtonian paradigm of medicine reduced us to a collection of physical parts that either worked or didn't work properly, much like a machine. Energy was relegated an incidental role in this universe.[4,6]

This perspective gave rise to the fractured lens through which we (and our doctors) viewed our world, our psychology, our bodies, and our maladies. There are still significant holdovers from the Newtonian world that we don't think much about. The ear, nose, and throat specialist, for example, does not treat GI problems, and the psychiatrist does not treat infections.

Clearly specialization and a more microscopic perspective are helpful in treating the complexity of the body. However, the Newtonian-inspired medical perspective lost sight of the whole person and the interrelated systems that work together for overall health. This system also ignored the importance of interpersonal relationships and our connection to nature itself.

Similarly, we have attempted to treat addiction but not its invisible forces or the underlying issues it springs from. We have also attempted to treat addiction without treating the entire person who is addicted. We have focused on the disease, overlooking an individual's integrity as a holistic being with innate self-regulating abilities. The totality of ourselves, our innate nature as energetic beings—as whole and integrated systems operating in a field of interconnected energies—has been largely overlooked.

## QUANTUM REALITY AND A HOLISTIC VIEW

When quantum physics was born at the beginning of the 20th century, fundamental changes occurred in our concept of reality. Beyond mechanistic reality governed by cause and effect, other forces were also at work. These invisible forces were governed by probability, synchronicity, and interconnectedness. This body of science acknowledged the world of energy.

In 1801 Thomas Young's famous double slit experiment proved not only that matter and energy are interchangeable, but also that human consciousness affects which state it can be.[7] He proved that *thought influences matter.* He demonstrated this by showing that light changes its form and can manifest as an energy wave or a particle of energy. Even more astounding was the discovery that human thought exerts an influence on these mysterious events.[8] The impact on our understanding of health, illness, and healing would dramatically change; human consciousness became an undeniable factor. This would later be understood in the science of epigenetics.

Most of us are relatively unaware of quantum science, even though it plays a large part in our everyday life. Without this science there would be no digital age, cell phones, super computers, nuclear power, or MRIs. Only recently has quantum science gotten a more noticeable foothold into mainstream health care. The advent of functional medicine, for example, bridges the worlds of matter and energy to that of the body and mind. Shamanism, however, has been rooted in this knowledge for thousands of years, long before quantum physicists arrived on the scene. We realize now that the science of shamanism *is* the science of quantum physics and that the shaman is an energy technician working in the realm of the soul.

## THE QUANTUM REALITY OF SHAMANISM

The shaman works with energy, which is the building block and organizer of everything in the universe including the human body and mind. Holding such knowledge, the shaman sits on the equal sign of Einstein's famous equation, $\Sigma = mc^2$, with one foot in the material world and one foot in the energetic realm.[9] From the shaman's vantage point, the seen and the unseen are intricately connected. If there is a physical symptom then there is an energetic correlation. The practice of shamanism mediates between them, accessing information from the physical and the non-physical worlds. The shaman can interact with the unseen world of energy and influence physical reality.

## THE LUMINOUS BODY

Healing in every culture and every medical tradition before ours was accomplished by moving energy.

—*Albert Szent-Gyorgyi, Nobel Laureate in Medicine*

In shamanic language, we understand the morphogenetic field to be the luminous energy field, the luminous body, or the energy body.[12] Most are not familiar with the luminous body, primarily because they have never learned to pay attention to it—similar to the middle toe on your left foot, which you have probably not thought about much until reading this sentence. We never pay specific attention to this part of the body, but it is there serving a function. Similarly, we are mostly unaware of the immune system and other subtle systems in the body; however, they are present and each serves a vital function. The same is true for the luminous body.

The luminous body is an atomic field surrounding the physical body. It organizes and regulates the cells of the physical body. It is a sea of living energy that stores information about everything that has ever influenced it. This field serves as the blueprint to the physical body, the mind, and the soul. Therefore, the coherence and vitality of this field directly influence the health and vitality of the body, mind, and soul. Trauma, suffering, generational patterns, toxins, abuse, abandonment, addiction, toxic relationships, hatred, shame, humiliation, and any number of toxic emotions all negatively influence the information in this field of energy.

Nature has provided us with automatic cleansing mechanisms for the luminous body. However, disturbances in the luminous field caused by trauma or other toxicities, which shaman call "imprints," can impede the detoxification process. If unable to cleanse itself, the luminous body integrates and imprints toxic pattern into its field of information, creating a chronic energetic disturbance. Imprints can permanently affect the field's delicate patterns of organizing information, affecting its regulating influence on the body and mind. Trauma, and the reliving of trauma in the limbic brain, changes the blueprint of the luminous field. This changed information informs the cells that they organize, which creates disease.

The luminous field affects the body much in the way a magnet will organize metal filings sprinkled on a flat surface. Without the magnet, the metal filings are randomly dispersed, much like sprinkled pepper. With a magnet under the surface, however, the metal filings organize into a pattern dictated by the magnetic field.

The shaman knows that disease will appear in the luminous energy field before it manifests in the physical body or in patterns of dysfunctional behavior.[11] The shaman also knows that attempting to heal disease without working with the luminous body is not complete healing. The body's blueprint will still carry the instructions for disease if the luminous body is not addressed. Imagine moving metal filings on a flat surface with your hand. You effectively change the previous pattern, but when the magnet is reapplied, it draws the metal back into the previous organizational pattern. This is what happens when the luminous body is not healed. It will eventually draw the body—which may have made some improvements—back to the structure of its blueprint. If unhealed, the luminous body's blueprint will still contain the template of the original disease. This helps explain why addiction is chronic and incurable when only treated at the level of the mind and energetic-level issues are not addressed.

Many of us have ineffectively tried to heal our physical or mental maladies with chemical remedies such as prescription drugs or self-medication. The result has often been a worsening condition we cannot escape from.

The same frustrating process occurs in addiction recovery efforts. Addicts attempt to change external factors such as the people, places, and things that trigger them in order to be well. This approach can be helpful in the early stages of addiction recovery. However, once we loosen our grip or let our guard down, we relapse if no fundamental changes have occurred inside us. Without core change, our metal filings of addiction re-organize themselves back into the disease structure.

Shamanic healing reorganizes the blueprint of the luminous energy field, reorganizing disturbances that have created illness and patterns of behavior that perpetuate illness. Once the energetic signature of disturbances are cleared, healing on the physical, mental, and emotional levels becomes possible. According to the theoretical physicist David Bohm, we are an *unbroken wholeness*.[13] Shamanic healing seeks to restore balance in that unbroken wholeness.

## WHAT THIS MEANS FOR ADDICTION RECOVERY

In the Western disease model, addiction is a chronic malady of the brain reward, motivation, memory, and related circuitry. There is lifelong management with disease remission maintenance protocols.[14] The disease is evidenced by impaired control over behavior, preoccupation with the substance/behavior, dependence/tolerance/withdrawal, and continued use despite negative consequences.

In this medical model, an addict is viewed as a victim of a genetically predetermined disease. The addict is also portrayed in our culture as the perpetrator of any number of transgressions against self, family, community, and society. Addiction permeates and transforms the addict and his life with obvious effects. As onlookers we can see the physical toll it takes, and with interaction we come up against other manifestations. Obsession and thought distortions are apparent; they are acutely evident in relationships and communication during stress and conflict. Behaviorally, we easily observe compulsive self-destruction as the addict returns again and again to addictive behaviors that cause negative consequences to pile up from all directions. Emotionally there is turmoil, chaos, pain, and instability. Finally, we see that the spark of life has slipped away. We see that particularly in the eyes of the addicted, and we hear it in their expressions of hopelessness, resignation, and helplessness. We also *feel* the absence of soul and spirit. Part of them is dead, and the rest will follow if they do not heal.

The shamanic wellness model is based on reestablishing connection to the regulating forces of the quantum field and restoring the body's self-regulation mechanisms. To accomplish this, the root causes of addiction must be healed at the essential level. The shaman works with an integrative approach—addressing all aspects of the unified energy field: body, mind, soul, and spirit. Shamanism understands that in a unified energy field any malady affects the whole, disconnecting us from the vital life force and divine intelligence that we, as energetic beings, need for health and well-being. In the field of addiction and codependency treatment, shamanism offers the possibility of *full recovery* from addiction and related co-occurring disorders.

Shamanic addiction treatment offers us a *health-centric* rather than *disease-centric* life after active addiction. With shamanic healing, we are no longer in remission, fearing relapse. Instead we experience deep healing at the essential level of quantum reality. We go beyond addiction to a fully recovered life.

### UNDERSTANDING THE SHAMAN'S VIEW OF ADDICTION

AA's Bill Wilson said that alcohol was only a symptom of a deeper malady.[15] This is congruent with the shamanic perspective of addiction. The shaman knows that in order to heal, a person must heal the original or underlying wound that caused an illness. That wound created an imprint in the luminous field that keeps organizing a painful reality in the body and the mind.

The shaman views all illness, including addiction and codependency, as the result of wounding. Energetically, this means that the luminous body is somehow disrupted and does not receive pristine information from the source as well as it should. Looking for the root cause of illness, the Shaman seeks the *original* wound, not its latest version, as it repeats itself throughout one's life. The original wound is considered the moment of separation and dissociation that expelled us from the sacred place of wholeness. It is our "fall from grace" if you will. We lose our natural state of possibility and creativity and fall into pure survival mode, only partially maintaining our connection with the larger field's vibrancy.

As in all events we encounter, it is not the facts of an event itself but rather our *interpretation* of the facts that wounds us. When we believe our survival is threatened or our integrity is severely compromised, an imprint is made in the luminous body and a neuro-connection in the limbic brain. Our energy body and in turn our external lives re-organize themselves around the terror and pain of the traumatic moment.[16] From this survival state, we create false beliefs about ourselves and the world around us. These false beliefs are reactionary, fear based, and safety oriented. They are not reflective of our true nature or our core values. As time progresses, they are not even reflective of our immediate circumstances. In essence, we are detached from our true nature, caught in a frozen moment of chaos and fear.[17] In this state, we are also cut off from pure and basic vital life-source energy. The original wounding event may be in our awareness, but the underlying beliefs that develop are buried in the unconscious mind. For example, Bob made no connection to his mother or the pressure he felt in caring for her.

From this traumatic state of separation and dissociation from vital life energy, we experience chronic pain and develop coping strategies to compensate for our compromised and depleted existence. The majority of this process happens in the unconscious mind. People rearrange their lives around these unsustainable and unconscious coping strategies. They can often function for decades (although with great difficulty) until the reality of unsustainability catches up with them. For some, mind-altering substances or behaviors become their best coping mechanism. This is the foundation of addiction.

## CORE HUMAN WOUNDING: THE ARCHETYPAL WOUNDS

> Your mind will adjust the body's biology and behavior to fit with your beliefs.
>
> —*Bruce Lipton*

From the Western medical perspective, there are only a few types of people and many ways of being sick. We need only look at the *Diagnostic and Statistical Manual for Mental Disorders* to see the countless labels medicine uses to categorize human behavior and suffering.[2] This approach lends itself to a fragmented and mechanized treatment approach. From the shamanic perspective there are many kinds of people and only a few ways to be sick. The shaman knows that disconnection from our inner nature will result in sickness.

While there are countless circumstances that inflict individual suffering, these translate into a small number of core traumas, or archetypal wounds, common to all humans. These are the themes of the original wounds that underlie our illnesses. They become the largely unconscious source of many of our sabotaging beliefs.

We re-experience these core wounds through countless iterations throughout our lives until they are healed. We naturally focus on the latest episode—losing a job, being left by a partner, feeling rejected, or somehow being wronged. However, the latest episode is often just a spinoff of the original trauma and its related beliefs that lie invisibly embedded in the energy system and the limbic brain. These archetypal wounds leave the following beliefs for us to contend with:

1. **Unworthiness:** I am not lovable. I do not deserve good things. I am not good enough.
2. **Abuse:** I am hurt physically or mentally. I am unsafe. I am a victim. Others are dangerous. The world is dangerous.

3. **Abandonment:** No matter what I do or who I am, I will eventually be left alone. People always leave me.
4. **Trust:** The world is an unsafe place. I am always waiting for the other shoe to drop. I can't let anyone close.
5. **Betrayal:** I am the victim of disloyalty.
6. **Separation:** I am abandoned by God. I am cut off from source energy. I have been "kicked out of the garden." I am always an outsider. I am alone. I am lonely.

From the traumatic impact forward, and until its healing, we live separated from the sacred from our authentic self, yearning for it consciously or not and "abandoned" or "orphaned" into an unsafe self with unsafe others in an unsafe world. The consequences of this abject state are pervasive and can be devastating, even fatal, when the path of addiction is chosen as a remedy.

The nature of intoxication offers us a momentary reprieve from the pain of our wounds and their related beliefs. Intoxication is at least a temporary solution. Respite from life's pain seems to be a place of ease and comfort, until this unsustainable coping mechanism backfires and creates more suffering. With unhealed wounds and in the madness of addiction, we are left to yearn for healing and a return to wholeness. The path of addiction was the result of searching for wholeness. Eventually, its illusion dissipates and we realize we are still living in painful and debilitating separation.

In any illness, shamanism looks for the essential trauma and the original wound, causing further disorder, disturbances, imbalances, and problems as time goes on. In the shamanic healing of addiction, a traumatic wound is viewed as the root of addiction and the driving force behind it. The wounding that precipitated addiction may be an ancient one in an individual's lifespan; it may even have been long forgotten, slipping into the unconscious. Nevertheless, once there the wound, if unhealed, continues to be felt throughout one's life in powerful ways.[18,19,20]

We want to be reborn in the addiction and return to a "state of grace" or to experience a comfort we might not even have had but yearn for nonetheless. In the dependency on our addictive drugs or processes, we seek the comfort of another type of dependency—one in which we feel safe, whole, and protected—like what the ideal childhood would have been. We somehow seek an attachment with that which is greater and more powerful than us. As children seek the loving protector, addicts mistakenly seek the embrace of their addictions. In doing so, they attempt to heal their profound attachment disorders that have developed in their original wounds.[21,22] From the shamanic perspective, we must heal the root in order to extricate ourselves from the pattern. Our sense of detachment is our separation from the supportive and life-giving quantum field.

## THE MECHANISM OF TRAUMA

We cannot talk about addiction nor recover from it without addressing the trauma that first created the conditions for it. We have long known that trauma and addiction are existential and clinical companions. Even active addiction itself is a traumatic event that contains a series of other traumatic events. For example, addicts encounter violence in the drug culture, and their vulnerability can be easy prey. They may become homeless, isolated, infected, impoverished, or incarcerated. And these are just the outer trappings of their plight.

Powerful and intricate dynamics occur between trauma and addiction so that each reinforces the other. Consequently, we have to address them simultaneously for best results. If we attempt to treat one without treating the other, they will pull themselves back together again so their symbiosis continues. Trying to split trauma and addiction apart in a fragmented treatment approach is an impossible task.[23-25] Trauma and addiction are intertwined and may in fact be essentially the same condition with many stages in the life of an addict.

Trauma is the pivotal and personally primal point in the life of an addict. It is the point at which wholeness—or the sense of self that is intact, safe, and authentic—is lost.[26] With traumatic impact, our brains split functioning off from the normal homeostasis that supports ordinary life.[17] The brain abruptly switches to fight, flight, or freeze in response to a threat—real or symbolic—as a defense mechanism strictly for self-preservation. This system overrides the higher command functions of the brain responsible for reasoning.[17,27,28] We sacrifice reasoning for response time when living in the terrified limbic brain during trauma.

While there are universal, archetypal wounds that we are all vulnerable to, it is the *personal experience* of an event that determines its traumatic impact.[29] We see this in groups of people who have experienced the same adversity. Some will develop PTSD, for example, and some will not. Consequently, the *degree* of traumatic impact is not determined by the "facts" of an event, but by one's reaction.[30] We have to know the personal post-trauma narrative. In shamanic intervention, we seek out the personal story of an individual's original wounding.

The brain does not distinguish between real and imagined threats or danger. It produces the same chemicals during a traumatic event or the remembering of the event. *As you leaned in to tuck me in, it may have been a shadow, for example, but if I perceived it as a knife in your hand, that is what counts.* Our interpretations of sensory information as threatening cause us to relive the trauma both consciously and unconsciously if it is unresolved. The beliefs spawned in the traumatic moment become powerful drivers for the rest of our lives.

In shamanic understanding, therefore, as in psychotherapy, we cannot assume how objective events have affected an individual—which have precipitated soul loss, a shamanic term for dissociation[31] and which have not, for example. What has wounded an individual lies within that individual's psyche. We have to explore the internal architecture of the psyche to find the originally wounding circumstance that continues its trauma echo throughout someone's life. The shaman seeks the narrative of the original wound—its story—in order to facilitate healing.

To help understand how traumatic experience creates permanent disturbances in the energy field, it is helpful to draw some comparisons to basic brain anatomy. Trauma is stored in both. It also helps to understand a bit more about the fight, flight, or freeze reactions we have during trauma. The most ancient part of the brain is the brain stem, which is responsible for survival and basic body functioning. This part of the brain is so powerful that, in the case of life-threatening blood loss, for example, it triages which organs receive blood flow, directing blood to organs of higher priority. The brain stem is charged with the responsibility of keeping us and our species alive.

The limbic brain developed later in our evolution. It is the brain of base human emotions and is known as the brain of the four Fs: feeding, fornicating, fighting, and fear. This part of the brain is strictly opportunistic and exists to meet slightly more complex needs such as procreation and interpersonal relationships, for example. Traumatic memories and disempowering beliefs are stored here. Since there is no sense of time, those memories are relived in real time when they are triggered, no matter how old they are. Both the brain stem and the limbic areas of the brain are unconscious and outside of our awareness. Much later in our evolution, the neo-cortex evolved, which is the brain of higher reasoning.

## SHAMANIC RESOLUTION OF COMPLEX TRAUMA

> Your mind will adjust the body's biology and behavior to fit with your beliefs.
>
> —*Bruce Lipton*

From a shamanic perspective, complex issues translate very simply: the cause of maladies is not always obvious, and an original wounding, if unhealed, will create problems in later life. From the shamanic perspective a wounding, or trauma, is the beginning of disease. We know that if unresolved, incidents of early trauma predict the likelihood of subsequent substance use and other mental health problems.[32] Additionally, we have deep knowledge of unhealed addiction and unhealed trauma both crossing generational lines, possibly for many generations.[18]

Best practice dual diagnosis programs come close to addressing the co-occurring and underlying forces of trauma in addiction. However, they typically offer language and thought-based therapies that lead to *insight* and an ability to verbalize an *intellectual understanding* of the problems. Recovery maintenance tools are typically more cognitive exercises as well. A language- and thought-based "healing" reinforces the separation of mind, brain, and body—again acting as if we are a more machine-like composition of parts instead of the unified energetic beings that shamans and quantum reality know us to be.[5]

Cognitive remedies are far different than the experiential- and energy-based ones of shamanic intervention that treat the whole person beyond language and thinking. The differing results are astounding: we go into cautious remission in mainstream treatment, but we fully recover from addiction in shamanistic healing. Another way of saying this is that insight and understanding are like *reading about* healing, while shamanistic healing is the *experience of healing*. Healing is the result when we apply energy-based and holistic restorative interventions to a disharmonious field of energy. In order to heal from addictions, we must treat the whole person.

Without treating trauma, which is the core of addiction, addiction is always ours; we have a chronic and relapsing disease.[33] We are told that we can never be free of it—that we can hold it in abeyance or, barring that, we can relapse. Even without symptoms of addiction, we are cautioned in recovery to live a disease-centric life, watching for signs of its presence because we are certain that it will be there. Traditional addiction treatment attributes this to the cunning nature of addiction; a predatory disease entity that never sleeps and is always gaining power and stealth.

Shamanic healing, on the other hand, treats addiction in the energy field of our quantum reality. Addiction is cured rather than caged by our constant vigilance or lulled to sleep in its complacency. The past, present, and future is healed through shamanic addiction intervention. We no longer have to live a life that revolves around an addictive illness. The present and the future become ours to live with a health-centric focus. The addictionogenic blueprints of our pasts can be resolved with shamanic healing, and they will no longer be able to govern us.[34]

When the traumatic core of addiction is not addressed, the trauma energies that precipitated the addictive process remain either active or dormant but not resolved. They lay like "time bombs" in the personal energy field awaiting ignition. Once triggered, even years later, their energy knots, disturbances, intrusions, or misplacements begin to manifest addiction again, using the blueprints of the original energetic disturbance.[10,11,34]

This is the cunning nature of addiction that lies in wait to pounce upon us. It is the unhealed addiction, however, the one healers could not see in its true reality in the quantum universe. Newtonian-based medicine relegates these time bombs and their blueprints to "genetics" and genetic determinism. We are left without the ability to conceive of transformation; our biological fates have been sealed in that paradigm. A quantum-based and shamanic view, however, says that epigenetics are a more correct way to view our biological "fates"—that there are countless possibilities of how a gene can be expressed and that we can even switch them off.[35,36]

Shamanic healing, therefore, restores the connection to the vital life force of the biosphere. It mobilizes the innate dynamics of our own healing processes. The origins of addiction, its workings and what is needed to heal it, have a common theme running throughout shamanic intervention: that we are whole and energetic beings, a unified field of energy; and we suffer when that field is disturbed as much as when our connection to the larger field is disrupted. Shamanism brings an understanding of nature: the nature of ourselves and the nature of our own brains to addiction treatment. The shamanic perspective includes the healing of the soul, which is part of our essential nature.

## THE COLLECTIVE SOUL SICKNESS

> It is no measure of health to be well adjusted to a profoundly sick society.
> —Jiddu Krishnamurti

From the shamanic perspective, holistic addiction treatment goes beyond the individual and accounts for the influence of external factors beyond the family and friends of the addict. They account for a quantum world where everything affects and interacts with everything else, consciously or unconsciously. We see this in many of the young addicts who are in constant rage, often without reason. While it is easy to project this anger onto their circumstances, on some imperceptible level they all feel hopelessness and despair about the planet they are inheriting. While unaware of the specifics, they feel a sense of doom.

In the quantum model, the shaman know that our individual health and well-being are not only affected by what others in the system are doing around us but also what they are thinking and feeling. Addicts often report themselves to be sensitive and particularly susceptible to the energetic influence of the biosphere. Said another way, the individual is affected by the workings of the collective unconscious. This is humanity's collective psychology that works across systems we are all a part of—families, groups, cultures, nations, and the world.

Carl Jung described the collective unconscious as the deepest and most fundamental layer of the psyche. The content of the collective unconscious is inherited rather than developed through our personal experiences.[37] This accounts for our common human characteristics despite our cultures or places of origin, for example. The similarities in myth all over the world are another example of the collective unconscious.

## The Shadow

The collective unconscious gives rise to the shadow aspect of humanity. The shadow comprises those things we do not wish to be, the unpleasant qualities in ourselves that we wish to hide, and those things we want to dissociate ourselves from.[38] These shadow characteristics are split off and disowned collectively much like the process of individual soul loss. In the collective unconscious of our groups and systems, however, the soul sickness and soul loss are also collective. The group becomes fragmented and sick.

The personal and collective processes mirror one another, manifesting as fractals. What lives in our own deep psychic structure becomes constellated in the world. What is disowned becomes someone else's responsibility. We might, for example, disown anger, strivings for power, aggression, blame, or guilt. Because we wish to disown these psychic contents, however, we project them out into the world, attributing them to others and making ourselves blameless for them: *I am not angry, but you are. I am not aggressive, but you are.*

We not only project as one person to another but collectively as a group and onto other collectives. We villainize certain ethnic, racial, or political groups, for example. We make ourselves victims, believing the shadow aspects we have projected constellate the "enemy" and are harming, oppressing, and victimizing us.[39]

Some North American native tribes, for example, have recognized this phenomenon as *Wetiko* or *Wendigo*. These phenomena are considered to be the spirit of cannibalism, greed, and excess, consuming the lives of others and their cultures through power and evil. Sometimes called a "psychosis," *Wetiko* is said to be contagious—a mindset that can spread and "infect" masses of people.[40]

The core of *Wetiko's* "insanity" is the delusion that beings are separate. In a delusion of separation, people can be pitted against one another in competition, dominated through power and control, and hated, killed, enslaved, and exploited.[41] This sets up and perpetuates an atmosphere of extreme consumerism: a symbolic cannibalism.

The spirit of consumerism has generalized to the world's resources—for example, minerals, forests, people, and animals are used and depleted. The media reinforces collective soul loss through fostering consumerism. Also, portrayals of a fragmented humanity through war, violence, and political strife are consistently "fed" to us in the media. Such focus sets up the belief in separation and competition. In many ways, our collective soul loss is a narcissism that views other beings and the earth as objects of gratification.

People who have managed to sustain interdependence have remained healthier. They continue to understand the value of community and cooperation. In a manner of speaking, they have not contracted *Wetiko* and are not "under the spell" of the consumption of others and the world.

Humans are beings of community by instinct. Survival of the species has depended upon interdependence, mutual support, and cooperation. Beyond survival, however, our biology is built to reinforce interdependence. We have an emotional and spiritual need for belonging and attachment. Our early mother-child bond generalizes to other attachments in triggering feelings of well-being through the endogenous opioid system.[42]

Shamanism has fostered the view that all life—plants, animals, people, and earth—is connected, valuable, and equally important. Shaman have served their communities traditionally—intervening during natural crises such as droughts and famine, for example. There are shaman that work with the world at large to restore balance in the greater unified field that supports us all. The importance of healing not only the personal self but also its greater field lies in the interconnectedness of life and its energetic basis. To treat the addict holistically, it is important to understand the influence of the collective upon the individual, most of which is unconscious.

## Conclusion

We live in a time of exciting technological advances in science and medicine. At the same time, more people are suffering from addiction and co-occurring disorders than ever before. People are using stronger recreational drugs at an earlier age, and the use of prescription drugs is rising for every demographic. The evidence points to the fact that traditional treatment, which has served us well until now, needs to take a broader view of the whole person. *Insanity is repeatedly doing the same thing and expecting a different result.* This is a popular saying often used in addiction treatment to demonstrate the futility of ongoing drug use. It is time we adopted this phrase to include the treatment of drug addiction. The old fragmented model of drug rehabilitation is incomplete. We are more than a body and a mind. We are holistic beings with a soul and a spirit.

I have worked as a shamanic energy medicine practitioner for the last 12 years exclusively treating addiction and co-occurring disorders. From my direct experience and observation, a treatment protocol that is not holistic is substantially less likely to succeed. Shamanic protocols are now being validated by mainstream science. In other words, science and spirituality are merging to say the same thing. The following chapter will discuss this connection by reviewing Ibogaine, a West African shrub that has been used in shamanic rituals for centuries and is currently under FDA review in a modified form as a treatment for addiction. We are much more than we think we are, and we interact and are informed by an unnamable source of energy. Bill Wilson referred to addiction as a spiritual disease. The shaman know that the remedy for this disease is also spiritual.

### REFERENCES

1. The Commonwealth Fund. Davis K, Stremikis K, Schoen C, Squires D. *Mirror, Mirror on the Wall, 2014 Update: How the U.S. Health Care System Compares Internationally.* http://www.commonwealthfund.org/publications/fund-reports/2014/jun/mirror-mirror. Accessed August 19, 2015.

2. American Psychiatric Association. *Diagnostic and Statistical Manual of Mental Disorders.* 5th ed. Arlington, VA: American Psychiatric Publishing; 2013.

3. Rakel D. Philosophy of integrated medicine. In: Rakel D. *Integrative Medicine: Expert Consult.* 3rd ed. Philadelphia, PA: Elservier; 2012: 2–11.

4. Lipton B. The new physics: planting both feet firmly on thin air. In: Lipton B. *The Biology of Belief: Unleashing the Power of Consciousness, Matter and Miracles,* Carlsbad, CA: Hay House; 2008:65–92.

5. Capra F. *The Web of Life—a New Scientific Understanding of Living Systems.* New York: Anchor; 1996.

6. Mindell A. *Quantum Mind: The Edge Between Physics and Psychology.* Portland, OR: Deep Democracy Exchange; 2012:151–164.

7. Rosenblum B, Kuttner F. The two-slit experiment: the observer problem. In: Rosenblum B, Kuttner F., eds. *Quantum Enigma: Psychics Encounters Consciousness.* New York: Oxford University Press; 2011: 87–100.

8. Schwartz J, Begley S. The quantum brain. In: Schwartz J, Begley S, eds. *The Mind and the Brain: Neuroplasticity and the Power of Mental Force.* New York: HarperCollins; 2002: 264–268.

9. Chopra D. In the rishi's world. In: Chopra D, ed. *Quantum Healing: Exploring the Frontiers of Medicine.* New York: Bantam; 1989:164–182.

10. Sheldrake R. *A New Science of Life: The Hypothesis of Morphic Resonance.* Rochester, VT: Park Street; 1999.

11. Sheldrake R. *The Presence of the Past: Morphic Resonance and the Memory of Nature.* Rochester, VT: Park Street; 2012.

12. Waller PF. The shamanic method. In: Waller PF, ed. *Shamanic Wisdom Meets the Western Mind: An Inquiry into the Nature of Shamanism.* Newark, DE: Sirius-C Media Galaxy; 2014:37–94.

13. Lemkow A. *The Wholeness Principle: Dynamics of Unity Within Science, Religion, and Society.* Wheaton, IL: Quest; 1990.

14. American Society of Addiction Medicine. Terminology Related to Addiction, Treatment, and Recovery. http://www.asam.org/docs/default-source/publicy-policy-statements/1-terminology-atr-7-135f81099472bc604ca5b7ff000030b21a.pdf?sfvrsn=0 2011. Accessed August 20, 2015.

15. Alcoholics Anonymous. *Alcoholics Anonymous.* 4th ed. New York: A.A. World Services; 2001.

16. Levine P, Frederick A. Shadows from a forgotten past. In: Levine P, Frederick A, eds. *Waking the Tiger: Healing Trauma.* Berkeley, CA: North Atlantic; 1997:15–21.

17. van der Kolk B. Running for your life: the Anatomy of survival. In: van der Kolk B, ed. *The Body Keeps Score: Brain, Mind, and Body in the Healing of Trauma.* New York: Viking; 2014:51–73.

18. Bradshaw J. *Healing the Shame that Binds You.* Deerfield, FL: Health Communications; 2005.

19. Herman J. Terror. In: Herman J., ed. *Trauma and Recovery: The Aftermath of Violence—from Domestic Abuse to Political Terror.* New York: Basic Books; 1997:33–50.

20. van der Kolk B. What's love got to do with it? In: van der Kolk B, ed. *The Body Keeps Score: Brain, Mind, and Body in the Healing of Trauma.* New York: Viking; 2014:136–148.

21. Flores P. *Addiction as an Attachment Disorder.* Lanham, MD: Rowman and Littlefield; 2004.

22. Gill R. *Addictions From an Attachment Perspective: Do Broken Bonds and Early Trauma Lead to Addictive Behaviours? (The John Bowlby Memorial Conference Monograph Series).* London: KARNAC; 2014.

23. Back S, Brady K, Sonne S, Verduin M. Symptom improvement in co-occurring PTSD and alcohol dependence. *Journal of Nervous and Mental Disease.* 2006;194:690–696.

24. Berenz E, Coffey S. Treatment of co-occurring posttraumatic stress disorder and substance use disorders. *Current Psychiatry Reports.* 2012;14(5):469–477.

25. Minkoff K. Best practices: Developing standards of care for individuals with co-occurring psychiatric and substance use disorders. *Psychological Services.* 2001;52(5):597–599.

26. Firman J. *The Primal Wound: A Transpersonal View of Trauma, Addiction, and Growth (S U N Y Series in the Philosophy of Psychology).* Albany: State University of New York Press; 1997.

27. van der Kolk B. The body keeps the score: approaches to the psychobiology of posttraumatic stress disorder. In: van der Kolk B, ed. *Traumatic Stress: The Effects of Overwhelming Experience on Mind, Body and Society.* New York: Guilford; 1996:214–241.

28. Levine P, Frederick A. How biology becomes pathology: freezing. In: Levine P, Frederick A, ed. *Waking the Tiger: Healing Trauma.* Berkeley, CA: North Atlantic; 1997:99–108.

29. Herman J. *Trauma and Recovery.* New York: Basic Books; 1992.

30. Berger R. *Stress, Trauma, and Posttraumatic Growth: Social Context, Environment, and Identities.* New York: Routledge; 2015.

31. Moss R. Understanding soul loss. In: Moss R, ed. *Dreaming the Soul Back Home: Shamanic Dreaming.* Novato, CA: New World Library; 2012:61–78.

32. Khoury L, Tang YL, Bradley B, Cubells JF, Ressler KJ. Substance use, childhood traumatic experience, and posttraumatic stress disorder in an urban civilian population. *Depress Anxiety.* 2010;27(12):1077–1086.

33. Jellinek EM. *The Disease Concept of Alcoholism.* Mansfield Centre, CT: Martino; 2010.

34. Sheldrake R. *Morphic Resonance—The Nature of Formative Causation.* Rochester, VT: Park Street; 2009.

35. Francis RC. *Epigenetics: How Environment Shapes Our Genes.* New York: W.W. Norton; 2011.

36. Gilbert S, Epel, D. *Ecological Developmental Biology Integrating Epigenetics, Medicine and Evolution.* Sunderland, MA: Sinauer Associates; 2008.

37. Jung CG. The concept of the collective unconscious. In: Jung CG, ed. *The Archetypes and the Collective Unconscious: Collected Works of C.G. Jung Vol. 9 Part 1.* New York: Bollingen; 1959:42–53.

38. Zweig C, Abrams J. *Meeting the Shadow: The Hidden Power of the Dark Side of Human Nature*. New York: Penguin; 1991.
39. Perera S. The scapegoat complex and ego structure. In: Perera S, ed. *Scapegoat Complex: Toward a Mythology of Shadow and Guilt (Studies in Jungian Psychology By Jungian Analysts)*. Toronto: Inner City; 1986: 44–72.
40. Levy P. *Dispelling Wetiko: Breaking the Curse of Evil*. Berkeley, CA: North Atlantic; 2013.
41. Forbes JD. *Columbus and Other Cannibals: The Wetiko Disease of Exploitation, Imperialism, and Terrorism*. New York: Seven Stories; 2008.
42. Winkelman M. Community rituals: social relations and well-being. In: Winkelman M, ed. *Shamanism: A Biopsychosocial Paradigm of Consciousness and Healing*. Santa Barbara, CA: Praeger, ABC-CLIO; 2010:223–227.

# 24

## Ibogaine: History, Pharmacology, Spirituality, & Clinical Data

### BENJAMIN SHAPIRO

## Introduction

Ibogaine is an indole alkaloid derived from the African shrub *Tabernathe iboga* that has garnered increasing attention over the last 60 years due to its broad anti-addictive properties as well as its potential to treat depression, epilepsy, and act as a CNS stimulant.[1,2,3,4] Ibogaine is categorized as an atypical hallucinogen or oneriogen, differentiating it from classic hallucinogens, empathogens, and dissociative anesthetics all of which operate through a single or dual monoaminergic and/or glutamatergic mechanisms.[5] Like other oneriogens it has the potential to induce a dreamlike state of consciousness resembling REM sleep.[6] We included ibogaine here as a separate chapter to serve as a detailed compliment to the preceding shamanism chapter and to provide a comprehensive understanding of the complex biological, medical, legal, and spiritual elements of this botanical.

The United States Controlled Substances Act currently categorizes ibogaine as Schedule 1 drug. Substances in Schedule 1 have been deemed to possess high abuse potential, lack accepted medical use in treatment, and/or fail to meet accepted safety for use under medical supervision criteria. The use, manufacture, distribution, or dispensing of Schedule 1 substances is illegal in the United States unless federally authorized, thus any therapeutic use in the United States is prohibited. Ibogaine is explicitly or categorically classified as illegal in several other Western countries as well, including France, Italy, Sweden, Switzerland, Belgium, Ireland, the United Kingdom, Norway, Finland, and Israel.[7] However, it is under limited regulation in Germany and remains unregulated in Canada, Mexico, and most other countries. Strong grassroots interest in its therapeutic potential in treating addiction has advanced the regulation and use of ibogaine, resulting it being legalized for use in Brazil in 2016 and the establishments of legal ibogaine treatment clinics in Mexico, Canada, the Netherlands, South Africa, Costa Rica, New Zealand, the Caribbean, and illegally underground in the United States and throughout Europe.[8]

# Background

*Tabernathe iboga* has been used in spiritual practice and as a stimulant in Central and West African tribal communities for centuries, particularly in Gabon.[9] Low-dose extracts of iboga reportedly enable hunters to stay awake and motionless while stalking prey, allowing them to stave off fatigue, hunger, and thirst. Higher doses are used as part of initiation rites and religious rituals of Bwiti and Mbiri cults where it is believed to empower users to "talk" with ancestors of the spirit world and invoke visions of death and rebirth.[10,11,12] Curiously, use in high doses in indigenous tribal rites is preceded by a days-to-weeks-long hypnotic rite where the user is isolated from normal life, conspicuously diminishing exposure of the user to stressors that incidentally could impact its toxicity. The user reconciles through ritual the risk of death involved in its use.[13] Spiritual practice involving *Tabernathe iboga* is invoked when an individual has a problem with the deceased. The resulting state, as recorded by ethnologists, qualifies as a near-death experience.[14,15]

At the turn of the 20th century, French pharmacologists discovered *Tabernathe iboga* and isolated and named its primary psychoactive alkaloid "ibogaine" and identified stimulant effects, anesthetic effects, and probable hallucinogenic effects in animals.[16] It was shelved for another 30 years until French investigators Rothlin, Raymond-Hamet, and Delourme-Houde embarked on a detailed pharmacologic investigation, ultimately identifying the substance's potential as a hallucinogen and stimulant in humans. Contemporaneous with these experiments, isolated ibogaine hydrochloride started being manufactured and distributed in France under the trade name "Lambarene" (named after the city in Gabon where Albert Schweitzer had his dispensary). Lambarene was marketed at 5 to 8 mg doses to be used in intervals of 3 to 4 times per day as a "neuromuscular stimulant, indicated in cases of depression, asthenia, in convalescence."[17,18]

Ibogaine began circulating in the illegal market in the United States in the 1960s, prompting the FDA to classify it as a Schedule 1 substance. Howard Lotsof, an American amateur pharmacologist, stumbled across ibogaine recreationally while seeking out a cure for his own heroin dependence in 1963. He became a champion of ibogaine use and started the Dora Weiner Foundation and later the Global Ibogaine Therapy Alliance to pursue the development of it as a therapeutic after he was given a gift of iboga by the president of Gabon in the early 1980s.[19] He acquired 5 patents for ibogaine between 1985 and 1992 for treating a broad array of substance abuse, including cocaine, amphetamine, alcohol, nicotine, and opiate abuse, and then brought the compound to Amsterdam for research purposes. The pilot data from this and another peer-reviewed research led the US Food and Drug Administration (FDA) to approve a Phase 1 clinical trial of ibogaine for the treatment of substance abuse in 1991.[20] However, in 1995 all federally funded human trials were discontinued due to the emergence of fatalities, findings of neurotoxicity in rats, and disputes over intellectual property ownership. Development of ibogaine as therapeutic shifted to grassroots efforts beginning with the opening of treatment centers in Panama in 1994 and in St. Kitts in the West Indies in 1995 (the latter started by a professor and patentholder at the University of Miami).

The collective study and use of ibogaine in the face of widespread prohibition or lack of regulation has been termed a "vast uncontrolled experiment" by the director of National Institute on Drug Abuse (NIDA).[21] By 2005, 30 to 40 clinics worldwide were administering and/or studying ibogaine, having treated an estimated 5,000 patients.[22] However, in 2014 NIDA initiated preclinical testing in addiction for the ibogaine derivative, 18-Methoxycoronaridin (18-MC) due to its lower toxicity and purported similar benefits.[23]

## Chemistry

Ibogaine is the primary representative among the estimated 100 known iboga alkaloids—a class of indolomonoterpenes produced by a small number of plants of the family Apocynaceae.[24] The principle metabolite of ibogaine in humans is noribogaine, which is both produced by the demethylation of ibogaine by hepatic cytochrome CYP2D6 in the gut wall and liver and is also present in the root bark of *Tabernathe iboga* and its preparations.[25] These two compounds are two of seven sibling alkaloids found in *Tabernathe iboga*, all of which may be toxic to humans.

Ibogaine's underlying chemical structure is naturally occurring and thus cannot be patented, except with regard to use. However, its synthetic congener, 18-MC, has been patented and is being investigated as an anti-addiction agent as well as a therapeutic agent for leishmaniasis by Savant HWP, a small pharmaceutical company in San Carlos, California. At least 5 synthetic analogs of ibogaine have been discovered and are also being explored for possible alternative treatments for pain and/or cannabinoid receptor CB1 agonists that may have promise in treating obesity, metabolic syndrome, and related disorders.[26]

## Pharmacology

The actions of ibogaine vary depending on the dose. Lower doses in the range of 8 to 12mg/kg are used as a stimulant to enhance performance or to facilitate psychotherapeutic or spiritual insight consistent with its oneriogenic activity.[27] The oneriogenic state has been hypothesized to result from an over-activation of the temporal lobe and the hippocampus and is associated with a 8 to 12 Hz rhythm of in the inferior olive, leading to enhanced excitation in cerebellar Purkinje cells.[28] This state typically precedes through 3 stages: first an initial dream state arises 1 to 3 hours after ingesting and lasts 4 to 8 hours; second, a reflective state lasting 8 to 20 hours ensues, and finally a residual stimulation state ensues, lasting up to 72 hours post-ingestion.[29] Higher doses, ranging 15 to 25mg/kg are used in addiction and are more likely to produce adverse affects (see the section "Toxicity").

The mechanisms of action of ibogaine and its primary metabolite noribogaine in the CNS remain complex and incompletely understood. Ibogaine's highest affinity is its agonism at σ1 and σ2 receptors and antagonism at α3β4 nicotinic and NMDA receptors.[30] It is also an agonist at μ and κ opioid receptors, which, along with σ1 and σ2 agonism and α3β4 nicotinic angonism, are likely to be responsible for its withdrawal-attenuating effects.[31] Ibogaine also has indirect effects on dopamine in the nucleus accumbens and on serotonin receptors, but it does not act as an acetylcholinesterase inhibitor as has been previously claimed.[32,33] It's primary metabolite noribogaine is a κ opioid receptor agonist and lacks most other activities of its parent.[34] 18-MC is a synthetic derivative of ibogaine invented in 1996 that retains ibogaine's α3β4 nicotinic and μ and κ opioid receptor antagonism. Ibogaine, noribogaine, and 18-MC block opioid and nicotine-induced dopamine increase in the nucleus accumbens, while only ibogaine enhances cocaine-induced increase accumbal dopamine.[35]

Microinjection of ibogaine into the ventral tegmental area (VTA) of rodents causes increased expression of glial cell line-derived neurotropic factor (GDNF).[36] Increased GDNF activity in the VTA mediates the action of ibogaine on ethanol consumption and likely other substances of abuse.[37] Noribogaine induces an analogous robust increase in GDNF in the VTA of rodents; yet, the synthetic derivative 18-MC fails to do so, suggesting that 18-MC and ibogaine/noribogaine act by different mechanisms and at different sites of action.[38] Other studies indicate that the anti-addictive actions of 18-MC that diminish morphine, cocaine, nicotine, and alcohol self-administration in rats, result from its antagonist activity at cholinergic α3β4 nicotinic receptors and reflect decreased signaling in the habenulo-interpeduncular pathway.[39,40,41] Early research indicated that 18-MC modulates dopamine release in the nucleus accumbens, but not by via the mesolimbic pathway where the habit-forming properties of substances of abuse are thought to emerge. 18-MC modulates a separate reward system, the dorsal diencephalic conduction system, which interacts with the mesolimbic pathway. The greater significance of this finding strongly suggests that cholinergic neurons in the habenulo-interpeduncular pathway participate in reward mechanisms responsive to morphine and likely to other drugs of abuse and may be untapped targets to treating substance dependence, particularly nicotine.[42]

# Preclinical Trials

## IBOGAINE

Decades of trials in animal models of addiction have demonstrated ibogaine's potential as an anti-addiction agent. Ibogaine attenuates opiate withdrawal in rodents and primates and reduces self-administration of morphine, cocaine, amphetamine, methamphetamine, and nicotine.[43,44,45,46,47,48,49,50,51] Ibogaine decreases ethanol intake by rats in two-bottle choice and operant self-administration paradigms as well as reduces operant self-administration in relapse models.[52]

## 18-MC

18-MC has been found to have similar effects attenuating addiction behavior in animals as ibogaine, decreasing self-administration of morphine, nicotine, and alcohol in rats after systemic injection as well as ameliorating withdrawal signs.[53,54] Dosage effects in rats differ depending on the substance. 18-MC dose-dependently reduced alcohol intake at all doses of study (10, 20, and 40mg/kg) and all levels of alcohol intake. However, only high dosing of 18-MC impacted lower-than-median nicotine self-administration, with lower dosing of 18-MC and higher nicotine self-administrations not demonstrating significant impact.[55] Consistent with its action in the habenulo-interpeduncular pathway, 18-MC has been shown to reduce nicotine-induced dopamine release in the nucleus accumbens of rats.[56]

# Human Trials

## IBOGAINE

Human trials of ibogaine effect have been limited but include several case series and two 12-month uncontrolled observational trials. All accounts consistently demonstrate rapid remission of acute withdrawal symptoms following a single administration that is sustained in the absence of further ibogaine treatment or opioid use. Studies differ in their findings with regard to impacts on abstinence and toxicity.

In an early case series ending in 1993, Alper and colleagues[57] describes outcomes of 33 patients treated over 31 years, all of whom meet criteria for opiate dependence. Subjects received 6 to 29 mg/kg of ibogaine, typically starting 10 hours after the last opiate use, or 24 hours if the subject was receiving methadone. Seventy-six percent of subjects were free of subjective complaints at 48 hours and made no attempts to use opiates over 72 hours. Subjects reported relief of opiate withdrawal symptoms within 1 to 3 hours. At least 5 subjects displayed drug-seeking behavior at or beyond 72 hours, but medium and long-term outcomes were not assessed. This study was pivotal in ibogaine's history after a 24-year-old female subject receiving 29mg/kg ibogaine developed respiratory arrest 18 hours after administration and died (see "Toxicity" section). This fatality in 1993 became pivotal, along with identification of cerebellar toxicity in rats and a dispute over intellectual property, in the NIDA decision in 1995 to abandon approval for a clinical trial, subsequently marginalizing the study of and use of ibogaine throughout the developed world.

Mash and colleagues[58,59] lead a more rigorous assessment of 27 subjects in St Kitts with cocaine and/or opiate dependence. Assessment included the Addiction Severity Index, the Beck Depression Inventory, and measures of cravings over 4 weeks following treatment. Subjects received from 1 to 9 fixed doses of either 500, 600, or 800 mg. Ibogaine was well tolerated by all subjects and produced substantial decline in self-reported depression and cocaine and opiate cravings, as well as other measures of abuse. Drug craving diminished at 36 hours after treatment and remained considerably reduced throughout 4 weeks of follow-up.

A retrospective case series completed in 2013 by Schenberg et al[60] of 75 individuals with alcohol, cannabis, and/or cocaine dependence treated in Paraná, Brazil, found a median length of abstinences after one ibogaine treatment of 5.5 months and 8.4 for multiple treatments. Subjects typically received an initial dose of 17 mg/kg and additional doses between 7.5 and 20 mg/kg in the event they had late emergence of intense cravings, relapse, or engaged in drug-related behavior. The increase in median abstinence from 5.5 to 8.4 months for additional ibogaine treatment supports more recent arguments that participating in more than 1 ibogaine session may be beneficial in achieving long-term abstinence.[61] Abstinence was common and reported as 61%; however, a variety of relapse patterns emerged and due to variations in follow-up, there are limitations in interpreting outcomes. Unique in this trail, all subjects were required to be abstinent of substance use for 30 to 60 days prior to treatment with ibogaine due to concerns about potential toxicity of ibogaine in the immediate withdrawal period. While this raises concerns about possible selection bias toward less severe cases, the authors argue that these subjects were representative of the clinic population and most were already treatment-refractory. Notably, the lack of opiate-dependent subjects limits the generalizability of this study: both in ascribing benefits to ibogaine as well as assessing its risk.

In 2012, under the auspices of the Multidisciplinary Association for Psychedelic Studies (MAPS), Brown, et al completed an uncontrolled observational study of 30 opiate-dependent subjects over 12 months at an ibogaine clinic in Baja, Mexico.[62] Their primary endpoint was length of time from treatment until first relapse and they employed various measures of addiction behavior, withdrawal, and depression. No adverse events arose during or after treatment. Thirty-three percent of subjects relapsed in the first month, 60% relapsed within the second month, and 80% relapsed within the first 6 months, leaving 20% to remain sober at 6 months and beyond. The investigators concluded that ibogaine is an addiction "interrupter" and not a "magic bullet."

In 2014 Noller et al completed an observational study of ibogaine in opiate-dependent users sponsored by MAPS in New Zealand.[63] Investigators emphasized establishing ibogaine's treatment outcome durability over 12 months in a setting where ibogaine has been legalized for prescription since 2009. Assessment instruments were similar to prior MAPS protocol by Brown, et al (above). Consistent with preceding studies, evidence showed significant attenuation of withdrawal, including sustained reduction in drug craving and drug use with a number of cases maintaining cessation of use at 12 months. Depression measures remained lower at 12 months, and 55% reported reduced use of other drugs and 36% reduced alcohol use. The authors note that subjects often characterize the improvement in their depression as due to ibogaine providing insight into their circumstance and not just mediating withdrawal symptoms or improving mood. Of broader concern, however, was that one subject died with the coroner's report indicating that death was likely due to arrhythmia following ibogaine ingestion, echoing events in the study by Alper et al in 1993.

## 18-MC AND NORIBOGAINE

Several safety studies and a single dose trial have been completed by investigators in New Zealand to further characterize clinical use and potential benefit of the primary active metabolite of ibogaine: noribogaine. A CYP2D6 inhibition study using paroxetine found that exposure to ibogaine and noribogaine was twice as great in subjects with CYP2D6 inhibited, suggesting that CYP2D6 genotyping or phenotyping are essential prior to ibogaine dosing and may require 50% or greater dosage reduction.[64] In a contemporaneous study, Glue et al noted that single oral doses of noribogaine ranging from 3 to 60 mg/day were safe and well tolerated in healthy volunteers up to 216 hours out from last dosing.[65] A randomized, placebo-controlled single dose trial in 2016 of 60, 120, or 180 mg of noribogaine in patients established on methadone opioid substitution therapy found a concentration-dependent increase in QTc (0.17 ms/ng/mL) up to 42 milliseconds in 180-mg group, which was deemed clinically concerning. The authors noted that noribogaine showed a non-statistically significant trend toward decreased total score in opioid withdrawal ratings, most notably at the 120-mg dose, but essentially noribogaine did not delay onset of or ameliorate measures of opiate withdrawal.[66]

The development and human testing of 18-MC remains in the early stages under the direction of Savant HWP pharmaceuticals.

# Toxicity

Ibogaine toxicity ranges from mild treatment-associated transient side effects to potential fatality: the latter of which has been the major impediment to further research and development of ibogaine as a therapeutic. Acute effects can include nausea, ataxia, emesis, tremors, headaches, changes in light perception, and confusion.[67] At least one episode of emesis is not uncommon following administration and should not be mistaken for the emergence of withdrawal symptoms. Treatment may also include a prophylactic dose of an antiemetic.

Concerns about possible lasting toxicity first arose in animal data after cerebellar damage was observed in rats treated with ibogaine at a high dose of 100 mg/kg and has been demonstrated repeatedly.[68] These findings were not supported by trials in monkey at similar doses.[69] Contrary argument has been made for use of ibogaine as a neuroprotectant to limit excitotoxicity.[70] Neurotoxicity that does result is likely to occur at much greater doses than needed for its anti-addictive effects and may be mediated by the sigma type-2 receptor.[71]

At least 21 ibogaine-related deaths have been reported from 1990 to 2014.[72] At least 19 have died within 1.5 to 76 hours of administration. The primary cause of death remains under debate. Autopsy has not supported a syndrome of neurotoxicity but rather most frequently has supported underlying medical comorbidities or concurrent use of other substances.[73] Genetic polymorphisms in cytochrome P450 enzyme CYP2D6 also raised potential concerns, given there are over 70 variants up to 10% of some ethic populations are poor metabolizers resulting in serum levels of ibogaine and its primary metabolite noribogaine being increased twofold.[74] It is also important to note that in at least 5 of the 21 (24%) previously documented fatalities, the substance ingested was not ibogaine HCl but either dried root or an alkali extract.[75]

Ibogaine toxicity in humans may occur through a variety of mechanisms. Research since the 1970s has indicated that ibogaine enhances opioid signaling and potentiates the lethality of opioids, although not through direct agonism or antagonism at the opioid receptor.[76] Subsequent clinical reports demonstrated ibogaine prolongs the QT interval and can produce potentially lethal polymorphic ventricular tachyarrhythmias, such as torsade's de pointes.[77,78,79] Ibogaine and noribogaine both block the hERG subunit of the at delayed rectifier cardiac potassium channel, causing this arrhythmia. In contrast, 18-MC causes less hERG inhibition, lending it lower toxicity in humans.[80] Currently the presence of Long-QT syndrome is the most widely accepted explanation of ibogaine fatality.[81,82] Given this various cardiac risk factors should be considered in the use of ibogaine, noribogaine, and 18-MC, including female gender, a prolonged baseline QT interval, bradycardia, hypomagnesaemia, hypokalemia, preexisting cardiovascular disease, hERG mutations, drug-drug interactions, and cytochrome P450 enzyme CYP2D6 variants.[83] Of note, QT prolongation may already present and up to 7 days following cessation in heavy alcohol and cocaine users, thus active substance use alone may pose a risk factor.[84,85]

## Future Directions

Ibogaine and its derivatives have driven a host of new research and the promise of alternative and more effective treatments for substance detoxification and cessation of use. Essential questions remain unanswered and continue to plague the study and use of ibogaine and noribogaine in humans. Is the risk of fatality and associated QT prolongation lower with different substances of abuse versus opioids? Can the risk of QT prolongation and toxicity be diminished? Is the risk of QTc prolongation lower in substance users 30 to 60 days into abstinence and low enough to justify clinical use? Does the decreased hERG inhibition with 18-MC adequately diminish risk of QTc prolongation and overall fatality and justify clinical use?

Despite many questions that remain unanswered, the study of ibogaine and its derivatives has considerably advanced our understanding of substance abuse, even its basic science. Increased understanding of the role habenulo-interpeduncular pathway in reward is likely to improve therapeutic interventions for SUDs, particularly in nicotine dependence. Study of ibogaine has fostered understanding σ1, σ2, and α3β4 nicotinic receptor activities in the CNS and may offer new ways to manage addiction, depression, and other mental illness. Furthermore, the decentralized and illicit use of therapeutics has offered a method of studying illness and therapeutics outside the established FDA model and has maintained focus on the agent when it otherwise may have shifted elsewhere. Lastly, ibogaine is a prominent part of the continued grassroots efforts to understand and legitimize clinical applications of ethnobotanical and recreational mind-altering substances. We are in a renaissance period in research on clinical applications of hallucinogens and other psychedelics: innovations are taking place that will dramatically change the landscape of psychiatry and substance abuse treatment and will require a commensurate and complicated change in regulation.

### REFERENCES

1. Alper KR, Lotsof HS, Frenken GM, Luciano DJ, Bastiaans J. Treatment of acute opioid withdrawal with ibogaine. *American Journal on Addictions*. 1999;8(3):234–242.
2. Glick SD, Maisonneuve IM. Development of novel medications for drug addiction: the legacy of an African shrub. *Alzeheimer's Disease: A Compendium of Current Theories*. 2000;909:88–103.

3. Schneider JA, Sigg EB. Neuropharmacological studies on ibogaine, an indole alkaloid with central-stimulant properties. *Alzeheimer's Disease: A Compendium of Current Theories.* 1957;66(3):765–776.

4. Leal MB, de Souza DO, Elisabetsky E. Long-lasting ibogaine protection against NMDA-induced convulsions in mice. *Neurochemical Research.* 2000;25(8): 1083–1087.

5. Garcia-Romeu A, Kersgaard B, Addy PH. Clinical applications of hallucinogens: a review. *Experimental and Clinical Psychopharmacology.* 2016;24(4):229–268.

6. Schultes RE, Hofmann A. Plants of the Gods: Origins of Hallucinogenic Use. New York: McGraw-Hill; 1979.

7. Global Ibogaine Therapuetic Alliance. Ibogaine Legal Status. The Global Ibogaine Therapy Alliance. Web site. https://www.ibogainealliance.org/ibogaine/law/. Accessed April 28, 2017.

8. Ibid.

9. de Rios MD, Grob CS, Baker JR. Hallucinogens and redemption. *Journal of Psychoactive Drugs.* 2002;34(3):239–248.

10. Popik P, Layer RT, Skolnick P. 100 years of ibogaine: neurochemical and pharmacological actions of a putative anti-addictive drug. *Pharmacological Reviews.* 1995;47(2):235–253.

11. Glick SD, Maisonneuve IM. Development of novel medications for drug addiction: the legacy of an African shrub. *Alzeheimer's Disease: A Compendium of Current Theories.* 2000;909:88–103.

12. Fernandez JW. Bwiti: an ethnography of the religious imagination in Africa. Princeton, NJ: Princeton University Press. 1982.

13. Ibid.

14. Maas U, Strubelt S. Fatalities after taking ibogaine in addiction treatment could be related to sudden cardiac death caused by autonomic dysfunction. *Medical Hypotheses.* 2006;67(4):960–964.

15. Strubelt S, Maas U. The near-death experience: a cerebellar method to protect body and soul-lessons from the Iboga healing ceremony in Gabon. *Alternative Therapies in Health and Medicine.* 2008;14(1):30–34.

16. Schneider JA, Sigg EB. Neuropharmacological studies on ibogaine, an indole alkaloid with central-stimulant properties. *Alzeheimer's Disease: A Compendium of Current Theories.* 1957;66(3):765–776.

17. Popik P, Layer RT, Skolnick P. 100 years of ibogaine: neurochemical and pharmacological actions of a putative anti-addictive drug. *Pharmacological Reviews.* 1995;47(2):235–253.

18. Glue P, Lockhart M, Lam F, Hung N, Hung CT, Friedhoff L. Ascending-dose study of noribogaine in healthy volunteers: pharmacokinetics, pharmacody- namics, safety, and tolerability. *Journal of Clinical Pharmacology.* 2015;55:189–194.

19. Hevesi D. Howard Lotsof dies at 66; Saw drug cure in a plant. *New York Times.* http://www.nytimes.com/2010/02/17/us/17lotsof.html Accessed April 27, 2017.

20. Global Ibogaine Therapuetic Alliance. Our Founder: Howard Lotsof—The Global Ibogaine Therapy Alliance. The Global Ibogaine Therapy Alliance. Web site. https://www.ibogainealliance.org/about/howard-lotsof/. Accessed April 28, 2017.

21. Vastag B. Addiction research. Ibogaine therapy: a 'vast, uncontrolled experiment.' *Science.* 2005;308:345–346.

22. Ibid.

23. Koenig X, Kovar M, Rubi L, et al. Anti-addiction drug ibogaine inhibits voltage-gated ionic currents: A study to assess the drug's cardiac ion channel profile. *Toxicology and Applied Pharmacology.* 2013;273:259–268.

24. Lavaud C, Massiot G. The iboga alkaloids. *Progress in the Chemistry of Organic Natural Products.* 2017;105:89–136.

25. Ibid.

26. Ibid.

27. Alper KR, Beal D, Kaplan CD. A contemporary history of ibogaine in the United States and Europe. *Alkaloids Chemical and Biology.* 2001;56:249–281.

28. Maas U, Strubelt S. Fatalities after taking ibogaine in addiction treatment could be related to sudden cardiac death caused by autonomic dysfunction. *Medical Hypotheses.* 2006;67(4):960–964.

29. Galea S, Lorusso M, Newcombe D, Walters C, Williman J, Wheeler A. Ibogaine: be informed before you promote or prescribe. *Journal of Primary Health Care.* 2011;3(1):86–87.

30. Alper KR, Stajić M, Gill JR. Fatalities temporally associated with the ingestion of ibogaine. *Journal of Forensic Science.* 2012;57(2):398–412.

31. Garcia-Romeu A, Kersgaard B, Addy PH. Clinical applications of hallucinogens: a review. *Experimental and Clinical Psychopharmacology.* 2016;24(4):229–268.

32. Lavaud C, Massiot G. The iboga alkaloids. *Progress in the Chemistry of Organic Natural Products.* 2017;105:89–136.

33. Glick SD, Rossman K, Wang S, Dong N, Keller RW, Jr. Local effects of ibogaine on extracellular levels of dopamine and its metabolites in nucleus accumbens and striatum: interactions with D-amphetamine. *Brain Research.* 1993;628(1–2): 201–208.

34. Maillet EL, Milon N, Heghinian MD, Fishback J, Schürer SC, Garamszegi N, Mash DC. Noribogaine is a G-protein biased κ-opioid receptor agonist. *Neuropharmacology.* 2015;99:675–688.

35. Glick SD, Maisonneuve IM, Szumlinski KK. 18-Methoxycoronaridine (18-MC) and ibogaine: comparison of antiaddictive efficacy, toxicity, and mechanisms of action. *Alzheimer's Disease: A Compendium of Current Theories.* 2000;914:369–386.

36. McGough NN, Ravindranathan A, Jeanblanc J, et al. Glial cell line-derived neuro-trophic factor mediates the desirable actions of the anti-addiction drug ibogaine against alcohol consumption. *Journal of Neuroscience.* 2005;25(3):619–628.

37. Ibid.

38. Carnicella S, He DY, Yowell QV, Glick SD, Ron D. Noribogaine, but not 18-MC, exhibits similar actions as ibogaine on GDNF expression and ethanol self-administration. *Addict Biology.* 2010;15(4):424–433.

39. Rezvani AH, Overstreet DH, Yang Y, Maisonneuve IM, et al. Attenuation of alcohol consumption by a novel nontoxic ibogaine analogue (18-methoxycoronaridine) in alcohol-preferring rats. *Pharmacology Biochemistry and Behavior.* 1997;58(2): 615–619.

40. Glick SD, Maisonneuve IM, Szumlinski KK. 18-Methoxycoronaridine (18-MC) and ibogaine: comparison of antiaddictive efficacy, toxicity, and mechanisms of action. *Alzeheimer's Disease: A Compendium of Current Theories.* 2000;914: 369–386.

41. Glick SD, Ramirez RL, Livi JM, Maisonneuve IM. 18-Methoxycoronaridine acts in the medial habenula and/or interpeduncular nucleus to decrease morphine self-administration in rats. *European Journal of Pharmacology.* 2006;537(1–3):94–98.

42. Ibid.

43. Cappendijk SL, Fekkes D, Dzoljic MR. The inhibitory effect of norharman on morphine withdrawal syndrome in rats: comparison with ibogaine. *Behav Brain Research.* 1994;65(1):117–119.

44. Cappendijk SL, Dzoljic MR. Inhibitory effects of ibogaine on cocaine self-administration in rats. *European Journal of Pharmacology.* 1993;241(2–3):261–265.

45. Dzoljic ED, Kaplan CD, Dzoljic MR. Effect of ibogaine on naloxone-precipitated withdrawal syndrome in chronic morphine-dependent rats. *Archives Internationales De Pharmacodynamie Et De Therapie.* 1988;294:64–70.

46. Glick SD, Rossman K, Rao NC, Maisonneuve IM, Carlson JN. Effects of ibogaine on acute signs of morphine withdrawal in rats: independence from tremor. *Neuropharmacology.* 1992;31(5):497–500.

47. Popik P, Layer RT, Fossom LH, et al. NMDA antagonist properties of the putative antiaddictive drug, ibogaine. *Journal of Pharmacology and Experimental Therapeutics.* 1995;275(2):753–760.

48. Aceto MD, Bowman ER, Harris LS, May EL. Dependence studies of new compounds in the rhesus monkey and mouse (1991). *NIDA Research Monograph Series.* 1992;119:513–558.

49. Glick SD, Kuehne ME, Raucci J, et al. Effects of iboga alkaloids on morphine and cocaine self-administration in rats: relationship to tremorigenic effects and to effects on dopamine release in nucleus accumbens and striatum. *Brain Research.* 1994;657(1–2):14–22.

50. Maisonneuve IM, Keller RW Jr, Glick SD. Interactions of ibogaine and D-amphetamine: in vivo microdialysis and motor behavior in rats. *Brain Research.* 1992;579(1):87–92.

51. Pace CJ, Glick SD, Maisonneuve IM, et al. Novel iboga alkaloid congeners block nicotinic receptors and reduce drug self-administration. *European Journal of Pharmacology.* 2004;492(2–3):159–167.

52. He DY, McGough NN, Ravindranathan A. Glial cell line-derived neurotrophic factor mediates the desirable actions of the anti-addiction drug ibogaine against alcohol consumption. *Journal of Neuroscience.* 2005;25(3):619–628.

53. Rezvani AH, Cauley MC, Slade S, et al. Acute oral 18-methoxycoronaridine (18-MC) decreases both alcohol intake and IV nicotine self-administration in rats. *Pharmacology Biochemistry and Behavior.* 2016;150–151:153–157. doi: 10.1016/j.pbb.2016.10.010.

54. Glick SD, Maisonneuve IM, Szumlinski KK. 18-Methoxycoronaridine (18-MC) and ibogaine: comparison of antiaddictive efficacy, toxicity, and mechanisms of action. *Alzeheimer's Disease: A Compendium of Current Theories.* 2000;914:369–386.

55. Kuehne ME, He L, Jokiel PA. Synthesis and biological evaluation of 18-methoxycoronaridine congeners: potential antiaddiction agents. *Journal of Medicinal Chemistry.* 2003;46(13):2716–2730.

56. Glick SD, Maisonneuve IM, Visker KE, Fritz KA, Bandarage UK, Kuehne ME. 18-Methoxycoronardine attenuates nicotine-induced dopamine release and nicotine preferences in rats. *Psychopharmacology (Berl).* 1998;139(3):274–280.

57. Alper KR, Lotsof HS, Frenken GM, Luciano DJ, Bastiaans J. Treatment of acute opioid withdrawal with ibogaine. *American Journal on Addictions.* 1999;8(3):234–242.

58. Mash DC, Kovera CA, Pablo J. Ibogaine in the treatment of heroin withdrawal. *Alkaloids Chemical and Biology.* 2001;56:155–171.

59. Mash DC, Kovera CA, Pablo J. Ibogaine: complex pharmacokinetics, concerns for safety, and preliminary efficacy measures. *Alzeheimer's Disease: A Compendium of Current Theories.* 2000;914:394–401.

60. Schenberg EE, de Castro Comis MA, Chaves BR, da Silveira DX. Treating drug dependence with the aid of ibogaine: a retrospective study. *Journal of Psychopharmacology.* 2014;28(11):993–1000.

61. Brown TK. Ibogaine in the treatment of substance dependence. *Current Drug Abuse Reviews.* 2013;6(1): 3–16.

62. Brown, TK, Mojeiko V, Gargour K, Jordan M. Observational study of the long-term efficacy of ibogaine-assisted treatment in participants with opiate addiction. 2012. http://www.maps.org/research-archive/presentations/Brown_GITA_Vancouver_Oct2012_iboga_comm_rev.pdf

63. Noller GE, Frampton CM, Yazar-Klosinski B. Ibogaine treatment outcomes for opioid dependence from a twelve-month follow-up observational study. *American Journal of Drug Alcohol Abuse.* 2018;44(1):37–46.

64. Glue P, Winter H, Garbe K. Influence of CYP2D6 activity on the pharmacokinetics and pharmacodynamics of a single 20 mg dose of ibogaine in healthy volunteers. *Journal of Clinical Pharmacology.* 2015;55(6):680–687. doi: 10.1002/jcph.471.

65. Glue P, Lockhart M, Lam F, Hung N, Hung CT, Friedhoff L. Ascending-dose study of noribogaine in healthy volunteers: pharmacokinetics, pharmacodynamics, safety, and tolerability. *Journal of Clinical Pharmacology.* 2015;55(2):189–194.

66. Glue P, Cape G, Tunnicliff D. Ascending single-dose, double-blind, placebo-controlled safety study of noribogaine in opioid-dependent patients. *Clinical Pharmacology Drug Development.* 2016;5(6):460–468.

67. Schenberg EE, de Castro Comis MA, Chaves BR, da Silveira DX. Treating drug dependence with the aid of ibogaine: a retrospective study. *Journal of Psychopharmacology.* 2014;28(11):993–1000.

68. Aceto MD, Bowman ER, Harris LS, May EL. Dependence studies of new compounds in the rhesus monkey and mouse (1991). *NIDA Research Monograph Series.* 1992;119:513–558.

69. Mash DC, Kovera CA, Buch BE, et al. Medication development of ibogaine as a pharmacotherapy drug dependence. *Alzeheimer's Disease: A Compendium of Current Theories.* 1998;844: 274–292.

70. Olney JW. Use of ibogaine in reducing excito-toxic brain injury. US patent 5 629 307. 1997;1–13.

71. Glick SD, Maisonneuve IM. Mechanisms of anti-addictive actions of ibogaine. *Alzeheimer's Disease: A Compendium of Current Theories.* 1998;844:214–226.
72. Noller GE, Frampton CM, Yazar-Klosinski B. Ibogaine treatment outcomes for opioid dependence from a twelve-month follow-up observational study. *American Journal of Drug Alcohol Abuse.* 2017 Apr 12:1–10.
73. Ibid.
74. Bertilsson L, Dahl ML, Dalén P, Al-Shurbaji A. Molecular genetics of CYP2D6: clinical relevance with focus on psychotropic drugs. *Brirish Journal of Clinical Pharmacology.* 2002;53(2):111–122.
75. Alper KR, Stajić M, Gill JR. Fatalities temporally associated with the ingestion of ibogaine. *Journal of Forensic Science.* 2012;57(2):398–412.
76. Ibid.
77. Hoelen DW, Spiering W, Valk GD. Long-QT syndrome induced by the antiaddiction drug ibogaine. *New England Journal of Medicine.* 2009;360,308–309.
78. Dettmer MR, Cohn B, Schwarz E. Prolonged QTc and ventricular tachycardia after ibogaine ingestion [(XXXIII International Congress of the European Association of Poisons Centres and Clinical Toxicologists [EAPCCT]). *Clinical Toxicology.* 2013;51, 285.
79. Shawn LK, Alper K, Desai SP, et al. Pause-dependent ventricular tachycardia and torsades de pointes after ibogaine ingestion (2012 Annual Meeting of the North American Congress of Clinical Toxicology [NACCT]). *Clinical Toxicology.* 2012;50, 654.
80. Koenig X, Kovar M, Rubi L, et al. Anti-addiction drug ibogaine inhibits voltage-gated ionic currents: A study to assess the drug's cardiac ion channel profile. *Toxicology and Applied Pharmacology.* 2013;273, 259–268.
81. Maas U, Strubelt S. Fatalities after taking ibogaine in addiction treatment could be related to sudden cardiac death caused by autonomic dysfunction. *Medical Hypotheses.* 2006;67(4):960–964.
82. Koenig X, Hilber K. The anti-addiction drug ibogaine and the heart: a delicate relation. *Molecules.* 2015;20(2):2208–2228.
83. Ibid.
84. Kino M, Imamitchi H, Morigutchi M, Kawamura K, Takatsu T. Cardiovascular status in asymptomatic alcoholics, with reference to the level of ethanol consumption. *British Heart Journal.* 1981;46(5):545–551.
85. Levin KH, Copersino ML, Epstein D, Boyd SJ, Gorelick DA. Longitudinal ECG changes in cocaine users during extended abstinence. *Drug Alcohol Depend.* 2008;95(1–2):160–163.

# SECTION IV

# Challenges

# 25

## Group Therapy and Support in Addiction Treatment

### RICK GINSBERG

In North America, the introduction and usage of the healing circle is most frequently attributed to the Woodland Native American tribes of the Midwest.[1] Sitting in a circle and passing a sacred object to denote each person's turn to speak, participants in a healing circle aim to tackle individual and community problems as they seek wisdom, solutions, and direction.

The human experience of participating in groups to foster healing in one's self, another person, or in one's community, has roots that extends back to early civilizations.[1] As inherently social mammals, human beings group together for many reasons including protection and shared strength and resources. But using the group to heal is a particular subset of this human proclivity for togetherness, which is of particular interest when treating addictive disorders within an integrative medicine model.

Integrative medicine, by its very nature, is itself a type of pooling and collaboration of a health-care professional community's resources and collective knowledge to treat an individual; it is a veritable grouping of helpers focused on a particular problem and is thus an apt field and methodology within which to discuss the effects of other therapeutic groups: those primarily of patients themselves, on one of the most pernicious individual and community problems worldwide—addiction.

Group therapy is a therapeutic modality often cited as pioneered by J. H. Pratt, a Boston physician who provided tubercular patients who could not afford more extensive institutional care with classroom instruction on home care, subsequently discovering the emotional benefits of the group experience in treating disease.[2] Its usage has greatly expanded during the past 110 years and has addressed issues as diverse as grief,[3] PTSD,[4] depression,[5,6] personality disorders,[7] relationship concerns,[8] and chronic diseases such as cancer.[9]

Group therapy is the most commonly used psychological therapeutic modality for drug and alcohol abuse in community treatment settings.[10] It is utilized for many reasons, including the assumption that it is cost effective compared to individual treatment and that certain aspects of the group experience provide particular therapeutic advantages compared to individual therapy.[10] Group support, most prominently characterized by AA, Narcotics Anonymous (NA), and other 12-step programs is utilized by millions of people worldwide and is the most widely used group support format.[11] In integrative medicine models in which a multitude of practitioners and community-based services can be involved creating increases in cost that need to be managed, it is likely that health-care provider and patient will quickly come into contact with group modalities for psychological care when treating addiction.

This chapter will provide integrative medicine health-care professionals with clear definitions of the different types of mental health group interventions that are the most empirically validated in treating substance abuse and addiction. It will also present a model for professionals to utilize when assessing the quality and appropriateness of group interventions for their patients. In an effort to minimize confusion about the myriad of group interventions available for this population, definitions will be provided and issues of confounding variables will be discussed to provide guidance on how to avoid misattributing efficacy to certain therapeutic factors and to increase the likelihood of positive outcomes by combining known successful factors.

For the purpose of this discourse a few definitions will be of assistance. "Intervention" will be used to designate any course of action that a patient is asked, mandated, prescribed, suggested, or compelled to engage in by his or her own self-referral, to address a particular problem. "Modality" will be used to describe the specific type, or format, of psychological therapeutic intervention (e.g., individual, group—be it group therapy or group support, family, couples, inpatient, outpatient). The term "group therapy" will be defined as a group of more than two individuals who are undergoing specific psychological treatment following specific theory, protocol, and information led by a professional health-care provider. Family therapy and couples therapy are not included in this definition. "Treatment content" will be used to describe the particular theoretical and practical elements of a therapeutic intervention regardless of modality (e.g., behavioral, psychodynamic, mindfulness based, cognitive, etc.). The term "group support" will be defined as a group of more than two individuals who are engaged in a setting in which a focus on commonality, empathy, and disclosure are the primary methods of interaction and in which the group is not led by a professional health-care provider but rather by someone from the community, a group member, or a paraprofessional. Finally, the term "common factors" will reference variables that differing therapeutic modalities and group support share.

The chapter aims to answer some fundamental questions: Are group interventions of any kind for individuals with substance-related and addictive issues effective compared with individual interventions? How can group therapy be differentiated from group support for this population? And how does it compare in terms of effectiveness?

## Group Therapy for People with Substance-Related and Addictive Disorders

The vast majority of treatment provided to people with substance-related and addictive disorders is done so in a group therapy format.[12,13] This is especially true in residential treatment, hospital, and community mental health settings that provide programmatic offerings.[14–16]

Given that researchers have noted numerous non-clinical factors (such as financial resources and lack of availability of individual treatment) are often primary reasons for patient assignment to group modalities regardless of one's condition,[17] and that there exist substantial challenges in appropriately and accurately assessing the effectiveness of group therapy including measurement of progress, flawed models used to analyze results, and confounding variables inherent in the group therapy process itself,[12] one has reason to pause in attributing the ubiquity of group therapy treatment for substance-related and addictive disorders to either its effectiveness or appropriateness.

Problems that have plagued group therapy research in the treatment of other medical and psychological issues parallel that for group therapy research in the treatment of substance-related and addictive disorders. Many researchers have noted that despite the fact that the vast majority of treatment provided to people struggling with substance abuse is delivered in group therapy format, most research done with this population focuses solely on individual interventions.[12,13] It is true that group therapy interventions for people with substance abuse problems have been found to significantly decrease depression and increase adherence to abstinence for patients in residential addiction treatment settings,[18] improve sexual self-efficacy and problem-solving skills among women with addictions compared to no-treatment controls,[19] and reduce heavy drinking and alcohol-related consequences among college women.[20] But many of these studies are flawed as well with regard to their methodologies, and as such their results need to be interpreted with caution.

In fact, a frequently cited meta-analytic review of treatment outcome studies from the early 1980s to the early 2000s, one that used group therapy and other interventions for people with substance-related and addictive disorders, found merely 24 substance abuse treatment outcome studies comparing group therapy and other experimental conditions.[13] Other researchers have emphasized that only three of Weiss, Jaffe, and deMenil's studies compared individual and group therapy for people with substance abuse directly.[21] In general, the meta-analysis demonstrated that while treatment made significant differences in participants' outcomes, there were no reliable differences in outcome between therapeutic groups with different treatment content, and there were no significant differences found between interventions delivered in group and individual modalities. Following up on Weiss et al's (2004) findings, Sobell and colleagues found only 1 other study[22] during the period reviewed that compared group therapy and individual therapy for substance abuse problems (and none in the following 5 years) and that the results of this study also found no significant differences between group and individual modalities. They also note that of these 4 studies 2 were "not pure comparisons"[21] as patients in them received other treatment immediately prior to the studies. Sobell and colleagues wisely highlight the fact that in order to accurately determine the effectiveness of group treatment, it must be properly compared to individual treatment by using the same treatment content and randomizing treatment groups while including a control group and call for such randomized clinical trials (RCTs). Their own RCT study providing group and individual cognitive-behavioral treatment to over 200 people abusing alcohol and over 50 people abusing drugs found that while there were significant reductions in alcohol and drug usage during treatment and at a 12-month follow-up, there were no significant differences between group and individual treatment.[21]

While it is true, as Weiss and colleagues state that the dearth "of research on this topic stems, in part, from the inherent difficulties in conducting meaningful research on group therapy"[13] referencing in particular the difficulty in controlling what happens in a group setting when there are a number of participants involved, it is incumbent upon the research community to determine ways to adequately study this complex issue. To not do so makes researchers, clinicians, and the public alike vulnerable to reach potentially misleading conclusions about the effectiveness (or lack thereof) of group therapy treatment. Indeed, one study indicates the complexity in researching group interventions with people who are abusing substances, especially in regard to participant problem variability, and provides initial indicators as to the potential hidden benefits of group therapy for patients who have substance-related and addictive disorders that may not immediately be revealed in the reviews and empirical studies done by Weiss et al and Sobell et al without looking more closely at any particular subject pool and related data. Examining patients with dual diagnoses of borderline personality disorder and substance abuse, the researchers compared two treatments, group and individual based, in a manualized behavioral treatment program. While both approaches had significant effects on reducing borderline personality disorder symptoms, results indicated that patients with clinical depression had not only more severe borderline symptoms to begin with but also had more severe substance-related and addictive issues. These patients were the only subgroup to show reductions of substance abuse, but they only did so in the group modality.[23]

Studies indicating that there are no differences between group and individual therapy in the treatment of people with substance-related and addictive disorders may lead one to conclude that there is nothing curative involving the group process and that improvement is solely a factor of treatment content; and beyond that, as some studies show, the treatment content does not particularly matter either. The only benefit of using groups is to save vital resources such as time and money within treatment programs.

## Group Support for People with Substance-Related and Addictive Disorders

Group support can, and does, occur in many settings, styles, and formats, creating grassroots healing environments run by participants or laypeople. Group support also eschews more formalized treatment (at least temporarily) in order to offer those in need a helping hand to make their lives better. As one set of researchers explained, "Across the country, in hospitals, churches, empty offices, and even shopping malls, small groups of individuals assemble to cope collectively with their unique challenges."[24] and "through such groups, millions of Americans attempt to overcome addiction."[24]

In general, researchers have found that peer-led groups have positive but qualitatively different effects on participants[25] and that "many view self-help organizations as an important complement or alternative to formal services provided by professionals"[25] They have also noted that such group support experiences contribute significantly to positive alcohol-related outcomes.[26,27]

AA, NA, and other 12-step programs are not only the most frequently used group support treatments for substance-related and addictive disorders, they are by far the most frequently utilized treatment for such conditions overall.[28] According to the Substance Abuse and Mental Health Services Administration, of the 4.1 million people who received treatment for alcohol or illicit drug use in 2012, 2.3 million of them sought assistance from a self-help group such as AA or NA.[29] Groups such as AA, NA, and other 12-step programs "have served as the primary, if not only, source of behavior change for many, as adjuncts to formal treatment, or as a form of continuing care and community support following treatment. These groups are highly accessible and are available at no cost in communities throughout the world, thus serving as important and readily available resources in substance abuse recovery."[29] Nearly 2 decades after Morgenstern, Labouvie, McCrady, Kahler, and Frey noted that "in spite of its availability, the 12-step model remains one of the most controversial, least understood, and least evaluated approaches for treating substance use disorders,"[30] we know much more about this group support's effectiveness. But it remains just as controversial.

For many years, studies have found 12-step programs to have mixed and varied results.[30] But several meta-analytic reviews have illustrated that AA has been effective increasing rates of abstinence[31-34] and reducing alcohol use,[35] and that similar 12-step programs have been effective in increasing rates of abstinence and decreasing usage of illicit drugs.[35-39] These are results that have been found with not only adults but with participants as young as teenagers.[40]

Quasi-empirical studies have illustrated some important long-term effects, including participants in AA having significantly better alcohol-related outcomes at 1- and 8-year follow-up compared with people who did not participate.[26] Also shown were significantly higher degrees of abstinence 24 months after treatment and[41] significantly positive changes in alcohol-related problems at 1- and 2-year follow-ups.[42] And significantly more successful abstinence was also seen at an 18-month follow-up.[43]

AA attendance appears to also have an effect on other conditions, including mood disorders and chronic pain. A study of over 250 early AA participants found that at 3, 6, 9, 12, 18, and 24 months, depression decreased, and AA attendance predicted later reductions in depression.[44] Group support resulted in significantly less pain, less stress, less desire for opiods, and less likelihood of developing opiod-use disorder than the group therapy intervention.[45]

Concerned with research that has tried to infer causal effects from studies that have found correlational results between involvement in AA and abstinence, McKellar, Stewart, and Humphreys sought to examine three hypotheses, that (1) AA involvement yielded better alcohol outcomes, (2) better alcohol outcomes yielded AA involvement, and (3) that a good prognosis yielded both AA involvement and better alcohol outcomes and that AA involvement and better alcohol outcomes promoted each other. By examining a sample of over 2,300 men with alcohol dependency at 1- and 2-year follow-ups, they found that 1 year of AA affiliation predicted lower alcohol-related problems at 2-year follow-up, but alcohol related problems at 1 year did not predict AA affiliation at 2-year follow-up, suggesting that the researcher's first hypothesis, that AA involvement yields better alcohol outcomes, is the most accurate conclusion.[42]

Because of AA's success, researchers have called for an integration of therapeutic approaches such as individual therapy[46] and group therapy[47] with 12-step involvement for some patients with substance-related and addictive disorders. This seems to be a strategy inherently embraced by AA's participants, as AA found that before coming to AA 59% of participants received some type of treatment or counseling related to their drinking, 58% received such treatment after their involvement in AA; and 84% of those who received additional treatment explained that it played an important part in their recovery.[11]

At least 1 study has already confirmed the utility of such integration. In a large-scale study investigating over 3,000 patients involved in 15 programs at the US Department of Veterans Affairs it was found that involvement in AA or cognitive behavioral therapy groups significantly improved alcohol-related outcomes as did a combination of AA and CBT groups: results that were sustained at 1-year-follow-up.[48] While some studies have found results indicating CBT to be more effective than 12-step facilitation, they have not found that adding a 12-step component to another treatment impedes patient progress.[47]

An important study examining the effectiveness of 12-step participation for individuals with substance-related and addictive disorders is the National Institute on Alcohol Abuse and Alcoholism study named "Project Match," the largest and most costly alcoholism treatment trial ever conducted, with over 1,700 participants across greater than 5 clinical sites. This randomized clinical research study provided participants with 12 weeks of treatment in either Cognitive Behavioral Therapy (CBT), Motivational Enhancement Therapy (MET), or Twelve Step Facilitation (TSF). The TSF intervention is an individual therapy approach in which the fundamentals of alcoholism as a long-term disease are addressed, the basic philosophy of AA is introduced along with the first five steps, and a client is encouraged to attend AA meetings. Outcomes were measured in percentage of days abstinent and drinks per drinking day.[49] Initial data analyses revealed that all treatments performed equally well in significantly reducing problematic drinking behaviors, providing one of the most robust indicators that at least the philosophies of AA were as clinically effective as other therapies.[50,51] At a 3-year follow-up it was subsequently found that clients who participated in TSF were significantly more likely to be abstinent (36%) than those in the MET (27%) and CBT (24%) groups, illustrating the potential benefits of an intervention that encourages AA principles and involvement.[52] It should be noted, however, that these results illustrate TSF effectiveness and not solely group support received in the actual involvement of AA.

While it appears that today most treatment providers in the United States encourage 12-step participation,[53] the approach is not without its critics and controversy. There are likely many reasons for this, including that 12-step programs such as AA and NA are run by participants and laypeople as opposed to trained healthcare professionals; they take an abstinence-only approach to substance use that leaves no room for those interested in attempting moderation; traditionally 5 of the 12 steps directly reference God (and use a male designation for God), and several others indirectly address spirituality; AA tends to view people's struggles in terms of defects in their characters;[54] and randomized controlled trials and other rigorous scientific testing of the intervention is lacking. Many of these issues have recently reached the public through highly visible debates by researchers and journalists in popular psychology books[55] and publications in mainstream magazines including *The Atlantic, New York Magazine, Pacific Standard,* and *Forbes.*[56–59]

However, as limited as some of the research is on AA, NA, and other 12-step programs, and as objectionable as critics might find aspects of its philosophy, there exists more than enough evidence to suggest that this form of group support for substance-related and addictive disorders warrants respect as a popular, long-standing, and effective grassroots movement addressing a problematic issue. It certainly merits a continued close examination by researchers, practitioners, and participants alike; and a strong consideration as a viable and potentially important aspect of treatment for people with substance-related and addictive disorders.

In this spirit, researchers have begun looking at specific elements and mechanisms within AA and other 12-step programs that are a cause for its success and that could enable clinicians, sponsors, meeting leaders, and participants themselves to tailor healing group experiences to the needs of individuals in order to maximize the intervention's efficacy.[35,39,60] Studies have examined components of the AA experience that may affect outcome including the differentiation between AA "attendance" and "AA involvement," creating scales that measure a person's degree of interaction within the group;[61] participant emotional readiness for AA;[62] and the impact that having an AA sponsor plays.[35,63] In the latter studies, having an AA sponsor early in one's involvement with the intervention (but not later) has been correlated with significantly greater success with abstinence[35,63] and AA participation.[63]

Another group support intervention that has gained popularity over the past 20 years is Smart Recovery, or self-management and recovery training. Similar to AA and other 12-step approaches, Smart Recovery groups are primarily run by paraprofessional facilitators who complete a 30-hour, 8-week, online training curriculum.[64] Smart Recovery groups are cognitive-behaviorally oriented, mutual support groups that emphasize empowerment and recovery through the advance-ment of skills in 4 domains: building and maintaining motivation; coping with urges; managing thoughts, feelings, and behaviors; and living a balanced life[64,65] Additionally, the Smart Recovery movement encourages participants to use this group support in coordination with whatever treatments they feel are useful, including 12-step programs such as AA and other therapeutic interventions.[64] While researchers have noted the paucity of research on the effectiveness of Smart Recovery groups,[66] some initial beneficial results have been found including high levels of participant satisfaction;[66] benefits of Smart Recovery group cohesion and homework assignments in activating positive alcohol-related behaviors outside of group;[65] improving alcohol- use behaviors, life satisfaction, overall health and em-ployment status;[67] and increasing percentage of days abstinent while decreasing mean drinks per episode.[68]

Perhaps the most conspicuous mechanism in AA, other 12-step support groups, and Smart Recovery groups that should be examined more closely is the nature of the group support experience and group process that occurs within meetings: this is above and beyond any of the more content-based information conveyed regarding the 12-step, cognitive-behavioral approaches, or addiction in general. Similar to group therapy, group support can have a certain degree of therapeutic content that varies in structure from group to group. For example, some AA groups are more focused on doing "step work" and/or reading and interpreting what is commonly referred to as "the big book," otherwise known by its formal name: *Alcoholic Anonymous: The Story of How Many Thousands of Men and Women Have Recovered from Alcoholism* written by AA co-founder Bill Wilson in 1939. Others are more focused on participants sharing stories and providing support to each other.[69,70] However, there is an undeniable interpersonal group interaction that occurs throughout all group support interventions that has yet to be closely studied as to its role in the efficacy of the intervention. These factors, common in many group therapies as well, need to be examined as to their effect on positive outcomes for people with substance-related and addictive disorders.

## Assessing and Working with Group Therapy and Group Support Interventions—A Model for Integrative Health-Care Professionals

In 1990 the Institute of Medicine suggested that treatment for SUDs should be broadened beyond specialty programs to include a wide range of health-care professionals including medical, mental health, and social service providers.[71] This notion fits well with the philosophy behind integrative medicine, defined as "healing-oriented medicine that takes account of the whole person (body, mind, and spirit), including all aspects of lifestyle. It emphasizes the therapeutic relationship and makes use of all appropriate therapies, both conventional and alternative."[72] It is also telling that according to AA, of those who received other treatment prior to coming to AA, 74% said it played an important role in getting them to AA; 57% were referred to AA by a health-care professional, and 75% of participants' doctors know they have used AA.[11] Health-care professionals play a critical role in the development and maintenance of effective treatment protocols for patients with SUDs and addiction; integrative medicine practitioners may be some of the professionals who have the ideal skills for this role.

Yet among confusing research, an even more complex and variable competitive health-care market, and patient attitudes, opinions, and desires, it can be hard to know how to best proceed when it comes to group interventions for patients with substance-related and addictive disorders. Group support and group therapy interventions can be found in a multitude of ways, and some of the best are often discovered by having strong working relations with health-care professionals both within and outside of one's specialized field. Physicians, psychologists, psychiatrists, psychiatric nurses, social workers, and complementary medicine service providers of all types should be speaking to each other about the group support and group therapy options in the community that are known to be the most effective for (and widely used by) people with SUDs and addictive-related disorders. Similarly, health-care providers should not overlook the knowledge about resources among health-care support and administrative professionals, as it is frequently people such as front office staff in a variety of locations who informally hear from patients and their families about the subjective, qualitative nature of patients' and their families' experiences with particular group interventions. Inpatient addiction facilities and units, intensive outpatient programs (IOPs), and addiction professionals in both the private and public sectors are likely to have suggestions for efficacious therapy groups, while people involved in the AA, NA, and Smart Recovery communities are the best resources for understanding the types and characteristics of nearby group support meetings. Health-care providers and patients alike can visit the AA website (http//www.aa.org), type in a zip code, and be provided a list of AA offices near that location that can provide a directory of local meetings, and similar resources are available at on the Smart Recovery website (http://www.smartrecovery.org). A health-care provider should feel comfortable taking the initiative to ask about particular meetings including details about format and general group member demographics.

Below, is a process aimed to be practical in terms of guiding integrative care specialists in how to best determine the most appropriate group intervention under such circumstances.

Upon learning of a potential group intervention for a patient with a substance-related or addictive disorder, a health-care provider must first determine if the referral is based on clinical or non-clinical factors (e.g., convenience, finances, availability, etc.) and to determine the patient's fit with a group intervention approach based on clinical grounds. If it is determined that a patient could clinically benefit from such an intervention, the patient must be assessed as to her or his readiness for group treatment through a clinical interview that queries attitudes about group work and motivation to engage in the intervention. Assessing available group interventions, a health-care provider must then determine if these interventions fall into a group therapy or group support category, and if the former, the particular treatment content being presented. With this initial information, the general overall quality of the intervention should be able to be ascertained. The health-care provider should ask him or herself whether the group seems able to provide adequate opportunities for growth, learning, and healing.

Once the health-care provider feels comfortable with the group and understands how it could benefit the patient, it's important to "sell" the intervention in a genuine manner. Using knowledge of research indicating how such groups can be helpful, it's important to take a "treatment of choice" approach that honestly informs the patient that group work is, indeed, the preferred and most used treatment for his or her SUD or addiction. Because there is sometimes a great deal of trepidation in

**Table 25.1    An Integrative Health-Care Provider Approach to Group Therapy and Group Support for Patients with Substance-Related and Addictive Disorders**

| Step | Approach |
|------|----------|
| 1. | Determine reason for referral to group intervention |
| 2. | Assess patient readiness for group intervention |
| 3. | Determine if group therapy or group support |
| 4. | Define group treatment content (if applicable) |
| 5. | Initially assess overall quality of intervention |
| 6. | "Sell" intervention to patient by taking a "treatment of choice" approach and neutralizing any perceived stigma and eliminating misconceptions of group work with facts |
| 7. | Help patient blend group intervention with individual and/or other interventions (if applicable) |
| 8. | Communicate with professional group therapy provider (if applicable) |
| 9. | Communicate with patient after group intervention has begun and continue throughout group intervention to assess fit, efficacy |
| 10. | Define, monitor, and measure any negative or positive substance related outcomes |
| 11. | Communicate with other practitioners involved in patient care to determine effect, efficacy of group intervention |
| 12. | Help patient make any necessary adjustments to initial group intervention |
| 13. | Assess when adjunct, alternative to, or termination of, initial group intervention is necessary and refer / adjust treatment plan accordingly |

patients about engaging in group, a patient and informative approach that helps people understand how and why such groups work is called for, as well as a warm, positive attitude that offers encouragement and hope. This will benefit the process of referral and patient engagement. If there are existing or potential individual interventions, it will be important to help the patient understand that the two modalities can work in tandem and to guide them in understanding how the meshing of these modalities can occur and the potential benefits of doing so. Step 7 calls for communicating with the professional health-care provider of the group intervention if one exists, although this can occur anytime during the process for continuity of care.

Once the intervention has begun, it will be important for the health-care provider to follow up with the patient to determine the fit between specific patient and specific group and to help the patient make small adjustments to his or her behavior in order to get the most out of the experience. Beginning measurements of the group intervention's efficacy by examining substance-related outcomes can occur and can move into more sophisticated and extensive measurements as the patient's involvement with the group progresses. Communicating with other practitioners involved in the patient's treatment will be critical at this time in order to determine if (and how) the group intervention is affecting outcomes. Similarly, 12-step sponsors can be consulted in this manner with appropriate disclosure agreements. Adjustments to the patient's involvement with the group intervention may need to be made, as group membership and facilitator changes often occur: and as she or he progresses, different therapeutic needs will arise. Eventually the group intervention might need to be used in conjunction with another type of treatment (if this has not yet occurred), or else the group involvement may need to be replaced or discontinued. At this point, it will be helpful for a health-care provider to assist the patient in transitioning to different therapeutic interventions and to actively build upon skills and improvement gained during the group intervention.

Utilizing and building upon the research done in the areas of group therapy and group support, integrative medicine health- care providers can become central components in assisting their patients' use of (and benefit from) these promising interventions and therapeutic elements. In doing so, they will be able to serve as integral players in promoting much-needed further research in this area and ultimately—perhaps more importantly—assist patients with substance-related and addictive disorders in finding the specific beneficial circles of healing that can contribute to their health, happiness, and well-being.

## REFERENCES

1. Mehl-Madrona L, Mainguy B. Introducing healing circles and talking circles into primary care. *The Permanente Journal.* 2014;18(2): 4–9.
2. Shally-Jensen, M. *Mental Health Care Issues in America; An Encyclopedia.* ABC-CLIO; Santa Barbara, Ca., 2013.
3. Ogrodniczuk J, Piper W, McCallum M, Joyce A, Rosie J. Interpersonal predictors of group therapy outcome for complicated grief. *International Journal of Group Psychotherapy,* 2003; 52:511–535.
4. Schnurr P, Friedman M, Foy D, et al. Randomized trial of trauma-focused group therapy for posttraumatic stress disorder: Results from a Department of Veterans Affairs cooperative study. *Archives of General Psychiatry.* 2003;60(5):481–489. doi:10.1001/archpsyc.60.5.481.
5. Hunter S, Witkiewitz K, Watkins K, et al. The moderating effects of group cognitive–behavioral therapy for depression among substance users. *Psychology of Addictive Behaviors.* 2012;26(4):906–916.
6. Ready D, Sylvers P, Worley V, et al. The impact of group-based exposure therapy on the PTSD and depression of 30 combat veterans. *Psychological Trauma: Theory, Research, Practice, And Policy.* 2012;4(1):84–93.

7. Gratz K, Tull M. Extending research on the utility of an adjunctive emotion regulation group therapy for deliberate self-harm among women with borderline personality pathology. *Personality Disorders: Theory, Research, and Treatment*. 2011;2(4):316–326.

8. Marmarosh C, Holtz A, Schottenbauer M. Group cohesiveness, group-derived collective self-esteem, group-derived hope, and the well-being of group therapy members. *Group Dynamics: Theory, Research, and Practice*. 2005;9(1):32–44.

9. Classen C, Butler L, Koopman C, et al. Supportive-expressive group therapy and distress in patients with metastatic breast cancer a randomized clinical intervention trial. *Archives of General Psychiatry*. 2001;58(5):494–501.

10. *Principles of Drug Addiction Treatment: A Research Based Guide*. 3rd ed. National Institute on Drug Abuse; Bethesda, Md., 2012. Web site. http://www.drugabuse.gov/publications/principles-drug-addiction-treatment-research-based-guide-third-edition/drug-addiction-treatment-in-united-states/types-treatment-programs.

11. Pamphlet-48. *Alcoholics Anonymous 2014 Member Survey*. New York: AA World Services; 2014.

12. Morgan-Lopez A, Fals-Stewart W. Analytic complexities associated with group therapy in substance abuse treatment research: problems, recommendations, and future directions. *Experimental and Clinical Psychopharmacology*. 2006;14(2):265–273.

13. Weiss R, Jaffee W, deMenil V, et al. Group therapy for substance use disorders: what do we know? *Harvard Review of Psychiatry*. 2004;12(6):339–350.

14. Scheidlinger S. The group psychotherapy movement at the millennium: some historical perspectives. *International Journal of Group Psychotherapy*. 2000;50(3):315–339.

15. Walters S, Ogle R, Martin J. Perils and possibilities of group-MI. In: Miller W, Rollnick SS, eds. *Motivational Interviewing: Preparing People to Change*. New York: Guilford; 2002:377–390.

16. Lorentzen S, Ruud T, Gråwe R. Group therapy in community mental health centres: a Norwegian survey. *Nordic Psychology*. 2010;62(3):21–35.

17. Quintana S, Kilmartin C, Yesenosky J, Macias D. Factors affecting referral decisions in a university counseling center. *Professional Psychology: Research And Practice*. 1991;22(1):90–97.

18. Hunter S, Witkiewitz K, Watkins K, Paddock S, Hepner K. The moderating effects of group cognitive–behavioral therapy for depression among substance users. *Psychology of Addictive Behaviors*. 2012;26(4):906–916.

19. Nooripour R, Apsche J, de Velasco B, Aminizadeh M. Effectiveness of self-efficacy group therapy on problem solving skill and sexual self-efficacy in addicted women. *International Journal of Behavioral Consultation And Therapy*. 2014;9(1):35–38.

20. Kenney S, Napper L, LaBrie J, Martens M. Examining the efficacy of a brief group protective behavioral strategies skills training alcohol intervention with college women. *Psychology of Addictive Behaviors*. 2014;28(4):1041–1051.

21. Sobell L, Sobell M, Agrawal S. Randomized controlled trial of a cognitive-behavioral motivational intervention in a group versus individual format for substance use disorders. *Psychology of Addictive Behaviors*. 2009;23(4):672–683.

22. Duckert F, Johnsen J, Amundsen A. What happens to drinking after therapeutic intervention? *British Journal of Addiction.* 1992;87(10):1457–1467.
23. Santisteban D, Mena M, Muir J, McCabe B, Abalo C, Cummings A. The efficacy of two adolescent substance abuse treatments and the impact of comorbid depression: Results of a small randomized controlled trial. *Psychiatric Rehabilitation Journal.* 2015;38(1): 55–64.
24. Davison K, Pennebaker J, Dickerson S. Who talks? The social psychology of illness support groups. *American Psychologist.* 2000;55(2):205–217.
25. Goering P, Durbin J, Sheldon C, Ochocka J, Nelson G, Krupa T. Who uses consumer-run self-help organizations?. *American Journal of Orthopsychiatry.* 2006;76(3):367–373.
26. Washington O, Moxley D. Promising group practices to empower low-income minority women coping with chemical dependency. *American Journal of Orthopsychiatry.* 2003;73(1):109–116.
27. Beehler S, Clark J, Eisen S. Participant experiences in peer- and clinician-facilitated mental health recovery groups for veterans. *Psychiatric Rehabilitation Journal.* 2014;37(1):43–50.
28. Moos R, Moos B. Long-term influence of duration and frequency of participation in Alcoholics Anonymous on individuals with alcohol use disorders. *Journal of Consulting and Clinical Psychology.* 2004;72(1):81–90.
29. Results from the 2013 National Survey on Drug Use and Health: Summary of National Findings. Substance Abuse and Mental Health Services. Web site. http://www.samhsa.gov/data/sites/default/files/NSDUHresultsPDFWHTML2013/Web/NSDUHresults2013.pdf
30. Morgenstern J, Labouvie E, McCrady B, Kahler C, Frey R. Affiliation with Alcoholics Anonymous after treatment: a study of its therapeutic effects and mechanisms of action. *Journal of Consulting and Clinical Psychology.* 1997;65(5):768–777.
31. Emrick C, Tonigan J, Montgomery H, Little L. Alcoholics Anonymous: What is currently known?. In: McCrady B, Miller W, eds. *Research on Alcoholics Anonymous: Opportunities and alternatives.* Piscataway, NJ: Rutgers Center of Alcohol Studies; 1993:41–76.
32. Forcehimes A, Tonigan J. Self-efficacy as a factor in abstinence from alcohol/other drug abuse: A meta-analysis. *Alcoholism Treatment Quarterly.* 2008;26:480–489.
33. Tonigan J. Benefits of Alcoholics Anonymous attendance: replication of findings between clinical research sites in Project MATCH. *Alcoholism Treatment Quarterly.* 2001; 19: 67–77.
34. Tonigan J, Toscova R, Miller W. Meta-analysis of the literature on Alcoholics Anonymous: Sample and study characteristics moderate findings. *Journal of Studies on Alcohol.* 1995; 57: 65–72.
35. Tonigan J, Rice S. Is it beneficial to have an Alcoholics Anonymous sponsor? *Psychology of Addictive Behaviors.* 2010;24:397–403.
36. Carroll K, Nich C, Ball S, McCance E, Frankforter T, Rounsaville B. One-year follow-up of disulfiram and psycho-therapy for cocaine-alcohol users: Sustained effects of treatment. *Addiction.* 2000;95:1335–1349.

37. Gossop M, Stewart D, Marsden J. Readiness for change and drug use outcomes after treatment. *Addiction*. 2007;102:301–308.
38. Weiss R, Griffin M, Gallop R, et al. The effect of 12-step self-help group attendance and participation on drug use outcomes among cocaine-dependent patients. *Drug and Alcohol Dependence*. 2005;77:177–184.
39. Rynes K, Tonigan J. Do social networks explain 12-step sponsorship effects? A prospective lagged mediation analysis. *Psychology of Addictive Behaviors*. 2012;26(3):432–439.
40. Kelly J, Myers M, Brown S. A multivariate process model of adolescent 12-step attendance and substance use outcome following inpatient treatment. *Psychology of Addictive Behaviors*. 2000;14(4):376–389.
41. Fiorentine R. After drug treatment: are 12-step programs effective in maintaining abstinence? *American Journal of Drug & Alcohol Abuse*. 1999;25:93–116.
42. McKellar J, Stewart E, Humphreys K. Alcoholics Anonymous involvement and positive alcohol-related outcomes: cause, consequence, or just a correlate? A prospective 2-year study of 2,319 alcohol-dependent men. *Journal of Consulting And Clinical Psychology*. 2003;71(2):302–308.
43. McCrady B, Epstein E, Kahler C. Alcoholics Anonymous and relapse prevention as maintenance strategies after conjoint behavioral alcohol treatment for men: 18-month outcomes. *Journal of Consulting and Clinical Psychology*. 2004;72(5): 870–878.
44. Wilcox C, Pearson M, Tonigan J. Effects of long-term AA attendance and spirituality on the course of depressive symptoms in individuals with alcohol use disorder. *Psychology of Addictive Behaviors*. 2015;29(2):382–391.
45. Garland E, Manusov E, Froeliger B, Kelly A, Williams J, Howard M. Mindfulness-oriented recovery enhancement for chronic pain and prescription opioid misuse: results from an early-stage randomized controlled trial. *Journal of Consulting and Clinical Psychology*. 2014;82(3):448–459.
46. Knack W. Psychotherapy and Alcoholics Anonymous: an integrated approach. *Journal of Psychotherapy Integration*. 2009;19(1):86–109.
47. Maude-Griffin P, Hohenstein J, Humfleet G, Reilly P, Tusel D, Hall S. Superior efficacy of cognitive-behavioral therapy for urban crack cocaine abusers: main and matching effects. *Journal of Consulting and Clinical Psychology*. 1998;66(5):832–837.
48. Ouimette P, Finney J, Moos R. Twelve-step and cognitive-behavioral treatment for substance abuse: a comparison of treatment effectiveness. *Journal of Consulting and Clinical Psychology*. 1997; 65(2):230–240.
49. Project MATCH Research Group. Project MATCH: rationale and methods for a multisite clinical trial matching patients to alcoholism treatment. *Alcoholism: Clinical and Experimental Research*. 1993;17(6).
50. Project MATCH Research Group. Matching alcoholism treatments to client heterogeneity: treatment main effects and matching effects on drinking during treatment. *Journal of Studies on Alcohol*. 1998;59(6).
51. Project MATCH Research Group. Matching alcoholism treatments to client heterogeneity: Project MATCH posttreatment drinking outcomes. *Journal of Studies on Alcohol*. 1997;58(7).

52. Project MATCH Research Group. Matching alcoholism treatments to client heterogeneity: project MATCH three year drinking outcomes. *Alcoholism: Clinical and Experimental Research.* 1998;22(6).

53. Kelly JF, Yeterian JD, Myers MG. Treatment staff referrals, participation expectations, and perceived benefits and barriers to adolescent involvement in twelve-step groups. *Alcoholism Treatment Quarterly.* 2008;26:427–449.

54. Step Six. Alcoholics Anonymous. Web site. http://www.aa.org/assets/en_US/en_step6.pdf

55. Dodes L. *The Sober Truth: Debunking the Bad Science Behind 12-Step Programs and the Rehab Industry.* Boston: Beacon Press; 2014.

56. Glaser G. The irrationality of Alcoholics Anonymous. *The Atlantic,* April 2015.

57. Singal J. Why Alcoholic Anonymous works. *New York Magazine,* March 2015.

58. Szalavitz M. After 75 years of Alcoholic Anonymous, it's time to admit we have a problem. *Pacific Standard,* February 2014.

59. Munro D. Inside the $35 Billion Addiction Treatment. *Forbes,* April 2015.

60. Subbaraman M, Kaskutas L. Social support and comfort in AA as mediators of "Making AA easier" (MAAEZ), a 12-step facilitation intervention. *Psychology of Addictive Behaviors.* 2012;26(4):759–765.

61. Tonigan J, Connors G, Miller W. Alcoholics Anonymous Involvement (AAI) scale: reliability and norms. *Psychology of Addictive Behaviors.* 1996;10(2):75–80.

62. Kingree J, Simpson A, Thompson M, McCrady B, Tonigan J, Lautenschlager G. The development and initial evaluation of the Survey of Readiness for Alcoholics Anonymous Participation. *Psychology of Addictive Behaviors.* 2006;20(4):453–462.

63. Bond J, Kaskutas L, Weisner C. The persistent influence of social networks and Alcoholics Anonymous on abstinence. *Journal of Studies on Alcohol.* 2003;64:579–588.

64. Smart Recovery. Web site. http://www.smartrecovery.org

65. Kelly PJ, Dean FP, Baker AL. Group cohesion and between session homework activities predict self report of SMART Recovery groups. *Journal of Substance Abuse Treatment.* 2015;51:53–58.

66. Kelly PJ, Raftery D, Dean FP, Baker AL, Hunt D, Shakeshaft A. Comparing treatments for dual diagnosis: twelve-step and self-management and recovery training. *Drug Alcohol Review.* 2016.

67. Brooks AJ, Penn PE. Comparing treatments for dual diagnosis: twelve-step and self-management and recovery training. *American Journal of Drug and Alcohol Abuse.* 2003;29(2):359–383.

68. Hester RK, Lenberg KL, Campbell W, Delaney HD. Overcoming addictions: a web-based application, and SMART recovery, and online and in-person mutual help group for problem drinkers, part 1: three-month outcomes of a randomized controlled trial. *Journal of Medical Internet Res.* 2013;15(7).

69. Anonymous. *Alcoholics Anonymous: The Story of How Many Thousands of Men and Women Have Recovered from Alcoholism.* 4th ed. New York: A.A. World Services; 2001.

70. *The AA Group: Where It All Begins.* New York: Alcoholics Anonymous World Services; 2005.

71. Institute of Medicine. Broadening the base of treatment for alcohol problems. Washington, DC: National Academy Press; 1990.

72. What is Integrative Medicine? Dr. Andrew Weil, MD. Web site. http://www.drweil.com/drw/u/ART02054/Andrew-Weil-Integrative-Medicine.html.

# 26

## Integrative Approaches to Healing

### E. HITCHCOCK SCOTT AND GEORGE E. MUÑOZ

The etiology of chemical addiction is multiclausal and multifactorial, spanning socioeconomic classes, cultures, and families. While there are known commonalities and vulnerabilities with regard to those with addiction, there are times it appears as if bad luck played Russian Roulette with one family member in particular while excluding the rest for seemingly nonsensical reasons.

The currently held view is that drug use is part of a brain disease encompassing physical, mental, and spiritual aspects. Historically, however, chemical addiction has been viewed as a moral problem by the general public, health professionals, and government agencies.

Government agencies dedicated to research and the treatment of drug and alcohol addiction as a disease entity include the National Institute of Drug Abuse (NIDA) and the National Institute on Alcohol Abuse and Alcoholism (NIAA). Both departments, as well as the federal bureaucracy, were initiated out of the Department of the Treasury in the post-Prohibition era. This fact presents an interesting societal commentary as to where problems of drug and alcohol abuse were relegated: drug and alcohol abuse problems were views with respect to government oversight and preview (i.e., its monetary effect on tax collection).

We have made progress in our understanding of addiction. NIDA's 2008 definition of chemical addiction compares the disorder to other medical problems, "Addiction is a chronic, often relapsing, brain disease . . . like other chronic, relapsing diseases such as diabetes, asthma, or heart disease."[1] Research supporting the neurological components of addiction has been helpful with the amelioration of societal scorn, contempt, and discrimination toward those with addiction as if morally weak rather than ill.

Tragically, the number of those with chemical substance abuse problems are increasing. Chemical addiction's morbidity and mortality are also on the rise with pharmaceutical abuse as well as with street drugs. Street drugs today are more accessible, less expensive, more highly addictive, more toxic, and potent than ever before. The United States has been immersed in a widespread heroin epidemic with significant numbers of overdoses and deaths previously unseen by coroners. Despite the risk of harm and death, young people are still using these dangerous drugs in rising numbers. A 2001 study found that the most popular functions for use were using to: relax (96.7%), become intoxicated (96.4%), keep awake at night while socializing (95.5%), enhance an activity (88.5%), and alleviate depressed mood (86.6%).

## Primary Medical Issues Related to Addiction

Advances in molecular mechanisms of gene analysis, gene-wide association, and specific gene probes have yielded advances in both animal models and human constructs to identify the complex neurobiology of brain circuitry. Addiction-related behaviors have been altered by more than 100 mouse gene knockouts and transgenic lines revealing the molecular complexity and multiplicity of pathways that may lead to addictions.

Translational medicine advances are on the brink of yielding personalized genomic information to treat individual patients. According to Anton, et al in their review of epigenetic status in clinical application realms, the future view is broad and "progress in the pharmacogenetics of addictions would reduce morbidity and mortality through better prevention and treatment. Progress is at this point limited and narrow in specificity. For example, the specific effect of the μ-opioid receptor polymorphism (OPRM1; Asn40Asp) Asp40 to predict favorable naltrexone treatment response in alcoholism was recently replicated offering a narrowly defined clinical tool. In contrast, integrated pharmacogenetics of addictions would require an understanding of interacting effects in multiple biological mechanisms involved in tolerance, craving, anxiety, dysphoria, executive cognitive function, and reward."[2]

Neanderthal DNA associated with depression persists today, as well as other ancient genomes initially selected for survival, whose primary purpose is no longer as essential. Nonetheless, these ancient genes can affect neurobiology, changes in mood, nutrition including B-vitamin absorption, and innate immunity through Toll receptors. Ancient Neanderthal genes have also been documented to increase tobacco addiction.[3]

The concept that we are genetically and energetically linked to our ancestors is true biologically and on various other planes when discussing and understanding our lineage as deeper than merely our immediate family and several recent layers of generations. The underpinning of these and other yet-to-be uncovered genomic clusters led to the concepts in medical anthropology of studying family issues, curses, and addictions from the viewpoint of maternal or paternal lineage.

Maternal inheritance can be housed within mitochondria that hold their own separate genetic code, interacting with metabolism, energy (ATP production), endocrine functions, and immunity and inflammatory states. Given these revelations of the importance of mitochondria in inheritance and the myriad functions noted above, mitochondrial health is an important integrative target to focus upon in mental health, wellness, and metabolic issues related to addiction.

Silencing ancient genomes and pro-inflammatory gene expression including NFkB, that no longer serve us today in our modern existence and promoting pathways and anti-informatory metabolic process are essential to maintaining a balanced neurohormonal and immune signaling. Obesity is the prototypic, pro-inflammatory metabolic state that exhibits both clinically active and silent inflammatory states.[4] The same is true of the active addict with secondary metabolic derangements.

## Secondary Medical Issues Related to Addiction

The secondary medical conditions associated with addiction have been reviewed and discussed in the "Functional Approaches" chapter in detail from that perspective. We will briefly review them here and reference chapter 18 when appropriate. As previously noted, active addiction irrespective of substance is a massively pro-inflammatory state. Consequently, any condition that already is characterized by inflammation (metabolic syndrome, CV disease, hypertension at the endothelial level) would be activated or worsened in active addiction due to the cumulative effects at the cellular, cytokine, metabolomic, and genomic levels of transcription and secondary immune and endocrine effects.[5-7] These systems are complex, but well-defined cross talk between them is acknowledged and referenced as to the "cumulative disease burden" effect in systemic rheumatic illness. The same concept is applicable to active addiction, as all these underlying and background medical conditions share the same common pathways irrespective of exact primary inciting event, hence in active addiction the secondary or worsened metabolic derangements and organ damage could be thought of "as the cumulative disease burden of addiction," affecting quality of life, morbidity, and mortality perhaps in a younger cohort of patients than the non-addicted counterparts. Some important and interesting points merit mention such as that the effect of cigarette smoking and alcohol (4%) exceeded illicit drug (0.8%) in cumulative disease burden metrics in the early 2000s but the gap is closing nearly 20 years later.[7] Globally, from public health perspectives, alcohol effects on health metrics was highest in Andean South America, Eastern Europe, and southern sub-Saharan Africa. For North America, smoking and secondhand effects were primary effectors of detrimental public health outcomes. Increased body mass index, global obesity rise and "dietary risk factors and physical inactivity collectively accounted for 10·0% (95% UI 9·2–10·8) of global DALYs in 2010" (DALYs represent deaths and disability adjusted life years).[8] Closely linked to obesity and increased processed sugar consumption is the notion that sugar in and of itself possesses addictive physiologic, behavioral, and neuro-pharmacologic properties with clear scientific constructs to substantiate this claim.[9,10] The recovering individual and their physician need to factor this reality into their lifestyle and nutritional patterns in addition to the reason that already exists for reductions in raising insulin levels, subsequent insulin resistance, and progression to pro-inflammatory metabolic syndrome and frank Type-2 diabetes. These are all potential results of active addiction as comorbid conditions and all amenable to interventional steps as part of the wellness recovery prescription.

Neurologic sequela of active addiction including neuropathy and neurocognitive dysfunction are large areas of clinical and scientific interest worth mentioning. While the specific insult to peripheral nerves may be dependent on the substance to some degree, certain general concepts prevail including micronutrient deficiency and increased oxidative stress. The classic situation found with alcohol abuse demonstrates the following in the summary by Chopra and Tiwari who state: "In addition to thiamine deficiency, recent studies indicate a direct neurotoxic effect of ethanol or its metabolites." Axonal degeneration has been documented in rats receiving ethanol while maintaining normal thiamine status. Human studies have also suggested a direct toxic effect, since a dose-dependent relationship has been observed between severity of neuropathy and total life time dose of ethanol. The exact mechanism behind alcoholic neuropathy is not well understood, but several explanations have been proposed. These include activation of spinal cord microglia after chronic alcohol consumption, activation of mGlu5 receptors in the spinal cord, oxidative stress leading to free radical damage to nerves, release of proinflammatory cytokines coupled with activation of protein kinase C, involvement of extracellular signal-regulated kinases (ERKs) or classical MAP kinases, involvement of the opioidergic and hypothalamo-pituitaryadrenal system. Some other studies have indicated that chronic alcohol intake can decrease the nociceptive threshold with increased oxidative stress and release of proinflammatory cytokines coupled with activation of protein kinase C.[11] Treatment of alcohol neuropathy including thiamine, B vitamins, B12, alpha lipoic acid, glutathione, acetyl-L carnitine. Vitamin E and myo-inositol (phospholipid) have all been recommended or studied in clinical treatment.[11] The use of drugs including anti-convulsants (gabapentin) and anti-depressants (amitriptyline) are widely prescribed. Moderate to high doses (2 to 6 grams daily) of omega-3 EPA/DHA are also utilized in this setting to stabilize the phospholipid cellular raft system in peripheral, central nerves, and immune cells.

# Psychosocial Influences Related to Addiction

Concepts including family of origin, trauma, genetics, and genomics are important factors for discussion in addiction and secondary behaviors. With respect to gene function, it appears that "addictive drugs induce adaptive changes in gene expression in brain reward regions, including the striatum, representing a mechanism for tolerance and habit formation with craving and negative affect that persist long after consumption ceases."[12] Studies have demonstrated that the combination of environment and genetics contributes to the phenomenon of addiction.

The Virginia Twin Study revealed that in early adolescence the initiation and use of nicotine, alcohol, and cannabis are more strongly determined by familial and social factors, but these gradually decline in importance during the progression to young and middle adulthood when the effects of genetic factors become maximal, declining somewhat with aging.[13] Additionally, the availability of drugs plays a factor in frequency of addiction by age and paradoxical findings have been noted: "The moderate to high heritability of addictive disorders are paradoxical because addictions initially depend on the availability of the addictive agent and the individual's choice to use it. The availability of addictive agents is determined by culture, social policy, religion, economic status, and narco-trafficking, and it changes across time and space."[14]

# Definition of Healing

According to the *Oxford English Dictionary*, healing is, "the process of making or becoming sound or healthy again."[15] When speaking about healing in the realm of addiction and recovery, the path required to help an individual process the real or perceived prior trauma primarily of their life, or transgenerational, and to learn to release the psychic wound at all levels of their being (physical, mental, and spiritual) is a possible encompassing definition.

The MEDLINE electronic database reveals no single MeSH heading for "healing." Instead, it added qualifiers associated with the spiritual and religious aspects of illness and recovery related to psychology and alternative medicine. It could be surmised that modern medicine considers holistic healing beyond its orthodoxy, leaving the promotion of healing to practitioners of alternative or aboriginal medicine nonscientific, non-medical practitioners described by anthropologists.[16]

Thomas Agnew describes healing as a transcendence of suffering. Agnew further attests, "The confusion concerning healing in medicine is evidenced by the lack of consensus about its meaning. Science values operational definitions. Yet, medicine promotes no operational definition of healing nor does it provide any explanation of it mechanisms, save those describing narrow physiological processes associated with curing disease. Most medical literature addressing holistic healing and using the word in the title never defines the term."

## An Inclusive Integrative Medicine Model of Healing

Addiction, when understood as a chronic illness involving a person in totality—physically, neurologically, emotionally, and spiritually—moves beyond the current medical model for effective treatment. The current medical model for diagnosis, treatment, and service delivery has a focus on acute care. Acute ailments happen suddenly, tend to be sharp or severe, and although serious are typically brief in duration. Chronic illnesses, however, exist and continue (or can have a recurring pattern) over an extended period of time that could be multiple years or life-long in duration (O'Brien, 2016, 67).[17] The problem is that with traditional medicine the focus of addiction as only a physical and neurological problem can become reductionistic and, therefore, less effective than a holistic approach.

Traditional Western medicine can be limited in scope, with a myopic focus on the physical body to the exclusion of other essential aspects of health and wholeness. When considering an inclusive integrative model of medicine, it is important to consider why conventional models of addiction treatment fall short. Thomas Agnew states:

> Medicine is traditionally considered a healing profession, and modern medicine claims legitimacy to heal through its scientific approach to medicine. Themarriage of science and medicine has empowered physicians to intervene actively during disease, to effect cures, to prevent illness, and to eradicate disease. In the wake of such success, physicians, trained as biomedical scientists, have focused on the diagnosis, treatment, and prevention of disease. In the process, cure, not care, became the primary purpose of medicine, and the physician's role became 'curer of disease' rather than 'healer of the sick.' Healing in a holistic sense has faded from medical attention and is rarely discussed in the medical literature.[16]

By contract, the integrative medicine construct attends to the entirety of an individual. "Integrative medicine (IM) is healing-oriented medicine that takes account of the whole person including all aspects of lifestyle. It emphasizes the therapeutic relationship between practitioner and patient, is informed by evidence, and makes use of all appropriate therapies."[18]

Aligning the mental, physical, and spiritual aspects of the person toward a healing paradigm is one of the objectives in an integrative recovery plan for the treating physician and health-care providers. This alignment requires discussion, planning, and interfacing a care team assessment that accounts for the radial and psychosocial aspects of chronic care of the recovering individual. This assessment is similar to what is applicable in a chronic care setting when applying an integrative are team model to Inflammatory Bowel Disease and autoimmune conditions such as Rheumatoid Arthritis which are also complex, chronic, and associated with flares and remissions. The Psychosocial Radial Tool as studied and validated by Marci Reiss and Dr. Sandborn, evaluates finances, family, mental health, work, schooling, transportation factors, and ability to access care and meds needed for full treatment. Identifying the at-risk individual early is critical for the health-care team to identify and intervene in preventing future compliance or care gaps, and in the case of addiction, relapse and repeated hospitalization treatment center admissions, overdoses and ER visits, and mortality potential.[19] In effect, this increases the value proposition while identifying highest risk individuals likely to relapse from identifiable psychosocial causes which could be mitigated in many instances.

## Integrating Treatment for Adverse Childhood Experiences in Addiction Recovery

Healing means to restore, make whole, or return to optimum condition. At the very least healing means relief; an ability to cope and function while bearing a difficult challenge.[1] The definition of healing, if taken in the context of emotional and spiritual constructs, expands the meaning from the obvious and simplistic to the most subtle and comprehensive. When speaking about healing in the realm of addiction treatment—if sufficiently comprehensive—recovery is able to reach levels beyond a return to prior functioning.

It is difficult to imagine, even with scientific data to support the link, how real or imagined childhood adverse experiences contribute to problems with substance abuse, sometimes decades later. It has become a well-circulated myth that people outgrow their experiences of childhood trauma and can rise above them unscathed. Due to mythmaking, it is difficult for many to imagine why it is important to address early negative childhood experiences and family dynamics for addiction treatment.

Trauma, from the Greek root, simply means "wound." Our human wounds happen on a continuum of intensity and impact. An adverse experience as an adult will have very different and often more profound consequences for a child—even if it appears to be exactly the same type of event. Early childhood developmental issues, including comprehension or lack of it, and healthy or unhealthy attachments to caregivers, can either exacerbate or ameliorate a potentially wounding event.

There are many kinds of wounds: emotional, physical, mental, sexual, and spiritual, (and/or energetic). There are adverse experiences that are associated with a dynamic rather than direct abuse. Parental marital discord, parental mental illness, criminal activities, and substance abuse are able to cause harm to a child's healthy development, even if only indirectly.

With data collected from the Adverse Childhood Experiences study (ACE) and the Center for Disease Control (CDC) from as early as 1900, is was found that people who reported "> 5 ACEs were 7–10-fold more likely to report illicit drug use problems, addiction to illicit drugs, and parenteral drug use," compared to those who reported no ACEs (A-page1). In this study, ACEs range from: (1) physical, emotional, or sexual abuse in childhood, (2) parental conflict, and (3) household members' dysfunction such as criminality, mental illness, and substance abuse.

In a workshop provided by one of the co-authors of this paper for 9 medical doctors, at least 4 of the 9 participants admitted an experience of childhood or young adult rape. At least one admitted that he or she had never shared their experience with anyone until that day. Sadly, profound trauma is revealed, more often than not, to this author in various professional settings. Therefore, should we find it surprising that there are professionals in the field of medicine who deny the reality of how negative childhood experiences contribute to a myriad of problems in adulthood? The lines of impactful connection, from childhood to adulthood, appear to be invisible and, in some cases, the connections are most invisible to health practitioners who have a history of unacknowledged trauma themselves.[20]

In many addiction programs, an industry that is burgeoning quickly and sometimes irresponsibly, the intake forms do not ask about trauma. Even if they do ask, the questions are minimal and superficial. In addition, intake staff is generally inadequately trained to ask about trauma, or to respond appropriately to disclosures—which can sometimes be the first time trauma has been revealed openly—from the patients. Too often, patients admit that after multiple failed treatments, someone finally asked about trauma or abuse. The greatest tragedy is that there are patients who do not survive to be asked the question.

Even with a thorough and comprehensive intake form, coupled with a skilled interviewer, there are problems with collecting an accurate adverse childhood experience history from clients with addiction. There are problems with patient shame and embarrassment. It is not uncommon for patients to erroneously think that the childhood trauma was and is their own fault, rather than the responsibility of an adult caretaker. In addition, there are familial loyalties and inordinate trauma bonds with the perpetrator, fostering false histories. In some families, keeping secrets has become ingrained into all forms of communication, to the point of making it difficult to collect basic accurate medical information. Lack of education, denial and minimization may also distort accurate reporting of trauma and abuse.

Just as patients minimize their intake of alcohol, illicit or non-prescribed chemicals, they minimize trauma and abuse. Also, there are reports of documented childhood trauma that is not remembered by the victim when asked later in life.

In other words, the patient may not remember early childhood trauma adequately to report it.

It is important to identify abuse early in the recovery process to prepare the patient for what may emerge on the post-sobriety date. Once the numbing substance is withdrawn, suppressed or repressed information is more likely to surface. For newly sober patients, early childhood trauma may surface in ways that sabotage recovery if the patient is unprepared. The purpose of concurrent treatment of adverse childhood experiences with addiction treatment is not to enable a patient to avoid accountability, but, instead, help them with resources, adequate support, and proper treatment.

## Interventions for Healing Addictions and Trauma

### MENTAL AND EMOTIONAL

The purpose in the recovery process is to achieve a balanced state that embodies and supports well-being. Mental and emotional healing embodies a clearance of painful memories that have created mental, emotional, autonomic nervous system, and energetic blocks. These blocks interfere with a free flow of energy, clarity of thinking and being, and a balanced serene state. The integrative medicine construct of attending to the entirety of an individual, not merely the traditional Western approach (with a primary attention to the physical body), calls for attention to all aspects of health and dis(ease), states of the mind, and psyche. Attending to the mind and mood of a patient involves more than reflex prescribing of anti-depressants and anxiolytics as the panacea for patient symptoms. The implications of decreased emotional well-being, sometimes predating the addictive processes, show up as mental health concerns such as stress, depression, and anxiety. These in turn can contribute to physical ill-health such as digestive disorders, sleep disturbances, and general lack of energy, plus an escalation of self-medicating behaviors.

Healing for addiction and trauma includes a process of gently challenging the cognitive distortions and errors that have helped maintain a dysfunctional abuse of mood altering chemical substances. These errors of cognition are addressed via CBT. CBT has a validated and proven record in the treatment of a variety of disorders including, but not limited to, addiction, anxiety, and depressive disorders. Although the research regarding the efficacy of cognitive behavioral therapies is being challenged, the utility of this approach remains a mainstay in the treatment of addictions.

Patients arrive to treatment defending their substance abuse with common and understandable types of dysfunctional logic such as, "I am not alcoholic, I only drink a six pack a night, my father drank a case." A similar cognitive distortion with regard to trauma might be, "I was only molested by my grandfather once. . . it isn't a big deal." A comprehensive intake process, along with education, helps the patient in collaboration with the health practitioner identify problems and issues to be addressed via an individualized treatment plan. Individualized treatment plans for patients, who may need more specialized treatment approaches, beyond CBT, may include Eye Movement Desensitization Reprocessing (EMDR), Somatic Experiencing (SE), hypnotherapy, creative arts psychotherapies (including music/sound/toning/singing/chanting; dance and movement; journal/story/script/poetry writing), psychodrama, psychoanalysis, ego-state therapies, EFT-tapping techniques.

Patients may also seek guidance and treatment from more unconventional approaches including energy healing, medical touch (the nursing model of energy medicine), Reiki, acupuncture, and shamanic traditions (the medical anthropology model). Whichever modality or combination is sought, the end goal is to achieve a state of healing, balance, and wholeness to eradicate primary emotional links as an addiction trigger. Mainstream mind body interventions such as, meditation, prayer, interacting with nature, yoga, Tai Chi, qigong, or guided imagery are recommended to reduce stress and anxiety and improve the neurologic balance of the autonomic nervous system and secondary neuroendocrine balance.[21]

These modalities, especially when carefully selected and used in conjunction with each other, are able to help the patient see their lives through a different lens, macro and micro, in ways that open up the patient to new awareness and insights. These healing processes may also engender new experiences of relief, ones not due to chemical abuse, giving a glimpse of hope to the most despairing.

By addressing cognitive distortions and dissonance, triggers to using, lifestyle choices, trauma, mental health issues, plus emotional, energetic, and autonomic system blocks, a free flow of energy, as well as, a clarity of thinking and being is able to be created, sometimes for the first time in the patient's life. This allows the patient to experience a sense of balance and states of serenity that enhances potential for long-term sobriety.

Whatever the processes used for healing, enhanced emotional well-being is seen to contribute to upward spirals in increasing coping ability, self-esteem, performance and productivity at work, and even longevity. Emotional well-being is also one of two aspects of personal well-being that can be measured in quantitative quality of life assessments, the other being "life evaluation," the evaluation of one's life in general against a scale. At its core, emotional well-being has been noted to decrease common maladies and reduce mortality and death rates.

## Physical Healing

The physical and medical challenges, primary and secondary, for the newly sober addict can be varied and not necessarily uniform but may include: (1) malnutrition and nutritional deficiency states, (2) proinflammatory metabolic state, (3) post-traumatic injuries with secondary neurologic and orthopedic sequelae, (4) chronic liver disease from drug polypharmacy, (5) viral hepatitis and its secondary effects, (6) type-2 diabetes, (7) metabolic syndrome and secondary endocrine disorders including hypothyroidism or other primary neuroendocrine dysfunction (either predating addiction or related to chronic opiate use), (8) dehydration, and (9) neurological damage due to toxic substance abuse.

Healing the physical body requires a comprehensive general medical evaluation, which includes a physical exam, blood work, and neurological and genetic testing. There needs to be special attention to the secondary pro-inflammatory conditions, prevalent in the general population but that are accelerated or aggravated by the using patterns of active addiction. The use of general supplements with anti-inflammatory benefits including omega-3 fish oils in therapeutic doses of 2 to 4 grams daily (EPA/DHA), Vitamin D3 to reach optimal serum levels of 50 to 70 mg/ml along with methylation support of B vitamins (B1, B6, B12) and neurologic support specific supplements such as magnesium citrate 200 to 250 mg nightly, CoQ10 100 to 200 mg daily, and anti-inflammatory botanicals including turmeric 500 to 1000 mg bid and ginger root 500 mg bid are all appropriate to consider as part of a comprehensive addiction and recovery supplement offering. Specifics about the role of detox protocols and GI functional medicine approaches are discussed specifically in the "Functional Approaches to Addiction" chapter (chapter 18).

## Exercise

Exercise is another important component to physical well-being in recovering individuals. The numerous benefits of exercise have been reviewed extensively in the literature and include the obvious cardiovascular, cancer reduction, and fantastic metabolic benefits as well as the mental, mood, and euphoric effects that accompany moderate exercise. Again, moderation is the key so as not to substitute a healthy activity and transform it into an obsessive one that could become associated with dysphoric and distorted body image or compulsivity with food. Consistent, regular patterned and disciplined self-care that aligns itself with the mind, body, spirit paradigm 30 to 60 minutes, 5 days per week (total 150 to 200 minutes weekly) is the recommended duration by the American Heart Association.

## Spending Time Engaging with Nature

There are many ways, traditional and non-traditional, to enhance and sustain spirituality, such as prayer, meditation, visiting sacred sites, or taking time to be in nature.

Most of us live in urban environments, too often filled with a landscape of cement, metal, and glass. Many of us are bombarded with electrical and cellular energy to the point of creating physical problems, such as disrupted sleep.

Some of the greatest shamans and planetary healers insist that an interactive engagement with nature and Mother Earth (as the planet is referenced), is key to the emotional, physical, and spiritual balance we have lost.

Lack of contact with mother nature, trees, grass, sand, oceans, hills, mountains, and animals creates an energetic void within us. Since we are part of the planetary ecosystem, and not above it, our balance depends on the planet's health as well. In this sense, the healing of humans and the earth is bi-directional and utterly dependent upon each other. For holistic health, we need contact with nature on a regular basis. Walking in parks, mediating next to a tree, and gardening are some urban nature options.

Planning vacations with "nature time" is often a great personal and family activity. Time in nature reduces stress, can be great fun, and it is an aid for wellness. Spending time alone in nature to commune with oneself, or a higher power, may allow us to find answers to deep personal existential questions. Seeking spiritual guidance via meditation and prayer is inherent in all spiritual disciplines and transpersonal practices. Carl Jung, first brought Native American and Eastern traditions of healing to Western psychotherapy, and with regard to addiction treatment the practice remains.

## Restorative Sleep

Restorative sleep is also an important part of the physical and mental recovery aspects. Problems with sleep are common for those with problems of addiction and/or a history of trauma. Sleep problems for those who have just begun addiction and trauma recovery can fluctuate on either side of the spectrum of too much sleep, not enough sleep, or a wide-ranging variation of the two.

Sleep disturbances are further associated with increasing proinflammatory states with elevation of CRP, IL-6, and TNF all further adding to the already disturbed metabolomic milieu of the hyperinflammatory changes seen in drug addiction states that can persist beyond drug discontinuation. Addressing sleep hygiene and attending to disorders such as Obstructive Sleep Apnea (OSA) reduce the cytokine and disturbed endocrine responses that follow primary insomnia and OSA.

Adequate amounts (7 to 8 hours) with enough deep REM is the ideal but not always achievable naturally, especially in early detox and recovering individuals. The use of sleeping aids as prescribed by the addiction specialist in acute detox settings will obviously be different from the approach taken in the outpatient setting in short- and long-term recovery. Effective supplements that aid sleep include magnesium citrate, melatonin sustained release in lowest possible doses, and calming teas such as chamomile. Valerian root 400 to 900 mg before sleep is a consideration, although valerian root is not the best recommendation for those with racing thoughts or a loose association with reality.

Homeopathic recommendations could include Coffea cruda, 9C, 15C, or 30C, 5 to 10 caplets sublingual before sleep. Practitioners should individualize the use of these botanicals, which could have a sedative effect that may not be desirable by many recovering individuals. Developing a healthy practice of good sleep hygiene includes (1) elimination of excessive lighting and electronics (light exposure before sleep reduces endogenous melatonin secretion), (2) the reduction of stimulants such as caffeine, nicotine, and media.[25] A mental cool down period that begins 30 to 60 minutes before planned sleep is a useful ritual approach. It may be important to add healing scents to create a relaxing environment. Daily self-reflection, meditation, and/or breath work are useful activates to perform to maximize the calming benefit of reduction in catecholamine, improved heart rate variability, and decreased sympathetic tone from the day's stress.[22]

## Spirituality and Forgiveness

Definitions of spirituality are contradictory. The 12-step definition of spirituality is divorced from traditional religions in part so that members of all faiths—including atheism—might feel welcome. For the purpose of this chapter, spirituality means attention to the human spirit, rather than an ideology or religion. Twelve-step programs, influenced by the Oxford Group, describe spirituality as a felt sense and trust of a higher power or divine presence. Spirituality might also be described as an existential search for meaning or higher purpose. A spiritual search, instead of adherence to a religious doctrine, might manifest as a disciplined practice of listening to inner direction, for the purpose of positive change.

The definition spirituality for a person in addiction and trauma recovery is dynamic and idiosyncratic to each individual person. Patients often arrive at the front door of a treatment facility with a feeling of despair. Despair manifests in various ways. Sometimes the despairing addict acts belligerently, "I don't need you, I don't need God, just leave me alone." Other times patients have spent years pleading for help, and they are tired of asking, because they think their prayers have not been answered.

Spiritual vulnerability is best addressed with tender and nonjudgmental attention by staff members. It is important to refrain from talk of a specific religion to circumvent, at least temporarily, defensiveness associated with a history of religious abuse.

Just as the intake forms need to ask about trauma, the intake forms need to have questions about early childhood experiences of religion or spirituality. During intake a lot can be learned about possible betrayal by religious leaders, family members, and/or a child's possible misperceptions of the meaning of a tragedy, as if punishment by God. Other times meaningful spiritual experiences that have been forgotten or dismissed can be remembered, validated, and integrated as inspiration into the patient's future life.

The act of forgiveness is a letting go of blame, judgment, or condemnation. When forgiveness is achieved the person may feel relief and a resolution of resentments, obsessive rumination, and/or a desire to punish the self or the other.

The role of forgiveness in the recovery process, for addiction, trauma, and dual diagnoses, is both fascinating and critical. There is usually a significant chaotic history preceding the entry point to recovery. The using history, whether short or long, is often defined as the "story." This story may have roots in fact, and it may also be a partially fictional construction, designed to protect the self from the pain of reality or accountability. This story, as told in treatment, is comprised of using behavior, and the primary and secondary consequences. The consequences of addiction include the emotional, physical, financial, familial, and possibly legal baggage, as well as the psychic spiritual wounds, all of which have accumulated exponentially overtime.

Achieving a healing state resides on forgiveness, self-forgiveness and the forgiveness of others, the recovering addict may have blamed. Forgiveness needs to happen, whether or not the judgments are accurate or misperceived. Skipping, ignoring, or avoiding this essential aspect of healing may delay or retard the potential of an individual to experience liberation. With forgiveness, of the self and the other, the chains of excessive anger, self-loathing, and blame are diminished or resolved completely. It is also important to note that a premature or pretend act of forgiveness may not achieve the same depth of healing, if any at all, yet taking action can start the process and pave the way to later resolution.

This aspect of psychologic health clearly impacts both the physical as well as the mental aspects of health and well-being. How to achieve forgiveness may require professional guidance, mentorship, journal writing, hypnotherapy, art therapy, and specialized approaches such as RADIX, sacred drama, or ceremony. Whatever is needed in this regard should be overseen by a professional, possibly an interfaith pastoral counselor or certified spiritual director, guiding the therapeutic soul work.

Twelve-step approaches incorporate a forgiveness element, and direct approaches other than 12-step may achieve the same result as therapeutic interventions. Other practices that are able to foster spiritual healing and forgiveness include: CBT, group interventions, family therapy, shamanic nature-based ceremonies, and other established as well as non-traditional modalities.

Irrespective of how forgiveness is facilitated, specific neuroanatoamy correlates have been identified associated with the act of forgiveness. Conclusions in this study included the following: "In summary, our study explored for the first time the neural correlates of forgiveness. We observed a link between forgiveness and subjective relief, which supports its use in therapeutic settings as an aid for the promotion of mental health. We observed activation in a brain cortical network responsible for perspective taking processes, appraisal and empathy, suggesting that these processes may play an important role in the adaptive extinction of negative affect and prevention of potential aggressive and socially unacceptable behavior."[23]

## Life and Soul Purpose

Recognizing one's individual life purpose is an important element that is not taught or emphasized in traditional education, even in advanced professional realms. Life meaning has been documented, in peer-reviewed studies, to be part of the critical construct for quality of life metrics by the World Health Organization. Other important elements critical for quality of life and sobriety are stress reduction, spirituality, 12-step programs, and strong social support. The cause of addiction is multifactorial and the same may be said of the lifelong recovery process that extends far beyond abstinence, detox, and the discontinuation of alcohol or drug/substance use.[24]

Creating a synchronous life with alignment of the life purpose allows an ease of movement of energy. Malalignment hinders flow, enhances recurrent hurdles and creates or is associated with a much more difficult path. The use of self-recognition, meditation for guidance and mentorship and professional therapy are some ways to check for the presence of alignment. In shamanic traditions, concepts such as destiny retrieval are used to aid in picking correct life choices that are energetically aligned to the soul's purpose. These are not usual and customary Western concepts and therefore are not taught or discussed in traditional medical training. It is through the prism of medical anthropology that we have an opportunity to learn about these wisdom based traditions embedded within the cosmology and teachings of ancient civilizations applicable still today even in our own technocratic cultural existence.

The Western civilization model for life purpose is based on picking career paths based on interest, or ability, or perhaps financial factors, and less frequently on global or social impact. Integrating an individual life or soul's purpose for the average individual(s) is neither addressed nor contemplated consciously. The indigenous cultures of the Americas do, however, address these concepts and teach that an alignment of the life or soul's purpose creates the necessary balance to achieve happiness and a global effectiveness for the greater good and planet. Ancient cultures have used these spiritually based principals anchored in the concepts that humans are part of the greater energetic cosmology of the planet and that an interconnectedness exists. Whether this is a global consciousness or not, the truth is we are physically sharing the planet earth and its resources. According to the shamanic traditions, humans hold no higher position or place than the planet or its animal inhabitants.

The cosmology of the Quero of the high Andes, descendants of the Inca, believe bringing into balance means thinking and acting in a way that includes the entire collective, the Pachamama, or Mother Earth.[25] Alignment of one's path with a synchronous life purpose enhances the balance of work, family, career, volunteer choices, future activities, donation of time, money, and resources—which makes sense based upon on this unique alignment. Recognizing and learning of the existence of these patterns is an awakening not necessarily guaranteed to everyone, only those who seek it.

Inherent in leading a life of purpose, meaning, and embodied with emotional well-being is the challenge to balance various aspects of life demands that include work or professional activities with personal time involving family, relationships and just one's own personal downtime to decompress. Not surprisingly, recovering individuals can be overzealous in their work life and therefore recognizing the need for balance is important to sustain an emotionally balanced life. While this challenge may be easier said than done, focus on one's personal emotional, mental, physical, and spiritual needs helps align the work compass with the boundaries toward learning and practicing self-care in all areas.

Ancient spiritual traditions appear to be a perfect construct to challenge and address the extreme compartmentalization of contemporary man. These spiritual approaches are clearly important as culture-specific interventions but do not have to be limited to ethnic groups. For those who have a history of religious abuse, the exploration of world religions and spiritual practices may help circumvent, repair, or resolve the rift between self and spirit. There is no correlation between one specific religion or belief system with regard to long-term sobriety; the important aspect appears to be the presence of a spiritual practice of some form.[26]

The use of the Traditional Native American Interventions, as represented by the medicine wheel's interpretation of the mental, physical, spiritual, and emotional aspects of the human psyche, is a useful paradigm to depict imbalances and consequent dysfunction in decision making that hold true in active addiction patterns.[27]

Balancing personal life and work life is a process worth perfecting. Workaholic behavior, another obsessive-compulsive activity, while transiently useful takes its toll on relationships, creates isolation, and decreases opportunities to participate in healthy activities. Working toward this balance in short-, mid-, and long-term recovery plans makes sense for the recovering individual. Furthermore, in a cohort study in Japan of 757 participants showed that workaholic patterns decrease positive health metrics while not significantly improving performance outcomes.[28] This is a lose-lose scenario.

# Giving Back

The Helper Theory Principle (HTP), as noted in AA, has been found to be effective in reducing the egocentrism commonly noted in those who have developed problems with alcoholism drug addiction.[29] The HTP model has been used as part of the treatment protocol for various issues such as depression and multiple sclerosis, and it has been targeted for use in youth-related drug rehabilitation and treatment formats. HTP has anthropologic roots, has transcultural relevance from the "wounded healer" model written about from the North American Indian traditions, and extrapolated to AA in the literature.[30] The progression of HTP to volunteer work and mentoring are natural progressions consistent with levels of the HTP activity model.

Picking one's "cause" or charity or expression of gratitude then becomes a personalized choice that follows the HTP model. This enhances personalization of life meaning once again and is in balanced coordination with an overall plan for emotional, physical, and spiritual health.

Becoming an empowered, healed individual by using the past wound or trauma experience to leverage and utilize the attained knowledge with self-realized concepts such as "this can be overcome" and "I can heal" is one step. The trick is then to use this inner truth for the good of others. The wounded cuts a path of healing for others who are stuck in the mire of their psychic injury and cannot always, on their own, see the forest for the trees. Joseph Campbell wrote in his book *The Hero with a Thousand Faces* a story of the wounded warrior becoming the greatest healer—a story that manifests and recurs thematically over and over through the millennia, transculturally embodying this transformational process. It is the mythic journey. Life creates the impetus of transformation via a mentor—a "supernatural being or "God(dess)"—and through the depths (addiction bottom) the magical transformation occurs. This phase of atonement follows the transformative metamorphosis that cycles into the return of the formerly wounded. The process leads to a transferable self-healing, capable of being bestowed upon others who also seek the knowledge and are on their own quest. Thus, the wounded healer concept is born.[31] The concept of the "original wound" in an individual's road to recovery is worthy of mention. Joseph Campbell's construct of the mythologic healing journey moves from the wounded state through a metamorphosis and subsequent transformative, mentor-driven awakening that embodies the universal past wound healing process.

In one's mythic life journey, the "weakness" or "wounded state" allows a severe liability to be transformed into a formidable strength when proper consciousness, acceptance, and responsibility are seized by the individual in their individual life's vision quest. The person, whether through a 12-step program or not, has the capacity to embody this same transformative paradigm. If one utilizes a 12-step approach, the recovering person can recount their past experiences, accept their personal role, and take responsibility while seeking a new path. In effect, this is the transformative mythic journey applied to a 12-step model. The degree to which a recovering individual embraces the aspect of helping others creates the opportunity to transform the original wounded sick and suffering addict to an empowered messenger of hope for others. This process is a self-embodiment of the death-rebirth lifecycle enumerated by ancient civilizations and within the cosmology of many indigenous peoples about which Campbell and others have written. Jungian archetypes of the super consciousness have been referenced and used with modern psychologic and psychiatric models of therapy and hinge upon some of these healing images to communicate universal conscious and subconscious imagery. For the recovering individual, following this pattern of personalized life details is one possible route to consider in the journey of healing the original wound of their life experience and even of family of origin.

## Creating a Healing Treatment Plan or Journey

Creation of the healing treatment plan or journey is a personal and individualized process that considers the type of addiction, age, comorbid clinical situations including potential dual diagnosis and comorbid medical conditions we have previously discussed. The journey of the recovering patient is a long-term plan, not merely a short-term one involving acute detox and a 90-day treatment. Long-term treatment has a role in selected cases, but long-term planning of the corresponding life journey is an optimal consideration for all recovering patients, their physician and recovery health team. Ongoing adjustments to increase, modify, or change directions of the plan require the treating physician(s), patient, family, and recovery team to utilize ongoing assessment tools. Identifying the life purpose of the individual as part of that plan formulation enhances the focus to create a dual recovery and life recovery process that is dynamic.

The surgeon general of the United States, General Vivek Murthy, has made emotional well-being one of his priorities and spoke about its importance at the Aspen Ideas Festival in 2016. He outlined exercise, meditation, and gratitude exercises along with meaningful social connections as key elements in developing and maintaining emotional well-being and enhancing its preventative benefits for both physical and mental health and happiness.[32]

Maintenance practices for emotional well-being and balance include these practices and strategies. The addition of stress management strategies utilizing mind-body therapies, consistent and regular meditation, yoga, spirituality, guided imagery, biofeedback, and hypnosis are all tools previously noted and effective for recovery and addiction patients[15,26] as well as the general populations for preventative medicine benefits. Daily self-reflection, meditation, and or breath work are useful activates to perform during this time to maximize the calming benefit of reduction in catecholamine, improved heart-rate variability and decreased sympathetic tone from the day's stress.

## Conclusion

Comprehensive integrated treatment, as defined by our chapter, creates a capacity for healing that reaches levels beyond a mere return to prior functioning. We acknowledge that this is a life-long pathway that requires proactive and dynamic participation by the patient and the health professional.

### REFERENCES

1. NIDA. NIDA Info Facts: Understanding Drug Abuse and Addiction. 2008.
2. Anton RF, Oroszi G, O'Malley S, Couper D, Swift R, Pettinati H, Goldman D. An evaluation of mu-opioid receptor (OPRM1) as a predictor of naltrexone response in the treatment of alcohol dependence: results from the Combined Pharmacotherapies and Behavioral Interventions for Alcohol Dependence (COMBINE) study. *Archives of General Psychiatry.* 2008;65(2):135–144. doi: 10.1001/archpsyc.65.2.135.
3. Vernot, B, Akey JM, *Resurrecting surviving neanderthal lineages from modern human genomes. Science.* 2014;343(6174):1017–1021.
4. Sears B, Ricordi C, Anti-inflammatory nutrition as a pharmacological approach to treat obesity. *Journal of Obesity.* 2011 (2011), Article ID 431985, 14 page. doi:10.1155/2011/431985.
5. Fan AZ, et al. Patterns of alcohol consumption and the metabolic syndrome. *The Journal of Clinical Endocrinology and Metabolism.* 2008;93(10):3833–3838.
6. Bau PFD, Bau CH, Rosito GA, et al. Alcohol consumption, cardiovascular health, and endothelial function markers, 2007. *Alcohol.* 2007;41(7):479–488.
7. Rehm J, Taylor B, Room R, Global burden of disease from alcohol, illicit drugs and tobacco. *Journal of Drug and Alcohol Review.* 2006;25(6):505–513.
8. Lim SS, Vos T, Flaxman AD, et al. A comparative risk assessment of burden of disease and injury attributable to 67 risk factors and risk factor clusters in 21 regions, 1990–2010: a systematic analysis for the Global Burden of Disease Study. *The Lancet.* 2010;380(9859):2224–2260.
9. Lyle M-H. The reclassification of sugar as a drug. *Lethbridge Undergraduate Research Journal.* 2006;1(1).
10. Rada P, Avena MN, Hoebel GB. Daily bingeing on sugar repeatedly releases dopamine in the accumbens shell. *Neuroscience.* 2005;134:737–744.
11. Chopra K, et al. Alcoholic neuropathy: possible mechanisms and future treatment possibilities. *British Journal of Social and Clinical Pharmacology.* 2012;73(3):348–362.

12. Bevilacqua, L, Goldman, D., Genes and addiction. *Clinical Pharmacology Theraphy.* 2009;85(4):359–361.

13. Kendler KS, Schmitt E, Aggen SH, Prescott CA. Genetic and environmental influences on alcohol, caffeine, cannabis, and nicotine use from early adolescence to middle adulthood. *Archives of General Psychiatry.* 2008;65(6): 674–682.

14. Goldman D, Oroszi G, Ducci F. The genetics of addictions: uncovering the genes. *Nature Reviews Genetics.* 2005;6(7):521–532.

15. Oxford Dictionary. 2017. Definition of healing. https://en.oxforddictionaries.com/definition/healing/

16. Egnew TR. LICSW the meaning of healing: transcending suffering. *Annals of Family Medicine.* 2005;3(3):255–262.

17. O'Brien RP. *Eco-Health & the Continuum of Care.* Boston: The Center for English Language Arts; 2016.

18. https://integrativemedicine.arizona.edu/

19. Reiss M, Sandborn WJ. The role of psychosocial care in adapting to health care reform. *Clinical Gastroenerology and Hepatology.* 2015;13(13):2219–2224.

20. Dube SR, Felitti VJ, Dong M, Chapman DP, Giles WH, Anda RF. Childhood abuse, neglect and household dysfunction and the risk of illicit drug use: The adverse childhood experience study. *Pediatrics.*2003;111(3):564–572.

21. Ricciardi E, Rota G, Sani L, et al. How the brain heals emotional wounds: the functional neuroanatomy of forgiveness. *Frontiers in Human Neuroscience.* 2013;7:839. doi:10.3389/fnhum.2013.00839.

22. Naiman R. Insomnia. In: Raykel, D., *Integrative Medicine* 3rd ed. Elselvier: Philadelphia, PA, 2012: 65–76.

23. Ricciardi E, Rota G, Sani, L, et al. How the brain heals emotional wounds: the functional neuroanatomy of forgiveness. *Frontiers in Human Neuroscience.* 2013;7:839. doi:10.3389/fnhum.2013.00839.

24. Laudet A, Morgen K, White WL, et al. The role of social supports, spirituality, religiousness, life meaning and affiliation with 12-step fellowships in quality of life satisfaction among individuals in recovery from alcohol and drug problems. *Alcohol Treat Q.* 2006;24(1–2):33–73.

25. Villoldo A. *Shaman, Healer.* 1st ed. New York: Harmony House; 2000.

26. Warne D. Alcoholism and substance abuse. In: Rakel D., *Integrative Medicine.* 3rd ed. Philadelphia, PA: Elsevier Saunders; 2012:746–756.

27. McGaa EEM. *Mother Earth Spirituality: Native American Paths to Healing Ourselves and Our World.* San Francisco: Harper & Row; 1989.

28. Shimaz A. How does workaholism affect worker health and performance? The mediating role of coping. *International Journal of Behavioral Medicine.* 2010;17(2):154–160.

29. Pagano M, Post S, Johnsons SM. Alcoholics anonymous-related helping and the helper therapy principle. *Alcohol Treat Q.* 2010;29(1):23–34.

30. White WL. The history of recovered people as wounded healers: from Native America to the rise of the modern alcoholism movement. *Alcoholism Treatment Quarterly*. 2000;18:1–23.
31. Campbell J. *The Hero with a Thousand Faces*. Princeton, NJ: Princeton University Press; 1949.
32. Facing Addiction in America: The Surgeon General's Report on Alcohol, Drugs, and Health, https://addiction.surgeongeneral.gov/surgeon-generals-report.pdf

# 27

## Integrative Approaches to the Management of Chronic Pain and Substance Abuse

LYNETTE M. PUJOL, BETTINA HERBERT, CYNTHIA M. A. GEPPERT, AND KAREN E. CARDON

### Introduction

This chapter is a merging of 2 prior works in the Weil Medical Library series: the respective pain chapters from *Integrative Psychiatry* and from *Integrative Pain Management.* The unique perspective represents the spectrum of clinical options available in approaching chronic pain of non-cancer origin in this unique at-risk population. Neither chapter alone is sufficient to cover the complexity of issues related to the recovering individual. Evidence-based options are offered for chronic pain management and the blended approach gives the clinician a framework with which to approach chronic pain management in addiction and recovery realms. Our hope is to deliver the best integrative approaches for care of these complex patients who require a high degree of individualized care in their approach to pain, addiction, and recovery.

There is no area of medicine in which integrative pain management is more crucial than in the treatment of comorbid addiction. Historically there has been a deleterious separation of the pain and addiction communities with little common ground in clinical training, fundamental assumptions, approaches to patient treatment, or even medical language. Health-care professionals have for decades been caught in the gulf that divided the two camps. In the late 1990s hospitals and regulatory agencies began to emphasize that pain was the "5th vital sign" and admonished clinicians for providing inadequate relief of chronic pain.[1] At the same time, practitioners were sent the public health message to join the campaign to prevent drug abuse and the diversion of controlled substances.[2] Attempts to close the gap between the 2 groups began with the landmark agreement of the American

Academy of Pain Medicine, the American Pain Society, and the American Society of Addiction Medicine on consensus definitions of basic terms, such as addiction, dependence, and tolerance.[3] The consensus definition of addiction is as follows:

> Addiction is a primary, chronic, neurobiological disease, with genetic, psychosocial, and environmental factors influencing its development and manifestations. It is characterized by behaviors that include one or more of the following: impaired control of drug use, compulsive use, continued use despite harm, and craving.[4]

The epidemic of opioid addiction and overdose deaths provided tragic momentum to the movement to integrate pain and addiction, education, practice, and research. In this chapter, we describe the problems that arise when the patient with co-occurring pain and addiction is treated in separate, parallel, or even sequential models of care and the benefits of a comprehensive, continuity-of-care approach. We suggest that the most advantageous center for this cooperative care is the primary-care setting, where the majority of patients with chronic pain and addiction are seen.[5]

Additionally another overall goal of this chapter is to expand the number of tools available to physicians for regaining perceived higher self-efficacy and self-regulation and to reduce the impact of pain and suffering of patients with chronic pain and addiction. Selected integrative medicine modalities for the treatment of chronic nonmalignant pain will be reviewed. Modalities were chosen primarily because of empirical support, although some reviewed here are promising areas of treatment or research.

## Pain and Addiction

There is no scholarly consensus on the prevalence of co-occurring chronic pain and addiction. Estimates vary widely depending on study methodology and setting, ranging from 3% to 30%.[6] In considering options for the integrative treatment of pain and addiction, the practitioner must recognize that there is a scarcity of reliable evidence-based guidance. Wachholtz et al, in a comprehensive review of both psychological and pharmacological treatments for pain and opioid addiction, concluded that "there are extremely few empirically validated treatments."[6] Fortunately, there is burgeoning clinical and basic research on treatment of pain and addiction, expert opinion, and consensus guidelines to support the best practice recommendations presented here.[7]

Emerging evidence as well as clinical experience shows that separate silos or series of pain and addiction treatment are at best frequently unsuccessful and at worst sometimes harmful. In primary care, scarcity of time, lack of access to pain and addiction training and expertise, clinician discomfort, poor reimbursement, and lack of referral sources generate and perpetuate the ghettoization of treatment.[8] When only the chronic pain is treated, especially with a purely pharmacological approach, the patient with an unappreciated current or historical SUD may develop aberrant behavior or dependence on the prescribed medications, particularly opioids and ben-zodiazepines.[9] Conversely, patients with comorbid pain and addiction who receive only substance-use treatment are highly likely to relapse and resort to the use of alcohol or cannabis, or they purchase opioids illicitly in an attempt to relieve their pain.[10] Pseudoaddiction is a paradigmatic example of the limitations and adverse consequences stemming from segregated programs providing fragmented care.[11] The beleaguered PCP under time pressure prescribes an inadequate pain regimen to the patient with legitimate neck or back pain. The patient with uncontrolled pain overtakes the drug and, running out early, requests a refill. The PCP, fearing legal or professional sanctions and with an inadequate knowledge base for how to handle such a situation, stops the prescription and refers the patient to substance-use treatment. At this point, the patient may travel a variety of undesirable public health and psychosocial trajectories, such as borrowing drugs from family or friends, resorting to alcohol or street drugs, unemployment and disability, and associated interpersonal and familial stresses and strains that further weaken the social fabric.[12] Box 27.1 illustrates this dynamic.

Similarly, failure to appropriately assess and aggressively treat anxiety, depression, and other common comorbid psychiatric conditions in this population can lead to self-medication with prescribed and illicit drugs and alcohol, poor response to standard therapies, and reluctance to participate in physical, rehabilitative and psychological therapies.[10,13] Pain practitioners, especially those relying mainly on interventional modalities, often lack the requisite knowledge and skill to diagnose, treat, and monitor addiction or psychiatric conditions. Addiction medicine and psychiatry professionals may not have the competence or comfort to identify and care for chronic pain complaints, even if they have facility with mental health conditions.[10] The result, to paraphrase W.B. Yeats, is that "things fall apart, the patient center does not hold"[14] and individual patients and their families may feel confused, demoralized, and frustrated with the lack of coordination of care and the adverse consequences such as frequent emergency department visits, multiple providers, excess of procedures and costs, drug interactions, and polypharmacy. In such divided houses of treatment, nonadherence, treatment failures, professional suspicion and tension, and death from unintentional overdose or suicide may be more likely.[15]

## Approach to the Patient

For there to be a joining of pain and addiction forces in the primary-care setting, 2 formidable walls blocking the construction of a therapeutic physician-patient relationship must be broken down: deficient knowledge and stigmatizing attitudes. There is a dearth of education in both pain and addiction in health professionals' training.[16,17] Unfortunately, despite the scientific understanding of pain, addiction, and psychiatric disorders as treatable chronic diseases, they remain stigmatized conditions in our society.[18] Within medical culture, pain and addiction patients are considered "difficult," a word that can express a practitioner's lack of confidence in treating these challenging patients and/or pejorative and judgmental views of these patients.[19] Those with clinical expertise working with this population have learned that empathic listening, compassionate but clear and consistent limit setting, and acceptance of patient vulnerability—balanced with the ability to be accountable—can lead to rewarding clinical interactions and enhanced self-efficacy on the part of both patient and practitioner.[20]

Yet both addiction and pain management have evolved to be inherently interprofessional collaborations of multiple specialties including nursing, pharmacy, medicine, psychology, social work, anesthesia, physical medicine, chiropractic, among many others. Leading scientific and professional organizations such as the Institute of Medicine have designated inter- and multidisciplinary pain management as the best practice for patients with chronic noncancer pain (CNCP).[21] Similarly, it is now widely recognized that coordinated, integrated treatment of comorbid substance use and mental health conditions is the optimal form of treatment.[22] It is logical to presume that integrative care would also be the most promising form of care for patients with co-occurring chronic pain, addiction, and psychiatric disorders. One of the few outcome studies to test this presumption is a 2003 study by Currie et al of a ten-week pain management group for patients with chronic pain and SUDs. The forty-four patients who participated in the group demonstrated improvement in pain, emotional distress, coping style, and reduction in medication.[23] A recent article demonstrates how integrative treatment can be provided within a primary-care setting. Brensilver et al describe a primary-care clinic at an academic medical center that shows the benefits for patients of a collaborative effort of primary care physicians, addiction medicine, and behavioral medicine operating within a medical home model.[24] Within a Veterans Affairs Medical Center, we have established a clinic within primary care, the Co-Occurring Disorders Clinic (CODC), which provides integrated care for patients with comorbid CNCP, addiction, and psychiatric problems from a chronic disease perspective. CODC reported outcome data for 143 veterans with chronic pain and opioid dependence managed with buprenorphine/naloxone. Ninety-three patients were successfully retained in treatment and reported modest but statistically significant improvements in pain levels.[25]

## Assessment of Pain

A thorough assessment of pain should precede and guide treatment planning. Conventional assessment involves a physical and a detailed musculoskeletal, neurologic, and mental status evaluation.[26] Pain intensity is generally measured in the clinical setting using a Numerical Rating Scale[27] ranging from 0 (no pain) to 10 (pain as bad as it can be). Common time points for measurement are the patient's current pain, and the most and least pain experienced during a 1-week period prior to the assessment. The following aspects of the pain experience are important to assess: the frequency and description of pain; patterns of pain; alleviating and exacerbating factors; previous treatments and their efficacy; current treatments and their efficacy; current physical, social, emotional, and occupational functioning; current coping techniques; and expectations for treatment.[28] Standardized instruments for the measurement of pain, mood, and functioning may also supplement the evaluation.

Assessment from an integrative medicine perspective includes standard assessment, as well as a whole person assessment. Some evaluations for integrative modalities are dependent on the treatment for which the person is evaluated. For example, traditional Chinese acupuncture involves a system of belief whereby energy is moved along meridians in the body. Therefore, assessment from this perspective would include an evaluation for blocked energy and a recommendation for its movement.

## Assessment and Management
## of Chronic Pain in Addiction

Nothing is more debated in the treatment of chronic noncancer pain than the role of opioids, and it is even more controversial in patients with historical or current addiction. Although addiction to stimulants, alcohol, nicotine, and other drugs is certainly of concern in the CNCP patient, opioids have been the subject of the most recent research and will be the primary focus of this overview. Our clinical experience supports the view of those experts who contend that opioid medications can be safely and beneficially used in a subgroup of patients with co-occurring pain and addiction.[7] Key to the responsible use of opioids in this population is the use of reliable screening tools as part of a comprehensive history; opioid *agreements* that cover rights and responsibilities of *both* the practitioner and patient as distinct from opioid *contracts* that can be unilateral, paternalistic, and coercive; regular and routine monitoring through toxicology screens, pill counts, and checking of

**Box 27.1 Risk Management for Opioids in Co-occurring Pain and Addiction**

- Obtain a full addiction/substance use history
- Obtain family history, including substance-use disorders
- Obtain psychiatric history, including anxiety, depression, history of suicide attempts
- Use validated risk tool to formally assess risk (SOAPP-R°, COMM°)[34,35]
- Urine toxicology, frequency adjusted to risk
- State prescription drug monitoring program checks, frequency adjusted to risk
- Pill counts, frequency adjusted to risk
- Participation in relapse prevention, 12-step programs, or other substance treatment

prescription monitoring programs. Research shows low utilization of these risk-assessment and reduction techniques among primary care practitioners.[29] A multidisciplinary opioid-renewal clinic co-located in primary care demonstrated the efficacy of these strategies in reducing aberrant behavior.[30] Although the evidence is not definitive, consensus guidelines favor the use of long-acting opioid preparations dosed in a scheduled rather than as-needed manner as providing more sustained pain relief with less likelihood of reinforcing aberrant behavior.[7,31] Box 27.1 outlines risk management strategies for chronic pain and addiction.

For those patients who develop or present with opioid dependence that have been unable to control their use of prescription opioid agonists even with close monitoring, there is early research demonstrating the efficacy of buprenorphine/naloxone for selected patients with chronic noncancer pain and opioid dependence.[25]

Nonopioid adjunctive medications are frequently neglected but important alternatives in this population, especially for neuropathic conditions. Disorders such a fibromyalgia that are challenging to treat and have substantial psychosomatic components and frequent concomitant substance use often respond well with fewer side effects or risk of addiction to anticonvulsants, such as pregabalin and gabapentin; antidepressants such as venlafaxine and duloxetine; and topicals such as lidocaine.[32]

Neither medications nor interventional procedures alone are sufficient for the efficacious treatment of chronic pain and addiction.[33] Among psychological modalities, CBT, both individual and group, has the strongest track record for CNCP and addiction as distinct disorders and would be expected to also be beneficial in patients with the combined conditions.[20] Primary goals of CBT in each of these cohorts is behavioral activation to combat depression; relaxation to manage anxiety; prosocial rewarding pursuits as alternatives to passivity, withdrawal, and use of substances; and fostering of self-confidence and competence that can replace externalizing and passive-aggressive coping styles.

## Integrative Approach to Chronic Pain

Below is a selective overview of several integrative approaches to the treatment of chronic pain, including research where available to describe efficacy. In using an integrative approach with patients, the goal is to create a larger understanding of the mind/body and its relationship to pain with an effort to create harmony and functionality.

## Mind–Body Interventions

### PSYCHOPHYSIOLOGIC INTERVENTIONS

Diaphragmatic breathing, progressive and autogenic relaxation, and biofeedback are modalities that involve making the patient aware of the ability to exert control over physiologic processes of they are not normally aware of (e.g., skin temperature, muscle tension, respiration). Progressive muscle relaxation involves tensing and relaxing various muscle groups.[36] Autogenic relaxation involves sensing tension or tightness in various muscle groups and mentally "letting go" of the tension while engaging in diaphragmatic breathing. Biofeedback uses a device or computer to give information about these functions. Psychophysiologic interventions are critical for patients with pain, since patients tend to hold muscles tight around the pain site, bracing against painful sensations. This bracing produces increased muscle tension and pain. These techniques can also aid sleep and reduce emotional reactivity. Outcomes for relaxation and biofeedback are generally positive for patients with chronic pain conditions. A recent review of relaxation strategies for acute and chronic pain found a significant, positive effect on pain in 8 of 15 studies reviewed.[36] A dose-response relationship occurred, with more studies showing effectiveness when relaxation was taught and practiced over several sessions.[37] When combined with relaxation training, individuals with migraine and or tension-type headaches show a 50%–55% success rate in reducing pain.[38] A review of mind–body therapies found that relaxation and thermal biofeedback are effective for recurrent migraine headaches and relaxation and electromyography biofeedback are effective for recurrent tension headache.[39]

### GUIDED IMAGERY

Guided imagery may be paired with diaphragmatic breathing and/or autogenic relaxation techniques. Imagery may be distracting in nature (e.g., a beach or meadow); focused (e.g., imagining white blood cells destroying cancer cells); or as a form of mental rehearsal (e.g., performing physical therapy exercises).[40]

In a meta-analytic review, imagery techniques were shown to be helpful in reducing painful sensations and had the highest rates of efficacy among 12 placebo-controlled trials of other cognitive interventions.[41] Guided imagery studies with older adults show good preliminary results when paired with relaxation[42] or alone.[43]

## HYPNOSIS

Hypnosis is defined as "a state of inner absorption, concentration and focused attention" by the American Society of Clinical Hypnosis. Hypnosis for pain generally involves the suggestion of pain reduction but may also involve a variety of positive outcomes (e.g., increased activity). A National Institutes of Health Technology Panel found strong support for hypnosis in the reduction of pain (NIH, 1996). Hypnosis has been found to improve recovery time after surgery when it is learned and performed preoperatively and to improve postsurgical pain.[39] A review and a meta-analysis found that hypnosis was an effective analgesic for many types of experimental and clinical pain conditions,[44] including chronic pain from headache, cancer, fibromyalgia, osteoarthritis, lower back pain, tempromandibular pain disorder, disability-related pain, and mixed chronic pain problems.[45] When hypnosis was compared with relaxation therapy for osteoarthritis, both groups improved, but the hypnosis group was the only one that maintained improvement at 3 months.[46] No differences were found at the 6-month mark.

## Mindfulness Meditation

Mindfulness meditation involves paying attention to the present moment with a nonjudgmental attitude and fosters disengagement from strong attachments to thoughts and emotions.[47] Mindfulness meditation has been studied as a part of the Mindfulness-Based Stress Reduction (MBSR) program, an 8-week group that teaches the technique. MBSR has been found to be helpful for patients with a variety of chronic pain conditions,[48] with a 4-year follow-up showing pain improvement in 60–72% of participants.[49] Two reviews of MBSR found that MBSR has positive outcomes in stress, anxiety, depression, and pain.[50,51] MBSR was recently studied for a group of older adults with chronic lower back pain. Compared to a wait-list control group, participants in the 8-week program had significant improvement in pain acceptance and in physical functioning, although the groups did not differ in pain ratings.[52]

Mindfulness-Based Art Therapy (MBAT) is a relatively new intervention that combines MBSR with art therapy. This program has been shown to be successful with women with breast cancer in decreasing psychological distress and enhancing quality of life.[53,54] Although no studies to date have implemented MBAT for persons with chronic pain, this therapy remains promising for this population.

## COGNITIVE BEHAVIORAL THERAPY

CBT is used to describe a broad array of cognitive and behavioral techniques that derive from different therapeutic models. Cognitive therapy[55] posits that automatic thoughts, underlying dysfunctional assumptions, cognitive distortions, and emotion interact in a reinforcing cycle that leads to psychopathology.[56] These thoughts influence mood and behavior. For example, a person with pain might wake up noticing increased pain. An automatic thought might be, "It's going to be a bad pain day." This thought can lead to negative mood and increasingly negative cognitions such as, "I'm going to have to cancel everything today. I can't do anything any more." The cycle perpetuates increased negative emotion and potentially maladaptive behavior (e.g., staying in bed all day).

Behavioral treatment methods for pain grew from operant research. Fordyce described the application to pain, focusing on pain behaviors, such as guarding, limping, taking medication, and resting.[57] Fordyce posited that contingencies in the environment maintained pain behaviors and that changing reinforcement would change attention to painful experiences. For example, an overly solicitous spouse might be taught to give less attention to pain behaviors and more attention to times of increased physical activity, thereby decreasing the frequency of pain behavior and increasing the frequency of more adaptive strategies.

A number of cognitive and behavioral strategies are combined in CBT. Behavioral strategies, such as helping a patient learn to pace activities and teaching relaxation techniques, are common. Numerous studies have found CBT effective for patients with chronic pain. A meta-analysis of 25 randomized controlled trials of CBT compared to wait-list control conditions found improved pain, mood, coping, pain behavior, and social interactions. When compared to alternative treatments, CBT participants had greater improvements in pain, coping, and pain behavior.[58]

CBT with patients with pain conditions is an active therapy that is generally short term (usually 6–12 weeks). It has demonstrated effectiveness with pain, as well as with depression and anxiety, both of which may affect people with pain. Patients are expected to be active participants in therapy and are often assigned "homework" to facilitate accomplishing therapeutic goals.[56] Therapeutic goals might be reducing pain, depression, anxiety or stress, and/or increasing daily activity, sleep, pain-coping skills, and purpose in life. Difficulties in relationships caused by changes brought on by pain may also be the focus of intervention. Identifying and changing maladaptive thoughts, emotions, and behaviors are central to the process of change in CBT.

## CONTEXTUAL CBT

A newer approach to working with patients with pain is contextual CBT.[59] The therapy addresses a criticism of CBT, namely that thinking about thoughts or physical sensations and trying not to focus on them only makes them stronger. Avoidance is conceptualized as potentially helpful in the short term but ultimately ineffective. A common application for people with pain conditions is physical exercise or activity; that is, avoiding activity can reduce painful sensations and rein- force inactivity, ultimately producing a maladaptive response to painful sensations.

CCBT aims to help patients with pain by moving away from attempts to manage or control pain and toward acceptance of the present reality of thoughts, emotions, behaviors, and physical sensations. First steps involve helping the person review historical efforts to control or manage painful sensations. Awareness of responses by significant others is also discussed. Mindful awareness and exercises that in- troduce the concept of noticing in the present moment are central to the pro- cess of defusing cognitions.[59] Through the course of therapy, patients practice experiencing emotions without need for a response. Additionally, the therapy includes a values-based action component in which the person with pain clarifies his or her values and begins to make value-based life choices.[59]

## PAIN-COPING STRATEGIES

There is a large literature on the use of pain-coping strategies, which are assessed by several coping measures. Some ways of coping with pain are guarding the af- fected painful part, resting, taking medication, ignoring painful sensations, using coping self-statements (e.g., "I can handle the pain"), praying and hoping the pain will be better, increasing activities, diverting attention from the pain, and catastrophizing. Coping has been linked to some pain treatment outcomes but not strongly to others such as exercise.[60] A recent follow-up study compared scores on coping and belief measures at posttreatment, and 1 year following treatment in a multidisciplinary pain treatment program. The investigators found that increasing disability and depression at follow-up was positively associated with increased use of resting, guarding, and asking for assistance, catastrophizing, and the belief that one is disabled by pain.[61]

# Body-Mind Therapies

The Platonic-Cartesian mind-body duality model, with separate specialties to treat 1 entity, has shaped the biomedical profession. Most mental health professionals do not touch their patients, and most physical medicine specialists, such as osteopathic physicians, chiropractors, physical therapists, and other hands-on care providers do not provide counseling. The patient must know enough to consult both, separately, for what is essentially a unified issue. In day-to-day practice, the two specialists often do not confer or collaborate, even though it is now well known that pain is a physical and psychological event, as reviewed above. Within the integrative model, mind and body are inseparable, which is why addressing psychological distress is almost universal to any integrative medicine treatment plan. With regard to pain issues, there are therapeutic approaches under the umbrella of CAM that address body and mind primarily through manual manipulation of the physical structure (i.e., manipulative and body-based therapies), and we review a few that have particular relevance to integrative medicine.

## OSTEOPATHIC MANIPULATIVE TREATMENT

For patients with 1 or multiple chronic neuromusculoskeletal or visceral conditions (osteoarthritis, cervicalgia, osteoporosis, lower back pain, irritable bowel syndrome, neurodegenerative disease), consulting an osteopathic physician trained in osteopathic manipulative treatment (OMT) may be a useful approach. In the United States, but not in Canada or Great Britain, osteopaths (DOs) have the same medical training as allopaths (MDs) with an additional emphasis on anatomical structure, physiology, and manipulation. There are some philosophical distinctions; for example, osteopathy contends that a body's structure affects its function, and, given proper alignment, the body will heal itself as much as possible. Good body biomechanics are integral to maintaining health. It is noted that OMT is not a component of many osteopathic physician practices, most of which now resemble allopathy more than classic osteopathic practice.

The emotional component of pain is part of osteopathic philosophy, and some manipulative techniques may produce cathartic emotional releases.[62] OMT provides many soft tissue (fascial) techniques that aim to effect changes that may be deep and long lasting. Manipulation, as part of a whole treatment approach, may be delivered either directly, up to and through tissue or joint restriction, or indirectly, following the direction of ease. The latter approach gradually allows the body (fascia, joint, muscle, bone, organ, spine) to release. Some of the most frequently used techniques include the following:

- *Myofascial release.* A technique designed that uses continual palpatory feedback to release myofascial tissues.[63]
- *Strain/counterstrain.* A system of diagnosis and indirect treatment in which somatic dysfunction is associated with a myofascial tenderpoint and treated by use of a passive position.[63]

- *Cranial osteopathy/craniosacral therapy.* A system of diagnosis and treatment that involves the primary respiratory system and balanced membranous tension.
- *Visceral manipulation.* A technique for releasing restrictions and adhesions in fascia suspending specific organs
- *Positional release.* A technique that uses leverage, ventilatory movement, and a fulcrum to mobilize a dysfunctional segment.[63]
- *Functional technique.* An indirect treatment that involves finding a dynamic balance point and applying a force, holding the postion or adding compression to allow for readjustment.[63]
- *High-velocity low amplitude (thrust).*Taking a joint up to its functional barrier and adding a slight force to restore range of motion.[63]

Osteopathic manipulative treatment has been found to be a useful modality for chronic pain. Three randomized trials of OMT have been conducted in the United States for individuals with chronic lower back pain.[64,65] Control groups generally received sham manipulation[65,66] or usual care.[64] Licciardone (2004) made 3 generalizations about these studies: (1) OMT appeared to reduce the use of other treatment modalities, such as medication and physical therapy; (2) OMT appeared more effective when compared to no-intervention controls and compared to sham manipulation control groups; and (3) clinical relevance of OMT may have been attenuated in these studies due to the relatively small number of subjects.

## MASSAGE

Therapeutic massage has been found to decrease pain, improve sleep, reduce muscle tension, and provide a sense of relaxation.[67] Massage can soften musculature and increase blood flow, promote restful sleep, release endorphins, and affect levels of catecholamines.[68] It is especially effective for pain relief when combined with exercise or physical therapy.

Massage has been tested in several randomized clinical trials, but all suffer from methodologic weaknesses.[69] A pilot study comparing MBSR or massage therapy to a standard care group for musculoskeletal pain found reduced pain unpleasantness and increased mental health status at 8 weeks.[70] Improved longer-term mental health status was found with MBSR compared to standard care. The authors concluded that massage was more effective at pain reduction and MBSR was more effective than massage in mood improvement.[70]

Contraindications for massage include deep vein thrombosis, burns, skin infections, eczema, open wounds, bone fractures, and advanced osteoporosis.

## POSTURAL/MOVEMENT RE-EDUCATION THERAPIES

Western movement approaches are often used by patients with chronic pain. Many share the therapeutic combination of passive therapy and active integration of that therapy using group classes, verbal cues, and gentle home exercises. Only a few of the more commonly used ones will be discussed here.

The Feldenkrais Method consists of a large variety of very gentle, simple exercises to develop new movement habits that are pain-free. The work consists of two parts: group movement lessons (Awareness Through Movement) and individual, hands-on sessions. Limited studies of the Feldenkrais Method suggest that it may be useful for anxiety, neck, and shoulder pain and both disability and anxiety in multiple sclerosis patients.[71]

The Alexander Technique, often used for chronic back and neck pain, uses verbal instructions and light touch to guide the patient to improve postural habits. Clinical trials are promising and small studies have also suggested benefits for reduction of both stress and chronic pain, enhanced relaxation as well as enhanced respiratory function.[72]

The Trager Psychophysical Integration approach also combines tablework and simple movement practices to release accumulated tension and help the patient learn ways of moving freely. Tablework consists of gentle movements to release restrictive holding patterns that create pain. Using "Mentastics," patients are taught to re-create the feelings of relaxation that they felt during the sessions. A recent study on the combination of the Trager Approach and acupuncture found that the treatment was effective in reducing shoulder pain in spinal cord injury patients.[73] It may also be effective in other musculoskeletal problems.

The Hellerwork practitioner, again, uses hands-on soft tissue manipulation techniques and educates the client about how to sit, stand, and walk in a more relaxed and comfortable way. Dysfunctional muscular holding patterns and diminished breathing may be addressed using therapeutic dialogue to address any emotional contribution.

## YOGA

Yoga is part of Ayurveda, an ancient medical system developed in India, that addresses the physical, mental, and spiritual aspects of the individual. There are many different forms of yoga practice, each of which emphasizes different skills, goals, and philosophies. For someone with pain, a gentle type is recommended. Postures may be adjusted to meet the needs and physical conditions of the student. Therapeutic yoga is the performance of postures for treating medical disorders.[74]

Though preliminary, there are a few studies that suggest useful applications of therapeutic yoga practice for lower back pain[75] and osteoarthritis of the knee.[76] Another pilot study in breast cancer patients notes improvements in quality of life[77] that indirectly influence the perception of pain. As such, it may be useful to consider it as part of an integrated approach.

## NUTRITION

Nutrition is a cornerstone of wellness and is utilized in integrative approaches to chronic conditions. The daily diet of the average American is deficient in fruit and vegetable consumption and excessive in meat, refined grain products, and desserts.[78] It is proposed that the results of this diet cause a biochemical reaction that creates a diet-induced proinflammatory state[78] and may contribute to inflammatory pain. Premature and accelerated atherosclerosis, thought to be related to chronic inflammation, has been found in patients with rheumatoid arthritis, increasing morbidity and mortality.[79]

Several nutrient groups have been identified and validated as anti-inflammatory.[80] Perhaps the best known is omega-3 fatty acids. Foods containing high levels of the anti-inflammatory omega-3 include coldwater oily fish such as wild caught salmon, herring, mackerel, and sardines as well as krill, walnuts, flaxseeds, soybeans, seeds and nuts, and some dark green leafy vegetables. There is also evidence to support the anti-inflammatory effects of other foods, such as green and white teas, extra virgin olive oil, and many phytonutrients. A gluten-free vegan diet has been shown to reduce LDL and oxidized LDL and raise atheroprotective natural antibodies against phosphorylcholine in patients with rheumatoid arthritis.[81]

Dietary examination may be useful in pain conditions where there is an inflammatory component, including joint pain, headaches, lower back pain, and neuroinflammation. An integrative nutritionist will help a patient identify what foods might exacerbate symptoms and which could be added to a diet that would eventually act to quell some of the inflammation. Some patients may wish to try a food elimination diet, followed by a food challenge.[82] Keeping a food and symptom diary is often an illuminating first step.

## SUPPLEMENTS

The use of dietary supplements among individuals with chronic pain has risen dramatically as the popularity of other CAM interventions has grown.[83,84] Patients are generally reluctant to report taking herbal preparations and/or supplements to their doctors, even though research finds physicians more open than anticipated by patients.[83]

A Cochrane Systematic Database review of herbal medicine for nonspecific lower back pain[85] found strong evidence for Harpagophytum Procumbens (Devil's Claw), with a daily dose of 50 mg or 100 mg to be better than placebo for short-term improvements in pain and rescue medications.[86] Another high-quality trial reviewed found Harpagophytum Procumbens to be equivalent to 12.5 mg per day dose of rofecoxib.[87] Moderate evidence was found for Salix Alba (White Willow Bark) at daily doses of 120 mg or 240 mg compared to placebo for short-term improvements in pain and rescue medication, and for Capsicum Frutescens (Cayenne) compared to placebo and other topical preparations.[85]

As many as a third of patients with osteoarthritis (OA) have used a supplement as a part of their treatment. Glucosamine sulfate has been shown to reduce symptoms and possibly slow disease progression.[88] Preliminary evidence shows chondroitin sulfate produces symptomatic relief and, possibly, structure-modifying effects, but it does not appear to have a significant benefit over that of glucosamine sulfate.[88,89] S-adenosylmethionine (SAMe) also decreases pain in osteoarthritis.[89] In addition to these, avocado soybean unsaponifiables show beneficial effects in OA according to a Cochrane systematic review.[90]

Most studies of nutraceuticals are performed with small numbers of subjects with standardized preparations, as opposed to those available over the counter.[91] More well designed, prospective studies are necessary to determine the safety and efficacy of a variety of nutraceuticals. Still, some reasonable evidence exists for some of these compounds.

## Energy Therapies

### ACUPUNCTURE

One of the most studied CAM modalities for pain is acupuncture. Acupuncture is an ancient Chinese practice and philosophy that involves the movement of life force, qi (pronounced "chee"), around meridians of the body. Disease or dysfunction is thought to result from a disturbance of the flow of energy. Acupuncture involves the insertion of small-gauge needles at various places on the body (e.g., ear, muscles) to rebalance qi.

Evidence for the efficacy of acupuncture for pain is strong for postoperative pain.[92] A meta-analysis found efficacy of acupuncture for lower back pain over sham acupuncture and no additional treatment.[93] Acupuncture has also been found effective for neck pain;[94] back pain;[93,95] headache;[96] knee osteoarthritis;[93]

migraine;[97] and fibromyalgia.[98,99] However, Staud (2007) points out that many of these trials have not been replicated.

The quality of randomized controlled trials has been questioned. In a study of more than 50 such trials, two-thirds received low scores for quality.[100] Part of the difficulty of conducting trials is that "sham" control groups do consistently better than inert placebo groups.[100] Although the evidence for lower back pain and OA of the knee are relatively strong, more research is needed to evaluate the effect of acupuncture for other pain conditions.[101]

## TAI CHI AND QIGONG

Both Tai Chi and Qigong are gentle movement practices that have been used for centuries in China. In addition to creating better balance with gentle exercise, these practices reduce stress and help relieve tension headaches.[102] When combined with education and relaxation training, they have also been shown to be effective for fibromyalgia,[103] chronic lower back pain,[104] and osteoarthritis.[105]

## PULSED ELECTROMAGNETIC THERAPY

Pulsed Electromagnetic Therapy ("PEMF") has been used for many years to aid in healing fractures. More recent data suggest pain reduction in rheumatoid arthritis, fibromyalgia,[106] and cervical and knee osteoarthritis.[107,108]

# Conclusion

The overarching assumption of treatment for integrative CNCP and addiction must be that these are relapsing, chronic conditions such as diabetes or depression that have physiological, psychological, social, and spiritual dimensions. Although the ideal objectives of pain management and substance-abuse treatment alone may be relief of pain and abstinence, respectively, the pragmatic goals of integrative treatment for co-occurring disorders are different. Reduction in global distress and improvement in overall functioning as a whole person with meaningful relationships and constructive endeavors should be the focus; this can be accomplished by framing and evaluating both disorders in a patient-centered, culturally congruent, age-attuned fashion. These recommendations are summarized in Box 27.2.

---

### Box 27.2 Summary Recommendations

- Provide integrated and integrative treatment for chronic pain and addiction and psychiatric disorders whenever possible.
- Strive for multi- and interdisciplinary management for co-occurring pain and addiction and psychiatric disorders through coordinated collaborative management when feasible or through referral and consultation with the PCP as coordinator of care.
- Consider non-opioid medications such as anti-depressants and anti-convulsants that may also address comorbid depression and anxiety for mild to moderate pain and addiction.
- Non-pharmacological modalities such as physical therapy and cognitive-behavioral therapy should be integral parts of any treatment plan for patients with co-occurring pain and addiction.
- Moderate-to-severe pain in patients with a SUD history that cannot be adequately controlled with other modalities warrants a trial of opioid medications.
- Risk assessment and monitoring tools should be the standard of care for all patients with co-occurring disorders, especially those on chronic opioid therapy.
- Complementary and alternative therapies are underutilized but potentially beneficial primary and adjunctive treatments for patients with chronic pain and addiction.

## REFERENCES

1. Ruoff GE. Assessing pain as the fifth vital sign. *Postgraduate Medicine.* 2002;112(1 Suppl):4–7.
2. Savage SR. Preface: pain medicine and addiction medicine—controversies and collaboration. *Journal of Pain and Symptom Management.* 1993;8(5):254–256.
3. Savage SR, Joranson DE, Covington EC, Schnoll SH, Heit HA, Gilson AM. Definitions related to the medical use of opioids: evolution towards universal agreement. *Journal of Pain and Symptom Management.* 2003;26(1):655–667.
4. Definitions Related to the Use of Opioids for the Treatment of Pain. A consensus statement of the American Academy of Pain Medicine, American Pain Society, American Society of Addiction Medicine. Accessed on August 25, 2015 at: http://www.asam.org/docs/publicy-policy-statements/1opioid-definitions-consensus-2-011.pdf?sfvrsn=0
5. Cheatle MD, Klocek JW, McLellan AT. Managing pain in high-risk patients within a patient-centered medical home. *Translational Behavioral Medicine.* 2012;2(1):47–56.

6. Wachholtz A, Ziedonis D, Gonzalez G. Comorbid pain and opioid addiction: psychosocial and pharmacological treatments. *Substance Use & Misuse.* 2011;46(12): 1536–1552.

7. Management of Opioid Therapy for Chronic Pain Working Group. *VA/DoD Practice Clinical Guideline for Management of Opioid Therapy for Chronic Pain.* Washington, DC: Department of Defense and Department of Veterans Affairs; 2010. Accessed on August 25, 2015 at: http://www.va.gov/painmanagement/docs/cpg_opioidtheray_summary.pdf

8. Barry DT, Irwin KS, Jones ES, et al. Opioids, chronic pain, and addiction in primary care. *Journal of Pain.* 2010;11(12): 1442–1450.

9. Miotto K, Compton P, Ling W, Conolly M. Diagnosing addictive disease in chronicpain patients. *Psychosomatics.* 1996; 37(3):223–235.
   Rosenblum A, Joseph H, Fong C, Kipnis S, Cleland C, Portenoy RK. Prevalence and characteristics of chronic pain among chemically dependent patients in methadone maintenance and residential treatment facilities. *JAMA.* 2003; 289(18): 2370–2378.

10. Lusher J, Elander J, Bevan D, Telfer P, Burton B. Analgesic addiction and pseudoaddiction in painful chronic illness. *Clinical Journal of Pain.* 2006; 22(3): 316–324.

11. Samet JH, Friedmann P, Saitz R. Benefits of linking primary medical care and substance abuse services: patient, provider, and societal perspectives. *Archives of Internal Medicine.* 2001; 161(1): 85–91.

12. Cheatle MD, Gallagher RM. Chronic pain and comorbid mood and substance use disorders: a biopsychosocial treatment approach. *Current Psychiatry Reports.* 2006;8(5):371–376.

13. Yeats WB. *The Collected Poems of W.B.Yeats.* 2nd rev. ed. New York: Scribner 1996.

14. Cheatle MD. Depression, chronic pain, and suicide by overdose: on the edge. *Pain Medicine.* 2011;12(Suppl 2):S43–S48.

15. Yanni LM, McKinney-Ketchum JL, Harrington SB, et al. Preparation, confidence, and attitudes about chronic noncancer pain in graduate medical education. *Journal of Graduate Medical Education.* 2010;2(2):260–268.

16. Miller NS, Sheppard LM, Colenda CC, Magen J. Why physicians are unprepared to treat patients who have alcohol- and drug-related disorders. *Academic Medicine.* 2001;76(5): 410–418.

17. Clark MR, Treisman GJ. From stigmatized neglect to active engagement. *Advances in Psychosomatic Medicine.* 2011;30:1–7.

18. Wasan AD, Wootton J, Jamison RN. Dealing with difficult patients in your pain practice. *Regional Anesthesia and Pain Medicine.* 2005;30(2):184–192.

19. SAMHSA. *Managing Chronic Pain in Adults with or in Recovery from Substance Use Disorders.* Rockville, MD: Substance Abuse and Mental Health Services Administration; 2011.

20. Institute of Medicine. *Relieving Pain in America: A Blueprint for Transforming Prevention, Care, Education, and Research.* Washington, DC: National Academic Press; 2011.

21. Minkoff K, Cline CA. Changing the world: the design and implementation of comprehensive continuous integrated systems of care for individuals with co-occurring disorders. *Psychiatr Clin North Am.* 2004;27(4):727–743.

22. Currie SR, Hodgins DC, Crabtree A, Jacobi J, Armstrong S. Outcome from integrated pain management treatment for recovering substance abusers. *Journal of Pain.* 2003;4(2):91–100.

23. Brensilver M, Tariq S, Shoptaw S. Optimizing pain management through collaborations with behavioral and addiction medicine in primary care. *Primary Care.* 2012;39(4):661–669.

24. Pade PA, Cardon KE, Hoffman RM, Geppert CM. Prescription opioid abuse, chronic pain, and primary care: a co-occurring disorders clinic in the chronic disease model. *J Subst Abuse Treat.* 2012;43(4):446–450.

25. Starrels JL, Becker WC, Weiner MG, Li X, Heo M, Turner BJ. Low use of opioid risk reduction strategies in primary care even for high risk patients with chronic pain. *J Gen Intern Med.* 2011; 6(9):958–964.

26. Pujol LAM, Katz NP, Zacharoff KL. *PainEdu.org Manual: A Pocket Guide to Pain Management.* (3rd ed.). Newton, MA: Inflexxion; 2007.

27. Cleeland CS, Ryan KM. Pain assessment: Global use of the brief pain inventory. *Annals of the Academy of Medicine.* 1994;23:129–138.

28. Menefee LA. Psychological evaluation of the patient with chronic pain (Chapter 16). In: Pappagallo M, ed. *The Neurological Basis of Pain.* New York: McGraw Hill; 2005:219–223.

29. Wiedemer NL, Harden PS, Arndt IO, Gallagher RM. The opioid renewal clinic: a primary care, managed approach to opioid therapy in chronic pain patients at risk for substance abuse. *Pain Medicine.* 2007;8(7): 573–584.

30. Chou R, Fanciullo GJ, Fine PG, et al. Clinical guidelines for the use of chronic opioid therapy in chronic noncancer pain. *Journal of Pain.* 2009;10(2):113–130.

31. Haanpaa ML, Gourlay GK, Kent JL, et al. Treatment considerations for patients with neuropathic pain and other medical comorbidities. *Mayo Clin Proc.* 2010;85(3 Suppl): S15–S25.

32. Turk DC, Swanson KS, Tunks ER. Psychological approaches in the treatment of chronic pain patients—when pills, scalpels, and needles are not enough. *Can J Psychiatry.* 2008;53(4):213–223.

33. Vickers AJ, Cronin AM, Maschino AC, et al. Acupuncture for chronic pain: individual patient data meta-analysis. *Archives of Internal Medicine.* 2012;172(19):1444–1453.

34. Butler SF, Fernandez K, Benoit C, Budman SH, Jamison RN. Validation of the revised Screener and Opioid Assessment for Patients with Pain (SOAPP-R). *Journal of Pain.* 2008;9(4): 360–372.

35. Butler SF, Budman SH, Fernandez KC, et al. Development and validation of the current opioid misuse measure. *Pain.* 2007;130(1–2):144–156.

36. Jacobson E. *Progressive Relaxation: A Physiological and Clinical Investigation of Muscular States and their Significance in Psychology and Medical Practice.* Chicago: University of Chicago Press; 1974.

37. Kwekkeboom KL, Gretarsdottir E. Systematic review of relaxation interventions for pain. *Journal of Nursing Scholarship*. 2006; 38(3): 269–277.

38. Arena JG, Blanchard E. Biofeedback therapy for chronic pain. In: Loser JD, Butler, S, Chapman, CR, Turk DC, eds., *Bonica's Management of Pain*. 3rd ed. Philadelphia: Lippincott, Williams, & Wilkins; 2001: 1759–1767.

39. Astin JA. Mind–body therapies for the management of pain. *Clinical Journal of Pain*. 2004;20:27–32.

40. Barrows KA., Jacobs BP. Mind–body medicine: An introduction and review of the literature. *Medicine Clinical of North America*. 2002;86: 1–15.

41. Fernandez E, Turk D. The utility of cognitive coping strategies for altering pain perception: a meta-analysis. *Pain*. 1989;38: 123–135.

42. Baird CL, Sands L. A pilot study of the effectiveness of guided imagery with progressive muscle relaxation to reduce chronic pain and mobility difficulties of osteoarthritis. *Pain Management Nursing*. 2004;5: 94–104.

43. Lewandowski WA. Patterning of pain and power with guided imagery. *Nursing Science Quarterly*. 2004;17:233–241.

44. Montgomery GH, Duhamel KN, Redd WH. A meta-analysis of hypnotically induced analgesia: How effective is hypnosis? *International Journal of Clin and Exper Hypnosis*. 2000; 48;138–153.

45. Jensen M, Patterson DR. Hypnotic treatment of chronic pain. *Journal of Behavioral Medicine*. 2006;29: 95–124.

46. Gay MC, Philippot P, Luminet O. Differential effectiveness of psychological interventions for reducine osteoarthritis pain: a comparison of Erikson. *European Journal of Pain*. 2002;6: 1–16.

47. Ludwig DS, Kabet-Zinn J. Mindfulness in medicine. *JAMA*. 2008;300:1350–1352.

48. Kabat-Zinn J, Lipworth L, Burney R. The clinical use of mindfulness meditation for the self-regulation of chronic pain. *Journal of Behavioral Medicine*. 1995;8:163–190.

49. Kabat-Zinn J, Lipworth L, Burney R. Four year follow-up of a meditation-based program for the self-regulation of chronic pain: Treatment outcomes and compliance. *Clinical Journal of Pain*. 1987;2: 157–173.

50. Baer RA. Mindfulness training as a clinical intervention: A conceptual and empirical review. *Clinical Psychology Science and Practice*. 2003;10: 125–143.

51. Grossman P, Neimann L, Schmidt S, Walach H. Mindfulness-based stress reduction and health benefits: A meta-analysis. *Journal of Psychosomatic Research*. 2004;54: 35–43.

52. Monroe NE, Greco CM, Weiner DK. Mindfulness meditation for the treatment of chronic low back pain in older adults: A randomized controlled pilot study. *Pain*. 2008;134: 310–319.

53. Monti DA, Peterson C. Mindfulness-based art therapy: Results from a two year study. *Psychiatry Times*. 2004;21: 63–66.

54. Monti DA, Peterson C, Kunkel EJ, et al. A randomized controlled trial of mindfulness-based art therapy (MBAT) for women with cancer. *Psycho-Oncology*. 2006;15: 363–373.

55. Beck AT. *Cognitive Therapy and the Emotional Disorders.* New York: International Universities Press; 1976.

56. Freeman A, Pretzer J, Fleming B, Simon KM. *Clinical Applications of Cognitive Therapy.* New York: Plenum; 1990.

57. Fordyce WE. *Behavioral Methods for Chronic Pain and Illness.* St. Louis, MO: Mosby; 1976.

58. Morley S, Eccleston C, Williams AC. Systematic review and meta-analysis of randomized adults, excluding headache. *Pain.* 1999;80:1–13.

59. McCracken LM. *Contextual Cognitive-Behavioral Therapy for Chronic Pain.* Seattle, WA: IASP; 2005.

60. Jensen MP, Turner JA, Romano JM. Changes in beliefs, catastrophizing and coping are associated with improvement in multidisciplinary pain treatment. *Journal of Consulting and Clinical Psychology.* 2001;69: 655–662.

61. Jensen MP, Turner JA, Romano JM. Changes after multidisciplinary pain treatment in patient pain beliefs and coping are associated with concurrent changes in patient functioning. *Pain.* 2007;13: 38–47.

62. Kuchera ML. Applying osteopathic principles to formulate treatment for patients with chronic pain. *Journal of the American Osteopathic Association.* 2007; 107(10 Suppl 6): ES28–ES38.

63. Educational Council on Osteopathic Principles and the American Association of Colleges of Osteopathic Medicine. *Glossary of Osteopathic Terminology Usage Guide.* Chevy Chase, MD; 2006; 11–13. http://www.aacom.org/people/councils/Documents/OsteopathicTerminologyGlossary.pdf.

64. Andersson GB, Lucente T, Davis AM, Kappler RE, Lipton, JA, Leurgans S. A comparison of osteopathic spinal manipulation with standard of care for patients with low back pain. *New England Journal of Medicine.* 1999;341:1426–1431.

65. Hoehler FK, Tobis JS, Buerger AA. Spinal manipulation for low back pain. *JAMA.*1981;245:1835–1838.

66. Licciardone JC, Stoll ST, Fulda KG, et al. Osteopathic manipulative treatment for chronic low back pain: a randomized controlled trial. *Spine.* 2003;28:1355–1362.

67. Field TM. Massage therapy effects. *American Psychologist.* 1998;53:1270–1281.

68. Monti DA, Yang J. Complementary medicine in chronic cancer care. *Seminars in Oncology.* 2005;32: 225–231.

69. Ernst E. Musculoskeletal conditions and complementary/alternative medicine. *Best Practice & Research in Clinical Rheumatology.* 2004;18(4): 539–556.

70. Plews-Ogan M, Owens JE, Goodman M, Wolfe P, Schorling J. A pilot study investigating mindfulness-based stress reduction and massage for the management of chronic pain. *Journal of General Internal Medicine.* 2005;20:1136–1138.

71. Lundblad I, Elert J, Gerdle B. Randomized controlled trial of physiotherapy and Feldenkrais interventions in female workers with neck-shoulder complaints. *Journal of Occupational Rehabilitation.* 1999;9(3): 179–194.

72. Ernst E, Canter P. The Alexander technique: A systematic review of controlled clinical trials. *Forsch Komplementarmed Research in Complementary and Classical Natural Medicine.* 2003;10: 325–329.

73. Dyson-Hudson T, Shiflett S, Kirshblum S, Bowen J, Druin E. Acupuncture and trager psychophysical integration in the treatment of wheelchair user's shoulder pain in individuals with spinal cord injury. *Archives of Physical Medicine.* 2000;82(8): 1038–1046.

74. Raub J. Psychophysiologic effects of Hatha Yoga on musculoskeletal and cardio-pulmonary function: a literature review. *Journal of Alternative Complementary Medicine.* 2002;8(6): 797–812.

75. Sherman K, Cherkin D, Erro J, Miglioretti D, Deyo R. Comparing yoga, exercise, and a self-care book for chronic low back pain: a randomized, controlled trial. *Annals of Internal Medicine* 2005;143(12): 849–856.

76. Kolasinski SL, Garfinkel M, Tsai AG, Matz W, Van Dyke A, Schumacher HR. Iyengar yoga for treating symptoms of osteoarthritis of the knees: a pilot study. *Journal of Alternative & Complementary Medicine.* 2005;11(4): 689–693.

77. Moadel AB, Shah C, Wylie-Rosett J, et al. Randomized controlled trial of yoga among a multiethnic sample of breast cancer patients: effects on quality of life. *Journal of Clinical Oncology.* 2007;25(28): 4387–4395.

78. Seaman DR. The diet-induced proinflammatory state: A cause of chronic pain and other degenerative diseases? *Journal of Manipulative and Physiological Therapeutics.* 2002; 25(3):168–179.

79. Naranjo A, Sokka T, Descalzo MA, et al. Cardiovascular disease in patients with rheumatoid arthritis: results from the QUEST-RA study. *Arthritis Research & Therapy.* 2008;10(2): R30. doi:10.1186/ar2383.

80. Goldberg RJ, Katz J. Meta-analysis of the analgesic effects of omega-3 poly-unsaturated fatty acid supplementation for inflammatory joint pain. *Pain.* 2007;129(1–2): 210–223.

81. Elkan AC, Sjoberg B, Kolsrud B, Hafstrom I, Frostegard J. Gluten-free vegan diet induces decreased LDL and oxidized LDL levels and raised atheroprotective nat-ural antibodies against phosphorylcholine in patients with rheumatoid arthritis: a randomized study. *Arthritis Research and Therapy.* 2008;10: R34. doi:10.1186/ar2388.

82. Drisko J, Bischoff B, Hall M, McCallum R. Treating irritable bowel syndrome with a food elimination diet followed by food challenge and probiotics. *Journal of the American College of Nutrition.* 2006;6:514–522.

83. Cauffield JS. The psychosocial aspects of complementary and alternative medicine. *Pharmacotherapy.* 2000;20(11): 1289–1294.

84. Fleming S, Rabago DP, Mundt MP, Fleming MF. CAM therapies among primary care patients using opioid therapy for chronic pain. *BMC Complementary and Alternative Medicine.* 2007;7:15. doi.10.1186/1472-6882-7-15

85. Gagnier JJ, vanTulder M, Berman B, Bombardier C. Herbal medicine for low back pain. *The Cochrane Database of Systematic Reviews.* 2008; 1.

86. Chrubasik S, Junck H, Breitschwerdt H, Conradt C, Zappe H. Effectiveness of Harpagophytum extract WS 1531 in the treatment of exacerbation of low back pain: a randomized, placebo-controlled, double-blind study. *European Journal of Anaesthesiology.* 1999;16:118–129.

87. Chrubasik S, Model A, Black A, Pollak S. A randomized double-blind pilot study comparing Doloteffin and Vioxx in the treatment of low back pain. *Rheumatology.* 2003;42:141–148.

88. Bruyere O, Reginster J.Y. Glucosamine and condroitin sulfate as therapeutic agents for knee and hip osteoarthritis. *Drugs and Aging.* 2007;24(7):573–580.

89. Gregory PJ, Sperry M, Wilson, AF. Dietary supplements for osteoarthritis. *American Family Physician.* 2007;77(2), 177–184.

90. Little CV, Parsons T, Logan S. Herbal therapy for treating osteoarthritis. *The Cochrane Database of Systematic Reviews.* 2008;1.

91. Clayton JJ. Nutraceuticals in the management of osteoarthritis. *Orthopedics.* 2007;30(8): 624–629.

92. National Institutes of Health Consensus Conference. Acupuncture. *Journal of American Medical Association.* 1998;280:1518–1524.

93. Manheimer E, White A, Berman B, Forys K, Ernst E. Meta-analysis: Acupuncture for low back pain. *Annals of Internal Medicine.* 2005;142:651–663.

94. He D, Veirsted KB, Hostmark AT, Medbo JL. Effects of acupuncture treatment on chronic neck and shoulder pain in sedentary female workers: A 6-month and 3-year follow-up study. *Pain.* 2004;109:299–307.

95. Weidenhammer W, Linde K, Streng A, Hoppe A, Melchart D. Acupuncture for chronic low back pain in routine care—a multicenter observational study. *Clinical Journal of Pain.* 2007;23:128–135.

96. Melchart D, Weidenhammer W, Streng A, Hoppe A, Pfaffenrath V, Linde K. Acupuncture for chronic headaches—an epidemiological study. *Headache.* 2006;46:632–641.

97. Vickers AJ, Rees RW, Zollman CE, et al. Acupuncture of chronic headache disorders in primary care: Randomized controlled trial and economic analysis. *Health and Technology Assessment.* 2004;8:1–35.

98. Deluze C, Bosia L, Zirbs A, Chantraine A, Vischer TL. Electroacupuncture in fibro-myalgia: results of a controlled trial. *British Medical Journal.* 1992;305:1249–1252.

99. Targino RA, Imamura M, Kaziyama HH, Souza LP, Hsing WT, Imamura ST. Pain treatment with acupuncture for patients with fibromyalgia. *Current Pain Headache Reports.* 2002;6:379–383.

100. Ezzo J, Berman B, Hadhazy VA, Jadad AR, Lao L, Singh, B. B. Is acupuncture effective for the treatment of chronic pain? A systematic review. *Pain.* 2000;86:217–225.

101. Staud R. Mechanisms of acupuncture analgesia: Effective therapy for musculo-skeletal pain? *Current Rheumatology Reports.* 2007;9:473–481.

102. Abbott R, Hui K, Hays R, Li M, Pan T. A randomized controlled trial of Tai Chi for tension headaches. *Evidence-Based Complementary and Alternative Medicine.* 2007;4(1):107–113.

103. Chen K, Hassett A, Hou F, Staller J, Lichtbroun A. A pilot study of external Qigong therapy for patients with fibromyalgia. *Journal of Alternative Complementary Medicine.* 2006;12(9):851–856.

104. Gallagher B. Tai Chi Chuan and Qigong: Physical and mental practice for functional mobility. *Topics in Geriatric Rehabilitation*. 2003;19(3):172–182.

105. Song R, Lee E, Lam P, Bae S. Effects of tai chi exercise on pain, balance, muscle strength, and perceived difficulties in physical functioning in older women with osteoarthritis: a randomized clinical trial. *Journal of Rheumatology*. 2003;30(9), 2039–2044.

106. Shupak N, McKay J, Nielson W, Rollman G, Prato F, Thomas A. Exposure to a specific pulsed low-frequency magnetic field: A double-blind placebo-controlled study of effects on pain ratings in rheumatoid arthritis and fibromyalgia patients. *Pain Research Management*. 2006;11(2):85–90.

107. *Hulme JM, Welch V, de Bie R, Judd M, Tugwell P. Electromagnetic fields for the treatment of osteoarthritis. Cochrane Database of Systematic Reviews 2002, Issue 1. Art. No.: CD003523. DOI: 10.1002/14651858.CD003523.*

108. Pipitone N, Scott D. Magnetic pulse treatment for knee osteoarthritis: A randomized, double-blind, placebo-controlled study. *Current Medical Research Opinion*. 2001;17(3):190–196.

# 28

## An Integrative Approach to Post-Acute Withdrawal and Relapse Prevention

WALTER LING, SHAHLA J. MODIR, AND GEORGE E. MUÑOZ

# 28.1

## Introduction

### WALTER LING, MD

Recovering from addiction is about staying off drugs and is known as relapse prevention. However, before patients can engage in relapse prevention as part of recovery, they must first get off the drugs—often referred to as detoxification ("detox"). While critically linked and seemingly part of the same process, getting off drugs and staying off drugs are, in reality, two entirely different processes. For treatment to succeed relapse prevention must follow detoxification. Detoxification—getting off drugs— deals with drug effects, which usually run their courses in a matter of days. On the other hand, relapse prevention—staying off drugs—concerns the neural adaptations from repeated drug exposure: the prolonged overstimulation of dopamine and other neurotransmitters involved in producing the euphoria sought by the person suffering from addiction and the learned drug use experiences that become incorporated into the drug use memories.[1,2] Success in relapse prevention is facilitated by proper management of drug withdrawal and the post-acute withdrawal period that follows detoxification.

The immediate clinical manifestations of drug withdrawal during detoxification are opposite those of the drug effects, such that excitation follows withdrawal from drugs that sedate, and lethargy follows withdrawal from drugs that stimulate. Symptoms can be so intense and pervasive that patients find it difficult to attend to anything else except the bodily discomfort and intense drug craving. Medications and acupuncture are often needed to ameliorate these clinical symptoms. As one senior clinician observed, patients are going through their "finite amount of suffering." It is unrealistic, futile, and frustrating during this time to insist that patients participate intensely in their recovery. Fortunately this phase is short-lived and merges imperceptibly into the period of post-acute withdrawal.

The post-acute withdrawal period is a time of tremendous challenge for patients and clinicians. Direct residual drug effects—aches and pains and the like—linger and new manifestations—anxiety, depression, lassitude, and craving—from the neurobiological readjustments are heaped on. It may seem counterintuitive at first that different drugs, which have different and even opposite effects on the brain, should cause similar brain changes, but in reality all drug exposures place similar demands on the brain to adapt. In the beginning, drugs and alcohol activate the reward system; this activation strengthens the "pleasure" response and weakens the fear response to potential harm, thus reducing cortical inhibition. Reduced cortical inhibition makes risky behaviors seem more rewarding and their potential harmful consequences less salient.[3] Eventually, and inevitably, a depleted reward circuitry dominates the clinical manifestations, its effects exaggerated by the concomitant loss of inhibitory control.[4] The extent of drug exposure and the severity of addiction determines the magnitude of the brain changes, and in recovery, the need to reverse and compensate for the neurobiological changes caused by repeated drug exposure.[5] It is what clinicians mean by the brain needing to heal.

The neurobiological underpinnings of these brain changes, neurochemically speaking, are the chronically elevated stress hormones: adrenaline and noradrenaline, cortisol, and amygdala corticotrophin releasing factor.[6] Clinically the manifestations are those of chronic stress: anxiety, depression, irritability, loss of energy, loss of interest, and a general sense of lassitude. Intense craving is triggered by daily life stress, by the presence of drugs, and even more intensely by cues that trigger drug memories.[7,8] Blood pressure can be persistently elevated and sleep is fitful and populated with drug dreams. Everything has a negative overtone to it. All these happen on top of a nervous system already exhausted by chronic drug exposure, a "stressed-out" subcortical neurocircuitry that is oversensitive to stress and underresponsive to cortical control.[9] The user often wishes for the return to the state of oblivion under the influence of drugs. Relapse, not surprisingly, is common. Understanding these underlying neurobiological mechanisms provides the foundation for pharmacological interventions described elsewhere in this chapter; these medications, in one way or another, are intended to mitigate the effects of the chronic stress responses.

Everyone intuitively knows that detoxification is only a necessary first step in recovery and, in itself, is insufficient for the treatment of addiction. However, in the United States detoxification is still the most widely used "treatment" for addiction, which is why relapse is so common. Many reasons, mostly excuses, have been offered to explain and justify the use of detoxification as treatment, from the patient with substance use disorder who may lack motivation, to the treatment system's lack of resources, to the urban myth that treatment doesn't work until you hit bottom, and so on. The truth is while detoxification may offer a number of potential benefits, staying off drugs is not one of them. Yes, detoxification is a necessary first step on the way to staying off drugs—relapse prevention—which is the real business of overcoming addiction. Detoxification is rightfully said to be the first step in the journey of recovery, and it is well said that a journey of a thousand miles begins with the first step. But in truth a thousand miles stepping in place gets you nowhere and does not make a journey. To make a journey there must be progress, moving from one step to the next. It is not easy; it is what relapse prevention is all about.

Relapse prevention, beyond withdrawing from the drugs of abuse and reestablishing homeostasis in the reward system, must address the existential question of why people take drugs in the first place. As Alan Leshner put it, people take drugs to feel good or, if they already feel good, to feel better. One way or the other, people take drugs because they like the effects of drugs on their brain. To put it another way, we can say people take drugs in pursuit of some form of happiness. Surely there is nothing wrong with the pursuit of happiness as such; it is an inalienable right embodied in our Declaration of Independence. However, the kind of happiness called hedonia, feeling good as a raw pleasure with no meaningful purpose, is not what the founding fathers had in mind. They were talking about happiness with virtue: happiness that makes you feel good being the person you are because you have done something meaningful and purposeful, the kind that relates to something you would be proud to tell your children and grandchildren about. Few patients in their addiction would really want to tell their kids how great they felt when they were stoned.

The good feeling produced by drugs takes place in the subcortical, animalistic if you will, brain reward circuitry without influence from the uniquely human, rational cortical brain.[6] Neurophysiologically, the user pays a heavy price for this good feeling. There are increases in blood pressure, respiration, blood sugar, and stress hormones like adrenaline and cortisol, and concomitant decreases in immune response.[10] Repeated exposure weakens the body and promotes illness, decreases the brain defense system, and increases its vulnerability to further stress.[11] Furthermore, people with addiction are prone to other adverse consequences related to their drug use—personal, occupational, social, and legal—which are additional sources of stress. It is axiomatic in neurological medicine that a poor brain reacts poorly to stress.

In contrast to hedonia, eudemonia is "pleasure with meaningful purpose." An activity with useful purpose promotes the sense of well-being. Simply put, it is feeling good by doing good. The difference between hedonia and eudemonia has to do with the level of brain involvement.[12] The higher cortical brain involved in eudemonia is what makes us uniquely human, giving us the sense of self, sense of right and wrong, morality, art, science, and the quest for meaning in our lives.

The post-acute withdrawal symptoms are experienced as anhedonia, which invariably follows hedonia, as surely as night follows day. The truly integrative approach to overcoming anhedonia and the sense of purposelessness during this time and to prevent relapse is to engage with people who are doing something good and meaningful and to strive to do good for others beyond one's self. This is not giving up self-interest; indeed, it is the best embodiment of being good to one's self. Engendering consideration for others is a critical step to regaining self-respect and self-worth necessary in the process of recovery. Doing good things, making someone else happy, reconnecting with family and friends and community, and finding happiness with purpose and meaning—those are the components of a truly integrative approach to staying off drugs and preventing relapse.

## REFERENCES

1. Saal D, Dong Y, Bonci A, Malenka RC. Drugs of abuse and stress trigger a common synaptic adaptation in dopamine neurons. *Neuron.* 2003;37(4):577–582.
2. Wise RA. Dopamine, learning and motivation. *Nature Reviews Neuroscience.* 2004;5(6):483–94.
3. Stalnaker T, Takahashi Y, Roesch M, Schoenbaum G. Neural substrates of cognitive inflexibility after chronic cocaine exposure. *Neuropharmacology.* 2009;56(Suppl 1):63–72.
4. Self DW, Nestler EJ. Relapse to drug-seeking: neural and molecular mechanisms. *Drug & Alcohol Dependence.* 1998;51(1-2):49–60.
5. Kauer JA, Malenka RC. Synaptic plasticity and addiction. *Nature Reviews Neuroscience.* 2007;8(11):844–858.
6. Niehaus JL1, Murali M, Kauer JA. Drugs of abuse and stress impair LTP at inhibitory synapses in the ventral tegmental area. *European Journal of Neuroscience.* 2010;32(1):108–117.
7. Miczek KA, Yap JJ, Covington HE. Social stress, therapeutics and drug abuse: preclinical models of escalated and depressed intake. *Pharmacology & Therapeutics.* 2008;120(2):102–128.
8. Volkow ND, Wang GJ, Fowler JS, et al. Addiction: beyond dopamine reward circuitry. *Proceedings of the National Academy of Sciences USA.* 2011;108(37):15037–15042.
9. Ungless MA, Argilli E, Bonci A. Effects of stress and aversion on dopamine neurons: implications for addiction. *Neuroscience & Biobehavioral Reviews.* 2010;35(2):151–156.
10. Roy S, Loh H. Effects of opioids on the immune system. *Neurochemical Research.* 1996;21(11):1375–1386.
11. Crews F. Immune function genes, genetics, and the neurobiology of addiction. *Alcohol Research.* 2012;34(3):355–361.
12. Wager T, Kang J, Johnson T, et al. A Bayesian model of category-specific emotional brain responses. *PLoS Computational Biology.* 2015;11(4):e1004066.

# 28.2

## Neurobiology of Post-Acute Withdrawal and Medical Treatment Ramifications

### SHAHLA MODIR, MD

Protracted withdrawal emerges after the acute symptoms of detoxification of a substance occur. For most drugs, acute withdrawal occurs in the first 5 to 10 days of abstinence. Following that is early abstinence, which lasts 2 to 3 weeks, during which time primary physical symptoms may wax and wane but more prominent are the symptoms of disturbed sleep, anxiety, and dysphoria. In the final phase, known as protracted abstinence, the actual symptoms vary to some extent by the drug of abuse, but there are common symptoms that can be part of any protracted withdrawal syndrome.[1] These symptoms are primarily related to neuroadaptive changes that have occurred in the brain and reflect a brain that is highly vulnerable to stress and has a reduced capacity to experience reward. In this phase, small stressors can produce an exaggerated negative affective state, craving and relapse. The capacity to enjoy reward, described as hedonia, is also impaired, with an attenuation of expected positive response to pleasurable life events. As a result, protracted abstinence and the affective shift that takes place with it are major factors in craving and relapse.[2]

One possible mechanism for changes in brain function relates to the induction of transcription factors like c-fos.[3] Acute use of cocaine, for example, induces this expression of c-fos, but within 12 hours levels normally return to baseline. However, in chronic users of cocaine, expression of c-fos was reduced in favor of a different transcription factor, activator protein A (AP-1), which is composed of delta fos-B. The upregulation of delta fos-B is long-lasting in chronic drug users and leads to an increase in the rewarding effects of cocaine and increases cocaine self-administration. Therefore, this longer-lasting change to delta fos-B has the potential to increase motivation for drug use for many weeks and months after the last use.[4]

During the protracted phase of abstinence, evidence from imaging studies shows increased sensitivity to drug cues.[4] This includes projections from the mesolimbic dopamine system including the prefrontal cortex or the "brakes" of the brain to the reward center known as the nucleus accumbens. Imaging studies also show poor functioning of the brain's executive function and inhibitory control network in the dorsolateral prefrontal cortex and cingulate gyrus and orbitofrontal cortex. This leads to poor impulse control and diminished inhibitory control under circumstances when the brain has even higher sensitivity to drug cues.[5]

Symptoms of prolonged abstinence from alcohol and sedative-hypnotics can include persistent anxiety and stress responsiveness. Increases in alcohol intake over initial baseline use and stress reactivity can persist for months. A rodent study done at 3 to 5 weeks after detoxification called the elevated plus maze (which measures anxiety behavior) showed the rodents had no anxiety at baseline, but anxiety responses were found in rats under mild stress if they had a history of alcoholism. When the rats were given a corticotrophin releasing factor (CRF) antagonist, this effect was reversed. Also, increases in alcohol self-administration were blocked by CRF antagonists, suggesting that cortisol releasing factor is another important component in increased reactivity to stress and relapse. It has been shown that CRF antagonists block stress-induced reinstatement and naltrexone, which blocks cue-induced reinstatement, does not block stress-induced relapse, reflecting two different mechanisms involved in protracted abstinence.[6]

In protracted withdrawal from opiates, often there are persistent physical symptoms such as temperature dysregulation, volatile blood pressure, increased respiratory rate, fatigue, increased pain sensitivity, and dysphoria.[7] There can be motivational symptoms that lead to diminished effort to make positive change or experience joy. This state of hyperalgesia has been shown to last up to 5 months.[8] Those in whom this symptom persists have been shown to have higher rates of cue-induced craving. Animal studies have shown, for example, that the first heroin dose may induce moderate hyperalgesia for 2 days, but the fifth injection of an equal dose can induce it for 6 days.[9] Daily opiate administration for 2 weeks can produce a slow decrease in the nociceptive threshold that can be observed for many weeks after the drug induction.[10] Brain changes associated with this effect involve the glutamate systems and a noncompetitive glutamate antagonist was shown to prevent long-term heroin-induced hyperalgesia.[9] The brain sites associated with motivational symptoms have been correlated to the nucleus accumbens and amygdala. This has been confirmed using data from conditioned place preference aversion in rodents. Studies have shown that in rodents who have lesions to the central nucleus of the amygdala, morphine withdrawal-induced place aversion is blocked. Also, CRF blockade in the central nucleus of the amygdala blocked conditioned place aversion produced by opiate withdrawal, as did blocking noradrenergic projections in the stria terminalis. Both CRF antagonists and alpha-1 noradrenergic antagonists decrease compulsive drug taking in rodents in a dose-dependent way.[11] Upregulation of delta fos-B is also found with chronic opioid use, leading to an increase in AP-1 and to an increase in the individual's sensitivity to the rewarding effects of morphine and relapse. In an electrophysiological study done on heroin-dependent subjects, event-related potentials in response to heroin cues during abstinence showed increased slow-wave components, which correlated with posttest craving levels, displaying continued drug cue saliency even months after abstinence.[12]

The treatment of protracted abstinence stems from the model that shows that the neuroadaptive changes from drug use decrease stress tolerance; enhance the brain's stress hormone system, including hypothalamic pituitary adrenal (HPA) axis regulation of cortisol; and diminish inhibitory and impulse control.[13,14] Medications aimed at reducing brain cortisol and noradrenergic tone have proven to be effective in decreasing relapse rates for both stress- and cue-induced relapse rates. This is likely because the medications act both on brain cortisol and in the prefrontal cortex to improve impulse control. Studies have shown that the alpha-2 adrenergic agonists clonidine, lofexidine, and guanfacine, given early in recovery during this period, reduce relapse rates for heroin, cocaine, alcohol, and nicotine use and decrease brain cortisol levels.[15-17] Also, the alpha-1 antagonist prazosin, which also decreases noradrenergic tone, has shown effectiveness in reducing stress-induced alcohol craving, anxiety, and negative emotions as well as decreasing alcohol use in alcohol-dependent individuals.[18] Rodent studies have shown that methadone and buprenorphine maintenance treatments block heroin-primed reinstatement of drug seeking but not stress-induced reinstatement. A recent study evaluated adding clonidine or placebo in patients taking buprenorphine and found that the addition of clonidine produced the longest duration of abstinence; through an ecological momentary assessment, the researchers showed the daily life stress was decoupled from opiate craving in the clonidine group versus placebo. Its effect was primarily on increasing the time to first relapse, but not the number of relapses.[19]

It is evident from the research just described that external life stress and the level of stress the brain maintains in the post-acute withdrawal period are both critically important factors in substance abuse relapse. Holistic interventions mentioned in detail throughout this book such as meditation, yoga, and exercise can be fundamental to a program of recovery by allowing the brain and body to decrease stress and heal.

## REFERENCES

1. Heilig M, Egli M, Crabbe JC, Becker HC. Acute withdrawal, protracted abstinence and negative affect in alcoholism: are they linked? *Addiction Biology.* 2010;15(2):169–184.

2. Koob G, Arneds M, Moal M. Alcohol. In: *Drugs, Addiction, and the Brain.* Waltham, MA: Elsevier; 2014:212–213.

3. Koob G, Arneds M, Moal M. Psychostimulants. In: *Drugs, Addiction, and the Brain.* Waltham, MA: Elsevier; 2014:128–129.

4. Nestler E. Molecular basis of long-term plasticity underlying addiction. *Nature Reviews Neuroscience.* 2001;2:119–128.

5. Koob GF, Volkow ND. Neurocircuitry of addiction. *Neuropsychopharmacology.* 2010;35(1):217–238.

6. Liu X, Weiss F. Additive effect of stress and drug cues on reinstatement of ethanol seeking: exacerbation by history of dependence and role of concurrent activation of corticotropin-releasing factor and opioid mechanisms. *Journal of Neuroscience.* 2002;22(18):7856–7861.

7. Simonnet G, Rivat C. Opioid-induced hyperalgesia: abnormal or normal pain? *NeuroReport.* 2003;14(1):1–7.

8. Koob G, Arneds M, Moal M. Opioids. In: *Drugs, Addiction, and the Brain.* Waltham, MA: Elsevier; 2014:152–154.

9. Koob G, Arneds M, Moal M. Opioids. In: *Drugs, Addiction, and the Brain.* Waltham, MA: Elsevier; 2014:162–168.

10. Laulin JP, Larcher A, Célèrier E, et al. Long-lasting increased pain sensitivity in rat following exposure to heroin for the first time. *European Journal of Neuroscience.* 1998;10(2):782–785.

11. Funk CK, Zorrilla EP, Lee MJ, et al. Corticotropin-releasing factor 1 antagonists selectively reduce ethanol self-administration in ethanol-dependent rats. *Biological Psychiatry.* 2007;61(1):78–86.

12. Nestler EJ, Malenka RC. The addicted brain. *Scientific American.* 2004;290(3):78–85.

13. Sinha R, Fox HC, Hong KA, et al. Effects of adrenal sensitivity, stress- and cue-induced craving, and anxiety on subsequent alcohol relapse and treatment outcomes. *Archives of General Psychiatry.* 2011;68(9):942–952.

14. Sinha R. New findings on biological factors predicting addiction relapse vulnerability. *Current Psychiatry Reports.* 2011;13(5):398–405.

15. Sinha R, Kimmerling A, Doebrick C, Kosten TR. Effects of lofexidine on stress-induced and cue-induced opioid craving and opioid abstinence rates: preliminary findings. *Psychopharmacology (Berlin).* 2007;190(4):569–574.

16. Fox HC, Seo D, Tuit K, et al. Guanfacine effects on stress, drug craving and pre-frontal activation in cocaine-dependent individuals: preliminary findings. *Journal of Psychopharmacology (Oxford, England).* 2012;26(7):958–972.

17. Fox H, Sinha R. The role of guanfacine as a therapeutic agent to address stress-related pathophysiology in cocaine-dependent individuals. *Advances in Pharmacology.* 2014;69:217–265.

18. Fox HC, Anderson GM, Tuit K, et al. Prazosin effects on stress- and cue-induced craving and stress response in alcohol-dependent individuals: preliminary findings. *Alcohol: Clinical & Experimental Research.* 2012;36(2):351–360.

19. Kowalczyk WJ, Phillips KA, Jobes ML, et al. Clonidine maintenance prolongs opioid abstinence and decouples stress from craving in daily life: a randomized controlled trial with ecological momentary assessment. *American Journal of Psychiatry.* 2015;172(8):760–767.

# 28.3

## Integrative Approaches to Relapse Prevention

### GEORGE E. MUÑOZ, MD

T he first section of this chapter distinguished hedonistic behavior from the higher callings of the "pursuit of happiness" envisioned by our forefathers. The second section examined neuropharmacology, defined both by detoxification time schedules and by substance. The interplay between dopamine and other neurotransmitters, the lack of cortical inhibition, and the resultant physiological changes that essentially equate to a chronic stress response were reviewed. This section is directed at the physician addiction specialist, the primary care doctor, and health care team involved in treating or supporting the patient in early recovery. The first two sections discussed the philosophy and the neuropharmacology, endocrinology, and secondary immune effects that occur during active addiction and the early phases of drug withdrawal. This section will explore behavioral and integrative approaches to relapse prevention, many of which have already been discussed in preceding chapters. The essence of this approach is for both the treatment team and the patient to have a plan to mitigate relapse risk, given the biology and secondary brain aspects previously discussed. While there is no perfect answer, some commonalities may exist as general suggestions in the whole-person, integrative approach. These concepts were covered in various prior chapters. In reviewing the current opinion of the brain disease model of addiction shown below by Nora D. Volkow et al. we can draw a parallel as to "how to approach relapse prevention" using this model.[1]

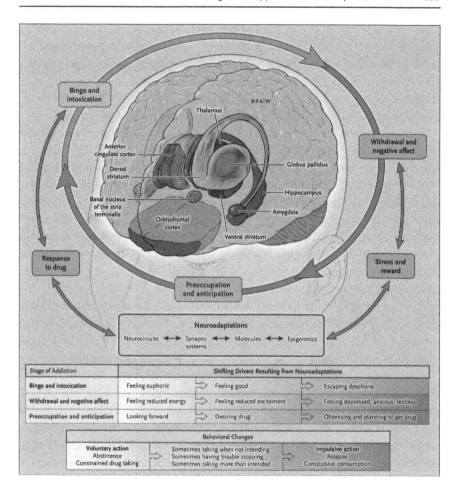

| Stage of Addiction | Shifting Drivers Resulting from Neuroadaptations | | |
|---|---|---|---|
| Binge and intoxication | Feeling euphoric | Feeling good | Escaping dysphoria |
| Withdrawal and negative affect | Feeling reduced energy | Feeling reduced excitement | Feeling depressed, anxious, restless |
| Preoccupation and anticipation | Looking forward | Desiring drug | Obsessing and planning to get drug |

| Behavioral Changes | | |
|---|---|---|
| Voluntary action Abstinence Constrained drug taking | Sometimes taking when not intending Sometimes having trouble stopping Sometimes taking more than intended | Impulsive action Relapse Compulsive consumption |

For the individual who is undergoing the many neuroadaptive, hormonal, metabolic, and emotional changes early in recovery, using an integrative model is important to initiating and maintaining abstinence. Combining an approach of psychosocial intervention that connects to the client (e.g., 12-step recovery, motivational enhancement, or cognitive-behavioral therapy) with this model makes operational sense as a fully integrative addiction approach. The use of mindfulness programs for relapse prevention has been studied by Glassner et al. and others.[2,3] The authors write that "in light of the known associations between stress, negative affect, and relapse, mindfulness strategies hold promise as a means of reducing relapse susceptibility." In this 12-week pilot study of 31 patients receiving mindfulness-based relapse prevention (MBRP) versus 30 with standard health education, the authors found that "MBRP effectively reduces negative affect and psychiatric impairment, and is particularly effective in reducing stimulant use among stimulant-dependent adults with mood and anxiety disorders."[2] Despite the small pilot numbers, this concept merits further evaluation with a larger cohort.

With respect to the use of exercise regimens as a stress reducer and adjunct in shifting drivers away from drug preoccupation, we can perhaps extrapolate from some animal data suggesting that, especially in cocaine addiction, the phase of exercise initiation can affect relapse incidence. In a rat model of cocaine addiction, animals that started exercising in the early phase of drug cessation had lower relapse rates than those that started exercising later. While we encourage that exercise be initiated at any time, with respect to relapse reduction plans, this preliminary model suggests that starting it in the early phase of abstinence should be considered as part of the overall prevention plan and may have greater potential for clinical benefit than exercise initiated later.[4] This is certainly an interesting concept when planning an overall relapse prevention schedule or plan. See other chapters in this book on the use of exercise and its benefits in addiction, as well as sections on mind-body exercises like yoga and meditation. It is vital to help the brain recover from stress using integrative tools along with a program of recovery.

Environment and stimulus control are also important parts of an addiction recovery program. As discussed earlier in this chapter, "euphoric recall" is a relevant part of relapse and response to drug-induced neuroadaptation. Volkow showed that the brain's reward system, when exposed to triggers for drugs of abuse, responds with a hyper-reward that exerts more dopaminergic reward stimulation than using the drug itself.[1] The impact of this cannot be underscored enough: choosing the right "people, places, and things" impacts the risk of relapse to addiction behavior. The implication is that it is critical to be in highly structured sober environment to help stabilize the brain during the early recovery stage. Thus, returning to an enabling household will lead to failure in most cases, even when other structured aftercare plans are in place, especially for patients with chronic drug relapse. It also means that spending more time in the structured sober environment will allow the client to acquire new coping skills and for the brain to heal. When it comes to situational triggers (people, places, and things), avoiding those major triggers in early sobriety aids in the recovery process. The cognitive therapy adage "It's better to be smart than strong" reminds the newly recovered person that, to maintain abstinence, it is the smart choice to avoid triggers. Naltrexone can also be a tool for patients with chronic relapse, as studies have shown that it reduces euphoric recall for opiates and alcohol.

With respect to the role of stress in the brain model, there are few intuitive and scientific animal data disputing the role of chronic stress as a factor in increasing and/or causing addiction behavior. The U.S. Surgeon General in his November

2016 report stated that addiction involves neurobiological processes not yet fully understood, but some have critiqued this report as deficient in some aspects, including the following:[5]

> The Report focuses much attention on the importance of stress in the development of drug addiction, and great prominence is given to the role of the stress neurohormone, corticotropin releasing factor (CRF), as the brain mechanism of drug withdrawal distress and cause of excessive drug use and relapse. There is little doubt that exposure to acute or chronic stress plays a significant role in drug addiction and relapse.[6,7] Furthermore, studies using animal models have demonstrated a critical role of CRF in stress-induced drug seeking, leading to the hypothesis that CRF plays a key role for in drug and alcohol dependence.[8] Yet to date, all attempts at developing CRF-based therapies for human addiction (or other psychiatric disorders) have been unsuccessful and major pharmaceutical companies have uniformly abandoned their development programs aimed at this target.[9,10] The fact that no reference to the known failures in targeting this mechanism was made in the Report provides the readers with an unbalanced picture of the state of research in this area.

This "deficiency" present an excellent opportunity for the field of integrative medicine to fill in the blanks, if you will, with a rubric and approach for a healing paradigm while the science catches up to the perceived molecular goals and mechanism sought. If the composite activities of mindfulness, stress reduction, healthy exercise, anti-inflammatory lifestyle, and targeted nutraceuticals augment or fill a present pharmaceutical gap in the treatment, the opportunity for increased value, lower costs, and fewer side effects is enhanced as well. Please see the chapter on nutraceuticals, exercise, and mind-body tools for further information.

Other approaches include the evaluation of event-related potentials using electrocorticography and personalizing the relapse program to help stratify those with a higher relapse potential from those with a lower one and understanding when and how to intensify interventions. This would be necessary to properly prioritize and leverage limited resources and control costs in larger systems or healthcare settings. This approach has been recommended as an adjunct within a multidisciplinary framework. The author notes that "there is a push to develop alternatives to psychotherapy- and medication-based approaches to addiction treatment." Two major cognitive factors have been identified that trigger relapse in addicted patients: attentional biases directed toward drug-related cues, which increase the urge to consume, and impaired response inhibition toward these cues, which makes it more difficult for addicted people to resist temptation. Recent studies on newly detoxified alcoholic patients have shown that by using the appropriate tasks to index these cognitive functions with event-related potentials

(ERPs), it is possible to discriminate between future relapsers and non-relapsers. These preliminary data suggest that the ERP technique has great clinical potential for preventing relapse in alcohol-dependent patients, as well as for addictive states in general. Indeed, ERPs may help to identify patients highly vulnerable to relapse and allow the development of individually adapted cognitive rehabilitation programs. The implementation of this combined approach requires an intense collaboration between psychiatry departments, clinical neurophysiology laboratories, and neuropsychological rehabilitation centers.[11] The potential pitfalls and limitations of this approach are also discussed and, while still preliminary, it merits further consideration and study as a potential tool.

Social support, adequate planning, and a structured daily regimen encompassing attendant care to the mind, body, and spirit are key parts of the relapse prevention paradigm. The use of art and music as adjunctive therapeutic approaches, ongoing outpatient psychosocial therapy, and patient education on specific aspects of the disease of addiction are all important aspects of the prevention protocol. Whether pharmacotherapy is used or required remains irrelevant to the need to attend to these self-care and lifestyle areas of personal well-being. Building strong social ties is important for recovering individuals and can be accomplished in in-person meetings such as 12-step programs, in online communities, and in formalized programs that encompass cognitive-behavioral therapy, motivational enhancement, drug counseling, and mindfulness training.

## REFERENCES

1. Volkow N, Koob G, MacLean T. Neurobiologic advances from the brain disease model of addiction. *New England Journal of Medicine*. 2016;374:363–371.
2. Glasner S, Mooney LJ, Ang A, et al. Mindfulness-based relapse prevention for stimulant-dependent adults: a pilot randomized clinical trial. *Mindfulness*. 2017;8(1):126–135.
3. Zemestani M, Ottaviani C. Effectiveness of mindfulness-based relapse prevention for co-occurring substance use and depression disorders. *Mindfulness*. 2016;7(6):1347–1355.
4. Lynch WJ, Beiter RM, Peterson AB, Abel J. Exercise during early, but not late abstinence, attenuates subsequent relapse vulnerability in a rat model. *Drug and Alcohol Dependence*. 2017;171:e124.
5. Badiani A, Berridge KC, Heilig M, et al. Addiction research and theory: a commentary on the Surgeon General's Report on alcohol, drugs, and health. *Addiction Biology*. 2018;23(1):3–5.
6. Shaham Y, Rajabi H, Stewart J. Relapse to heroin-seeking in rats under opioid maintenance: the effects of stress, heroin priming, and withdrawal. *Journal of Neuroscience*. 1996;16:1957–1963.

7. Badiani A, Belin D, Epstein D, et al. Opiate versus psychostimulant addiction: the differences do matter. *Nature Reviews Neuroscience*. 2011;12:685–700.

8. Heilig M, Koob GF. A key role for corticotropin-releasing factor in alcohol dependence. *Trends in Neuroscience*. 2007;30:399–406.

9. Schwandt ML, Cortes CR, Kwako LE, et al. The CRF1 antagonist verucerfont in anxious alcohol-dependent women: translation of neuroendocrine, but not of anticraving effects. *Neuropsychopharmacology*. 2016;41:2818–2829.

10. Shaham Y, de Wit H. Lost in translation: CRF1 receptor antagonists and addiction treatment. *Neuropsychopharmacology*. 2016;41:2795–2797.

11. Campanella S. Neurocognitive rehabilitation for addiction medicine: from neurophysiological markers to cognitive rehabilitation and relapse prevention. In: Ekhtiari H, Paulus MP, eds. Neuroscience for Addiction Medicine: From Prevention to Rehabilitation—Methods and Interventions. *Progress in Brain Research*. 2016;224:2–461.

# 29

## The Future of Addiction and Recovery Healing Arts

### SHAHLA J. MODIR AND GEORGE E. MUÑOZ

The future of science, medicine, technology and their applications are fascinating areas to explore and ponder. Visionary application and integration of emerging technologies in all areas of science are worth considering. This chapter is dedicated to peer into this future world of possibility by crossing the chasm of "in the box thinking" to the universe of possibilities. As quantum mechanics theory has shown us, objects exist in wave form, as do differential possibilities of realities in multiple time and space coordinates. Without getting too hypothetical, we will review some emerging innovations that will impact the field, some of which are in the initial phases of basic research but in an accelerated format.

## Repetitive Transcranial Magnetic Stimulation (rTMS) Therapy for Drug Addiction

### INTRODUCTION

Transcranial magnetic stimulation (TMS) uses an apparatus consisting of an electrical pulse generator and an electrically conductive coil element to non-invasively project a brief strong magnetic field pulse onto the brain. When these pulses are administered in rapid sequence the process is referred to as repetitive transcranial magnetic stimulation (rTMS).

Single-dual pulse TMS has been approved as a treatment modality for migraine headache. Repetitive TMS has been approved for the treatment of resistant major depression.[1] Recently completed small-scale investigative studies have evaluated the therapeutic utility of rTMS treatments in drug addiction.

## OVERVIEW

Repetitive TMS is a subject of intensive investigation within the neuroscience community. This interest began with the recognition that rTMS can induce electrical currents in human neurons via electromagnetic induction. Furthermore, rTMS treatments can be precisely targeted to affect discrete regions of the brain. These regions begin at the surface of the brain with a cross-sectional width as small as 25 mm and a typical penetration depth of 2 to 3 cm.

Within these regions, rTMS has been shown to induce depolarization of superficial cortical neurons with persistence of alteration in neural functionality in the region and interconnected areas beneath the coil.[10,18,36,38] These long-term changes in cortical function may produce inhibition or facilitation effects that vary depending on the specific intensity, frequency of stimulation, length of trains of pulses, and time interval between trains utilized in a particular study. In particular, high-frequency (5 to 10 Hz) rTMS usually causes cortical excitation and low-frequency rTMS (1 Hz) usually causes cortical depression. Once researchers realized they had a method to safely and non-invasively induce changes in small well-defined regions of the neocortex, studies began to investigate the effects of rTMS in patients suffering a wide variety of neurological and psychiatric disorders, including neurodevelopmental and neurodegenerative diseases, traumatic brain injuries, schizophrenia, OCD, depression, and addictive disorders, including drug addiction.

The first indications that rTMS may have therapeutic utility in drug addiction appeared with studies demonstrating decreased excitability in the motor cortex of cocaine- and nicotine-dependent subjects, increased excitability of the visual cortex in chronic MDMA users, and decreased excitability in the motor and the prefrontal cortex (PFC) in subjects with acute alcohol exposure.[5,6, 9,14,26,27,29,33,34,37,39,42]

Studies completed to date investigating the possible therapeutic efficacy of rTMS treatments in drug-addicted test subjects have targeted selected cortical regions believed to play an important role in the neuropathology of addiction.[15] Of primary interest is the dorsolateral prefrontal cortex (DLPFC), which is involved in decision making.[36] Addiction is associated with increased impulsivity and willingness to take risks, which in turn can lead to impaired decision making.[10] This suggests that rTMS may alter these decision-making processes by exciting the DLPFC, increasing its activity, and thereby increasing its inhibitory control function in drug-addicted subjects. This should increase the subject's ability to cope with drug craving, thereby decreasing drug-seeking behavior and reducing the likelihood of relapse.

## rTMS THERAPY IN SUBSTANCE USE DISORDER

To date there are 13 completed studies that have investigated high- frequency (5 to 10 Hz) rTMS as a potential treatment for drug dependency and one study investigating low frequency (1 Hz) effects on craving in methamphetamine users. These studies are summarized in Table 29.1.

Table 29.1 Studies Investigating High- and Low-Frequency rTMS as a Potential Treatment for Substance Use Disorder

| Study | N Subjects | Stimulation Site | Assessment | Findings |
|---|---|---|---|---|
| Johann et al. (2003)[25] | 11 | Left DLPFC | Craving, assessed by VAS | Reduction in craving |
| Eichhammer et al. (2003)[13] | 14 | Left DLPFC | Craving, assessed by VAS; cigarettes number | Reduction in consumption |
| Amiaz et al. (2009)[2] | 22, 26 | Left DLPFC | Craving, assessed VAS; cigarettes number | Reduction in craving, consumption, and dependence |
| Wing et al. (2012)[41] | 6, 9 | Bilateral DLPFC | Craving, assessed by TQSU | Reduction in craving |
| Rose et al. (2011)[37] | 15 | SFG | Craving, assessed by Shiffman-Jarvik questionnaire and cigarette evaluation Questionnaire | Reduction in craving (10Hz) |
| Li et al. (2013)[30, 31] | 14 | Left DLPFC | Fagerström Test for Nicotine Dependence (FTND) score | Decreased cue induced craving |
| Hayashi et al. (2013)[19] | 10 | Left DLPFC | Craving, assessed by VAS | Decreased cue induced craving |

## Table 29.1 Continued

| Study | N Subjects | Stimulation Site | Assessment | Findings |
|---|---|---|---|---|
| **Alcohol Use Disorder** | | | | |
| Mishra et al. (2010)[32] | 30, 15 | Right DLPFC | Craving, assessed by ACQ-NOW | Reduction in immediate craving; no effect on craving after 4 weeks |
| Hoppner et al. (2011)[22] | 10, 9 (females) | Left DLPFC | Craving, assessed by OCDS; Depressive symptoms, assessed by BDI; AB for neutral and alcohol related pictures | No reduction in craving and no effect on mood; increase AB for alcohol related pictures |
| Herremans et al. (2012)[20] | 36 | Right DLPFC | Craving, assessed by OCDS | No effect on immediate and long-term craving |
| De Ridder et al. (2011)[11] | 1 (female) | dACC | Craving, assessed by VAS | Reduction in immediate craving and consumption; relapse after 3 months with increased craving after 3 months |
| **Cocaine Use Disorder** | | | | |
| Camprodon et al. (2007)[8] | 6 | Bilateral DLPFC | Craving, anxiety, happiness, sadness, and discomfort, assessed by VAS | Reduction in craving (with right DLPFC rTMS); reduction in anxiety after right-sided rTMS; increase in happiness after right-sided and in sadness after left-sided rTMS; increase in discomfort equally by left- and right-sided stimulation |

*(continued)*

**Table 29.1 Continued**

| Study | N Subjects | Stimulation Site | Assessment | Findings |
|---|---|---|---|---|
| Politi et al. (2008)[35] | 36 | Left DLPFC | Clinical assessment of craving related symptoms | Reduction in craving |
| *Methamphetamine Dependence* | | | | |
| Li et al. (2013)[31] | 10,8 | Left DLPFC Low frequency | Craving, assessed by VAS | Increased cue-induced craving |

AB: attention blink; ACQ-NOW: alcohol craving questionnaire-now; BDI: Beck depression inventory; ACC: anterior cingulate cortex; DLPFC: dorsolateral prefrontal cortex; SFG: superior frontal gyrus; MOC: motor cortex; MT: motor threshold; OCDS: obsessive compulsive drinking scale; VAS: visual analogue scale; TQSU: Tiffany Questionnaire for Smoking Urges.

## DISCUSSION

The consensus of the authors of 6 published reviews that included some or all these studies is that rTMS is a promising treatment for drug addiction.[3,4,12,16,17,24]

One review (Bellamoli et al) subjected 11 of the studies to analysis and classification according to the system reported by Brainin et al[7] and concluded that rTMS falls within the level-B recommendation as "probably effective in the treatment of nicotine addiction."

Another review, a meta-analysis by Jansen that also included rTMS treatment studies for overeating disorders, concludes that there is clear evidence that non-invasive neurostimulation (including rTMS) of the DLPFC decreases craving levels in substance use disorder.

It is important to note that although all of the studies are individually too small and lacking in sufficient methodological rigor to provide a sufficient basis for the approval of rTMS as a clinical treatment modality in drug addiction, as a group they do provide a consistent and growing body of evidence demonstrating beneficial effects of rTMS therapy in drug addiction.

These pioneering studies have not only given a solid basis to proceed with further studies but have also laid the groundwork for much improvement in the design of future research utilizing rTMS. A comprehensive analysis of these early studies by Grall-Bronnec and Sauvaget (2014)[5] has identified critical issues in the technical and methodological design of human trials using rTMS and has proposed key recommendations to improve the sensitivity and reliability of future research protocols involving rTMS.

These studies have also helped delineate the neuroanatomical and neurochemical landscape of the neocortex and interconnected structures involved in drug addiction. In large part the initial targeting of the DLPFC in rTMS drug addiction therapy trials was based on earlier studies using neuroimaging and rTMS in animals and humans. These studies identified probable interconnected neuroanatomical regions mediating the three stages of the addiction cycle; binge/intoxication, withdrawal/negative affect, and craving.

The ventral tegmental area and ventral striatum appear to play a central role in the binge/intoxication stage, the extended amygdala in the withdrawal/negative affect stage, and a widely distributed network involving the orbitofrontal cortex-dorsal striatum, PFC, basolateral amygdala, hippocampus, and insula in craving. Disrupted inhibitory control appears to involve the cingulate gyrus, dorsolateral prefrontal, and inferior frontal cortices.[28]

Most authorities consider therapies designed to reduce craving and enhance inhibitory control to be the most promising strategy in treatment of drug addiction. Give the presumed importance of the DLPFC in these processes as, this region presented an ideal target for rTMS therapy for drug addiction trials. Based on the observation of reduction of craving in drug dependent test subjects, the results of the therapeutic trials completed to date provides some objective evidence in support of this proposed neurocircuitry of addiction.

## Genomics

Application of advanced and cusp genomic technologies are realms worth exploring as innovative approaches to the field of addiction. Borrowing from breakthrough basic scientific application that have already impacted research and future applications in the fields of cancer, immunology, and rheumatology, we can make a case for their use in addiction. With respect to genomics, the following are some interesting applications that may shape and change approaches.

1. **GWA—gene-wide association**. Use of this technology allows genetic studies to be performed and linked more efficiently, looking at the whole of the human chromosome. Associations of individual and family genetics will be enhanced along with targeting of specific genetic loci. This has been initiated in alcohol genetic studies and can be expanded to other substances to confirm whether different loci are involved or if loci are universal and substance agnostic. Targeting areas of the loci

that seem to be associated with impaired decision making is one possible strategy. Since genetic factors account for more than 50% of the variance in alcoholism liability it makes sense to pursue this avenue of exploration. Furthermore, opportunity of exploring the neuronal mechanisms through which genetic variation is translated into behavior exists. Fundamental to the detection of gene effects is also the understanding of the interplay between genes as well as genes/environment interactions that have been challenging areas to tease out and decipher with current research formats and technologic limitations.[43] This technology advancement and deployment in clinical and research use is one future avenue worth continuing to develop, as this approach may enhance current clinical decision making and influence future treatment selections.

# Biotech Applications

## DRUG DEVELOPMENT IN NEUROCIRCUITRY AND ADDICTION PHASES

As has been eloquently delineated by Koob and Mason in the *Annual Review of Pharmacology*:

> The identification of stages of the addiction cycle that are linked to neurocircuitry changes in pathophysiology includes the binge/intoxication stage, the withdrawal/negative affect stage, and the preoccupation/anticipation (craving) stage, which represent neuroadaptations in three neurocircuits (basal ganglia, extended amygdala, and frontal cortex, respectively) may be leveraged for pharmacologic exploration with specific anatomic and functional target effects. Furthermore, identification of excellent and validated animal models, the development of human laboratory models, and an enormous surge in our understanding of neurocircuitry and neuropharmacological mechanisms have provided a different view of addiction that emphasizes the loss of brain reward function and gain of stress function that drive negative reinforcement (the dark side of addiction) as a key to compulsive drug seeking.

These approaches will lead to future pharmacotherapy decisions based on anatomic correlates of this behavior and addiction phase theory integrating drug, anatomy, behavior, and decision making as clinical markers of addiction.

## Public Health and Prevention

An excellent review update on the neurobiology and addiction phase model correlates is discussed by Koob and others as well as key issues of public health policy integral in viewing addiction as a brain disease as it relates to legislation, insurance coverage, and national health policy. Prevention measure for higher-risk individuals, identified by family structure and/or genomics (especially in the adolescent phase of highest neuroplasticity and risk) is one strategy for the future of population addiction health prevention.[44,45] Utilizing data from structured electronic health records, with loaded risk metrics for addiction and relevant CPT diagnosis may all be analyzed by overlaying individual and family genomics that could help target higher-risk individuals, communities, school, and families with preventative educational, interventional, and whole-person stress-reduction techniques. Implementation of early addiction education and personalized genomic data for high-risk individuals, family clusters, and communities makes sense from a population and community prevention standpoint to reduce incidence and frequency of addiction by proactive interventional education and training. One futuristic model of reducing the risk of addiction (especially on susceptible brain pathways in youth with the highest neuroplasticity risk) is to target preadolescent and adolescent populations, as well as their heads of household and community leaders and implement a whole "community" approach that mirrors the "whole person" approach embodied by integrative medicine.

## Advanced Functional Imaging and Targeted Therapies

The neuroanatomic correlates associated with addiction behavior and stages, according to model theory, have already provided insight into addiction using a variety of advanced imaging. These include SPECT, fMRI, and Positron emission studies.[46] As imaging technology advances, so will the ability to peer into the detailed microanatomy of associated structures correlating to behavior and drug effect.[47,48] What may be in store for the future could be consideration of targeted therapies based on molecular, antibody, and immune binding sites involved in the neuroimmune and humoral pathways of addiction. Whether these are substance specific or agnostic remains to be seen, but we already have defined specific neuropharmacology differences in response to various drugs (i.e., cocaine). Vergara et al reports in *Neuro Image*[49] that "a general pattern of resting state hypo-connectivity among substance users compared to controls, as well as substance-specific patterns of resting state connectivity that may serve as targets for different types of intervention." Analysis of the immune effects of drug addiction and the global effects on hormone levels, function, and recovery (or a lack of pathway function) remain areas of addiction endocrinology that will need further exploration. Cocaine's specific immune deficiency effects have been described, but further research and implementation of this interactions merits further consideration. The role of cocaine in immune function is currently postulated to reside within dopamine receptors shared centrally in the CNS and by peripheral T-helper lymphocytes that may provide the neural immune cross-talk bridge to effect changes in both systems. This connection is a future pathway to explore in addiction treatment, research, and approach from both the biotech and the integrative addiction stand points.[50] Advanced imaging and immune-based probes will aid in endeavors such as PET imaging of the Dopamine 3 receptor and its associated behavioral context with targeted therapies.[51] New understanding that the CNS is not devoid of immunity function, anatomic access, and function has opened a plethora of novel approaches and theoretical concepts not previously entertained. The anatomy, compartmentalization, and background of such formulated thinking is reviewed by Engelhardt et al.[52] The coming of age of CNS inflammatory conditions and the interaction between mental health and their respective disorders are now connected by anatomy, immunology, and neuro-humoral function and via GWA and genetic probes genomics. Antibody-mediated imaging of inflamed areas of the brain in acute addiction now become "hot targets" during the induction phase of recovery. This is akin to the "induction phases" of treatment in the fields of oncology and rheumatology when the "inflammatory burden" or "disease burden" is the highest. Again, advanced imaging techniques coupled with advanced biomarkers for both inflammation and antibody-specific markers for individual substance/drug and their neurobiological effects (hormone markers, neurotransmitter metabolites [mu Amyloid protein, a marker for TBI and CBT in concussion]) may be used to follow treatment effects.[53] This is different than testing for substance presence in urine for reactively identifying relapse or a non-abstinent individual, as the underlying neurochemical, hormonal, and inflammatory aspects of addiction will be targeted to identify physiologic resistant individuals: this is including nuances not previously identifiable other than the labeling of the patient as "difficult," "chronic relapse," or a myriad of similar descriptors. Doing so will allow new treatment pathways focused on this resistance to be identified and preemptively employed with intention to reduce relapse rates as a new paradigm of addiction view and interventional treatment emerges as the field expands. The maturation of the subspecialized field of psychogenomics holds much promise in bridging the complexity of molecular genome and translational protein targets with associated complex behavior as seen in addiction and the behavioral disorders. Nestler reviews the burgeoning field and states in this review that

psychogenomics will probably be the last frontier of the functional genomics revolution. This is because of the complexity of the brain and the obstacles inherent in diagnosing and treating brain diseases, such as the enclosure of the brain within the skull and the lack of access to tissue from living patients. Within psychogenomics, however, the addiction field may lead the way, based on the relative ease of relating molecular events to meaningful animal models of the human disorders. The fields of genomics and proteomics provide tools of unprecedented power to identify genes and proteins that control complex behavior under normal and pathological conditions. Eventually, these discoveries can be exploited for clinical applications as diverse as improved treatments, diagnostic tests, and ultimately disease prevention and cure.[54]

Coupling of this advanced biotech approach with intensive whole- person, mind-body, psychologic, psychiatric individual and current group therapy and social supports (12-step, etc.), along with positive lifestyle choices, provides the totality of the integrative model that offers better outcomes than a singular approach attempting to treat the complex disease of addiction.

## Consumer Tech, Wearables, Relapse, Risk Management

A peek into the future would not be complete without a quick tour of what consumer technology and physician and health-care team technology might look like in addiction treatment.

As the portability of physiologic metrics, detection, and deployment increases along with circuitry miniaturization, medical smart wear will continue to evolve. Currently, thousands of medical apps exist for the consumer for mind-body meditation, exercise, nutrition, sleep, hydration, pulse, and other biometrics including oxygen saturation. Now one can organize this data into a single type of digital patient-reported outcome within a single app: the app could then transmit the data via Bluetooth to the medical organization or secure patient portal. This grouping of data is important to track both within the single patient as well as for population analysis within a practice or larger cohort. Again, this capability already exists and is being used (but perhaps not in an organized fashion). The use of technology has implications for public health, cost savings, and increasing access in mental and behavioral health areas and reviewed by Marsch and Lord.[55,56] As always, the issue of privacy versus the need for clinical informatics will be a sticking point as these technologies evolve and improve along with the privacy issues currently debated as technology and privacy become recurring social and political themes.

We foresee this type of wearable to aid and interact with both patient-medical and/or patient non-medical support groups. Each interaction may relate some qualitatively different data sets, but in both instances, it is patient centered, patient authorized, and maintains anonymity and privacy. Leveraging this type of technology use makes sense, as the data regarding the population at-risk pre-adolescents and the current number of youth being treated for addiction is increasing: from teenage addicts, to those in their early 20s and 30s. The millennial and premillennial generations use technology much more than older people; they use it because of convenience and to reduce costs. Examples of technology-based use in addiction have been studied in fairly resistant populations including cocaine[57] and methadone[58] and alcohol[59] populations. Phone apps including the system have proven effective as outpatient support tools. Hence, the approach to improve communication and accessibility should continue to be explored as a tool, especially in the younger and future cohorts.

## REFERENCES

1. American Psychiatric Association. *Diagnostic and Statistical Manual of Mental Disorders, Text Revision (DSM-IV-TR)*. 4th ed. Washington, DC: American Psychiatric Association; 2000.
2. Amiaz R, Levy D, Vainiger D, Grunhaus L, Zangen A. Repeated high-frequency transcranial magnetic stimulation over the dorsolateral prefrontal cortex reduces cigarette craving and consumption. *Addiction (Abingdon, England)*. 2009;104(4):653–660.
3. Barr MS, Farzan F, Wing VC, George TP, Fitzgerald PB, Daskalakis ZJ. Repetitive transcranial magnetic stimulation and drug addiction. *International Review of Psychiatry*. 2011;23(5):454–466. doi: 10.3109/09540261.2011.618827.
4. Bellamoli E, Manganotti P, Schwartz RP, Rimondo C, Gomma M, Serpelloni G. rTMS in the treatment of drug addiction: *An Update About Human Studies Behavioural Neurology*. *Behavioural Neurology*. 2014(2014), Article ID 815215, 11 pages. http://dx.doi.org/10.1155/2014/815215
5. Boutros NN, Lisanby SH, McClain-Furmanski D, Oliwa G, Gooding D, Kosten TR. Cortical excitability in cocaine-dependent patients: a replication and extension of TMS findings. *Journal of Psychiatric Research*. 2005;39(3):295–302.
6. Boutros NN, Lisanby SH, Tokuno H, et al. Elevated motor threshold in drug-free, cocaine-dependent patients assessed with transcranial magnetic stimulation. *Biological Psychiatry*. 2001;49(4):369–373.
7. Brainin M, Barnes M, Baron J-C, et al. Guidance for the preparation of neurological management guidelines by EFNS scientific task forces—revised recommendations 2004. *European Journal of Neurology*. 2004;11(9):577–581.
8. Camprodon JA, Martinez-Raga J, Alonso-Alonso M, Shih MC, Pascual-Leone A. One session of high frequency repetitive transcranial magnetic stimulation (rTMS) to the right prefrontal cortex transiently reduces cocaine craving. *Drug and Alcohol Dependence*. 2007;86(1):91–94.
9. Conte A, Attilia ML, Gilio F, et al. Acute and chronic effects of ethanol on cortical excitability. *Clinical Neurophysiology*. 2008;119(3): 667–674.

10. Daskalakis Z, Christensen B, Fitzgerald P, Chen R. Transcranial magnetic stimulation: a new investigational and treatment tool in psychiatry. *Journal of Neuropsychiatry and Clinical Neurosciences.* 2002;14(4):406–415.

11. De Ridder D, Vanneste S, Kovacs S, Sunaert S, Dom G. Transient alcohol craving suppression by rTMS of dorsal anterior cingulate: an fMRI and LORETA EEG study. *Neuroscience Letters.* 2011;496(1):5–10.

12. De Sousa A. Repetitive transcranial magnetic stimulation (rTMS) in the management of alcohol dependence and other substance abuse disorders. *Emerging Data and Clinical Relevance Basic Clin Neurosci.* 2013;4(3):271–275.

13. Eichhammer P, Johann M, Kharraz A, Binder H, Pittrow D, Wodarz N, Hajak G. High-frequency repetitive transcranial magnetic stimulation decreases cigarette smoking. *Journal of Clinical Psychiatry.* 2003;64(8):951–953.

14. Fitzgerald PB, Williams S, Daskalakis ZJ. A transcranial magnetic stimulation study of the effects of cannabis use on motor cortical inhibition and excitability. *Neuropsychopharmacology.* 2009;34(11):2368–2375.

15. Goldstein RZ, Volkow ND. Drug addiction and its underlying neurobiological basis: neuroimaging evidence for the involvement of the frontal cortex. *American Journal of Psychiatry.* 2002;159(10):1642–1652.

16. Gorelick DA, Zangen A, George MS. Transcranial magnetic stimulation in the treatment of substance addiction. *Annals of the New York Academy of Sciences.* 2014;1327: 79–93.

17. Grall-Bronnec M, Sauvaget A. The use of repetitive transcranial magnetic stimulation for modulating craving and addictive behaviours: a critical literature review of efficacy, technical and methodological considerations *Neuroscience & Biobehavioral Reviews.* 2014;47:592–613.

18. Hallett M. Transcranial magnetic stimulation: a primer. *Neuron.* 2007;55(2):187–199.

19. Hayashi T, Ko JH, Strafella AP, Dagher A. Dorsolateral prefrontal and orbitofrontal cortex interactions during self-control of cigarette craving. *Proceedings of the National Academy of Sciences of the United States of America.* 2013;110(11):4422–4427

20. Herremans SC, Baeken C, Vanderbruggen N, et al. No influence of one right-sided prefrontal HF-rTMS session on alcohol craving in recently detoxified alcohol-dependent patients: results of a naturalistic study. *Drug and Alcohol Dependence.* 2012;120(1–3):209–213.

21. Herremans SC, Vanderhasselt MA, De Raedt R, Baeken C. Reduced intra-individual reaction time variability during a Go-NoGo task in detoxified alcohol-dependent patients after one right-sided dorsolateral prefrontal HF-rTMS session. *Alcohol and alcoholism (Oxford, Oxfordshire).* 2013;48(5):552–557.

22. Hoppner J, Broese T, Wendler L, Berger C, Thome J. Repetitive transcranial magnetic stimulation (rTMS) for treatment of alcohol dependence. *The World Journal of Biological Psychiatry: The Official Journal of the World Federation of Societies of Biological Psychiatry.* 2011;12(Suppl 1):57–62.

23. Hyman SE, Malenka RC. Addiction and the brain: the neurobiology of compulsion and its persistence. *Nature Reviews Neuroscience.* 2001;2(10): 695–703.

24. Jansen JM. Effects of non-invasive neurostimulation on craving: a meta-analysis *Neuroscience & Biobehavioral Reviews*. 2010;37(10):2472–2480.

25. Johann M, Wiegand R, Kharraz A, et al. *Psychiatrische Praxis*. 2003;30(Suppl 2): S129–131.

26. Kähkönen S, Kesäniemi M, Nikouline V.V. et al. Ethanol modulates cortical activity: direct evidence with combined TMS and EEG. *NeuroImage*. 2001;14(2):322–328.

27. Kähkönen S, Wilenius J, Nikulin V.V, Ollikainen M, Ilmoniemi RJ. Alcohol reduces prefrontal cortical excitability in humans: a combined TMS and EEG study. *Neuropsychopharmacology*. 2003;28(4):747–754.

28. Koob GF, Volkow ND. Neurocircuitry of addiction. *Neuropsychopharmacology*. 2010;35(1):217–238.

29. Lang N, Hasan A, Sueske E, Paulus W, Nitsche MA Cortical hypoexcitability in chronic smokers? A transcranial magnetic stimulation study. *Neuropsychopharmacology*. 2008;33(10): 2517–2523.

30. Li X, Hartwell KJ, Owens M, et al. Repetitive transcranial magnetic stimulation of the dorsolateral prefrontal cortex reduces nicotine cue craving. *Biological Psychiatry*. 2013;73

31. Li X, Malcolm RJ, Huebner K. Low frequency repetitive transcranial magnetic stimulation of the left dorsolateral prefrontal cortex transiently increases cue-induced craving for methamphetamine: a preliminary study. *Drug and Alcohol Dependence*. 2013;133(2):641–646.

32. Mishra BR, Nizamie SH, Das B, Praharaj SK. Efficacy of repetitive transcranial magnetic stimulation in alcohol dependence: a sham-controlled study. *Addiction (Abingdon, England)*. 2010;105(1):49–55.

33. Nardone R, Bergmann J, Kronbichler M et al. Altered motor cortex excitability to magnetic stimulation in alcohol withdrawal syndrome. *Alcoholism*. 2010;34(4):628–632.

34. Oliveri M, Calvo G. Increased visual cortical excitability in ecstasy users: a transcranial magnetic stimulation study. *Journal of Neurology Neurosurgery and Psychiatry*. 2003;74(8):1136–1138.

35. Politi E, Fauci E, Santoro A, Smeraldi E. Daily sessions of transcranial magnetic stimulation to the left prefrontal cortex gradually reduce cocaine craving. *American Journal on Addictions/American Academy of Psychiatrists in Alcoholism and Addictions*. 2008;17(4):345–346.

36. Rachid F, Bertschy G. Safety and efficacy of repetitive transcranial magnetic stimulation in the treatment of depression: a critical appraisal of the last 10 years. *Clinical Neurophysiology*. 2006;36(3),:157–183.

37. Rose JE, McClernon FJ, Froeliger B, Behm FM, Preud'homme X, Krystal AD. Repetitive transcranial magnetic stimulation of the superior frontal gyrus modulates craving for cigarettes. *Biological Psychiatry*. 2011;70(8):794–799.

38. Rossini PM, Rossi S. Transcranial magnetic stimulation: diagnostic, therapeutic, and research potential. *Neurology*. 68(7):484–488.

39. Sundaresan K, Ziemann U, Stanley J, Boutros N. Cortical inhibition and excitation in abstinent cocaine-dependent patients: a transcranial magnetic stimulation study. *NeuroReport.* 2007;18;3:289–292.

40. Walsh V, Pascual-Leone A. Transcranial magnetic stimulation: a neurochronometrics of mind. Cambridge, MA: MIT Press; 2003.

41. Wing VC, Bacher I, Wu BS, Daskalakis ZJ, George TP. High frequency repetitive transcranial magnetic stimulation reduces tobacco craving in schizophrenia. *Schizophrenia Research.* 2012;139(1–3):264–266.

42. Ziemann U, Lonnecker S, Paulus W. Inhibition of human motor cortex by ethanol. *Brain.* 1995;118;1437–1446.

43. Goldman D, Ducci, F, Genetic approaches to addiction: genes and alcohol. *Addiction SSA.* 2008. 103(9): 1414–1428.

44. Koob G, Mason B. Existing and future drugs for the treatment of the dark side of addiction. *Annual Review of Pharmacology and Toxicology.* 2016;56:299–322.

45. Surgeon's General Report 2016. https://addiction.surgeongeneral.gov/chapter-7-vision-for-the-future.pdf

46. Volkow ND, Koob GF, et al. Neurobiologic advances from the brain disease model of addiction. *New England Journal of Medicine.* 2016;374:363–371.

47. Goldstein R, Volkrow ND. Dysfunction of the prefrontal cortex in addiction: neuroimaging findings and clinical implications. *Nature Reviews Neuroscience.* 2011;12(11):652–669.

48. Chung T, Tittgemeyer M, Feldstein Ewing, S. Introduction to the special issue: using neuroimaging to probe mechanisms of behavior change. *NeuroImage. 151, Elsveier,* 17 January 2017. doi:10.1016/j.neuroimage.2017.01.03

49. Vergara V, Liu J, Claus ED, Hutchison K, Calhoun VD. Alterations of resting state functional network connectivity in the brain of nicotine and alcohol users. *Neuroimage, Elsveier,* 17 January 2017;151:45–54. doi:10.1016/j.neuroimage.2016.11.012. Epub 2016 Nov 15.

50. Ersche KD, Döffinger R. Inflammation and infection in human cocaine addiction. *Current Opinion in Behavioral Sciences* 2017;13: 203–209.

51. Boileau I, Nakajama S, Payer D. Imaging the D 3 dopamine receptor across behavioral and drug addictions: positron emission tomography studies with [11 C]-(+)-PHNO. *European Neuropsychopharmacology.* 2015;25(9):1410–1420.

52. Engelhardt B, Vajkoczy P, Weller RO. The movers and shapers in immune privilege of the CNS. *Nature Immunology.* 2017;18:123–131.

53. Buttner A, Rohrmoser K, Mall G. Widespread axonal damage in the brain of drug abusers as evidenced by accumulation of β-amyloid precursor protein (β-APP): an immune-histochemical investigation. *Addiction.* 2006;101(9): 1339–1346.

54. Nestler EJ. Psychogenomics: opportunities for understanding addiction. *Journal of Neuroscience.* 2001;21(21): 8324–832.

55. Marsch LA, Lord S. Textbook of addiction treatment: international perspectives applying technology to the assessment. Prevention, Treatment, and Recovery

Support of Substance Use Disorder. Oxford University Press, New York, 2014, 1085–1092.

56. Marsch LA. Leveraging technology to enhance addiction treatment and recovery. *Journal of Addictive Diseases.* 2012, 31:3, 313–318.

57. Carroll KM, Kiluk BD, Nich C, et. al. Computer-assisted delivery of cognitive-behavioral therapy: efficacy and durability of CBT4CBT among cocaine-dependent individuals maintained on methadone. *American Journal of Psychiatry.* 2014;171(4):436–444.

58. Campbell ANC, Matthews AG, Nunes EV, et al. Internet-delivered treatment for substance abuse: a multisite randomized controlled trial. *American Journal of Psychiatry.* 2014;171:683–690.

59. Gustafson DH, McTavish FM, Chih MY, et al. A amartphone application to support recovery from alcoholism. A *Randomized Clinical Trial JAMA Psychiatry.* 2014;71(5):566–572.

# INDEX